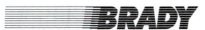

ninth edition

EMERGENCY MEDICAL RESPONDER

First on Scene

Christopher J. Le Baudour • J. David Bergeron

Medical Reviewer: Keith Wesley, MD
Legacy Author: Gloria Bizjak

Pearson

Boston   Columbus   Indianapolis   New York   San Francisco   Upper Saddle River
Amsterdam   Cape Town   Dubai   London   Madrid   Milan   Munich   Paris   Montreal   Toronto
Delhi   Mexico City   Sao Paulo   Sydney   Hong Kong   Seoul   Singapore   Taipei   Tokyo

Library of Congress Cataloging-in-Publication Data

Le Baudour, Chris.
    Emergency medical responder / Christopher J. Le Baudour, J. David
Bergeron; medical reviewer, Keith Wesley, MD; legacy author, Gloria
Bizjak. — 9th ed.
        p.; cm.
    Rev. ed. of: First responder / J. David Bergeron, Chris Le Baudour.
8th ed. c2009.
    Includes bibliographical references and index.
    ISBN-13: 978-0-13-512570-0
    ISBN-10: 0-13-512570-7
    1. Medical emergencies. 2. Emergency medical technicians.
    I. Bergeron, J. David, (date) II. Bergeron, J. David, (date) First responder.
    III. Title.
    [DNLM: 1. Emergency Medical Services. 2. Emergencies.
    3. Emergency Medical Technicians. 4. Emergency Treatment. WX 215]
    RC86.7.B47 2011
    616.02′5—dc22

                                                                    2011007444

Publisher: Julie Levin Alexander
Publisher's Assistant: Regina Bruno
Executive Editor: Marlene McHugh Pratt
Acquisitions Editor: Sladjana Repic
Assistant Editor: Jonathan Cheung
Senior Managing Editor for Development: Lois Berlowitz
Development Editor: Jo Cepeda
Director of Marketing: David Gesell
Marketing Manager: Brian Hoehl
Marketing Specialist: Michael Sirinides
Marketing Assistant: Crystal Gonzalez
Managing Production Editor: Patrick Walsh
Production Liaison: Julie Boddorf
Production Editor: Peggy Kellar
Senior Media Editor: Amy Peltier
Media Project Manager: Lorena Cerisano
Manufacturing Manager: Alan Fischer
Creative Director: John Christiana
Interior Designer: Kathy Mrozek
Cover Designer: Kathy Mrozek
Cover Photo: Ray Kemp
Composition: Aptara®, Inc.
Printing and Binding: Courier/Kendallville
Cover Printer: Lehigh-Phoenix Color/Hagerstown

Notice on Care Procedures

It is the intent of the authors and publisher that this textbook be used as part of a formal Emergency Medical Responder education program taught by qualified instructors and supervised by a licensed physician. The procedures described in this textbook are based upon consultation with first responder and medical authorities. The authors and publisher have taken care to make certain that these procedures reflect currently accepted clinical practice; however, they cannot be considered absolute recommendations.

The material in this textbook contains the most current information available at the time of publication. However, federal, state, and local guidelines concerning clinical practices, including, without limitation, those governing infection control and universal precautions, change rapidly. The reader should note, therefore, that new regulations may require changes in some procedures.

It is the responsibility of the reader to familiarize himself or herself with the policies and procedures set by federal, state, and local agencies as well as the institution or agency where the reader is employed. The authors and the publisher of this textbook and the supplements written to accompany it disclaim any liability, loss, or risk resulting directly or indirectly from the suggested procedures and theory, from any undetected errors, or from the reader's responsibility to stay informed of any new changes or recommendations made by any federal, state, and local agency as well as by his or her employing institution or agency.

Notice on Gender Usage

The English language has historically given preference to the male gender. Among many words, the pronouns *he* and *his* are commonly used to describe both genders. Society evolves faster than language, and the male pronouns still predominate our speech. The authors have made great effort to treat the two genders equally, recognizing that a significant percentage of Emergency Medical Responders are female. However, in some instances, male pronouns may be used to describe both males and females solely for the purpose of brevity. This is not intended to offend any readers.

Brady
is an imprint of

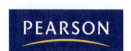

www.bradybooks.com

10 9 8 7 6 5 4 3 2 1
ISBN-10:   0-13-512570-7
ISBN-13:   978-0-13-512570-0

CONTENTS

SPECIAL FEATURES

PHOTO SCANS

Appendices

ALGORITHMS

As the authors of this textbook, we want to personally congratulate you on your decision to become an Emergency Medical Responder. Your decision to serve others, especially in times of great need, is one of the most rewarding opportunities that anyone can experience.

This textbook has been an important component of thousands of training programs over the past 30 years and has contributed to the success of hundreds of thousands of students just like you. The new Ninth Edition retains many of the features found to be successful in previous editions and includes some new topics and concepts that have recently become part of most Emergency Medical Responder programs. The foundation of this text is the new National Emergency Medical Services Education Standards for Emergency Medical Responder. This edition also includes the 2010 American Heart Association Guidelines for Cardiopulmonary Resuscitation, and First Aid.

Your decision to become an Emergency Medical Responder is significant. We believe strongly that being able to assess and care for patients requires much more than just technical skills. It requires you to be a good leader, and good leaders demonstrate characteristics such as integrity, compassion, accountability, respect, and empathy. We have enhanced components in the Ninth Edition that we believe will help you become the best Emergency Medical Responder you can be. One such component is the "First on Scene" scenarios woven throughout each chapter. In these scenarios, we throw you right in the middle of a real-life emergency and offer you a perspective that you will not get with any other training resource. You will see firsthand how individuals just like yourself make decisions when faced with an emergency situation. You will feel the fear and anxiety that is such a normal part of being a new Emergency Medical Responder. Not everyone you meet will make the best decisions, so we want you to consider each scenario carefully and discuss it with your classmates and instructor. At the end of each chapter is the "First on Scene—Run Review." Here you will have a chance to answer specific critical-thinking questions relating to the First on Scene scenario and consider how you might have done things differently.

One of the guiding themes that we used in the development of this textbook is "making connections." This theme has inspired a brand new feature for the Ninth Edition that allows us to better connect you with our very own Medical Director, Dr. Keith Wesley. This feature is called "From the Medical Director" and appears in each chapter. Through this feature, Dr. Wesley identifies key concepts and explains important details regarding everything from the role of the Medical Director to insights into the pathophysiology of specific medical conditions to the assessment and care of patients. We think that you will find his perspective as a Medical Director both informative and insightful.

Becoming an Emergency Medical Responder is just the first step in what is likely to be a lifetime of service. Just a warning to you: The feeling you get when you are able to help those in need is contagious. We encounter students all across the country who have discovered that their passion is helping others. We hope that we can be part of discovering your passion. We welcome you to EMS and a life of service!

Chris Le Baudour & J. David Bergeron

PREFACE

The publication of the Ninth Edition of *Emergency Medical Responder* marks the 30th anniversary of the publication of the first edition back in 1982. This new edition is being driven by a couple of significant events in the world of EMS education. The first is the release of the new National Emergency Medical Services Education Standards. These new standards represent the work of leading EMS educators across the nation as well as internationally. They are an important update from the last curriculum revision in 1995. Since that time, many things have changed relative to how we care for patients in an emergency. The majority of the changes are the result of evidence-based research conducted by many individuals and organizations.

The second event affecting the Ninth Edition is the release of the 2010 American Heart Association Guidelines for Cardiopulmonary Resuscitation, Emergency Cardiovascular Care, and First Aid. The guidelines represent research that has been conducted and assembled by an international group of experts over the past 10 plus years. Many of the changes that you will see in this edition will be reflective of the AHA 2010 guidelines for both resuscitation and first aid.

The contents of the Ninth Edition are summarized in this preface (below), with emphasis on what's new. Please note that the Ninth Edition also includes the following new features in every chapter:

- *Updated!* Chapter objectives have been completely revised and updated to reflect the new National Emergency Medical Services Education Standards.
- *Updated!* Key terminology for each chapter is now introduced within the list of chapter objectives, and they appear with definitions in the chapter margins beside the text where each term is used.
- *Updated!* "First on Scene" chapter scenarios have been updated to reflect the newest treatment guidelines.
- *New!* "Take Action" is a brand new feature at the end of each chapter with suggestions for how you the student can apply chapter concepts for practice and reinforcement.
- *New!* "From the Medical Director" is a new feature that appears throughout the book and includes insights and tips from our very own Medical Director, Dr. Keith Wesley.
- *New!* "Run Review" includes critical-thinking questions that ask you to evaluate the care provided during the "First on Scene" scenarios in each chapter. Here you get the opportunity to discover why the Emergency Medical Responders in the scenarios provided the care they did and to offer suggestions for improving that care.

Module 1

The first module sets the foundation for all of the modules that follow by introducing the basic concepts, information, and framework for someone entering the profession. The EMS system and the role of the Emergency Medical Responder within the system are introduced. Legal and ethical principles of emergency care are covered, as well as basic anatomy, physiology, and medical terminology.

What's New?

- *Updated! Chapter 1, Introduction to EMS Systems*, now includes updated definitions for the four levels of EMS personnel: Emergency Medical Responder, Emergency Medical Technician (EMT), Advanced Emergency Medical Technician (AEMT), and Paramedic. The 10 key components of an integrated EMS system as identified by the Highway Traffic Safety Administration (NHTSA) have been added. Added also is information on the Scope of Practice Model and the National EMS Education Standards, public safety answering points, continuous quality improvement, the role of the public health system, a description of disaster assistance, and the role of research in EMS.
- *Updated! Chapter 2, Legal and Ethical Principles of Emergency Care* has had the discussions on consent, competence, and advance directives expanded.
- *Updated! Chapter 3, Wellness and Safety of the Emergency Medical Responder* has had a discussion of the Emergency Medical Responder's baseline health status added, and discussions on immunizations and safety precautions, routes of exposure, and managing risks have been expanded.
- *Updated! Chapter 4, Medical Terminology, Human Anatomy, and Lifespan Development* has had a new section added: Lifespan Development. There also is an expanded discussion of medical terminology.

Module 2

The second module introduces many of the fundamental skills necessary to be an effective Emergency Medical Responder, covering the proper techniques for lifting, moving, and positioning ill and injured patients. It also addresses important principles related to effective verbal and written communication and documentation.

What's New?

- *Updated! Chapter 5, Principles of Lifting, Moving, and Positioning of Patients* has had the discussion on standard moves expanded to include the Trendelenburg, Fowler's, and semi-Fowler's positions; a new section on the restraining of patients added as well.
- *New! Chapter 6, Principles of Effective Communication*, is a chapter new to this edition. It introduces the common elements of effective communication as well as strategies to improve communication with diverse groups. The concept of therapeutic communication also is introduced as are some of the communication devices commonly used in EMS today.
- *New! Chapter 7, Principles of Effective Documentation*, is a chapter new to this edition. It introduces the patient care report and explains the importance and benefits of thorough and accurate documentation.

Module 3

There are only two chapters in Module 3, but they may be considered the most important. No patient will survive without an open and clear airway. Basic airway-management techniques are covered in detail, as is proper ventilation and oxygen administration.

What's New?

- *Updated! Chapter 8, Airway Management and Ventilation*, includes expanded material on assessing, opening, and maintaining a clear airway. There is expanded content related to the signs of adequate and inadequate breathing, as well as proper techniques for ventilating a patient with inadequate breathing.
- *Updated! Chapter 9, Oxygen Therapy*, has been moved from the optional appendices section to the main body of the text. It now has an expanded section on oxygen regulators, the Venturi mask, and blow-by oxygen delivery.

Module 4

This module is completely revised and contains all the most recent updates related to cardiopulmonary resuscitation (CPR) and the use of the AED.

What's New?

- *Updated! Chapter 10, Resuscitation and the Use of the Automated External Defibrillator*, has been completely updated to meet the 2010 guidelines and recommendations of the American Heart Association.

Module 5

Second in importance only to the module on airway management, this module is all about patient assessment and is the foundation for all the care Emergency Medical Responders will provide. It contains expanded information on obtaining vital signs and performing both a primary and secondary assessment of both medical and trauma patients.

What's New?

- *New! Chapter 11, Obtaining a Medical History and Vital Signs*, introduces basic principles of obtaining complete and accurate vital signs as well as the importance of trending. This chapter also offers many tips that will assist in developing proficiency with history taking, including the SAMPLE and OPQRST assessment tools.
- *Updated! Chapter 12, Principles of Patient Assessment*, offers an expanded section on both primary and secondary assessments, including performing an appropriate physical exam.

Module 6

This module covers many of the most common medical emergencies encountered in the field and how best to provide care for them. Much of the content has been expanded and includes the most up-to-date recommendations for patient care.

What's New?

- *New! Chapter 13, Caring for Cardiac Emergencies*, discusses some of the more common conditions that affect the heart's ability to pump adequately, the consequences that will often result, and the care that you as an Emergency Medical Responder will need to provide to support these patients.
- *New! Chapter 14, Caring for Respiratory Emergencies*, introduces the signs and symptoms of inadequate breathing, the common causes of inadequate breathing, and how Emergency Medical Responders care for these patients until more advanced help arrives.
- *New! Chapter 15, Caring for Common Medical Emergencies*, offers an overview of altered mental status, stroke, seizures, diabetes, poisoning, and overdose and the Emergency Medical Responder's emergency care.
- *New! Chapter 16, Caring for Environmental Emergencies*, provides an overview of a wide variety of conditions, including exposure to extremes of heat and cold, as well as bites, stings, and water-related and ice-related emergencies.

Module 7

This module addresses many of the more common emergencies related to trauma and bleeding. All the chapters have been expanded, offering more information on caring for victims of traumatic injury, including soft-tissue injuries, shock, and injuries to the head, chest, abdomen, and spine.

What's New?

- *Updated! Chapter 17, Caring for Soft-Tissue Injuries and Bleeding,* offers complete up-to-date information on bleeding control, use of a tourniquet, and hemostatic dressings and agents. It also offers new sections on multisystem trauma and detecting and managing internal bleeding.
- *New! Chapter 18, Recognition and Care of Shock,* covers the four primary categories of shock, the common types of shock, and how Emergency Medical Responders will be able to recognize and care for patients who are experiencing this life-threatening condition.
- *Updated! Chapter 19, Caring for Muscle and Bone Injuries,* includes more information related to the assessment of a suspected fracture, as well as the role and techniques for manual stabilization. Additional information has been added about the assessment of distal circulation, sensation, and motor function of an injured extremity.
- *New! Chapter 20, Caring for Head and Spine Injuries,* covers the common causes of head and spine injury as well as the proper techniques for assessment and care of someone who you suspect may have a head or spine injury.
- *New! Chapter 21, Caring for Chest and Abdominal Injuries,* discusses some of the more common injuries associated with the chest and abdomen, as well as how to properly assess and care for those injuries.

Module 8

This module covers the information related to what to expect during a normal pregnancy and childbirth. It also discusses many of the common emergencies related to pregnancy and childbirth, as well as the care of the infant and mother following delivery.

What's New?

- *Updated! Chapter 22, Care During Pregnancy and Childbirth,* has new information regarding the signs, symptoms, and care for predelivery emergencies, such as preeclampsia and eclampsia. New information also has been added regarding the proper care of the infant following delivery and the role of suctioning for the newborn.

Module 9

This module covers the unique differences in the special populations of the pediatric and geriatric patients. It also introduces assessment strategies for each group that are sure to help you provide a better assessment.

What's New?

- *Updated! Chapter 23, Caring for Infants and Children,* offers a new section on the Pediatric Assessment Triangle, as well as updated information on the AHA 2010 resuscitation guidelines.
- *Updated! Chapter 24, Special Considerations for the Geriatric Patient,* offers a new section on elder abuse and neglect and on the Emergency Medical Responder as an advocate for the elderly.

Module 10

This module covers many of the topics related to EMS operations, such as the phases of an emergency response, responding to a hazardous incident, and responding to multiple-casualty incidents. The principles of the incident management system (ICS) and triage also are addressed.

What's New?

- *Updated! Chapter 25, Introduction to EMS Operations and Hazardous Response,* offers a new section on isolation and protection and on decontamination of hazardous materials.
- *Updated! Chapter 26, Introduction to Multiple-Casualty Incidents, the Incident Command System, and Triage,* offers new sections on the medical, triage, treatment, transport, and medical staging groups in the Incident Command System.

Appendices

There are five appendices in this new edition: Patient Monitoring Devices, Principles of Pharmacology, Air Medical Transport Operations, Introduction to Terrorism Response and Weapons of Mass Destruction, and Answer Key.

What's New?

- *New! Appendix 1, Patient Monitoring Devices,* discusses some of the more common assessment and monitoring devices that the Emergency Medical Responder will likely encounter in the field.
- *Appendix 2, Principles of Pharmacology,* discusses some of the more common medications that the Emergency Medical Responder will likely encounter in

the field, as well as the indications, contraindications, and actions for each.

- *Appendix 3, Air Medical Transport Operations,* discusses the difference between rotor-wing and fixed-wing transport and when each is appropriate. Principles of establishing an appropriate helicopter landing zone are also discussed.
- *Appendix 4, Introduction to Terrorist Response and Weapons of Mass Destruction,* discusses the common devices and weapons used by terrorists and the signs and symptoms related to exposure.

New! Appendix 5, Answer Key, provides answers and rationales for the student for each of the end-of-chapter Quick Quizzes and First on Scene Run Reviews.

ACKNOWLEDGMENTS

I constantly remind my students that responding to the needs of others during an emergency is a team sport. It takes the efforts of many to render care efficiently and appropriately every time. Assembling a project such as this is no exception. Without the coordinated efforts of many people spread throughout the United States, this project could not have been possible. I'd like to acknowledge the key players who helped create the end product that you see before you.

I'd like to begin with Audrey Le Baudour, my personal assistant, copy editor, travel coordinator, and last but not least my wife, the one who keeps me organized, focused, and, most important, on schedule.

I'd like to extend a special thank-you to our photographer, Michal Heron, who has singlehandedly raised the bar for the way EMS is depicted in textbooks across this country. Michal, you bring something that no other artist brings when shooting for these books. Your work is clearly head and shoulders above the rest, and you really challenge authors to do it better.

I'd like to say thank you to editor in chief Marlene Pratt, acquisitions editor Sladjana Repic, and developmental editors Jo Cepeda and Lois Berlowitz for their invaluable editorial assistance and eye on quality. I'd also like to extend my appreciation to Jonathan Cheung and Monica Moosang and the entire sales team at Pearson Education, who provide the support and infrastructure to make these projects happen and get to those that need them. The skill and teamwork it takes to choreograph a project such as this is truly amazing.

Medical Director

Keith Wesley, MD FACEP

Our special thanks to Dr. Keith Wesley. His reviews were carefully prepared, and we appreciate the thoughtful advice and keen insight offered.

Dr. Keith Wesley is a board-certified emergency medicine physician and the EMS Medical Director for HealthEast Medical Transportation in St. Paul, Minnesota. He has served as both the State EMS Medical Director for Minnesota and Wisconsin and chair of the National Council of State EMS Medical Directors. Dr Wesley is the author of many articles and EMS textbooks and a frequent speaker at EMS conferences across the nation. He is an active EMS Medical Director who in addition to his HealthEast position provides medical oversight to the Chippewa Fire District in Chippewa Falls, Wisconsin; the EMT-Basic Services of Ashland and Bayfield counties; the Apostle Islands Lake Shore National Park; and United EMS Ambulance, a paramedic service in Wisconsin Rapids, Wisconsin.

Contributors

We would like to extend our sincere appreciation and thanks to the following individuals who contributed to the completion of the Ninth Edition! Thank you for your ideas, feedback, and contributions!

Lorenzo J. Alviso,

CHT, NREMT; Instructional Assistant, Santa Rosa Junior College EMT Program, Santa Rosa, CA

Lt. John L. Beckman,
AA, BS, FF/EMT-P; Fire Science Instructor, Technology Center of Dupage, Addison, IL

Brian Bricker,
EMT; Communications Manager, REACH Air Medical Services, Santa Rosa, CA

Lieutenant James Logan,
Memphis Fire Department

Erin Middleton,
NREMT; Instructional Assistant, Santa Rosa Junior College EMT Program, Santa Rosa, CA

Reviewers

We wish to thank the following EMS professionals who reviewed material for the Ninth Edition of *Emergency Medical Responder*. The quality of their reviews has been outstanding, and their assistance is deeply appreciated.

John P. Alexander, EMS-I; Adjunct Instructor, Connecticut Fire Academy, Windsor Locks, CT

Daniel Benard, BS, EMT-P-IC; EMS Program Director, Kalamazoo Valley Community College, Kalamazoo, MI

Art Breault, RN, NREMT-P, CIC; Emergency Medicine Outreach Coordinator, Albany Medical Center Hospital, Albany, NY

Rhonda K. Broekema, AAS, EMT-P, I/C; Consultant, Owner/Operator, Broekema Associates–Education, Schoolcraft, MI

Kevin H. Budig, NREMT-P; EMS Educator, North Memorial EMS Education, Robbinsdale, MN

Debra Cason, RN, MS, EMT-P; Associate Professor and Program Director, Emergency Medicine Education, UT Southwestern Medical Center, Dallas, TX

Larry Causby, NREMT-P, MS; EMS Training Coordinator, Cobb County Fire and Emergency Services, Marietta, GA

Joshua Chan, BA, NREMT-P; EMS Educator, Cuyuna Regional Medical Center, Crosby, MN

John Dugay, BS, NREMT-P, I/C; EMT-B & Continuing Education Programs Coordinator, McLaren Regional Medical Center, Flint, MI

Debbie Harrington, RN, AAS, EMT-P/CC/IC, NREMT-P, SANE; Instructor, Nursing/EMS Education, Roane State Community College, Knoxville, TN

E. Bunny Hearn, B.S., EMT; Captain/Instructor. Augusta County Fire-Rescue, VA

Deb Kaye, BS, NREMT-P; Director/Instructor, Dakota County Technical College, Sunburg Ambulance, Lakes Area Rural Responders, Rosemount, MN

Lawrence Linder, PhD (c), NREMTP; Independent EMS Instructor, Hillsborough Community College, Ruskin, FL

Jeff Och, RN, EMT-B; Carver, MN

Deb Preston, BS, RN; Manager, EMS Education, North Memorial Health Care, Robbinsdale, MN

Gary Reese, BS, NREMT-P; BLS Director, Crafton Hills College, Yucaipa, CA

Kenneth Sandlin, BS, AAS, NREMT-P; Engineer/Paramedic, EMS Instructor, Bentonville Fire Department, Northwest Arkansas Community College, Bentonville, AR

Brian J. Wilson, BA, NREMT-P; Education Director, Texas Tech Health Sciences Center School of Medicine, El Paso, TX

We also wish to express appreciation to the following EMS professionals who reviewed earlier editions of *Emergency Medical Responder*. Their suggestions and insights helped to make this program a successful teaching tool.

Cheryl Blazek, EMT-P; Southwestern Community College, Creston, IA

Brian D. Bricker, NREMT REACH Air Medical, Santa Rosa, CA

Leo M. Brown, Lafe Bush, EMT-P; NJ Administrative Deputy Chief, Longboat Key Fire Rescue, FL

David J. Casella, MEd, EMT-B; Osseo OEC Program, Osseo, MN

Henry Cortez, LP, AAS; Texas Emergency Response Training and Consulting, McAllen, TX

Christopher Ebright, BEd, NREMT-P; University of Toledo Division of EMS Education, Toledo, OH

James W. Fox, EMT-PS, EMS-I; EMS Assistant Coordinator, Des Moines Fire Department, Des Moines, IA

Les Hawthorne, BA, NREMT-P; EMS Coordinator, Southwestern Illinois College, Belleville, IL

Bernard Kay, BSME, EMT-D, North Seattle (WA) Community College

James S. Lion, Jr., AEMT-I; EMS Instructor, Erie County, EMT Lt, Williamsville Fire Department, NY

T.J. MacKay, Glendale Community College, Glendale, AZ

Michael O'Brien, MA, EMT-P; Illinois Medical Emergency Response Team, Chicago, IL

Robert D. Parker, BS, NREMT-P; Associate Professor of EMS, Johnson County Community College, Overland Park, KS

Wade Skinner, Adviser, Safety and Health, Kennecott Utah Copper Corp., Bingham Canyon, UT

Nerina J. Stepanovsky, PhD, RN, EMT-P; EMS Program Director, St. Petersburg College, St. Petersburg, FL

Photo Acknowledgments

All photographs not credited adjacent to the photograph or in the photo credit section below were photographed on assignment for Brady Prentice Hall Pearson Education.

PHOTO CREDITS: Page 6, Fig. 1.1.3: © 2005 Scott Metcalfe LLC. All Rights Reserved. Page 11, Fig. 1.2.1: © Craig Jackson/In the Dark Photography. Page 48, Fig. 3.7: © Craig Jackson/In the Dark Photography. Page 143, Fig. 8.6: Photograph courtesy of Laerdal Medical Corporation. Page 180, Fig. 9.7A: Photograph courtesy of Laerdal Medical Corporation. Page 326, Fig. 15.9B: © Edward T. Dickinson, MD. Page 329, Fig. 15.12: © Craig Jackson/In the Dark Photography. Page 536, Fig. 23.15A and Fig. 23.15B: © Robert A. Felter, MD. Page 559, © Ray Kemp/911 Imaging. Birthing photos in Ch. 22 by Kevin Link for Pearson Education.

Organizations

We wish to thank the following organizations for their assistance in creating the photo program for this edition:

Charles M. Schulz Sonoma County Airport, Santa Rosa, CA

Foothills Regional Park, Windsor, CA

Gamba Vineyards & Winery, Russian River Valley, Sonoma County, CA

REACH Air Medical Services, Santa Rosa, CA

Santa Rosa Campway, Inc., Santa Rosa, CA

Windsor Fire Protection Agency, Windsor, CA

Technical Advisers

Thanks to the following people for providing valuable technical support during the photo shoots for the Ninth Edition:

Scott Snyder, Paramedic

Ted Williams, Paramedic

Photo Shoot Coordinator: Audrey Le Baudour

MODELS (Alphabetical)

Lorenzo Alviso
Marian Andrews
Barbara Becker
Robert Becker
Bob Bjorkquist
Nancy Bradley
Marc Busalacchi
Nico Busalacchi
Renee Busalacchi
Deborah Chigazola
Shannon Coleman
Anne Donnels
Aubree Dowell
Hailey Frank
Jacob Frank
Kaden Frank
Michael Frank
Sylvia Frey
Jason Freyer
Gus Gamba
Dennis Gilson
Shawn Hanna

Brandon Hefele
Courtney Heinz
Scott Heinz
Andrew Henderson
Martin Huddleston
Aaron Hunt
John Imschweiler
Mike Johnson
Robert Johnson
Jason Jones
Stephanie Laslo
Audrey Le Baudour
Joanne Le Baudour
Jordan Le Baudour
Thomas Leach
Becky Lipe
Dennis McQueeny
Alex Meints
Cass Meints
Sara Meints
Taine Meints
Matthew Merritt
Erin Middleton

Christopher Mills
John Muela
Suzanne Murphy
Terrance Pesenti
Jason Piloni
Lea Poisson
Shane Redmond
Jerika Richardson
Lawee Roeum
William Seubert
Alex Shahi
Linda Shahi
Lucas Shimetz
Selam Solomon
Joan Sorensen-Schmidt
Joe Stokes
Rebecca Taylor
Shaun Vong
Kate Waldschmidt
Brad Wenner
Ted Williams

Photo and Digital Assistant: Brad Wenner

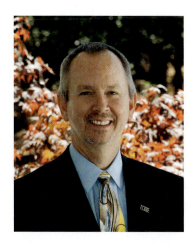

Chris Le Baudour

Chris Le Baudour has been working in the EMS field since 1978. In 1984, Chris began his teaching career in the Department of Public Safety—EMS Division at Santa Rosa Junior College in Santa Rosa, California.

Chris holds a master's degree in education with an emphasis in online teaching and learning as well as numerous EMS and instructional certifications. Chris has spent the past 28 years mastering the art of experiential learning in EMS and is well known for his innovative classroom techniques and his passion for both teaching and learning in both traditional and online classrooms.

Chris is very involved in EMS education at the national level as a board member of the National Association of EMS Educators and advises many organizations throughout the country. Chris is a frequent presenter at both state and national conferences and a prolific EMS writer. Along with numerous articles, he is the author of *Emergency Care for First Responders*, and coauthor of *EMT Complete—A Basic Worktext*, *Emergency Medical Responder—The Workbook*, and the *Active Learning Manual for the EMT Basic*. Chris and his wife, Audrey, have two children in college and reside in Northern California.

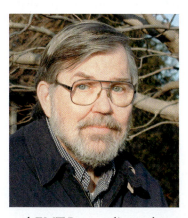

David Bergeron

David Bergeron has been active in the development of instructional and training programs for the emergency medical services (EMS) for over 35 years. His early work included "a front row seat" to the development of modern patient assessment and care inspired by the studies of Dr. R. Adams Cowley, Maryland Shock Trauma Center, Maryland Institute of EMS Systems, and Maryland Fire and Rescue Institute (MFRI).

David's work in instructional development for emergency medicine has included EMT-Basic, Emergency Medical Responder (First Responder), EMT-Intermediate, and EMT-Paramedic student and instructor programs. He is credited with writing the first comprehensive textbook for the first responder, for establishing the first behavioral objectives for EMTs, and for being the first to develop a full-course glossary for EMT instruction.

As well as serving as an instructional technologist on leading textbooks in emergency medicine, David has been on the teaching faculty of the University of Maryland, Longwood University, and numerous community colleges and schools of nursing. His publications include textbooks that have been translated into Spanish, Portuguese, French, German, Italian, Lithuanian, and Japanese.

His development of this current edition of *Emergency Medical Responder* has benefited from the work being done by many EMS systems and the creative co-authorships of Gloria Bizjak and Chris Le Baudour.

Resource Central

This online study aid provides chapter support materials and resources in one location. Students can prepare for class and exams with skills and objective checklists, multiple-choice exams, case-study activities, interactive exercises, games, an audio glossary, web links, animations and videos, study aids, chapter summaries in Spanish, and more! At the completion of select text sections, students are prompted to visit Resource Central to access valuable resources that enhance the material introduced in the textbook.

To access Resource Central, follow the directions on the Student Access Code Card provided with this textbook. If there is no card, go to www.bradybooks.com and follow the Resource Central link to Buy Access from there.

Workbook for *Emergency Medical Responder: First on Scene*, Ninth Edition

(0-13-512572-3)
This self-paced workbook features activities such as defining key terms, labeling, listing, matching, and answering short-essay questions. Personal development and application exercises are designed to reinforce key concepts. This workbook is available for purchase at **www.bradybooks.com.**

First Responder Certification Program

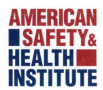

The American Safety & Health Institute (ASHI) is an association of safety and health educators providing nationally recognized training programs. ASHI's mission is to make learning to save lives easy. ASHI authorizes qualified individuals to offer First Responder training and certification programs for corporate America, government agencies, and emergency responders. To learn more about ASHI, visit **www.hsi.com/ashi.**

About the ASHI First Responder Certification Program

In the early 1970s, officials at the U.S. Department of Transportation National Highway Traffic Safety Administration (NHTSA) recognized a gap between basic first aid training and the training of Emergency Medical Technicians (EMTs). Their solution was to create "Crash Injury Management: Emergency Medical Services for Traffic Law Enforcement Officers," an emergency medical care course for "patrolling law enforcement officers." As it evolved, the course expanded to include other "First Responders"–public and private safety and service personnel who, in the course of performing other duties, are likely to respond to emergencies (firefighters, highway department personnel, etc.). The Crash Injury Management course provided the basic knowledge and skills necessary to perform lifesaving interventions while waiting for EMTs to arrive. The original program was never intended for training EMS personnel. Because the Crash Injury Management course was designed to fill the gap between basic first aid training and EMT, it was considered "advanced first aid training." In 1978, the Crash Injury Management course was renamed *Emergency Medical Services: First Responder Training Course* and was specifically targeted at "public service law enforcement, fire, and EMS rescue agencies that did not necessarily have the ability to transport patients or carry sophisticated medical equipment." Then in 1995, the course went through a major revision and its name was changed to *First Responder: National Standard Curriculum.* At that time, the First Responder was described as "an integral part of the Emergency Medical Services System." Later in 2006, a FEMA EMS Working Group recommended a new job title for first responders working within the EMS system-the **Emergency Medical Responder (EMR).** This title is meant to specify a state-licensed and credentialed individual responding within an EMS-providing entity, organization, or agency. Specifically, the use of the word "medical" in the EMR title is intended to help distinguish those persons who have successfully completed a state-approved EMR program from other first responders such as law enforcement officers, public health workers, and search & rescue personnel (to name a few).

The ASHI First Responder

The gap between basic first aid training and the training of EMS professionals that was recognized more than 30 years ago remains. There is still a need for an "advanced first aid course" for the original "first responder" target audience–non-EMS providers who, in the course of performing other duties, are likely (or expected) to respond to emergencies. These individuals, law enforcement officers, fire fighters, and other public and private safety and service personnel, are indeed an integral part of the overall EMS System. That is to say, part of a network of resources–people, communications, and equipment–prepared to provide emergency care to victims of sudden illness or injury. On the other hand, these individuals are not, and in most cases do not wish to be, state-licensed and credentialed EMS professionals. The original first responder program was intended to provide these "pre-EMS" responders with the basic knowledge and skills necessary for lifesaving interventions while waiting for the EMS professionals to arrive. That original intent–filling the knowledge and skill gap between basic first aid training and EMS–is the intent of ASHI's First Responder program. Additionally, because this program uses the same textbooks and related instructional tools as those used to train EMRs, it serves to encourage a continuum in care for the ill or injured person as he or she is transitioned from care provided by the first responder to care provided by the EMS professional.

Certification as an ASHI First Responder

Evaluation of knowledge and skill competence is required for certification as an ASHI First Responder. The learner must successfully complete the 50-question ASHI First

Responder Exam and demonstrate the ability to work as a lead first responder in a scenario–based team setting, adequately directing the initial assessment and care of a responsive and unresponsive medical and trauma patient.

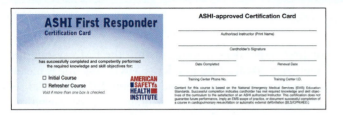

State Licensure and Credentialing

State EMS agencies have the legal authority and responsibility to license, regulate, and determine the scope of practice of EMS providers within the state EMS system. ASHI's First Responder program is designed to allow properly authorized Instructors to train and certify individuals as a first responder consistent with national curriculum requirements and education standards. It is not the intent of ASHI's First Responder program to cross the EMS scope of practice threshold. An individual that has been trained and certified as an ASHI First Responder is NOT licensed and credentialed to practice emergency medical care as an EMS provider within an organized state EMS system. EMS provider licensing and credentialing are legal activities performed by the state, not ASHI. Individuals who require or desire licensure and credentialing within the state EMS system as a First Responder or Emergency Medical Responder must complete specific requirements established by the regulating authority.

International Use of ASHI First Responder

Given the current state of globalization and the increasing international reach of ASHI-authorized Instructors, the ASHI First Responder program has expanded outside of the United States. As appropriate actions by First Responders alleviate suffering, prevent disability and save lives, ASHI encourages this international expansion, particularly in areas with emerging but undeveloped EMS systems. However, as in the United States, the scope of practice for medically trained persons is often subject to federal, state, provincial or regional laws and regulations. It is not the intent of ASHI's First Responder program to cross the EMS (or medical) scope of practice threshold in any country.

Health & Safety Institute (HSI)

Health & Safety Institute (HSI) unites the recognition and expertise of the American Safety & Health Institute (ASHI), MEDIC First Aid International, 24-7 EMS, 24-7 Fire, EMP Canada, First Safety Institute (FSI) and GotoAID to create the largest privately held emergency care and response training organization in the industry. For more than 30 years, in partnership with 16,000 approved training centers and 200,000 professional emergency care, safety and health educators, HSI authorized instructors have certified more than 19 million emergency care providers in the US and over 100 countries worldwide. HSI is an accredited organization of the Continuing Education Board for Emergency Medical Services (CECBEMS), the national accreditation body for Emergency Medical Service Continuing Education programs and a member of the American National Standards Institute and ASTM International, two of the largest voluntary standards development and conformity assessment organizations in the world. ASHI and MEDIC First Aid training programs are used to teach and certify first aid and emergency care providers in health care, business, industry, and the general public. ASHI and MEDIC First Aid training programs are nationally recognized and are endorsed, accepted, or approved by many state regulatory agencies and occupational licensing boards, including those licensing EMS providers, pharmacists, dental health professionals, child care providers, school teachers, and many others. Additionally, our programs meet the requirements established by a wide variety of accreditation organizations, professional associations, councils, academies and boards.

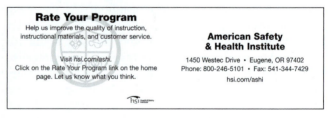

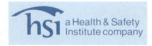

American Safety & Health Institute
1450 Westec Drive, Eugene, OR 97402.
PHONE 800-447-3177 FAX 541-344-7429

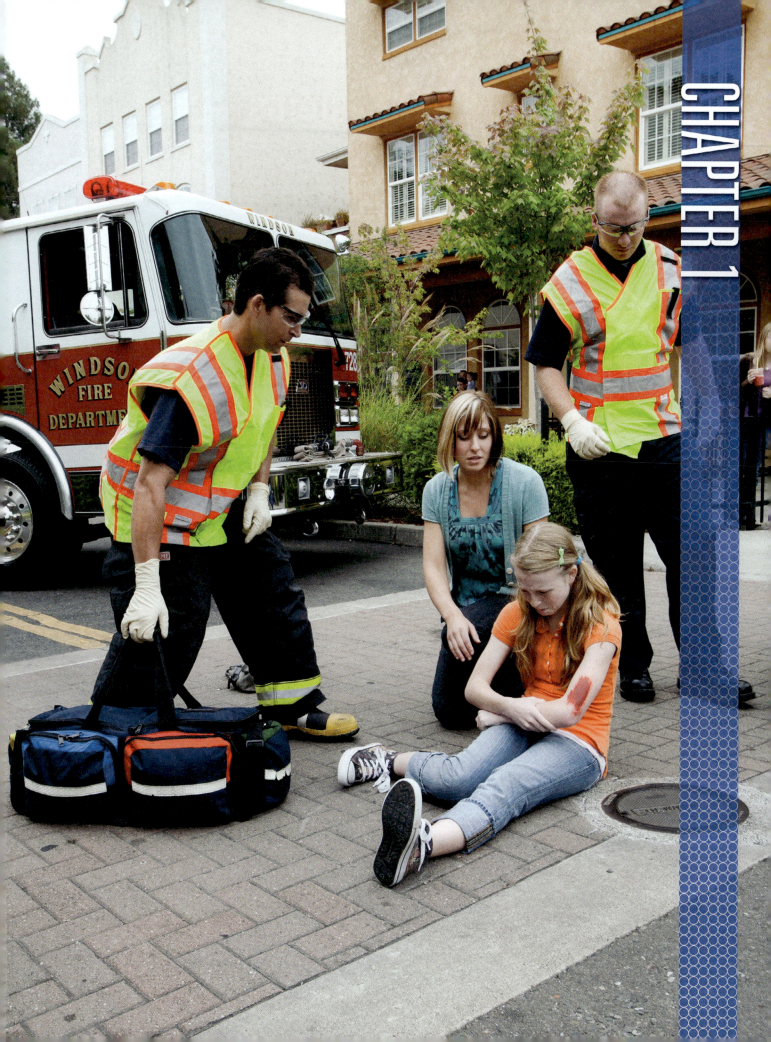

Introduction to EMS Systems

• Preparatory—EMS Systems, Research, Public Health

COMPETENCIES

• Uses simple knowledge of the EMS system, safety/well-being of the Emergency Medical Responder, medical/legal issues at the scene of an emergency while awaiting a higher level of care.
• Has an awareness of local public health resources and the role EMS personnel play in public health emergencies.

CHAPTER OVERVIEW

You have made a great choice in deciding to become a part of the EMS team and become trained as an Emergency Medical Responder. Thousands of people become ill or are injured every day, and physicians are seldom close by when they do. In fact, some time usually passes between the onset of an injury or illness and the delivery of medical care. Emergency medical services (EMS) systems have been developed for this very reason. The purpose is to get trained medical personnel to the patient as quickly as possible and to provide emergency care at the scene of the emergency and en route to the hospital. Emergency Medical Responders are an essential part of that EMS team.

Realizing that people will depend on you to provide assistance during an emergency can be overwhelming. To gain confidence in your knowledge and skills, it is very important that you learn and understand what is expected of you in this new role. When you do, you can act more quickly to provide efficient and effective emergency care.

To begin, this chapter will introduce you to EMS systems and to the roles and responsibilities of the Emergency Medical Responder.

OBJECTIVES

Upon successful completion of this chapter, the student should be able to:

COGNITIVE

1. Define the following terms:
   a. Advanced Emergency Medical Technician (AEMT) (p. 19)
   b. continuous quality improvement (CQI) (p. 15)
   c. Disaster Medical Assistance Team (DMAT) (p. 16)
   d. emergency care (p. 3)
   e. Emergency Medical Dispatcher (EMD) (p. 8)
   f. Emergency Medical Responder (EMR) (p. 7)
   g. emergency medical services (EMS) system (p. 4)
   h. Emergency Medical Technician (EMT) (p. 7)
   i. medical direction (p. 6)
   j. Medical Director (p. 5)
   k. National EMS Education Standards (p. 7)
   l. off-line medical direction (p. 9)
   m. on-line medical direction (p. 9)
   n. Paramedic (p. 7)
   o. protocols (p. 9)
   p. public health system (p. 16)
   q. public safety answering point (PSAP) (p. 8)
   r. research (p. 16)
   s. scope of practice (p. 8)
   t. Scope of Practice Model (p. 7)
   u. specialty hospital (p. 8)
   v. standing order (p. 9)

2. Explain the role of the National Highway Traffic Safety Administration (NHTSA) and its relationship to EMS. (p. 5)

3. Explain the role that the National EMS Education Standards and the National Scope of Practice Model play in shaping EMS around the country. (p. 7)

4. Differentiate the various EMS models in practice around the United States. (p. 8)

5. Differentiate the various components of an EMS system and describe the function of each. (p. 5)

6. Explain the role that state EMS offices, medical oversight, and local credentialing play in an EMS system. *(p. 8)*

7. Differentiate the four levels of EMS provider. *(p. 7)*

8. Explain the various methods used to access the EMS system. *(p. 8)*

9. Explain the various types of medical direction and how the Emergency Medical Responder might interact with each. *(p. 9)*

10. Differentiate the roles and responsibilities of the Emergency Medical Responder from other EMS providers. *(p. 7)*

11. Describe the characteristics of professionalism as they relate to the EMS provider. *(p. 14)*

12. Explain the role of the Emergency Medical Responder with regards to continuous quality improvement (CQI). *(p. 15)*

13. Explain how state/region specific statutes and regulations affect how an Emergency Medical Responder might function. *(p. 8)*

14. Explain the role of public health systems and their relationship to EMS, disease surveillance, and injury prevention. *(p. 16)*

15. Explain the role that Disaster Medical Assistance Teams (DMAT) play and how they integrate with EMS systems. *(p. 16)*

16. Explain the role that research plays in EMS and the ways that an Emergency Medical Responder might identify and support research. *(p. 16)*

PSYCHOMOTOR

17. Participate in simple research activities facilitated by the instructor.

AFFECTIVE

18. Value the importance of accepting and upholding the responsibilities of an Emergency Medical Responder.

19. Support the rationale for always maintaining a high degree of professionalism when performing the duties of an Emergency Medical Responder.

20. Value the importance of providing the best possible care for all patients regardless of cultural, gender, age, or socioeconomic status.

21. Model a desire for continuous quality improvement (CQI) both personally and professionally.

22. Value the importance of quality research and its connection to good patient care.

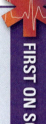

FIRST ON SCENE

It's a bright sunny spring day and you have just left what you feel was one of your best interviews yet. All that time playing on the computer and messing around with video games is starting to pay off. If all goes well, you will soon be working for a major video game development company right in your own hometown.

Things are looking up, and there is a noticeable bounce in your step as you descend the stairs to the visitor parking lot. Just as you reach the sidewalk, you hear a yell for help from across the lot. You hesitate for a moment and look around to see if anyone else hears what you hear. Again you hear a female voice yelling for help, but you cannot see anyone. You decide to investigate and go toward the direction of the call.

Two rows over, you see a middle-aged woman leaning over a young boy on the ground. He appears to be shaking, and there is a white, foamy substance coming from his mouth. The woman sees you and yells in a panicked voice for you to go call an ambulance.

"Yes, okay. I'll go back to the lobby and call for help. I'll be right back!" You make it back to the lobby in record time and in short bursts of words advise the receptionist that someone is down in the parking lot and to call 911. She does and alerts the building's Medical Emergency Response Team as well. With some hesitation, you return to the scene in the parking lot.

The EMS System

It is likely that people have been providing **emergency care** for one another since humans first walked the earth. While many of those early treatments would seem primitive by today's standards, what has not changed is the awareness that care of some kind is often needed. A formal system for responding to emergencies has only existed for a relatively short time (Table 1.1). It was during the American Civil War that the Union Army first began training soldiers to provide first aid to the wounded in the battlefield. These "corpsmen," as they were known, were trained to provide care for the most immediate life threats, such as bleeding. After their initial care, the injured were transported by

emergency care ▶ the prehospital assessment and basic care for the sick or injured patient; during care the physical and emotional needs of the patient are considered and attended to.

1790s	Napoleon's chief physician, Dominique Jean Larrey, develops a system designed to triage and transport the injured soldiers from the battlefield to established aid stations.
1805–1815	Dominique Jean Larrey formed the Ambulance Volante (flying ambulance). It consisted of a covered horse-drawn cart designed to bring medical care closer to the injured on the battlefields of Europe.
1861–1865	Clara Barton coordinates the care of sick and injured soldiers during the American Civil War.
1869	New York City Health Department Ambulance Service begins operation out of what was then known as the Free Hospital of New York, now Bellevue Hospital.
1915	First recorded air medical transport occurs during the retreat of the Serbian army from Albania.
1928	The concept of "on-scene care" is first initiated in 1928, when Julian Stanley Wise started the Roanoke Life Saving and First Aid Crew in Roanoke, Virginia.
1950–1973	The first use of helicopters to evacuate injured soldiers and deliver them to waiting field hospitals occurs in the Korean and Vietnam wars.
1966	The report entitled "Accidental Death and Disability: The Neglected Disease of Modern Society," commonly referred to as the "White Paper," is published. The study concludes that many of the deaths occurring every day were unnecessary and could be prevented through better prehospital treatments. The report resulted in Congress passing the National Highway Safety Act.
1973	Congress passes the Emergency Medical Services Act, which provides funding for a series of projects related to trauma care.
1988	The National Highway Transportation and Safety Administration (NHTSA) defines elements necessary for all EMS systems.
1990	The Trauma Care Systems and Development Act encourages development of improved trauma systems.
1995	An update to the EMT Basic and First Responder National Standard Curricula is released.
1996	The EMS Agenda for the Future outlines the most important directions for the future of EMS development.
1998	A recent update to the EMT Paramedic National Standard Curricula is released.
1999	The most recent update to the EMT Intermediate National Standard Curricula is released.
2000	NHTSA publishes the EMS Education Agenda for the Future—A Systems Approach.
2005	NHTSA publishes the National EMS Core Content.
2006	NHTSA publishes the National EMS Scope of Practice Model redefining the four levels of EMS certification and licensure.
2009	NHTSA publishes the new EMS Education Standards.

horse-drawn carriage to waiting physicians (Figure 1.1). Thus, the first formal ambulance system in the United States had begun.

The first civilian ambulance services began in the late 1800s with the sole purpose of transporting injured and ill patients to the hospital for care. It was not until 1928 that the concept of civilian "on scene" care was first implemented, with the organization of the Roanoke Life Saving and First Aid Crew in Roanoke, Virginia.

In 1966, the National Academy of Sciences released a report called the "Accidental Death and Disability: The Neglected Disease of Modern Society." That report revealed for the first time the inadequacies of prehospital care. It also provided suggestions for the development of formal EMS systems.

If hospital personnel had to wait for all patients to come to them, many people would die before getting medical care. Fortunately, it has become possible to extend lifesaving care through a chain of resources known as the **emergency medical services (EMS) system**

emergency medical services (EMS) system ▶ the chain of human resources and services linked together to provide continuous emergency care from the onset of care at the prehospital scene, during transport, and on arrival at the medical facility. In some localities, multiple EMS agencies work together as an EMS network.

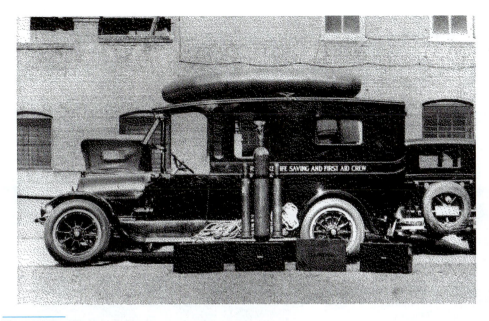

Figure 1.1 • Early ambulance.

(Scan 1.1). Once the system is activated, care begins at the emergency scene and continues during transport to a medical facility. At the hospital, a formal transfer of care to the emergency department staff ensures a smooth continuation of care. (Note that the emergency department may still be referred to as the emergency room or ER in some areas.)

The National Highway Traffic Safety Administration (NHTSA) has identified 10 key components of an integrated EMS system and assists states in developing and assessing those components. They are:

- *Regulation and policy.* To provide a quality, effective system of emergency medical care, each state must have in place legislation that identifies and supports a lead EMS agency. This agency has the authority to plan and implement an effective EMS system. It also can create appropriate rules and regulations for each recognized component of the EMS system.
- *Resource management.* Each state must have in place a centralized method to coordinate all system resources.
- *Human resources and training.* The lead state EMS agency must have a mechanism to assess current human resource needs. It also must establish a comprehensive plan for stable and consistent EMS training programs. EMS training programs must be monitored routinely to ensure that instructors meet certain requirements, the curriculum is standardized throughout the state, and valid and reliable testing procedures are utilized.
- *Transportation.* Each state must have a comprehensive transportation plan that includes provisions for uniform coverage, including written guidelines for air medical dispatch and a mutual aid plan.
- *Facilities.* A seriously ill patient must be delivered in a timely manner to the closest appropriate facility. The lead EMS agency must have a system for letting EMS personnel know which health-care facility is appropriate for each patient.
- *Communications.* The lead agency in each state is responsible for central coordination of EMS communications. The public must be able to access the EMS system with a single, universal emergency phone number, such as 911, and the communications system must provide for prioritized dispatch.
- *Public information and education.* Each state must develop and implement an EMS public information and education (PI&E) program. It should ensure that consistent, structured PI&E programs are in place. Such programs should enhance the public's knowledge of the EMS system, support appropriate EMS system access, demonstrate essential self-help and appropriate bystander care actions, and encourage injury prevention.

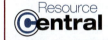

Educate yourself on the outlook of the profession with the EMS Agenda for the Future.

OBJECTIVES

2. Explain the role of the National Highway Traffic Safety Administration (NHTSA) and its relationship to EMS.

5. Differentiate the various components of an EMS system and describe the function of each.

Medical Director ▶ a physician who assumes the ultimate responsibility for medical oversight of the patient care aspects of the EMS system.

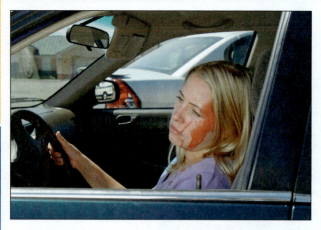

1.1.1 | EMS is made up of a highly specialized chain of resources. A crash scene.

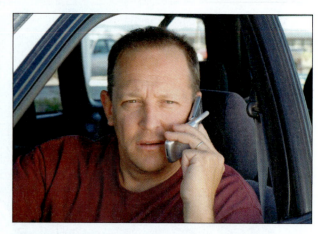

1.1.2 | A citizen calls 911.

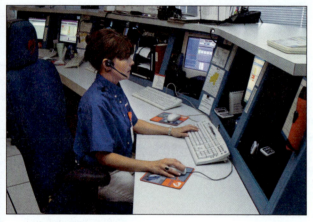

1.1.3 | The Emergency Medical Dispatcher allocates resources.
(© 2005 Scott Metcalfe LLC. All Rights Reserved)

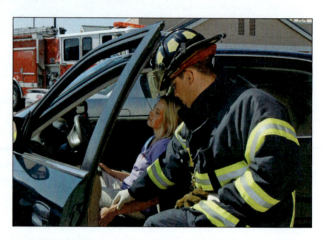

1.1.4 | An EMS Emergency Responder assists the patient.

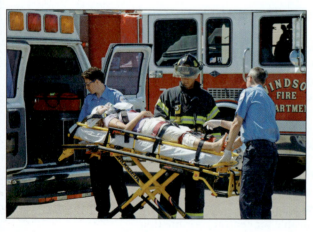

1.1.5 | EMTs continue treatment en route to the hospital.

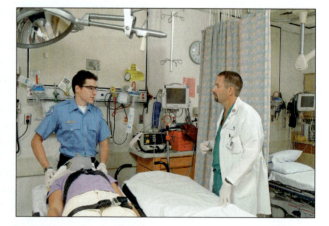

1.1.6 | The patient is transferred to the care of emergency department personnel.

medical direction ▶ the medical oversight provided for an EMS system or one of its components by a licensed physician.

- *Medical direction.* Each state must ensure that physicians are involved in all aspects of the patient care system. The role of the state EMS **Medical Director** must be clearly defined. It should have legislative authority and responsibility for EMS system standards, protocols, and evaluation of patient care. **Medical direction** for all EMS providers must be used to evaluate medical care as it relates to patient outcome, training programs, and medical direction.

- *Trauma systems.* Legislation should be in place for the development and implementation of the trauma care component of the EMS system. It should include designated trauma center triage and transfer guidelines, data collection and trauma registry definitions and mechanisms, mandatory autopsies, and quality improvement for trauma patients.
- *Evaluation.* Each state EMS system is responsible for evaluating the effectiveness of its services. A uniform, statewide data-collection system must exist to capture the minimum data necessary to measure compliance with standards. It also must ensure that all EMS providers consistently and routinely provide data to the lead agency. The lead agency performs routine analysis of that data. Your participation in the evaluation process will help drive the improvement of the EMS system and the care that patients receive.

The events that occurred on September 11, 2001, increased public awareness of the EMS system. They also brought to the public's attention rescue personnel who are called "first responders." Unfortunately, the public did not understand the difference between a rescuer who appears first on scene and an EMS first responder, a trained medical care provider. Serving as the lead coordinating agency for EMS on a national level, the National Highway Traffic Safety Administration (NHTSA) in late 2009 redefined and renamed all levels of EMS providers. These changes were included in two documents called the **Scope of Practice Model** and the **National EMS Education Standards**. In support, this textbook refers to the previous EMS first responder level of training as **Emergency Medical Responder**, or EMR for short.

Refer to Table 1.2 to see the new titles and to compare their roles and responsibilities. All are based on NHTSA's National Scope of Practice Model but may vary slightly from state to state and region to region. Your instructor will explain variations in your area. The framework for this book and all EMS training and education is guided by the National EMS Education Standards for Emergency Medical Responder training. Those standards are the culmination of many years of work and will serve as the basis for EMS education at all levels for many years to come.

Scope of Practice Model ▶ a national model that defines the scope of care for all levels of EMS training.

National EMS Education Standards ▶ the education and training standards developed by the National Highway Traffic Safety Administration (NHTSA) for all levels of EMS training.

Emergency Medical Responder (EMR) ▶ a member of the EMS system who has been trained to render first aid care for a patient and to help EMTs at the emergency scene.

OBJECTIVES

3. Explain the role that the National EMS Education Standards and the National Scope of Practice Model play in shaping EMS around the country.

7. Differentiate the four levels of EMS provider.

10. Differentiate the roles and responsibilities of the Emergency Medical Responder from other EMS providers.

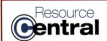

Read up on the new National EMS Education Standards for Emergency Medical Responders. Also, find out more about the levels of EMS Training.

Emergency Medical Technician (EMT) ▶ a member of the EMS system whose training emphasizes assessment, care, and transportation of the ill or injured patient. Depending on the level of training, emergency care may include starting IV (intravenous) lines, inserting advanced airways, and administering some medications.

Paramedic ▶ a member of the EMS system whose training includes advanced life support care, such as inserting endotracheal tubes and starting IV lines. Paramedics also administer medications, interpret electrocardiograms, monitor cardiac rhythms, and perform cardiac defibrillation.

TABLE 1.2 | Levels of EMS Training
Emergency Medical Responder (EMR)—This level of EMS training is designed specifically for the person who is often first to arrive at the scene. Many police officers, firefighters, industrial workers, and other public service providers are trained as Emergency Medical Responders. This training emphasizes scene safety and how to provide immediate care for life-threatening injuries and illnesses as well as how to assist ambulance personnel when they arrive
Emergency Medical Technician (EMT)—In most areas, an EMT is considered the minimum level of certification for ambulance personnel. The training emphasizes assessment and the care and transportation of the ill or injured patient. The EMT also may assist with the administration of certain common medications. (This was formerly called the EMT-Basic level of training.)
Advanced Emergency Medical Technician (AEMT)—An Advanced EMT is a basic-level EMT who has received specific additional training in specific areas, allowing some level of advanced life support. Some of the additional skills an Advanced EMT may be able to perform are starting IV (intravenous) lines, inserting advanced airways, and administering medications. (This was formerly called the EMT-Intermediate level of training.)
Paramedic—Paramedics are trained to perform what is commonly referred to as advanced life support care, such as inserting endotracheal tubes and starting IV lines. They also administer medications, interpret electrocardiograms, monitor cardiac rhythms, and perform cardiac defibrillation. (This was formerly called the EMT-Paramedic level of training.)

scope of practice ▶ the care that an Emergency Medical Responder, an Emergency Medical Technician, or Paramedic is allowed and supposed to provide according to local, state, or regional regulations or statutes. Also called *scope of care*.

Learn more about the National EMS Scope of Practice Model.

IS IT SAFE?

Many people are injured and even killed each year when they rush into an unsafe scene to help an injured victim. Take the time to stop and observe the scene before rushing in. Do your best to identify any obvious hazards that could endanger you or others arriving at the scene.

public safety answering point (PSAP) ▶ a designated 911 emergency dispatch center.

Emergency Medical Dispatcher (EMD) ▶ a member of the EMS system who provides prearrival instructions to callers, thereby helping to initiate lifesaving care before EMS personnel arrive.

specialty hospital ▶ a hospital with special designation that is capable of provide specialized services such as trauma care, pediatric care, or burn care.

EMS Models

The broad nature of the Scope of Practice Model and the National EMS Education Standards allow for a variety of EMS models. One model is called the "fire-based" EMS model. In a fire-based system, much of the EMS services and infrastructure are operated by a local fire department or consortium of departments within a region. Another model is referred to as "third-service." That model is typically operated by non-fire government entities such as cities, counties, or privately owned ambulance services. Another common system around the country is the hospital-based EMS system. Typically, it is operated by a large hospital or group of hospitals serving a particular region.

Regardless of the model, all EMS systems are designed to deliver the best care possible in the shortest amount of time.

Scope of Practice

The **scope of practice** identifies the duties and skills an EMS provider is legally allowed to perform. Quite often the scope of practice of any given level of EMS provider is defined by state and/or regional statutes and regulations. Those statutes and regulations also will define any related licensing, credentialing, and certification that may be needed. While a scope of practice typically is defined at the state level, quite often local counties and EMS agencies also will have a process for identifying and tracking EMS providers in the local system. It is becoming quite common today for a state or local EMS authority to require criminal background checks for anyone seeking certification or licensing to practice. Those processes all are designed to protect the patient and ensure the quality of patient care delivered within an EMS system.

Activating the EMS System

Once an emergency is recognized, the EMS system must be activated (Scan 1.1). Most citizens activate it by way of a 911 phone call to an emergency dispatcher, who then sends available responders—Emergency Medical Responders, **Emergency Medical Technicians (EMTs)**, and **Paramedics**—to the scene. Some areas of the country may not have a 911 system. In those areas the caller may need to dial a seven-digit number for the ambulance, fire, police, or rescue personnel.

The most desirable 911 service is referred to as an *enhanced* 911 system. It enables the communications center to automatically receive caller information, such as phone number and address, making it easier to confirm location and reconnect should the call be lost.

All 911 calls are automatically directed to a **public safety answering point (PSAP)**. Most primary PSAPs are law enforcement agencies with specially trained dispatchers. Some 911 dispatch centers are staffed with **Emergency Medical Dispatchers (EMDs)**, who receive special training. EMDs provide prearrival instructions to callers, thereby helping to initiate lifesaving care before EMS personnel arrive.

Once the EMS system is activated, resources such as personnel and vehicles are dispatched. EMS personnel then will provide care at the scene and during transport. They also deliver the patient to the most appropriate medical facility.

In-Hospital Care System

Most patients are taken to a hospital emergency department. There personnel stabilize all immediate life threats. Then the patient's care is transferred to the most appropriate in-hospital resources, such as the medical/surgical or intensive care units, or the patient is transferred to a more specialized hospital.

Some hospitals handle all routine and emergency cases but have a specialty that sets them apart. One **specialty hospital** is a trauma center, where specific services and surgery teams are available 24 hours a day. Some hospitals specialize in the care of certain conditions such as burns or cardiac problems. Other hospitals may specialize in a particular type of patient, such as pediatric and neonatal patients.

By the time you return to the scene, you can tell that the young boy has stopped shaking. Within seconds, a pair of women arrive and introduce themselves as Elizabeth and Nora, members of the company's Medical Emergency Response Team. They have equipment with them and seem to know what they are doing. Elizabeth kneels beside the patient and appears to be listening for something. Nora takes the woman aside and asks questions about the boy.

Medical Direction

Each EMS system has a Medical Director. He or she is a physician who assumes the ultimate responsibility for direction and oversight of all patient care. The Medical Director also oversees training and assists in the development of treatment **protocols**. Most EMS systems have prescribed protocols that describe how to manage the most common types of patients, such as patients with chest pain, cardiac arrest, difficult breathing, and severe allergic reaction. Emergency Medical Responders act as designated agents of the Medical Director. The physician cannot physically be present at every emergency. So, the EMS provides **standing orders**. These written orders are in the form of protocols, which authorize rescuers to perform specific skills in specific situations. For instance, the protocol for how to care for a patient who has chest pain may include a standing order for oxygen. Thus, the Emergency Medical Responder may provide oxygen to any patient who has chest pain based on that standing order. That kind of behind-the-scenes medical direction is called **off-line medical direction** (or *indirect medical direction*).

Procedures not covered by standing orders or protocols require the Emergency Medical Responder to contact medical direction by radio or telephone prior to performing a particular skill or administering care. Orders from medical direction given in this manner—by radio or phone—are called **on-line medical direction** (or *direct medical direction*). The primary role of medical direction is to ensure that the quality of care is standardized and consistent throughout the local EMS system.

As an Emergency Medical Responder at the scene of an emergency, you may have limited access to the Medical Director. It will be necessary for you to adhere to the training you receive or to follow the orders of on-scene EMS providers who have a higher level of training or certification.

Like all EMS personnel, you must only provide care that is within your scope of practice. The scope of practice is defined as the care an Emergency Medical Responder is allowed and supposed to provide according to local, state, or regional regulations or statutes. The scope of practice includes protocols and guidelines set in place by the local jurisdiction.

OBJECTIVE

9. Explain the various types of medical direction and how the Emergency Medical Responder might interact with each.

protocols ▶ written guidelines that direct the care EMS personnel provide for patients.

standing orders ▶ the Medical Director's specific instructions for the Emergency Medical Responder, Emergency Medical Technician, or Paramedic to provide care for specific medical conditions or injuries.

off-line medical direction ▶ an EMS system's standing orders and protocols, which authorize personnel to perform particular skills in certain situations without actually speaking to the Medical Director. Also called *indirect medical direction.*

on-line medical direction ▶ orders to perform a skill or administer care from the on-duty physician, given to the rescuer in person by radio or by phone. Also called *direct medical direction.*

From the Medical Director

Welcome to the World of EMS

Congratulations on choosing to expand your knowledge and become a part of the prehospital patient care team called EMS. Depending on where you live, you may or may not be required to have a medical director to authorize your actions. Regardless, it is important to understand the role medical directors play in allowing Emergency Medical Responders to function.

Medical directors are a committed group of physicians who review and approve your curriculum, patient care protocols, and evaluations of your performance. Throughout this text you will find notes "From the Medical Director" that have the goal of helping you better understand important points about EMS and your new profession. Welcome to the world of EMS!

The scope of practice may vary from state to state and region to region. Your instructor will inform you of any local protocols and policies that may define your scope of practice. Always follow your local protocols.

The Emergency Medical Responder

The lack of people with enough training to provide care before more highly skilled EMS providers arrive at a scene is the weakest link in the chain of the EMS system. Training Emergency Medical Responders will help correct this problem.

Emergency Medical Responders are trained to reach patients, find out what is wrong, and provide emergency care. They also are trained to move patients when necessary and without causing further injury (Scan 1.2). They are usually the first medically trained personnel to reach the patient. In all cases, an Emergency Medical Responder has successfully completed an Emergency Medical Responder course. Many police officers and firefighters are trained to this level. Industrial companies are beginning to train employees as Emergency Medical Responders as well. The more private citizens become trained as Emergency Medical Responders, the stronger the EMS system becomes.

Since the beginning of Emergency Medical Responder training programs, hundreds of thousands of people have completed formal training courses, with many going on to provide essential emergency care. The care that Emergency Medical Responders provide reduces suffering, prevents additional injuries, and saves many lives.

Roles and Responsibilities

Personal Safety

Your primary concern as an Emergency Medical Responder at an emergency scene is your own *personal safety*. The desire to help those in need of care may tempt you to ignore the hazards at the scene. You must make certain that you can safely reach the patient and that you will remain safe while providing care.

Part of an Emergency Medical Responder's concern for personal safety must include the proper protection from infectious diseases. All Emergency Medical Responders who assess or provide care for patients *must* avoid direct contact with patient blood and other body fluids. Personal protective equipment (PPE) that minimizes contact with infectious material includes the following:

- Disposable protective gloves
- Barrier devices, such as pocket face masks with one-way valves and special filters for rescue-breathing procedures
- Protective eye wear, such as goggles or face shields to avoid contact with droplets expelled during certain care procedures such as ventilating and suctioning
- Special face masks with filters that minimize contact with airborne microorganisms
- Gowns or aprons that minimize contact of splashed blood and other body fluids

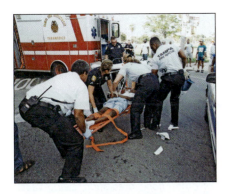

1.2.1 | Emergency Medical Responders may work on rescue squads and transport units.
(© Craig Jackson/In the Dark Photography)

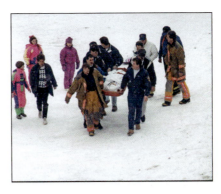

1.2.2 | They may be firefighter volunteers.
(© Craig Jackson/In the Dark Photography)

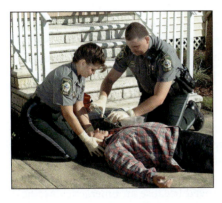

1.2.3 | Emergency Medical Responders may be law enforcement personnel, including state troopers, ATF, DEA, and FBI agents.

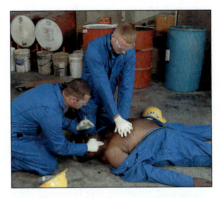

1.2.4 | They are homeland defense personnel, campus security police, shopping mall and factory security personnel, and industrial Medical Emergency Response Teams.

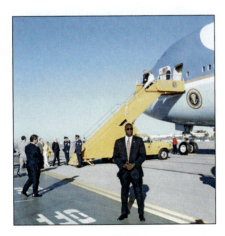

1.2.5 | Emergency Medical Responders are park rangers, lifeguards, athletic trainers, military combat lifesavers, and executive protection personnel such as Secret Service agents.

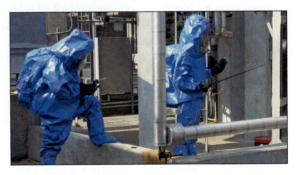

1.2.6 | Emergency Medical Responders are also rescue team specialists for specific disciplines, such as hazardous materials, confined space, swift water, ice, trench, high angle, cave, and urban rescues.

Personal Safety

Besides proper handwashing and the use of personal protective equipment to prevent being exposed to infectious agents, an additional and often overlooked precaution is to be vaccinated against some of the more common agents you may encounter. Blood has the potential of exposing you to hepatitis B and C while a person with a fever may expose you to pneumonia, meningitis, and influenza (the flu). There are vaccines available to immunize you against hepatitis B but not C. There are vaccines for meningitis, pneumonia, and influenza. The influenza vaccine is released yearly based on assumptions of what type of flu will be most prevalent. Being vaccinated against those agents provides you with one more layer of protection. In addition, being vaccinated may help you stay healthy during flu season when exposure may occur outside of your Emergency Medical Responder duties. Please consider getting vaccinated.

Typically, you will only need protective gloves and possibly face masks for most patient care situations. However, all the items listed on page 10 should be on hand so that you can protect yourself and provide care safely. (Find more about infectious diseases and personal protection in Chapter 3.)

Keep in mind that Emergency Medical Responders who are in law enforcement, the fire service, or industry may be required to carry out their specific job tasks before they provide patient care (such as controlling traffic, stabilizing vehicles, or shutting down machinery). If this applies to you, always follow department or company standard operating procedures.

Patient-Related Duties

Prior to receiving care, the injured or ill person is referred to as a *victim*. Once you start to carry out your duties as an Emergency Medical Responder, the victim becomes a *patient*. Your presence at the scene means that the EMS system has begun its first phase of care (Scan 1.3). True, the patient may need a physician at the hospital to survive, but the patient's chances of reaching the hospital alive are greatly improved because an Emergency Medical Responder has initiated emergency care. As an Emergency Medical Responder, you have six main patient-related duties to carry out at the emergency scene (Scan 1.3). They are:

- *Size up the scene.* Scene safety is your first concern, even before patient care. Evaluate how to protect yourself and the patient, and try to determine what caused the patient's injury or illness, how many patients there are, and what kind of assistance you will need. You must control the scene to protect yourself and the patients and to minimize additional injuries.
- *Determine the patient's chief complaint.* Gather information from the patient, from the scene, and from bystanders. Using the supplies you have, provide emergency care to the level of your training. Remember, emergency care deals with both illness and injury. It can be as simple as providing emotional support to someone who is frightened because of a crash or mishap. Or it can be more complex, requiring you to deal with life-threatening emergencies, such as providing basic life support measures for a heart attack victim. In later chapters, you will learn how to provide a combination of emotional support and physical care skills to help the patient until more highly trained personnel arrive.
- *Lift, move, or reposition the patient only when it is necessary.* You need to judge when safety or care requires you to move or reposition patients. When you must move a patient, use techniques that minimize the chance of injuring yourself.
- *Transfer the patient and patient information.* Provide for an orderly transfer of the patient and all patient-related information to more highly trained personnel. You also may be asked to assist such personnel and work under their direction.
- *Protect the patient's privacy, and maintain confidentiality.* This responsibility is not only a matter of good patient care but also a matter of legality.
- *Be the patient's advocate.* You must be willing to be an advocate for the patient and do what is best for him as long as it is safe to do so.

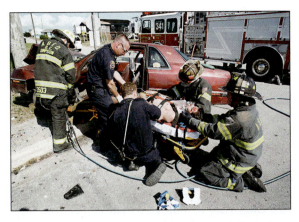

1.3.1 | One of the duties of an Emergency Medical Responder is to safely gain access to the patient. *(Photo by Nathan Eldridge)*

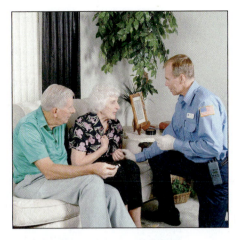

1.3.2 | Emergency Medical Responders must find out what is wrong with the patient.

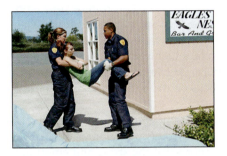

1.3.3 | Emergency Medical Responders lift or move patients when necessary without causing further injury.

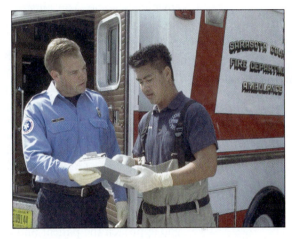

1.3.4 | The Emergency Medical Responder also transfers the patient and patient information to appropriate medical personnel, protects the patient's privacy and maintains confidentiality, and acts as the patient's advocate.

Traits

To be an Emergency Medical Responder you must be willing to take on certain duties and responsibilities. It takes hard work and study to be an Emergency Medical Responder. Since you must keep your emergency care skills sharp and current (Figure 1.2), you may be required to recertify or relicense periodically.

You also have to be willing to deal with people. Individuals who are sick or injured are not at their best. You must be able to overlook rude behavior and unreasonable demands, realizing that patients may act this way because of fear, uncertainty, or pain. Dealing with patient reactions is often the hardest part of the job. To do so in a professional manner is sometimes very difficult.

All patients have the same right to the very best of care. Your respect for others and acceptance of their rights are essential parts of the total patient care that you provide as an

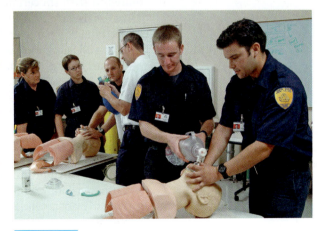

Figure 1.2 • Frequent training promotes a high standard of care for your patients.

Emergency Medical Responder. You must not modify the care you provide or discriminate based on your view of religious beliefs, cultural expression, age, gender, social behavior, socioeconomic background, or geographic origin. Every patient is unique and deserves to have his or her needs met by a consistent standard of care.

To be an Emergency Medical Responder, you must be honest and realistic. When helping patients, you cannot tell them they are okay if they are truly sick or hurt. You cannot tell them that everything is all right, when they know that something is wrong. Telling someone not to worry is not realistic. When an emergency occurs, there is truly something to worry about. Your conversations with patients can help them relax, if you are honest. By telling patients that you are trained in emergency care and that you will help them, you ease their fears and gain their confidence. Letting patients know that additional aid is on the way also will help them relax.

As an Emergency Medical Responder, there may be limits to what you can say to a patient or a patient's loved ones. Telling a patient that a loved one is dead may not be appropriate if you are still providing care for the patient. In such circumstances, it is often necessary for you to be tactful. Remember, people under the stress of illness or injury often do not tolerate additional stress well.

Being an Emergency Medical Responder requires that you control your feelings at the emergency scene. You must learn how to care for patients while controlling your emotional reactions to their injury or illness. Patients do not need sympathy and tears. They need your professional care.

As an Emergency Medical Responder, you have to be a highly disciplined professional at the emergency scene. You must not make inappropriate comments about patients or the horror of the incident. You must maintain your focus on the patient and avoid unnecessary distractions.

Providing appropriate care requires you to admit that the stress of responding to emergency scenes will affect you. You may have to speak with a counselor, or other EMS professionals, or a specialist within the EMS system to resolve the stress and emotional challenges caused by responding to emergencies.

No one can demand that you change your lifestyle to be an Emergency Medical Responder. However, first impressions are very important, and your appearance alone can earn a patient's confidence. So keep your uniform neat and clean at all times. Also, how you approach the patient and the respect you show are very important. Refer to the patient in a manner that is appropriate for his or her age. All elders should be referred to as Mr., Mrs., or Ms. In contrast, children respond well to their first names. The significance of how you refer to a patient can greatly affect the willingness of the patient to share information and feel comfortable in your care.

OBJECTIVE

11. Describe the characteristics of professionalism as they relate to the EMS provider.

Skills

In addition to learning the facts that are the foundation of emergency care, you will be required to perform certain skills as part of your Emergency Medical Responder training. Those skills vary from course to course. The list below is an example of the skills learned by the typical Emergency Medical Responder. You are not expected to memorize the list. Read it and check off each skill as you learn it in your course.

As an Emergency Medical Responder, you should be able to:

- Assess for and manage potential hazards at the scene
- Gain access to patients in vehicles
- Gain access to patients in buildings as well as in outdoor settings
- Evaluate the possible cause of an illness or injury
- Properly use all items of personal safety
- Conduct an appropriate patient assessment
- Gather accurate vital signs (pulse, respiration, skin signs, pupils)
- Properly document assessment findings
- Relate signs and symptoms to illnesses and injuries
- Evaluate and manage a patient's airway and breathing status
- Perform cardiopulmonary resuscitation (CPR) for adults, children, and infants

- Operate an automated external defibrillator (AED) for patients in cardiac arrest
- Control bleeding by using direct pressure, elevation, and tourniquets
- Assess and manage the patient who is showing signs of shock
- Assess and provide care for patients who have closed injuries and open injuries, including face and scalp wounds, nosebleeds, eye injuries, neck wounds, chest injuries, and abdominal injuries
- Perform basic dressing and bandaging techniques
- Assess and care for injuries to bones and joints
- Assess and care for possible head and face injuries
- Assess and care for possible injuries to the neck and spine
- Assess and care for possible heart attacks, strokes, seizures, and diabetic emergencies
- Identify and care for poisoning
- Assess and care for burns
- Assess and care for heat- and cold-related emergencies
- Assist a mother in delivering her baby
- Provide initial care for the newborn
- Identify and care for drug-abuse and alcohol-abuse patients
- Perform standard and emergency patient moves when required
- Perform triage at a multiple-patient emergency scene
- Work under the direction of an Incident Commander in an incident command system (ICS) or incident management system (IMS) operation
- Work under the direction of EMTs or more highly trained personnel to help them provide patient care, doing what you have been trained to do at your level of care as an Emergency Medical Responder

In some systems, Emergency Medical Responders may be required to perform some or all of the following:

- Deliver oxygen
- Apply or assist in applying a traction splint
- Apply or assisting in applying a cervical collar
- Assist with the application of a vest-type extrication device
- Assist in securing a patient to a long spine board (backboard) or other device used to immobilize a patient's spine

Equipment, Tools, and Supplies

Most Emergency Medical Responders carry very few pieces of equipment, tools, and supplies. Some may carry specialized kits for trauma emergencies, medical emergencies, and childbirth. It is easier to grab a small kit containing the items needed for the incident than to pick up and carry a large kit with everything in it. If you are assigned to a special event, such as a concert, sporting event, or a carnival, you may want to include items that will meet the needs of that event in addition to the standard dressings and bandages. For instance, if you were providing medical support for a football game, it would be appropriate to have cervical collars and a backboard handy, given the likelihood of a significant mechanism of injury.

In some localities, Emergency Medical Responders are expected to take a patient's blood pressure. In those cases, the kit would include a blood pressure cuff and a stethoscope. Some jurisdictions may have Emergency Medical Responders administer oxygen and suction the patient's mouth and nose when needed. In those jurisdictions, Emergency Medical Responders carry oxygen-delivery systems and suctioning equipment.

Continuous Quality Improvement

One of the goals of the evaluation component of an EMS system is a concept known as **continuous quality improvement (CQI)**. CQI is exactly what the name implies—a continuous improvement in the quality of the product or service being delivered. In the case of

OBJECTIVE

12. Explain the role of the Emergency Medical Responder with regards to continuous quality improvement (CQI).

continuous quality improvement (CQI) ▶ a continuous improvement in the quality of the product or service being delivered.

EMS, that product is patient care. As a trained Emergency Medical Responder working within an EMS system you will be accountable for and expected to participate in the CQI process.

If designed properly, a CQI program is based on the philosophy that every component within a system can be improved. It is a process that expects and allows everyone in the system to participate and contribute to improvement. It should focus on the systems and processes and less on the people within the system.

As an Emergency Medical Responder, you will be an important component of the CQI system and will be expected to submit accurate and complete patient care reports that will be audited by trained individuals. Those audits are meant to reveal many characteristics of the care being provided, including but not limited to types of illnesses and injuries, ages of patients, geographic location of calls, and many other factors.

You may be asked to participate in training or serve on a quality committee as part of the CQI process. Whatever your role or level of participate, everyone in the system plays an important part in the CQI process.

OBJECTIVES

14. Explain the role of public health systems and their relationship to EMS, disease surveillance, and injury prevention.

15. Explain the role that Disaster Medical Assistance Teams (DMAT) play and how they integrate with EMS systems.

16. Explain the role that research plays in EMS and the ways that an Emergency Medical Responder might identify and support research.

public health system ▶ local resources dedicated to promoting optimal health and quality of life for the people and communities they serve.

Disaster Medical Assistance Team (DMAT) ▶ specialized teams designed to provide medical care following a disaster.

research ▶ the systematic investigation to establish facts.

The Role of the Public Health System

Each country, region, and state has people and resources that serve as part of the **public health system**. Those resources are dedicated to promoting optimal health and quality of life for the people they serve. Public health systems help ensure the quality of life by monitoring the health of the population, providing health care, and educating the community about disease and injury prevention. They also serve to advance population-based health programs and policies.

Disaster Assistance

Each state has identified specific individuals already working in its EMS systems to participate in specialized teams designed to provide medical care following a disaster. This type of team is called a **Disaster Medical Assistance Team (DMAT)**. The individuals who make up DMATs are highly experienced, trained EMS personnel. They can be deployed on a moment's notice should a disaster strike anywhere in the United States. For example, DMATs from across the nation descended on New Orleans immediately following hurricane Katrina. DMATs arrive in an area following a disaster and are quickly integrated into the local EMS resources.

The Role of Research in EMS

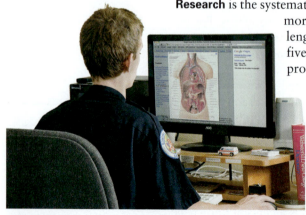

Research is the systematic investigation to establish facts (Figure 1.3). Each year more and more new research is being conducted and old research is being challenged. Several organizations around the globe have spent the past five years gathering and verifying research that is defining how EMS providers practice emergency care. In late 2010, the American Heart Association and the International Liaison Committee on Resuscitation (ILCOR) released new guidelines that will define how EMS providers will perform resuscitation and emergency care for the next several years. The military also has been conducting research that is influencing how EMS provides care for those who are ill or injured in the civilian world.

This book includes many of the changes in emergency care that are being recommended as a result of this new research. Be sure to play an active role in searching for, reading, and evaluating research that affects your job as an Emergency Medical Responder.

Figure 1.3 • Staying current with the latest research is an important aspect of good patient care.

Advances in Technology

In recent years there have been several advances in technology that have made the job of the EMS team more effective and efficient. One of the most important of those advances is the introduction of the global positioning system (GPS) to the civilian marketplace (Figure 1.4). GPS is becoming more common and is being installed in all types of public safety vehicles, such as police cars, fire engines, and ambulances. The use of GPS technology allows emergency personnel to more easily navigate to the location of the emergency, thus reducing response time. It also gives dispatch personnel the ability to track the location of emergency vehicles and to utilize resources more efficiently.

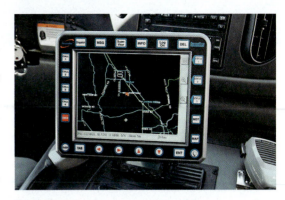

Figure 1.4 • A typical GPS device installed in an emergency vehicle.

It looks like the cavalry is arriving. There are so many vehicles with lights and sirens. First, there are two fire trucks. Then an ambulance shows up, and behind that is another SUV-type vehicle painted just like the ambulance. Before you know it, there is what seems like a dozen people all hovering over the young boy.

You stick around to observe the excitement and even forget for a minute why you are actually there. You hear Elizabeth give a report to the ambulance team about the boy and how she thought he might have had a seizure.

Wow, what an exciting day! You can't stop thinking about the poor boy and how he must have felt when he woke to see so many people hovering over him. The woman with the boy turns out to be his mother, and she takes the time to thank you for making sure the call to 911 was made quickly.

CHAPTER REVIEW

Summary

The emergency medical services (EMS) system is a chain of resources established to provide care to the patient at the scene of an emergency and during transport to the hospital emergency department. Review these key concepts related to working within an EMS system:

- There are four levels of EMS training: Emergency Medical Responder (EMR), Emergency Medical Technician (EMT), Advanced Emergency Medical Technician (AEMT), and Paramedic.

- EMS personnel are dispatched to the scene of an emergency when a dispatcher receives an emergency call. Dispatchers may be specially trained as Emergency Medical Dispatchers (EMDs) who offer pre-arrival care instructions to bystanders at the scene.

- Every EMS system is required to designate a Medical Director, a physician who assumes the ultimate responsibility for medical oversight of the patient care aspects of the EMS system.

- The Emergency Medical Responder's primary responsibility is personal safety. No one should enter or approach an emergency scene until it is safe to do so.

- An Emergency Medical Responder's main duties are scene safety, gaining access to the patient, assessing the patient and providing emergency care, moving patients (when necessary), transferring care to more highly trained personnel, protecting the patient's privacy, and being the patient's advocate.

- Emergency Medical Responders have a duty to maintain skills, keep up-to-date with the latest trends and research, and maintain a professional demeanor at all times.

- As an Emergency Medical Responder, you play an important part in the quality of the system you will be working in and may participate in specific duties related to the CQI process.

- More than ever before, research is defining the way that EMS personnel deliver care to patients. As an Emergency Medical Responder you have a duty to stay informed about the latest research findings.

Take Action

KNOW YOUR SYSTEM

1. No two EMS systems are exactly the same. To provide the best care possible, you must know what resources are available within your system. Find someone who is currently working with EMS and ask him or her the following questions:
   - Where are 911 calls answered?
   - Does the system utilize an *enhanced* 911 system?
   - Which of the four levels of EMS provider are recognized by your local EMS system?
   - What types of EMS model or models exist in your area or region: fire-based, third-service, or hospital-based?
   - Are there any specialty hospitals in your system?
   - Are there helicopter resources operating in your local system?

2. If possible, try to arrange a tour of a 911 dispatch center. A good place to begin is by asking your instructor. Most dispatch centers allow people to sit in and observe during certain times. This experience will give you a good appreciation for how the dispatch side of things work.

First on Scene Run Review

Recall the events of the "First on Scene" scenario in this chapter and answer the following questions, which are related to the call. Rationales are offered in the Answer Key at the back of the book.

1. Prior to calling 911, what important information should you have obtained from the woman who was with the boy? And why?

2. What equipment should the company's Medical Emergency Response Team have with them when responding to a call?

3. When treating this patient, how would each of the six patient-related duties apply?

4. How would protocols and standing orders apply to this call?

Quick Quiz

To check your understanding of the chapter, answer the following questions. Then compare your answers to those in the Answer Key at the back of the book.

1. Which one of the following is NOT a common component of an EMS system?

    a. Ambulances
    b. Hospitals
    c. Clinics
    d. Fire service

2. All care provided by EMS personnel within an EMS system is overseen by a(n):

    a. Medical Director.
    b. Fire Chief.
    c. Ambulance Supervisor.
    d. Nursing Supervisor.

3. Which one of the following BEST describes the role of the Emergency Medical Responder in an EMS system?

    a. Identifies hazards and transports patients
    b. Cares for immediate life threats and assists EMTs
    c. Secures the scene and serves as an Incident Commander
    d. Assists Paramedics with advanced skills

4. Emergency Medical Dispatchers receive training that allows them to:

    a. control the scene via the radio.
    b. triage patients via the radio.
    c. declare a mass-casualty incident.
    d. provide pre-arrival care instructions.

5. Which one of the following receives the highest level of training in an EMS system?

    a. Emergency Medical Responder
    b. Emergency Medical Technician
    c. Advanced Emergency Medical Technician
    d. Paramedic

6. Guidelines written by the Medical Director describe the care that EMS personnel provide for patients. Those guidelines are called:

    a. dispatching.
    b. protocols.
    c. on-line direction.
    d. prescriptions.

7. Which one of the following would MOST likely be considered a standing order?

    a. Stay clear of an unsafe scene.
    b. Run with lights and sirens.
    c. Begin CPR on a victim of cardiac arrest.
    d. Dispatch an ambulance to an emergency scene.

8. Protocols and standing orders are forms of:

    a. off-line medical direction.
    b. on-line medical direction.
    c. pre-arrival instructions.
    d. stand-by guidelines.

9. The care that an Emergency Medical Responder is allowed and supposed to provide according to local, state, or regional regulations or statutes is known as:

    a. scope of practice.
    b. standard of care.
    c. national standard curricula.
    d. Emergency Medical Responder care.

10. As a member of the EMS team, your primary role is one of:

    a. patient care.
    b. safety.
    c. transport.
    d. documentation.

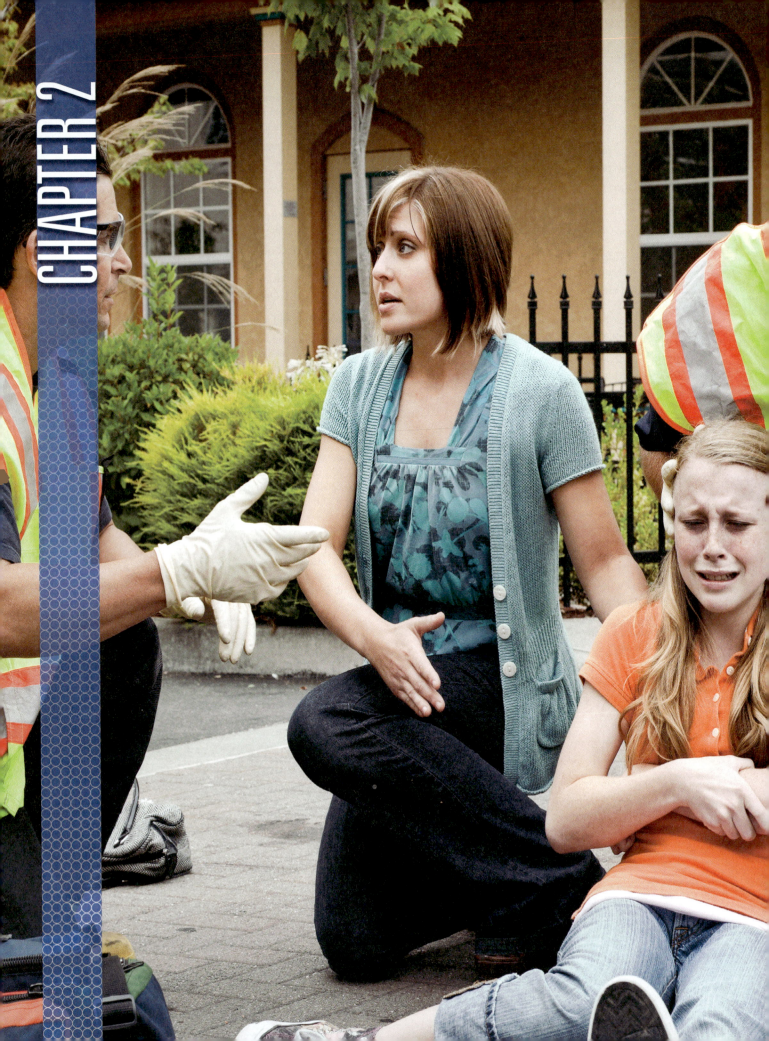

CHAPTER 2

Legal and Ethical Principles of Emergency Care

EDUCATION STANDARDS
- Preparatory—Medical/Legal and Ethics

COMPETENCIES
- Uses simple knowledge of the EMS system, safety and well-being of the Emergency Medical Responder, medical/legal issues at the scene of an emergency while awaiting a higher level of care.

CHAPTER OVERVIEW

As an Emergency Medical Responder, you must make many decisions when responding to an emergency and while caring for patients. Understanding the related legal and ethical issues will help you make the best decisions possible.

You may already have concerns about some legal and ethical issues. For example, does an off-duty Emergency Medical Responder stop to aid victims of an automobile crash? Should you release information about your patient to an attorney over the telephone? May a child with a suspected broken arm be treated, even if a parent is not present? What should you do if a patient who needs emergency medical care refuses it?

This chapter will provide you with an overview of the legal and ethical aspects of being an Emergency Medical Responder.

Upon successful completion of this chapter, the student should be able to:

COGNITIVE

1. Define the following terms:
   a. abandonment *(p. 30)*
   b. advance directive *(p. 27)*
   c. battery *(p. 26)*
   d. breach of duty *(p. 29)*
   e. civil law (tort) *(p. 29)*
   f. competence *(p. 24)*
   g. competent *(p. 24)*
   h. confidentiality *(p. 30)*
   i. consent *(p. 24)*
   j. criminal law *(p. 26)*
   k. duty *(p. 22)*
   l. duty to act *(p. 29)*
   m. emancipated minor *(p. 26)*
   n. ethics *(p. 23)*
   o. expressed consent *(p. 25)*
   p. Good Samaritan law *(p. 30)*
   q. Health Insurance Portability Accountability Act (HIPAA) *(p. 31)*
   r. implied consent *(p. 25)*
   s. informed consent *(p. 25)*
   t. mandated reporter *(p. 32)*
   u. negligence *(p. 29)*
   v. standard of care *(p. 23)*
   w. unresponsive *(p. 25)*
   x. values *(p. 24)*

2. Explain the concepts of "duty" and "breach of duty" as they relate to the Emergency Medical Responder. *(p. 29)*

3. Explain the term *ethics* and how it relates to the Emergency Medical Responder. *(p. 23)*

4. Explain the term *Good Samaritan law* and how these laws relate to the Emergency Medical Responder. *(p. 22)*

5. Explain the term *mandated reporter* and how it relates to the Emergency Medical Responder. *(p. 31)*

6. Differentiate the terms *scope of practice* and *standard of care*. *(p. 22)*

7. Compare and contrast the various types of consent utilized by the Emergency Medical Responder. *(p. 24)*

8. Explain the role of the Emergency Medical Responder for patients who refuse care. *(p. 26)*

OBJECTIVES

9. Differentiate civil and criminal litigation. *(p. 26)*

10. Explain the common elements of an advance directive. *(p. 27)*

11. Explain the role of the Emergency Medical Responder when confronted with an advance directive. *(p. 27)*

12. Explain the role of the Emergency Medical Responder with regards to patient confidentiality. *(p. 30)*

13. Explain the role of the Emergency Medical Responder with respect to evidence preservation when working in or around an actual or potential crime scene. *(p. 32)*

There are no psychomotor objectives identified for this chapter.

AFFECTIVE

14. Consistently model ethical behavior in all aspects of Emergency Medical Responder training and job performance.

15. Demonstrate compassion and empathy toward all classmates, coworkers, and simulated patients.

16. Participate willingly as a team member in all class/training activities.

17. Value the importance of maintaining patient confidentiality.

18. Demonstrate a desire to always do what is right for the patient.

FIRST ON SCENE

They're moving fast on the open road when Anthony yells, "Hold on!" and she feels his body tense under the smooth leather jacket. The motorcycle leans far to the right and then quickly back to the left, causing the tires to squeal and wobble as the bike comes to a clumsy stop. Sara looks over Anthony's shoulder and feels her stomach grow cold. Two deep gouges scar the asphalt all the way to the far side of the road where a small sports car is overturned and partially wrapped around a tree. Behind her, amazingly close to the black skid marks left by the motorcycle, a man is lying in a heap on the road.

In a matter of seconds, the entire Emergency Medical Responder class that Sara took two months ago flashes through her head.

"Stop," she says, quickly pulling her wind-whipped hair back into a ponytail. "That guy in the road needs help right now!"

Legal Duties

OBJECTIVE

4. Explain the term *Good Samaritan law* and how these laws relate to the Emergency Medical Responder.

duty ▶ the legal obligation to provide care.

Read up on EMS laws in the United States.

OBJECTIVE

6. Differentiate the terms *scope of practice* and *standard of care.*

Most of us have heard stories about people being sued because of something they did or did not do when they stopped to help someone at the scene of an emergency. Successful suits of this type are not very common. Most states have established laws called "Good Samaritan laws" that minimize exposure to liability and encourage passersby to provide emergency care to those in need. Those laws require the individual who is providing care to be doing so without compensation and to remain within a specified *scope of practice.*

Depending on the specific role that you play as an Emergency Medical Responder, you may have a legal and/or ethical duty to assist those in need. **Duty** is a legal term that simply means *that one is morally or legally obligated to provide care.* An Emergency Medical Responder who works normal shifts or is on-call as a volunteer and is expected to respond to dispatches has a legal duty to respond and provide care to those who are ill or injured. In addition to the duty to respond, you also have a duty, or obligation, to provide care as you have been trained and to the expected standard in your area, region, or state.

Scope of Practice

Recall from Chapter 1 that the term *scope of practice* refers to what is legally permitted to be done by some or all individuals trained or licensed at a particular level, such as an Emergency Medical Responder, Emergency Medical Technician (EMT), or Paramedic. The scope of practice, however, does *not* define what must be done for a given patient or in a particular situation.

The scope of practice for a layperson might be based on nothing more than common sense or an eight-hour first-aid class taken many years ago. However, the scope of practice for Emergency Medical Responders and other EMS personnel is based in part on the U.S. Department of Transportation's education standards for EMS and in most cases is more clearly defined by local and state statutes and regulations.

Standard of Care

The term **standard of care** is more subjective and deals with questions such as "Did you do the right thing, at the right time, and for the right reasons?" It is defined by several factors, such as scope of practice, common practice, current research, and sometimes juries. Just like the scope of practice, standard of care can and does vary from county to county, state to state, and region to region (Figure 2.1).

A standard of care allows you to be judged based on what is expected of someone with your training and experience working under similar conditions. Your Emergency Medical Responder course follows guidelines developed by the U.S. Department of Transportation as well as other authorities that have studied what is needed to provide the most appropriate standard of care required at your level in your region. You will be trained so that you can provide this standard of care. If the care you provide is not up to the expected standard, you may be held liable for your actions.

You may be required to communicate with your Medical Director by telephone or radio, and you will be expected to follow approved standing orders or protocols for your EMS system.

Keep written notes of what you do at the emergency scene, especially if a crime has occurred. You may be called on to provide this information at a later date. If your EMS system requires you to complete forms, submit reports, or sign patient transfer papers, complete those forms thoroughly and in a timely manner. Your documentation must be able to show that you provided an appropriate standard of care.

standard of care ▶ the care that should be provided for any level of training based on local laws, administrative orders, and guidelines and protocols established by the local EMS system.

Ethical Responsibilities

Ethics can be simply defined as "behavior." However, it is not any behavior, but behavior that is right, good, and proper. As an Emergency Medical Responder, you have an ethical obligation to behave in a way that puts your patient's needs before your own, so long as it is safe to do so. You have a responsibility to see that your patient receives the most appropriate medical care possible, even when he does not think he needs any care.

OBJECTIVE

3. Explain the term *ethics* and how it relates to the Emergency Medical Responder.

ethics ▶ the study of the principles that define behavior as right, good, and proper.

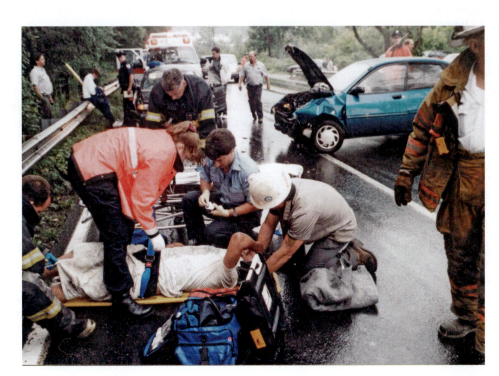

Figure 2.1 • Different emergency personnel may be assisting during an emergency, including police, firefighters, and EMTs. Each must practice the standard of care expected of his own level of training. *(© Mark C. Ide)*

Patient Advocacy

The term patient advocate *refers to putting the needs of the patient first. This can be difficult in situations where you know the patient personally and do not want him to feel inconvenienced or embarrassed. It is natural to want to be a friend, but when responding to an emergency, you must put aside your feelings and consider the patient's best interest medically.*

Resource Central

Learn more about the EMS Code of Ethics and how it applies to you.

values ▶ the personal beliefs that determine how a person actually behaves.

As an Emergency Medical Responder, you will be caring for people of all social, economic, and cultural backgrounds. You must maintain an open mind and develop an understanding of those differences. You have an ethical responsibility to treat all people equally and provide the highest standard of care for your patients.

Another ethical responsibility as a member of the EMS team is to maintain your skills and knowledge constantly. This includes keeping abreast of current research by reading professional publications and attending conferences when practical. It also means practicing your skills in order to maintain confidence and an appropriate level of competency. You must attend continuing education and refresher programs, because it is necessary to keep yourself ready to perform at all times. Remember, every patient deserves the best care possible.

It is also important for you to be honest in reporting the care you provided to a patient, even if a mistake was made. While all EMS providers should provide the appropriate care at all times, mistakes do happen. Errors should be reported immediately so corrective steps, if needed, may be taken as soon as possible.

Your behavior (ethics) is always being influenced by your personal core values. **Values** are core beliefs that you hold to be true. Doing the right thing is not always easy and can cause you internal struggles. Many groups and professions have a common set of shared values. Those values serve as a "moral compass" and help guide an individual's decision-making process. Because EMS personnel are frequently faced with making difficult decisions, several EMS groups, agencies, and institutions have adopted the following set of values:

- Integrity
- Compassion
- Accountability
- Respect
- Empathy

OBJECTIVE

7. Compare and contrast the various types of consent utilized by the Emergency Medical Responder.

consent ▶ the legal term that means to give formal permission for something to happen.

Consent

Consent is a legal term that means *to give formal permission for something to happen.* In the case of the Emergency Medical Responder, you must receive permission from each and every patient before you can legally provide care. The person providing consent must be legally competent to do so, and the consent may come in several forms.

Competence

competence ▶ the quality of being adequately or well qualified to make decisions both physically and intellectually.

competent ▶ properly or sufficiently qualified or capable of making appropriate decisions about one's own health or condition.

A discussion about consent would not be complete without a clear definition of the word *competence.* **Competence** is the patient's ability to understand what is going on around him, your questions, and the implications of the decisions he is making. In order for an Emergency Medical Responder to obtain consent or accept a refusal of care, he should establish that the patient is competent to make such decisions.

A patient may not be **competent** to make medical decisions in certain cases, such as being a minor, intoxication, drug ingestion, serious injury, or mental illness. To determine competency, the Emergency Medical Responder may begin by asking questions that a competent adult should be able to answer, such as where the patient is at the time, what day or month it is, and what has happened.

Approximately 15% of all people in the United States over the age of 65 demonstrate some degree of dementia. Dementia is the deterioration of specific mental capacities such as memory, concentration, and judgment. One of the most common causes of dementia is Alzheimer's disease.

An elderly patient with dementia may not fully comprehend the seriousness of his situation and may not want you to provide care. In other words, the elderly patient with dementia may not be competent to make decisions regarding his own medical care.

When presented with an elderly patient who is showing signs of disorientation, a short attention span, confusion, or hallucinations, obtain a detailed history from family members or caregivers. It will be important to determine if the patient's mental status is normal for him or if it has gotten worse since you arrived on the scene.

Do not allow patients who are showing signs of dementia to refuse care without further investigation into their normal state of mind. In most cases you will want to wait for the EMTs to arrive and take over care before you leave the scene.

Expressed Consent

An adult patient of legal age, when alert and competent, can give you consent to provide care. In Emergency Medical Responder care, a patient's consent is usually oral and commonly referred to as **expressed consent** (also referred to as *informed consent*). To qualify as expressed consent, the patient must be making an informed decision (Figure 2.2).

For a patient to make an informed decision, you need to advise the patient of the following:

- Your level of training
- Why you think care may be necessary
- What care you plan to provide
- Any consequences related to refusing care

You must receive consent before caring for any patient. A simple way to gain this consent may be by stating something like, "Hi, my name is Chris. I am an Emergency Medical Responder. May I help you?" A patient who is responsive may answer verbally or simply allow you to continue your care. Expressed consent does not need to be verbal. By *not* pulling away or stopping you, the patient is giving consent.

There are occasions when a child refuses care. By law only a parent or guardian of the child may give consent or refuse care. Of course, gaining the child's confidence and easing any fears should be a part of your care.

expressed consent ▶ a competent adult's informed decision to accept emergency care provided by an Emergency Medical Responder. Also referred to as *informed consent.*

informed consent ▶ See *expressed consent.*

unresponsive ▶ **having** no reaction to verbal or painful stimuli; previously referred to as *unconscious.*

implied consent ▶ a legal position that assumes that an unresponsive or incompetent adult patient would consent to receiving emergency care if he could. This form of consent may apply to other types of patients (e.g., the mentally ill).

Implied Consent

In emergency situations in which a patient is **unresponsive**, confused, or so severely ill or injured that expressed consent cannot be given, you may legally provide care based on **implied consent**. It is implied that the patient would want to receive care and treatment if he or she were aware of the situation and able to respond.

Since children are not legally allowed to provide consent or to refuse medical care, a form of implied consent is used in most states when parents or guardians are not on the scene and cannot be reached quickly. The law assumes that the parents would want care to be provided for their child (Figure 2.3).

The same holds true in cases involving the developmentally disabled and the mentally ill. It is assumed that the patient's parents or legal guardians would give consent for treatment if they knew of the emergency situation.

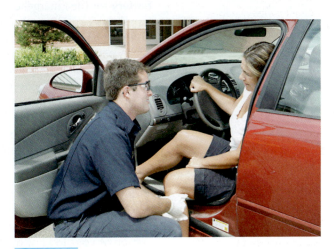

Figure 2.2 • Obtaining consent from an adult patient.

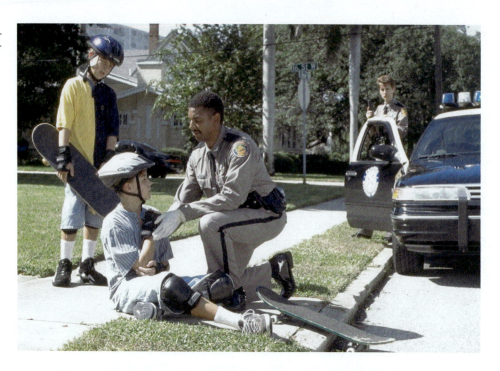

Emancipated Minor

emancipated minor ▶ a minor whose parents have entirely surrendered the right to the care, custody, and earnings and no longer are under any duty to support the minor.

Not all those under the age of 18 are considered minors in the traditional sense. There are some who have become legally emancipated and have been freed from control by their parents or legal guardians. **Emancipated minors** are legally allowed to make their own decisions regarding medical care. Minors may become legally emancipated if they are married, pregnant, a parent, a member of the armed forces, or financially independent and living away from home. It is rare that you might encounter an emancipated minor. Simply provide care as you would any other adult patient in the same situation.

Refusal of Care

criminal law ▶ the body of law dealing with crimes and punishment.

battery ▶ unlawful physical contact.

Alert and competent adults have the right to refuse care. Their refusal may be based on a variety of reasons, including their economic situation or religious views. They may even base it on a lack of trust. In fact, they may have reasons that you find senseless. For whatever reason, competent adults may refuse care. You may not force care on them, nor may you restrain them. Restraining or threatening to restrain a patient against his or her wishes could result in a violation of **criminal law** and result in a charge of assault and/or **battery** for the Emergency Medical Responder. Your only course of action is to try to gain a patient's confidence through conversation. If this fails and you feel the patient is at risk, you may have to call in law enforcement.

A patient does not have to speak to refuse your care. If the patient shakes his head to signal "no" or if he holds up his hand to signal you to stop, the patient has refused your help. Should the patient pull away from you, that also may be viewed as refusal of care.

It is important for you to understand the laws that govern patient refusal in your area. In many jurisdictions an Emergency Medical Responder may not leave a patient who is refusing care until someone with higher training has arrived and taken over care.

When your care is refused:

- Stay calm and professional and do your best to explain the situation to the patient.
- Inform them of the potential dangers of refusal.
- Use the aid of someone the patient trusts to try to convince them to accept care.
- Carefully document the refusal of care. Document your offer of help, your explanation of your level of training, why you think care is needed, the consequences of not accepting care, and the patient's refusal to accept your care. Also document the names

of anyone who witnessed your efforts to assist the patient. If your EMS system provides you with release forms, ask the patient to please read and sign the form. Make certain that you ask him if he understands what he has read before he signs the form.

A parent or legal guardian can refuse to let you care for a child. If the reason is fear or lack of confidence, simple conversation may change the individual's mind. In cases involving children, if the adult takes the child from the scene before EMTs arrive, you must report the incident to the EMTs or to the police. All states have special laws protecting the welfare of children. Know the laws in your state and jurisdiction regarding reporting such events. In all cases, know and follow local protocols.

continued ▶

Sara approaches the man lying in the road and finds him unresponsive. With each raspy breath, blood pours from his mouth and collects on the pavement in a shining pool. Unsure exactly what to do, she walks over to the overturned car, where she finds a woman, clad in a bright bikini top and cutoff jean shorts, pinned between the passenger door and the tree. "Hello?" Sara says. "Are you okay?"

The woman moans softly, but her eyes remain closed.

Anthony is now off the motorcycle and staring at the man in the road. "Come on!" he shouts to Sara. "My cell phone has no signal. Let's go find a pay phone!"

Advance Directives

There have been many high-profile medical cases over the years that involve the right to die and end-of-life decisions. These decisions are often left up to the surviving family members who do not always agree on the most appropriate action. Many of these cases can enter the court system and take many years to resolve. One solution to the dilemma of end-of-life decisions is a legal document referred to as an advance directive. An **advance directive** is a document that allows a patient to define in advance what his wishes are should he become incapacitated due to a medical illness or severe injury.

Advance directives are relatively simple documents that allow you to define your wishes or appoint another person to make decisions on your behalf. Advance directives commonly address such issues as:

- Designation of an agent to make decisions on your behalf
- Do not resuscitate (DNR) order
- Choice to prolong or not prolong life
- Pain relief
- Donation of organs

OBJECTIVES

10. Explain the common elements of an advance directive.

11. Explain the role of the Emergency Medical Responder when confronted with an advance directive.

advance directive ▶ a document that allows a patient to define in advance what his wishes are should he become incapacitated due to a medical illness or severe injury.

Do Not Resuscitate (DNR) Orders

At some time, you will come upon a patient who has a Do Not Resuscitate (DNR) order. It is typically in the form of a written document, usually signed by the patient and his or her physician. It states that the patient has a terminal illness and does not wish to prolong life through resuscitative efforts.

A DNR order is one type of *advance directive*, because it is written and signed in advance of any event where resuscitation may be undertaken (Figure 2.4). It is more than the expressed wishes of the patient or family. It is an actual legal document. In some cases, the patient will be wearing a DNR bracelet. This should not be mistaken for a medical identification bracelet, which gives information about medical conditions and/or allergies.

There are varying degrees of DNR orders, expressed through a variety of detailed instructions. For example, one DNR order might stipulate that resuscitation be attempted

OBJECTIVES

10. Explain the common elements of an advance directive.

11. Explain the role of the Emergency Medical Responder when confronted with an advance directive.

PREHOSPITAL DO NOT RESUSCITATE ORDERS

<u>ATTENDING PHYSICIAN</u>

In completing this prehospital DNR form, please check part A if no intervention by prehospital personnel is indicated. Please check Part A and options from Part B if specific interventions by prehospital personnel are indicated. To give a valid prehospital DNR order, this form must be completed by the patient's attending physician and must be provided to prehospital personnel.

A) _____ **Do Not Resuscitate (DNR):**
No Cardiopulmonary Resuscitation or Advanced Cardiac Life Support be performed by prehospital personnel

B) _____ **Modified Support:**
Prehospital personnel administer the following checked options:
_____ Oxygen administration
_____ Full airway support: intubation, airways, bag/valve/mask
_____ Venipuncture: IV crystalloids and/or blood draw
_____ External cardiac pacing
_____ Cardiopulmonary resuscitation
_____ Cardiac defibrillator
_____ Pneumatic anti-shock garment
_____ Ventilator
_____ ACLS meds
_____ Other interventions/medications (physician specify)
_____

Prehospital personnel are informed that (print patient name)_____
should receive no resuscitation (DNR) or should receive Modified Support as indicated. This directive is medically appropriate and is further documented by a physician's order and a progress note on the patient's permanent medical record. Informed consent from the capacitated patient or the incapacitated patient's legitimate surrogate is documented on the patient's permanent medical record. The DNR order is in full force and effect as of the date indicated below.

_____   _____
Attending Physician's Signature

_____   _____
Print Attending Physician's Name   Print Patient's Name and Location
                                               (Home Address or Health Care Facility)

_____
Attending Physician's Telephone

_____   _____
Date   Expiration Date (6 Mos from Signature)

Figure 2.4 • A DNR order is one example of an advance directive. Other examples include health-care proxies and living wills.

only if cardiac or respiratory arrest is observed but *not* attempted if the patient is found already in cardiac arrest. Another DNR order might specify that only assisted ventilations can be administered should the patient stop breathing, but if the heart stops, chest compressions are not to be provided.

The presence of a DNR order does not mean "do not care." As an Emergency Medical Responder, you have a duty to provide appropriate comfort and care within the bounds of the DNR. It is also within the patient's rights to withdraw the DNR order at any time.

Many states also have laws governing living wills. These are statements signed by the patient, commonly about the use of long-term life support and comfort measures such as respirators, intravenous feedings, and pain medications.

Advance Directives

Be sure to understand the laws in your state regarding living wills and DNR documents so that you can provide the patient with the most appropriate and compassionate care. If in doubt as to whether the documents presented to you are valid or pertain to the patient's condition, it is better to err on the side of treating him until EMS arrives.

Negligence

The basis for many civil (tort) lawsuits involving prehospital emergency care is **negligence**. Tort law involves a wrongful act, whether intentional or negligent, that causes an injury and can be addressed in civil court. *Negligence* is a term often used to indicate that either a care provider did not do what was expected or did something carelessly. However, from a legal standpoint, negligence is a complicated matter. For a lawsuit alleging negligence to be successful, the following four elements must be established:

- *Duty to act.* The Emergency Medical Responder had a legal duty to provide care.
- *Breach of duty.* Care for the patient was not provided to an acceptable standard of care.
- *Damages.* The patient was injured (damaged) in some way as a result of improper or lack of care.
- *Causation.* A direct link can be established between the damages to the patient and the breach of duty on the part of the Emergency Medical Responder.

In many cases, Emergency Medical Responders have a legal **duty to act**. Those functioning as part of a fire service, rescue squad, police agency, or formal response team may be legally obliged to respond and render care. This means that they are required, at least while on duty, to provide care according to their agency's standard operating procedures. In some localities, this duty to act also may apply to paid Emergency Medical Responders when they are off duty.

The concept of a "duty to act" can be less clear in the case of Emergency Medical Responders working in a business office or industrial environment. When in doubt, it is best to provide care and call for help.

Since the laws governing the duty to act vary from state to state, your instructor can inform you about the specifics in your state or region. In most cases, an Emergency Medical Responder is considered to have a duty to act once help is offered to a patient. If care is offered and then accepted by the patient, a legal duty to act has been established and the Emergency Medical Responder must remain at the scene until someone of equal or higher training takes over for them.

After a duty to act has been established, the second condition for negligence would be applicable if the care provided was substandard. The same would apply if the care rendered was beyond the scope of the Emergency Medical Responder.

Finally, if there was a duty to act and the standard of care was not met, a suit for negligence may be successful if the patient was injured (damaged) in some way due directly to the inappropriate actions of the Emergency Medical Responder. This is a complex legal concept, made more difficult by the fact that the damage may be physical, emotional, or psychological.

Physical damage is the easiest to understand. For example, if an Emergency Medical Responder moved a patient's injured leg before applying a splint and the standard of care states that the Emergency Medical Responder should have suspected a fracture and placed a splint on the limb, then the responder may be negligent if this action worsened the existing injury.

The same case becomes much more involved when the patient claims that the Emergency Medical Responder's inappropriate action caused emotional or psychological problems. The court could decide that the patient has been damaged and establish the third requirement for negligence.

OBJECTIVE

2. Explain the concepts of "duty" and "breach of duty" as they relate to the Emergency Medical Responder.

negligence ▶ a failure to provide the expected standard of care.

civil law (tort) ▶ a body of law that addresses and provides remedies for civil wrongs not arising out of contractual obligations.

breach of duty ▶ a violation of the basic duty to act; failure to provide care to an acceptable standard.

duty to act ▶ a requirement that Emergency Medical Responders in the police and fire service, at least while on duty, must provide care according to their department's standard operating procedures.

IS IT SAFE?

One of the most common places abandonment is likely to occur is in the emergency department of the hospital. This occurs when an Emergency Medical Responder or EMT arrives at the emergency department with a patient and then leaves without a proper hand off to an appropriate ED staff member. If that patient suddenly becomes worse and a proper hand off was not performed, it can be said that the Emergency Medical Responder or EMT abandoned the patient and therefore may be liable for any damages the patient may suffer. Never leave a patient anywhere without properly handing him over to the next level of care. And remember, a proper hand off includes a full verbal report.

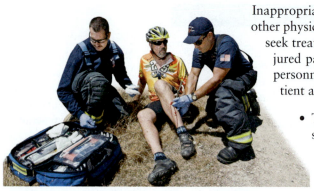

Figure 2.5 • Once care is initiated, the Emergency Medical Responder assumes responsibility for the patient until relieved by more highly trained personnel.

Inappropriate care does not always involve splinting, bandaging, or some other physical skill. As a general rule, you should always advise a patient to seek treatment by EMTs and to go to the hospital. If you tell an ill or injured patient that he does not need to be seen by more highly trained personnel, you could be negligent if you had a duty to act and the patient accepted your care, but:

- The standard of care stated that you should have alerted or had someone activate the EMS system to request an EMT response, and you failed to do so.
  - An avoidable delay in care caused complications that led to additional injury.

As stated above, a requirement for proof of negligence is the failure of the Emergency Medical Responder to provide care to a recognized and acceptable standard of care. There is no guarantee that you will not be sued, but a successful suit is unlikely if you provide care to an acceptable standard.

If your state has **Good Samaritan laws**, you may be protected from civil liability if you act in good faith to provide care to the level of your training and to the best of your ability. You will be trained to deliver the standard of care expected of Emergency Medical Responders in your area. Your instructor will explain the laws specific to your locality.

Good Samaritan laws ▶ a series of state laws designed to protect certain care providers if they deliver the standard of care in good faith, to the level of their training, and to the best of their abilities.

abandonment ▶ to leave a sick or injured patient before equal or more highly trained personnel can assume responsibility for care.

OBJECTIVE

12. Explain the role of the Emergency Medical Responder with regards to patient confidentiality.

KEY POINT ▼

Patient confidentiality does not apply if you are required by law to report certain incidents (such as rape, abuse, or neglect), if you are asked to provide information to the police, or if you receive a subpoena to testify in court. Maintain notes about each incident to which you respond, and keep a copy of any official documents filled out by you or responding EMTs.

confidentiality ▶ refers to the treatment of information that an individual has disclosed in a relationship of trust and with the expectation that it will not be divulged to others.

Abandonment

Once you begin to help someone who is sick or injured, you have established a legal duty and must continue to provide care until you transfer patient care to someone of equal or higher training (such as an EMT or physician). If you leave the scene before more highly trained personnel arrive, you may be guilty of abandoning the patient and may be subject to legal action under specific civil (tort) laws of **abandonment** (Figure 2.5).

Since you are not trained in medical diagnosis or how to predict the stability of a patient, you should not leave a patient even if someone with training equal to your own arrives at the scene. The patient may develop more serious problems that would be better handled by two Emergency Medical Responders.

Some legal authorities consider abandonment to include the failure to turn over patient information during the transfer of the patient to more highly trained personnel. You must inform those providers of the facts that you gathered, the assessment made, and the care rendered.

Confidentiality

Confidentiality is an important concept for those who deal with and care for patients. As an Emergency Medical Responder, you should not speak to your friends, family, and other members of the public (including the press and media) about the details of care you have provided to a patient. You should not name the individuals who received your care. If you speak of the emergency, you should not relate specifics about what a patient may have said, any unusual aspects of behavior, or any descriptions of personal appearance. To do so invades the privacy of the patient. Your state may not have specific laws stating the above, but most individuals in emergency care feel very strongly about protecting the patient's right to privacy.

Information about an emergency and patient care should only be released if the patient has authorized you to do so in writing or if you receive an appropriate request from a court or law enforcement agency. In all other cases, refer requests for patient information to your supervisor or other appropriate person.

Authorization is not required for you to pass on patient information to other healthcare providers who are a part of the continued care of the patient (Figure 2.6). This sharing

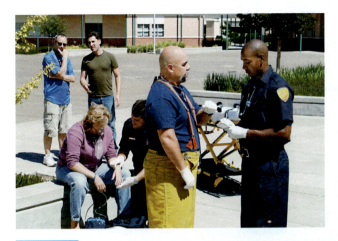

Figure 2.6 • To maintain patient confidentiality, discuss your patient only with those who will be continuing patient care.

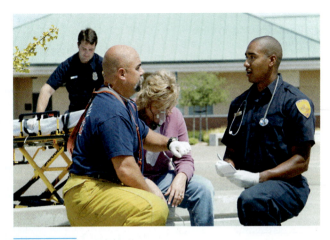

Figure 2.7 • During transfer, sharing of information with those involved in the care of the patient is a necessary and important part of good patient care.

of information with those involved in the care of the patient is a necessary and important part of good patient care (Figure 2.7).

There are laws, such as the **Health Insurance Portability and Accountability Act (HIPAA)** that went into effect in 2003, that dictate the extent to which protected health information can be shared. HIPAA gives patients more control over their own health-care information and limits the way that information is stored and shared with others. It also establishes strong accountability for the use and sharing of patient information.

A good rule of thumb regarding the sharing of patient information is, when in doubt, don't. Your instructor will explain in detail what types of information may be shared and in what situations.

Reportable Events

All 50 states have laws that define **mandatory reporters** and what types of events they must report. What differs from state to state is who is considered a mandatory reporter. For example, all Emergency Medical Responders must report certain events or conditions that they know or suspect have occurred. Those events may include such things as exposures to certain infectious diseases, suspicious burns, vehicle crashes, drug-related injuries, crimes that result in knife or gunshot wounds, child and elder abuse, domestic violence, and rape. Check with your instructor, chief officer, EMS division chief, or with state and federal agencies to learn which incidents are reportable in your area and to whom or to which agency you should report them.

Health Insurance Portability Accountability Act (HIPAA) ▶ a law that dictates the extent to which protected health information can be shared.

IS IT SAFE?

One of your legal and ethical obligations is patient confidentiality. Discuss with your instructor just what you can talk about and with whom before you accidentally share something that you should not. It is better to be safe than sorry. If in doubt, don't share!

OBJECTIVE

5. Explain the term *mandated reporter* and how it relates to the Emergency Medical Responder.

continued

FIRST ON SCENE

Sara realizes that she can't safely reach the woman pinned by the car and decides to try to help the man in the road. She shakes off her backpack, rummages through it, and pulls out two large beach towels. "Help me roll him onto his side," she says to Anthony. "Slow and careful!"

They are able to get the man onto his side and clear much of the blood from his mouth and nose. "Hey, here comes a car," Anthony says as he holds the man's head still. "Let's have them stay here with these people while we go get help."

"I've already started helping them," Sara says and grabs one of her oversized beach towels to flag down the oncoming car. "I can't leave now."

The approaching car slows to a stop and the windows are suddenly filled with round, curious faces. "Listen," Sara runs to the driver's side. "These people are really hurt. I need you to find a phone and call 911!"

Special Situations

Organ Donors

You may respond to a call where a critically injured patient is near death and has been identified as an *organ donor*. An organ donor is a patient who has completed a legal document that allows for donation of organs and tissues in the event of his or her death. A family member may give you this information, or you may find an organ donor card in a patient's personal effects. Sometimes this information is indicated on the patient's driver license.

Emergency care of a patient who is an organ donor must not differ in any way from the care of a patient who is not a donor.

Resource Central

Learn more about the Health Insurance Portability and Accountability Act (HIPAA) and how it affects you as a health care professional. Also, get more information about the role of EMS in organ donation.

Medical Identification Devices

Another special situation involves the patient who wears a medical identification device (Figure 2.8). This device—a necklace, arm or ankle bracelet, or card—is meant to alert EMS personnel that the patient has a particular medical condition, such as a heart problem, allergies, diabetes, or epilepsy. If the patient is unresponsive or unable to answer questions, this device may provide important medical information.

In some areas of the country the "Vial of Life" program is currently in use. This program includes a special vial where important medical information is stored and a window sticker that alerts EMS personnel to the presence of the vial. The vial is kept in the patient's refrigerator, where it can be found easily by rescuers.

OBJECTIVE

13. Explain the role of the Emergency Medical Responder with respect to evidence preservation when working in or around an actual or potential crime scene.

Crime Scenes

A *crime scene* is defined as the location where a crime has been committed or any place where evidence relating to a crime may be found. Many crime scenes involve injuries to people and therefore require the assistance of EMS personnel. If you suspect a crime has been committed, do not enter the scene until instructed to do so by law enforcement personnel.

When an Emergency Medical Responder is providing care at a crime scene, certain actions should be taken to preserve evidence. Make as little impact on the scene as possible, only moving items necessary for patient care. Take special care to note the position of

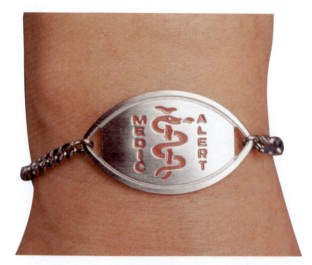
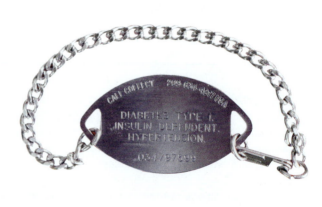

Figure 2.8 • The Medic Alert bracelet is one example of a medical identification device (front and back shown).

the patient and preserve any clothing you may remove or damage. Try not to cut through holes in clothing from gunshot wounds or stabbings. Remember to report any items you move or touch.

About 15 minutes later, just when Sara is beginning to think that the people in the car might have just kept on driving, she hears sirens approaching. "What a sweet sound!" she thinks. Within moments, the scene is filled with firefighters in bulky yellow coats and pants, carrying multicolored bags and shouting information to each other.

The man on the road is quickly loaded into an ambulance, which rushes away with sirens blaring. Sara turns and walks over to see what they are doing to help the trapped woman. The firefighters have peeled most of the car away using large, noisy power tools. Once the woman is finally freed, Sara sees that the woman's left leg is nearly severed at about midthigh.

With a sigh, Sara makes her way past the blood and bent pieces of the small car and finds Anthony over by the motorcycle. She hugs him and they both watch silently as the second ambulance pulls away and disappears around the same bend.

CHAPTER REVIEW

Summary

As an Emergency Medical Responder, you must become well informed regarding the legal and ethical responsibilities that come with your new role. Here is a summary of some of these key principles:

- You may have a legal duty to provide care and must do so within your scope of practice.

- You must maintain a high degree of integrity as well as ethical and moral standards when caring for patients.

- You have a responsibility to keep both your knowledge and skills up to date.

- You must obtain consent from each and every victim you encounter and be able to apply the principles of expressed and implied consent appropriately.

- It is especially important to properly manage and document all patients who refuse care and enlist the assistance of law enforcement when necessary.

- You could be accused of negligence if you do not provide an acceptable level of care or if you abandon your patient.

- You must respect the privacy and confidentiality of all patients and refrain from sharing information about patients unless legally allowed or required to do so.

Take Action

MY WISHES

Most states have a standard "advance directive" form that can be found online. Download this form and study it so that you can be familiar with what it looks like and what it contains. Take it one step further and complete the form with your own information. Going through the steps of deciding your own end-of-life choices is a good exercise for all EMS professionals. Share your wishes with family members and ask them to share theirs as well.

COMPANY VALUES

Ethics and values were briefly discussed in this chapter. Consider doing some research to determine if the company or agency that you work or volunteer for has a common set of shared values. If so, what are they, and do you feel you can embrace them? Perhaps they have a code of ethics. Find out what it says and ask yourself how such a document may have been developed. Compare these values with your own. Do they complement or perhaps conflict with one another? For a fun activity that allows you to identify your own personal core values go to: www.icarevalues.org.

First on Scene Run Review

Recall the events of the "First on Scene" scenario in this chapter and answer the following questions, which are related to the call. Rationales are offered in the Answer Key at the back of the book.

1. Why do you think Anthony wanted to leave?

2. Out of the patients listed, who is your first priority and why?

3. Should you leave the scene after you start treatment?

4. What information will you want to give the ambulance crew when they arrive on scene?

Quick Quiz

To check your understanding of the chapter, answer the following questions. Then compare your answers to those in the Answer Key at the back of the book.

1. Which one of the terms below is best defined as what an Emergency Medical Responder is allowed to do based on the U.S. Department of Transportation educational standards as well as state and local statutes and regulations?
   a. Standard of care
   b. Scope of practice
   c. Duty
   d. Negligence

2. Which one of the following is an example if an advance directive?
   a. Protocols
   b. Standing orders
   c. Do not resuscitate (DNR) order
   d. Medical direction

3. What type of consent is necessary from responsive, competent adult patients?
   a. Implied
   b. Applied
   c. Absentee
   d. Expressed

4. Which one of the following is NOT true about expressed consent?
   a. It is also known as informed consent.
   b. It must always be given verbally by the patient.
   c. It can be given by parents of minors on their behalf.
   d. The patient must be informed of your intentions.

5. You are caring for an overdose patient who is unresponsive. You are legally allowed to provide care based on what type of consent?
   a. Informed
   b. Expressed
   c. Assumed
   d. Implied

6. Which one of the following patients may legally refuse care at the scene of an emergency?
   a. 11-year-old boy who was hit by a car while riding his bicycle
   b. 26-year-old unresponsive overdose patient
   c. 46-year-old intoxicated driver of a vehicle involved in a collision
   d. 68-year-old alert woman having chest pain

7. Which one of the following is NOT an element required for a claim of negligence?
   a. Duty
   b. Absence of duty
   c. Damages
   d. Causation

8. Most states require Emergency Medical Responders and other EMS personnel to report incidents involving known or suspected:
   a. seizure activity.
   b. accidental overdose.
   c. child abuse or neglect.
   d. pregnancy.

9. You have been dispatched to a shooting with three possible victims. Before entering the scene, you should:
   a. ensure that the scene has been made safe by law enforcement personnel.
   b. ensure that the scene has been made safe by fire personnel.
   c. obtain permission from your supervisor.
   d. wait for the EMTs to arrive.

10. Which one of the following is MOST likely a breach of patient confidentiality by an Emergency Medical Responder?
    a. Provides detailed information about the patient to the nurse in the emergency department
    b. Returns to the station and shares details of the call with colleagues
    c. Shares details of the patient's condition with the EMTs who are taking over care
    d. Provides details about the emergency after being subpoenaed to the court

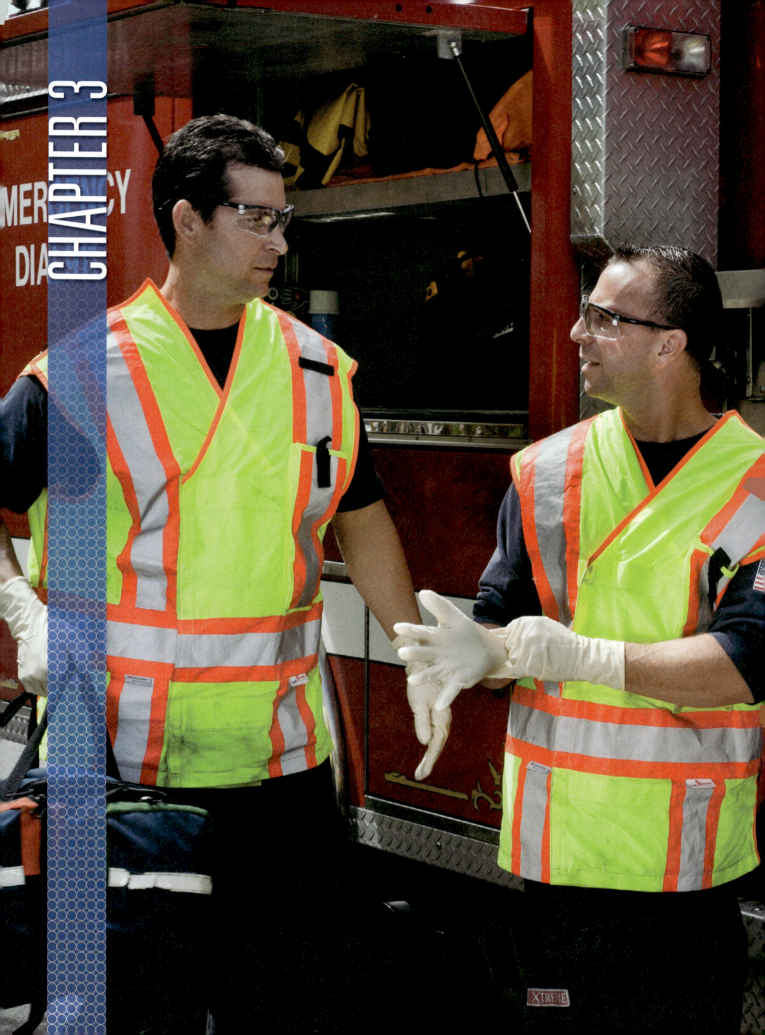

Wellness and Safety of the Emergency Medical Responder

EDUCATION STANDARDS
- Preparatory—Workforce Safety and Wellness
- Medicine—Infectious Diseases

COMPETENCIES
- Uses simple knowledge of the EMS system, safety/well-being of the EMR, medical/legal issues at the scene of an emergency while awaiting a higher level of care.

CHAPTER OVERVIEW

Caring for others in their time of need is an awesome responsibility and one that brings great rewards. It requires a considerable amount of mental, physical, and emotional conditioning that is sometimes difficult to balance due to the demands of the job. As you will soon learn, your personal well-being is an essential component for a long and healthy career in EMS. In this chapter you will be introduced to the steps necessary to keep yourself in top shape, some of the common stressors that can weaken your defenses, and strategies for keeping yourself healthy and safe during your career in EMS.

OBJECTIVES

Upon successful completion of this chapter, the student should be able to:

COGNITIVE

1. Define the following terms:
   a. baseline health status *(p. 38)*
   b. body substance isolation (BSI) precautions *(p. 38)*
   c. burnout *(p. 49)*
   d. CDC *(p. 42)*
   e. critical incident *(p. 47)*
   f. critical incident stress debriefing *(p. 51)*
   g. critical incident stress management (CISM) *(p. 51)*
   h. exposure *(p. 40)*
   i. hazardous materials incident *(p. 46)*
   j. infection *(p. 40)*
   k. multiple-casualty incident (MCI) *(p. 47)*
   l. NFPA *(p. 39)*
   m. OSHA *(p. 39)*
   n. pathogen *(p. 40)*
   o. personal protective equipment (PPE) *(p. 41)*
   p. standard precautions *(p. 38)*
   q. stress *(p. 47)*
   r. stressor *(p. 49)*
   s. universal precautions *(p. 38)*

2. Explain the importance of a baseline health assessment for new EMS providers. *(p. 38)*

3. Describe the various immunizations recommended for health-care providers. *(p. 38)*

4. Explain the term *standard precautions* as it relates to the Emergency Medical Responder. *(p. 39)*

5. Explain what body substance isolation (BSI) precautions are and when they should be used. *(p. 39)*

6. Identify the four routes by which pathogens enter the body. *(p. 40)*

7. List examples of personal protective equipment (PPE) and the purpose of each. *(p. 41)*

8. Explain the procedure the Emergency Medical Responder should follow after a possible pathogen exposure. *(p. 45)*

9. Describe common hazards at the scene of an emergency. *(p. 45)*

10. Explain the steps the Emergency Medical Responder should take to mitigate common scene hazards. *(p. 45)*

11. Explain the terms *stress* and *stressor* as they relate to the Emergency Medical Responder. *(p. 47)*

12. Describe several sources of stress commonly encountered by the Emergency Medical Responder. *(p. 47)*

13. Describe common physical, emotional, and psychological responses to stress. *(p. 49)*

14. Describe common responses to death and dying and strategies to assist oneself and others in coping with death. *(p. 50)*

15. Describe strategies for minimizing the affects of stress on the Emergency Medical Responder. *(p. 50)*

16. Describe the key components of critical incident stress management (CISM). *(p. 51)*

17. Differentiate between cleaning and disinfection, and state when each should be performed. *(p. 41)*

PSYCHOMOTOR

18. Demonstrate and describe proper handwashing technique.

19. Demonstrate and describe the proper application and removal of personal protective equipment (PPE).

AFFECTIVE

20. Maintain a high regard for safety in all aspects of Emergency Medical Responder training.

21. Value the importance of body substance isolation (BSI) precautions.

FIRST ON SCENE

Jake swallows the last of his hot chocolate, steps carefully across the rubber flooring, and glides back onto the smooth ice of the skating rink. He can't help but smile. Everything is perfect, from the crispness of the air to the sweet aftertaste of the chocolate and the warmth radiating from his exercising muscles. He glides toward a woman who is helping a small boy with wobbly ankles to skate—like a scene right from a Norman Rockwell painting. Just as he passes them, the woman pinwheels her arms and grabs for the railing that runs around the edges of the rink.

Jake digs his blades in for a quick stop, sending a spray of ice shavings into the air, and grabs for the woman's flailing arms. He just misses her fingers and watches as she crashes onto her back, her head bouncing off the ice with a hollow thud. She immediately sits up, laces both hands together on the back of her head, and begins to rock back and forth. Her cry of pain echoes across the rink.

"Are you okay?" Jake asks. He kneels next to her and places a hand on her shaking shoulder. "I'm an Emergency Medical Responder," Jake says. "May I help you?"

She doesn't respond but continues weeping and rocking. The boy is now sobbing, too, and trying to hold on to her jacket as he watches Jake fearfully. It's then that Jake notices blood falling in large round splatters onto the ice. "Oh, hey, you're bleeding."

The woman suddenly looks wide-eyed at Jake and then at the boy and scoots frantically backward away from both of them. "Stay away!" she cries between sobs. "Just stay away."

OBJECTIVE

2. Explain the importance of a baseline health assessment for new EMS providers.

baseline health status ▶ a pre-employment medical examination to determine overall health status prior to beginning a job.

standard precautions ▶ steps to take to protect against exposure to body fluids.

OBJECTIVE

3. Describe the various immunizations recommended for health-care providers.

universal precautions ▶ a component of standard precautions that involves the philosophy that all patients are considered infectious until proven otherwise.

body substance isolation (BSI) precautions ▶ practice of using specific barriers to minimize contact with a patient's blood and body fluids.

Personal Well-Being

It is not uncommon for an employer to require a medical exam before a person starts a new job. In most cases the purpose is to establish a **baseline health status**. It also will help you and your new employer to be certain that you are physically ready to handle the job.

As an Emergency Medical Responder, you will be exposed to risks that the average person is not. For example, you will be caring for patients who are ill and/or injured, which can expose you to a wide variety of diseases. You also will be exposed to the same unsafe scenes where people have been injured. You must be able to recognize those and other stressors unique to the EMS profession and learn how to manage them appropriately if you hope to stay healthy enough to help others.

Immunizations

One way Emergency Medical Responders can minimize the risk of acquiring an infectious disease is by becoming immunized. Vaccines are available for many common infectious diseases. While most people receive them as part of childhood wellness checks, additional vaccines are available to adults.

In 1992, OSHA mandated that all employees who have a reasonable risk of becoming exposed to blood or other potentially infectious materials (OPIM) must be offered hepatitis B vaccinations. Employers are required to offer the vaccine at no charge. However, employees have the option to decline.

New vaccines are being developed all the time that could greatly decrease the likelihood of acquiring an infectious disease. Be sure to educate yourself. Consult with your own physician before receiving vaccinations.

A list of the most common vaccines recommended for EMS personnel includes tetanus, hepatitis, measles, mumps, rubella, chicken pox, and influenza. Some are given only once in a lifetime. Others may need to be given more often. In addition, you may need to take a simple test to ensure that you are not a carrier of tuberculosis.

Prior to employment, you will likely be asked to have a thorough medical exam. A physical agility test may be needed as well. Regardless of what your employer might require, it is your responsibility to ensure that you are as prepared as you can be before beginning your job as an Emergency Medical Responder.

Standard Precautions

The term **standard precautions** refers to the guidelines recommended by the Centers for Disease Control and Prevention (CDC). They are used to reduce the risk of transmission of disease in the health-care setting. Combining **universal precautions** and *body substance isolation (BSI) precautions*, they are to be applied with all patients, no matter what the diagnosis or infection status.

Body Substance Isolation (BSI) Precautions

Body substance isolation (BSI) precautions are specific steps that help to minimize exposure to a patient's blood and body fluids. Examples of BSI precautions include wearing protective gloves, masks, gowns, and eyewear.

Consider the following situations:

- A police officer puts handcuffs on a suspect who has a small open wound on his hand.
- A firefighter finds his leather gloves soaked with blood after extricating a patient from a wrecked car.
- A lifeguard touches dried blood while cleaning equipment after an emergency.
- A sheriff's deputy is searching the front seat of a suspect's car and is stuck by a needle that the suspect dropped the night before.
- A firefighter, who is checking his equipment, handles a tool covered with blood from an earlier call.
- A security guard arrives first on the scene to care for a patient who has suddenly become ill and is exposed to the patient's heavy coughing spell.

In each situation, the Emergency Medical Responder may be at risk of exposure to an infectious disease. What BSI precautions should be taken in each case described above? At the start of each shift, Emergency Medical Responders should check their hands for breaks in the skin and cover the areas that are not intact. If unprotected hands come in contact with blood (wet or dry) or any other body fluids, they should be washed with soap and warm water or a commercially produced antiseptic hand cleanser (Figure 3.1).

Make sure you wear disposable gloves before touching any patient and before handling equipment that may have been exposed to blood and body fluids (Figure 3.2). Your hands are very vulnerable to exposure and should be protected any time there is a chance of contact with a patient's blood or other body fluid.

Wear glove, mask, and eye protection with any patient who is coughing, sneezing, spitting, or otherwise spraying body fluids. Finally, to dispose of blood-soaked equipment (including gloves), follow **OSHA** or **NFPA** guidelines.

Emergency Medical Responders frequently face unpredictable, uncontrollable, and life-threatening circumstances. Anything can happen in an emergency. You might make an

OBJECTIVES

4. Explain the term *standard precautions* as it relates to the Emergency Medical Responder.

5. Explain what body substance isolation (BSI) precautions are and when they should be used.

OSHA ► U.S. Occupational Safety and Health Administration.

NFPA ► National Fire Protection Association.

KEY POINT ▼

Even dried body fluids are potentially infectious. Take the appropriate measures to prevent contact.

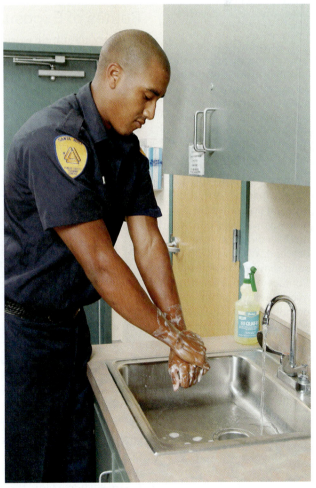

Figure 3.1 • Hand washing is one of the most effective means of minimizing the spread of infection.

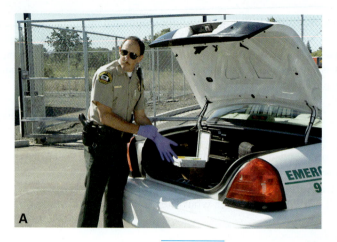 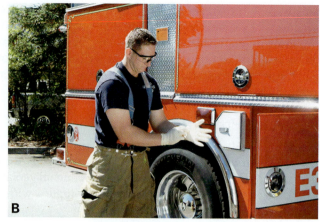

Figure 3.2 • (A) Even law enforcement officers need to take precautions when dealing with injured individuals in unknown situations. (B) In non-fire emergencies, firefighters should wear synthetic gloves under their leather gloves.

arrest or help a heart-attack victim. You might carry a child from a burning building. You might stop a brawl or help deliver a baby. Each situation has the potential to expose you to infectious diseases. Use good judgment. Always take proper protective precautions. By being consistent and thorough, you become a role model for your colleagues and peers.

Routes of Exposure

The very nature of work in EMS means that **exposure** to pathogens is likely. Under the right conditions, pathogens multiply and produce harmful effects. They enter the body in one of four ways:

- *Ingestion* – by swallowing
- *Injection* – through a needle stick, sting, or bite
- *Absorption* – through the skin
- *Inhalation* – breathed in through the lungs

You must be aware of each of the routes of exposure and learn the appropriate precautions to take when faced with a variety of known diseases.

Managing Risk

Some emergency personnel worry more about acquired immunodeficiency syndrome (AIDS) than they do about going into a burning building. The fact is that as a member of the EMS team, your chances of being infected with the human immunodeficiency virus (HIV), the virus that causes AIDS, are very slight. That is true even if you come in direct contact with infected blood or body fluids. You are at a much greater risk of contracting hepatitis B or C. About 250 health-care workers die each year from hepatitis or its complications, more than from any other infectious disease.

Regardless of the risk of **infection**, all EMS personnel must follow the rules for their own safety and the safety of others. The way disease is spread and develops is a subject so complicated that its study is a specialty unto itself. Do not guess at which standard precautions are necessary to take. Do not assume that you can determine easily on your own how to prevent disease. You have entered this course prepared to help care for illness and injury. You can begin by not becoming a patient yourself and by not spreading infections.

Infections are caused by organisms such as viruses and bacteria. Viruses cause illnesses such as colds, flu, HIV, and hepatitis. Bacteria cause sore throats, food poisoning, rheumatic fever, gonorrhea, and tuberculosis, to name a few. There are both viral and bacterial forms of pneumonia and meningitis. Viruses and bacteria also are called **pathogens**.

exposure ▶ a condition of being subjected to fluid or substance capable of transmitting an infectious agent.

OBJECTIVE

6. Identify the four routes by which pathogens enter the body.

KEY POINT ▼

Liquid or droplet exposure to skin, hair, gloves, clothing, and equipment requires you to find out from medical direction how to proceed. Washing with soap may not be enough. Contact with any unknown microbe or potential pathogen may require being seen by a physician.

infection ▶ the condition in which the body is invaded by a disease-causing agent.

pathogen ▶ an organism such as a virus or bacterium that causes infection and disease.

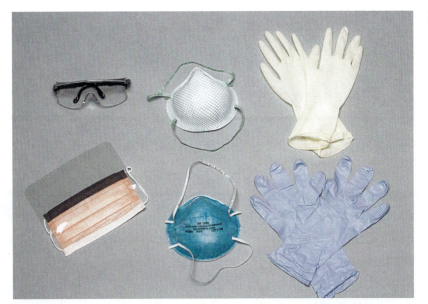

Figure 3.3 • Personal protective equipment (PPE).

The term *pathogen* refers to something that generates suffering (*patho-*, suffering; *-gen*, create or form). Pathogens are spread by exposure to body fluids such as blood and vomitus, as well as exposure to airborne droplets such as those that come from coughing, sneezing, spitting, or even breathing close to someone's face.

Infectious diseases are a real danger to EMS personnel. However, if you follow safety procedures and use the personal protective equipment provided by your agency, the risks can be minimized. Remember, you can transmit pathogens to the patient and the patient can transmit them to you unless you use **personal protective equipment (PPE)** (Figure 3.3):

OBJECTIVE

7. List examples of personal protective equipment (PPE) and the purpose of each.

personal protective equipment (PPE) ▶ equipment such as gloves, mask, eyewear, gown, turnout gear, and helmet that protects rescuers from infection and/or from exposure to hazardous materials and the dangers of rescue operations.

- *Synthetic gloves.* Inspect your hands before donning gloves and cover any broken skin. Put on your gloves before any contact with the patient. Put on a second pair of gloves if you are working around sharp objects, such as broken glass and metal edges at a collision scene. If the outer gloves are torn, the gloves underneath still provide a layer of protection. Wash hands and change gloves between patients. OSHA has stated that hand washing is one of the most important steps to take for infection control.
- *Face shields or masks.* Wear surgical-type masks for blood or fluid splatter. For fine particles of airborne droplets (coughing), wear a high-efficiency particulate air (HEPA) or N-95 respirator. In addition, a surgical-type mask may be placed on the patient if he is alert and cooperates (monitor respirations).
- *Eye protection.* The mucous membranes of your eyes can absorb fluids and are a route for infection. Use eyewear that protects them from both the front and sides.
- *Gowns.* Protect your clothing and bare skin when there is spurting blood, childbirth, or multiple injuries with heavy bleeding.

Since you cannot tell if patients have infectious diseases just by looking at them, it is important to wear personal protective equipment (PPE) for any contact with a patient. This includes wearing gloves at all times. In addition, wear face shields and eye protection whenever you may be exposed to splattering fluids or airborne droplets. This protection builds a barrier between you and the patient.

Your instructor will show you how to properly put on and use protective equipment in a way that maintains its cleanliness (Scan 3.1). You also will learn how and where to properly dispose of all used materials.

It is important that all reusable equipment be cleaned after each use to minimize the spread of disease. First, equipment must be cleaned thoroughly with soap and water to remove all visible blood, vomit, and other body fluids. Then it must be properly

OBJECTIVE

17. Differentiate between cleaning and disinfection, and state when each should be performed.

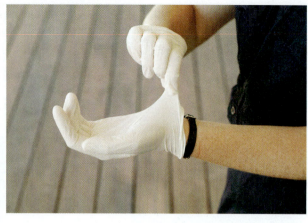

3.1.1 | Begin by grasping the outer cuff of the opposite glove.

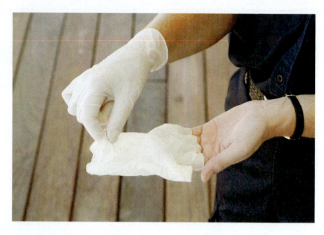

3.1.2 | Carefully slip the glove over the hand, pulling it inside out.

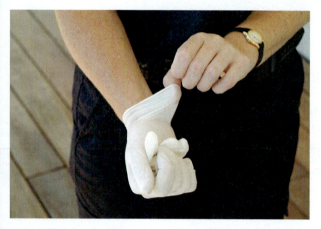

3.1.3 | Next, slip a finger of the ungloved hand under the cuff.

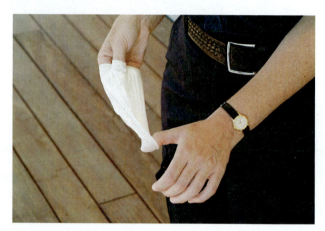

3.1.4 | Carefully slip it off, turning it inside out.

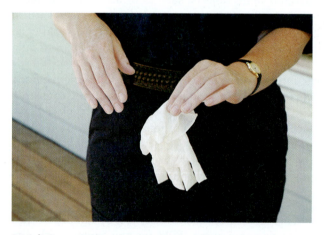

3.1.5 | Once removed, both gloves will end up inside out with one glove inside the other. This will contain any blood or body fluids.

disinfected using an appropriate solution. Cleaning with soap and water alone will not eliminate pathogens.

You must learn, understand the need for, and practice infection-control procedures to reduce your risk of infection. They are based on guidelines from OSHA and the **CDC**. Practicing them is part of your responsibility as an Emergency Medical Responder.

CDC ▶ Centers for Disease Control and Prevention.

Bloodborne and Airborne Pathogens

Infectious diseases range from such generally mild conditions as the common cold to life-threatening diseases such as tuberculosis. The four diseases of most concern to Emergency Medical Responders are (Table 3.1):

- Human immunodeficiency virus (HIV)
- Hepatitis
- Tuberculosis
- Meningitis

HIV is the pathogen that causes AIDS. As yet, there is no cure, but there are newly developed medications that help reduce the patient's symptoms. Even so, new medical developments should not prevent you from using personal protective equipment while caring for every patient. Keep in mind several facts about HIV. First, HIV does not survive well outside the body. It also is not as concentrated in body fluids as is the hepatitis B virus.

The routes of exposure to HIV are limited to direct contact with nonintact (open) skin or mucous membranes and with blood, semen, or other body fluids. Thus, it is very unlikely that a rescuer taking proper BSI precautions will get the disease on the job.

In contrast to HIV, hepatitis B (HBV) is a very tough virus. It can survive on clothing, newspaper, or other objects for days after infected blood has dried. HBV causes permanent liver damage in many cases and can be fatal. Several other forms of the disease, including hepatitis C, are less common than HBV but still present a risk to Emergency Medical Responders.

Tuberculosis (TB), a disease most often affecting the lungs, also can be fatal. Thought to have been nearly eradicated as recently as 1985, incidents of TB are on the rise once again. Even worse, new strains of the disease are resistant to treatment with traditional medications. Unlike HIV and HBV, TB is spread by aerosolized droplets in the air, usually the result of coughing and sneezing. Thus, TB can be contracted even without direct physical contact with a carrier. Use face masks with one-way valves for rescue breathing. Use a HEPA respirator or N-95 respirator when TB is suspected (Figure 3.4). These respirators greatly reduce the risk of exposure to this airborne disease.

Meningitis, an inflammation of the lining of the brain and spinal cord, is also a serious disease, especially for children. The most infectious varieties of meningitis are caused by bacteria. Meningitis is transmitted by respiratory droplets, like TB, but is far easier to contract. The disease may have a rapid onset (several hours to a few days) and needs quick treatment with antibiotics. Antibiotics taken after exposure to bacterial meningitis may prevent acquisition of the disease.

TABLE 3.1	Diseases of Concern to Emergency Medical Responders	
DISEASE	**HOW TRANSMITTED**	**VACCINE**
AIDS/HIV	Needle sticks, blood splash on mucous membranes (eye, mouth), or blood contact with open skin	No
Hepatitis B virus (HBV)	Needle sticks, blood splash on mucous membranes (eye, mouth), or blood contact with open skin; some risk during mouth-to-mouth CPR and exposure to contaminated equipment and dried blood	Yes
Tuberculosis (TB)	Airborne aerosolized droplets	No
Meningitis	Respiratory secretions or saliva	Yes, for one strain

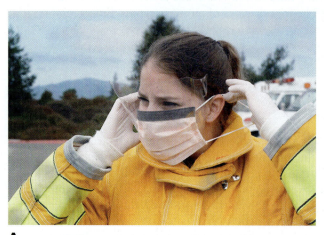

A.

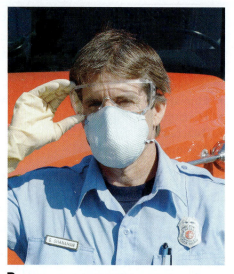

B.

Figure 3.4 • Wear either (A) a high-efficiency particulate air (HEPA) mask or (B) an N-95 respirator to minimize your chances of being exposed to an airborne pathogen.

Not all pathogens are well understood. In fact, there are new pathogens emerging all the time. The following is a list of well-known pathogens that in recent years have received significant attention from the CDC and the media:

- *Swine flu (H1N1).* This is a form of influenza. It is common in pigs and has been known to spread to humans. In 2009, the strain known as H1N1 became a pandemic among humans.
- *Severe acute respiratory syndrome (SARS).* First reported in Asia in 2003, the SARS virus quickly spread to more than 8,000 people in two dozen countries in North America, South America, Europe, and Asia. According to the World Health Organization (WHO), a total of 774 died before the SARS global outbreak of 2003 was contained.
- *West Nile virus (WNV).* A potentially serious illness, WNV is a seasonal epidemic in North America. It flares up in the summer and continues into the fall.
- *Avian flu.* This is a form of influenza that is common in birds. In rare cases it has been known to spread to humans, in which it causes a very high likelihood of death.
- *Methicillin-resistant Staphylococcus aureus (MRSA).* This bacterium is resistant to certain antibiotics, including oxacillin, penicillin, and amoxicillin. MRSA and other staph infections occur most frequently in hospitals and health-care facilities (such as nursing homes and dialysis centers) among people who have weakened immune systems.

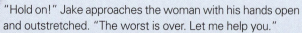

continued

FIRST ON SCENE

"Hold on!" Jake approaches the woman with his hands open and outstretched. "The worst is over. Let me help you."

She scoots back against the low carpeted wall that surrounds the rink and shakes her head. "I've got hepatitis," she whispers, tears still flowing from her red eyes. "Please just call an ambulance." Her dark hair and black jacket have been hiding the seriousness of the blood loss, but now that they are saturated, bright blood begins to pool quickly on the ice around her.

Jake hesitates and looks at his ungloved hands. There is a paper cut on the side of his left index finger. He looks from his hands to the woman's crying face. He turns and shouts to the advancing skate guard, "Call 911! Then bring me a first-aid kit."

Employee Responsibilities

An infection-control program will only work if EMS personnel learn and follow correct procedures. As an Emergency Medical Responder, you have an obligation to adhere to safe work practices in order to protect yourself, your family, and the public. Washing hands regularly, using gloves and other personal protective equipment, and making safe work practices a habit are good ways to start.

Following an Exposure

First and foremost, you need to understand the difference between an exposure and an infection. All infections come from an exposure to a pathogen. However, not all exposures result in an infection. In fact, the vast majority of exposures do not. To help protect yourself from becoming infected following an exposure, follow these simple steps:

- For an exposure to the skin, immediately wash the area with warm water and soap.
- If exposure is to the eyes, flush with clean water for 20 minutes.
- Document the details of the exposure on the appropriate form included in your employer's exposure-control plan.
- Report the exposure to your company/agency infection-control plan administrator.
- Schedule a follow-up medical evaluation with an appropriate health-care provider.

The follow-up evaluation will include an assessment of the exposure and the development of a plan of action to minimize the likelihood of an infection. In some cases it may include an immediate test for infection as well as post-exposure medications. Your health-care provider will help develop a plan of action based on the facts surrounding your exposure.

Scene Safety

Scene safety begins long before Emergency Medical Responders actually arrive at the scene. En route to the scene, get as much information from dispatch about the emergency as possible. The nature of the call will help to determine what type of personal protective equipment may be needed. It also will tell you what type of precautions to take as you approach the scene.

Dispatchers will not always have complete or accurate details about an incident. Often, those who report an emergency are excited, nervous, confused, in pain, or in a panic. They may even hang up before they finish giving all the details.

When approaching an emergency scene, always look around for hazards. One of your first decisions will be where to place the vehicle. (Should it be facing the scene to provide lighting? Should it be beyond the scene to provide quick and easy supply access and patient loading? Should it be on the street to block traffic? Should it be off the street to protect yourself and your partner?) When deciding where to position the vehicle, consider that placement must provide for access to equipment, efficient loading of the patient, and continued traffic flow where possible or at least rerouting of traffic around the scene.

Before approaching the patient, ensure scene safety for yourself, the patient, and bystanders. Look for the presence of weapons. Do not attempt to provide care if you see them. Contact law enforcement immediately. Also check for hazardous materials, toxic substances, downed power lines, or unstable vehicles at the scene. Environmental conditions such as icy and slippery roads, steep grades, rocky terrain, or heavy traffic and a crowd of onlookers must all be considered in your approach and care of your patient.

Violent situations may involve weapons—not just guns but knives or bats, boards, chains, and other items (Figure 3.5). All can be used to harm you, just as they harmed the victim. In

KEY POINT ▼

You may not withhold emergency care from a patient who you think may have an infectious disease. With the proper precautions, you can provide emergency care to people infected with HIV or HBV without putting yourself at risk. To date, there are no known cases of emergency workers contracting HIV or HBV during routine patient care using gloves and appropriate personal protective equipment. Emergency Medical Responders who practice infection control should feel confident that they are not risking their lives.

OBJECTIVES

8. Explain the procedure the Emergency Medical Responder should follow after a possible pathogen exposure.

9. Describe common hazards at the scene of an emergency.

10. Explain the steps the Emergency Medical Responder should take to mitigate common scene hazards.

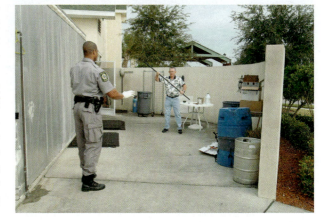

Figure 3.5 • Safety at the scene includes looking for weapons as you approach. Do not approach anyone who is armed with any type of weapon.

Exposures in the Home

The most common exposures occur in the home. It often happens when various cleaning products, when mixed together, produce dangerous fumes. Many home garages are full of hazardous materials that are often not properly labeled or stored.

hazardous materials incident ▶ the release of a harmful substance into the environment. Also called a hazmat incident.

addition, you must be aware of the potential for violence. If it exists, do not approach the scene until it is safe. When the scene is safe to enter, do not disturb evidence any more than you must while caring for the patient.

Crowds also can be potentially dangerous. When necessary, notify dispatch that you need assistance from law enforcement for crowd control, protection, and scene security.

Keeping yourself safe is your first responsibility. Once you can ensure your own safety, approach and take care of the patient.

Hazardous Materials Incidents

Some chemicals can cause serious illness or death, even if your exposure is brief. Some chemicals may be transported by truck or rail. Some may be stored in warehouses or used in local industries.

In a collision involving chemicals, damaged or leaking containers should be considered a hazard to the community and responding EMS personnel. A safe distance should be maintained, and the scene treated as a **hazardous materials incident**.

Placards identify hazardous materials with coded colors and numbers. All placard codes are listed in the U.S. Department of Transportation's *Emergency Response Guidebook*. This book should be placed in every emergency response vehicle. It provides important information about hazardous substances, as well as information on safe distances, emergency care, and suggested procedures in the event of a spill or chemical release.

You also would be wise to carry a pair of binoculars in your vehicle. Use them to identify hazardous materials placards from a safe distance, thus ensuring your own safety.

As an Emergency Medical Responder, your most important duties in a hazardous materials incident is to recognize potential problems and take action to preserve your own safety and that of others. (See more in Chapter 25.) You also should make sure a specially trained hazardous materials response team is notified (Figure 3.6). Leave the handling of the incident to them. Do not take any action other than to protect yourself, your patients, and bystanders. Many emergency response agencies require hazardous materials training at the awareness level. Your instructor can inform you of the requirements in your area.

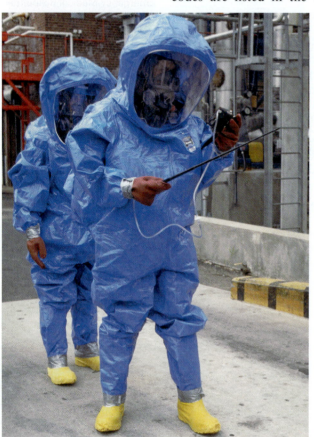

Figure 3.6 • Emergency Medical Responders should wait for hazmat teams to arrive at the scene of any hazardous materials incident.

Rescue Operations

Rescue scenes may include dangers from electricity, fire, explosion, hazardous materials, traffic, or water and ice. It is important to evaluate each situation and request the appropriately trained teams to assist. You may need the police, fire services, the utility company, or other specialized personnel. Never perform acts that you are not properly trained for. Secure the scene to the best of your ability. Then wait for the help you have requested to arrive.

Remember that whenever you are working at a rescue operation, you must use personal protective equipment. That may include turnout gear, protective eyewear, helmet, puncture-proof gloves, and disposable synthetic gloves.

Crime Scenes and Acts of Violence

Emergency Medical Responders may respond to scenes involving victims of violence or crimes. In some areas, EMS providers are issued bulletproof vests for their protection, along with personal protective equipment. No matter what area you work in, your first priority—even before patient care—is to be certain the scene is safe before you enter it.

Threatening people or animals, people with weapons, intoxicated people, and others may present problems that you are not prepared to handle. Recognize those situations. Then request the necessary help. Do not enter the scene until help arrives to secure it and make it safe for you to perform your duties.

Emotional Aspects of Emergency Medical Care

Emergency Medical Responders and Stress

Almost everyone must deal with some type of stress on a daily basis, whether driving in traffic, coping with work and family problems, meeting school and office deadlines, or waiting for an appointment. **Stress** is an emotionally disruptive or upsetting condition that occurs in response to adverse external influences. It is capable of affecting one's physical health. It can cause an increased heart rate, a rise in blood pressure, muscular tension, irritability, and depression.

Surveys and research reports over the past two decades have revealed that a large percentage of all adults suffer adverse health effects from stress. Recent research confirms that stress contributes to cardiovascular disease, stroke, diabetes, cancer, and arthritis, as well as to gastrointestinal, skin, neurological, and emotional disorders.

Another Side of Personal Safety

Stress is a concern for all Emergency Medical Responders. The job makes intense physical and psychological demands on your well-being. Police officers, firefighters, and disaster response personnel must respond quickly to emergencies and react appropriately to situations in which lives are at risk. The need to make immediate decisions about patient care is a big responsibility. They know that a mistake caused by their reaction to stress can cause harm to patients as well as to other rescuers.

Two of the best ways to minimize the stress associated with responding to emergencies and caring for patients are to work closely with other, more experienced responders and to practice your skills often.

Causes of Stress

Emergencies are stressful events, some more than others. The following are examples of very stressful situations, or **critical incidents**, encountered in EMS. The stress of any one of these events can continue long after the event is over. They include:

- *Multiple-casualty incidents.* An emergency that involves multiple patients is referred to as a **multiple-casualty incident (MCI)**. MCIs range from a motor-vehicle crash that injures two drivers and a passenger to a large tropical storm that causes injury to hundreds of people (Figure 3.7).
- *Pediatric patients.* Emergencies involving infants or children are considered some of the most stressful that EMS providers—even the most experienced ones—are required to handle (Figure 3.8).

OBJECTIVE

11. Explain the terms *stress* and *stressor* as they relate to the Emergency Medical Responder.

stress ▶ an emotionally disruptive or upsetting condition that occurs in response to adverse external influences. Stress is capable of affecting physical health. It can increase heart rate, raise blood pressure, and cause muscular tension, irritability, and depression.

OBJECTIVE

12. Describe several sources of stress commonly encountered by the Emergency Medical Responder.

critical incident ▶ any situation that causes a rescuer to experience unusually strong emotions that interfere with the ability to function either during the incident or after; a highly stressful incident.

multiple-casualty incident (MCI) ▶ a single incident that involves multiple patients. Also called a mass-casualty incident.

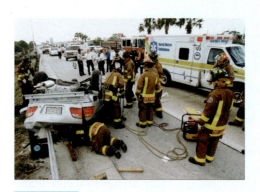

Figure 3.7 • A range of stressful reactions can result from working at emergency scenes such as a multiple-vehicle collision.
(© Craig Jackson/In the Dark Photography)

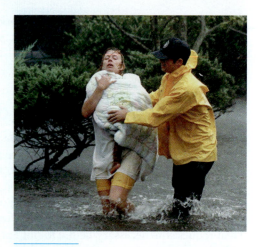

Figure 3.8 • Emergencies can be stressful to all responders and care providers.

- *Untimely death.* It can be difficult for a health-care provider to deal with the death of a patient, and even more so if the patient is young or someone the provider knows. The death or injury of another provider, even if you do not personally know that person, also can cause a stress response (Figure 3.9).
- *Violence.* Not only is it difficult to witness violence against others, but it is also dangerous. Take steps to protect yourself when responding to a violent situation or when a situation suddenly becomes violent.
- *Abuse and neglect.* As an Emergency Medical Responder, you may be called upon to provide care for an infant, child, adult, or elderly patient who exhibits signs of abuse or neglect. Remember that abuse and neglect occur in all social and economic levels of society.

Remember, although everyone responds to stress a little differently, stress and the reactions to it are common to all emergency personnel. It pays to stay aware of the stress factors you are exposed to every day, as well as your immediate and long-term reactions to them. Just as important is the ability to recognize stress in your coworkers. Keep an eye out and offer assistance as appropriate.

Figure 3.9 • The death of a member of the emergency services team is an emotional event.
(© Chip East/Reuters Newmedia Inc./Corbis)

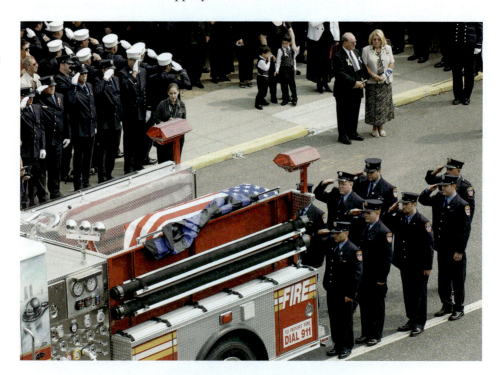

Burnout

EMS personnel are trained to handle difficult situations, but **stressors**—factors that cause wear and tear on the body's physical or mental resources—can take their toll. Stressors in EMS work can be as obvious as a fatal collision or the unexpected death of a child. Sometimes, however, stress can accumulate over months or even years of responding to ordinary injuries and illnesses.

Some EMS providers suffer from **burnout**, a reaction to cumulative stress or to multiple critical incidents. Emergency Medical Responders are at increased risk for burnout because of the demands and activities of the job. The signs of burnout include a loss of enthusiasm and energy replaced by feelings of frustration, hopelessness, low self-esteem, isolation, and mistrust. Many factors contribute to burnout. They include multiple or back-to-back emergency events involving serious medical problems, injuries, or death; facing public hostility; struggling with bureaucratic obstacles; long hours; and putting up with poor working conditions.

Shift work, 12 or 24 hours at a time, can be a significant source of stress, particularly when combined with other stress factors. This pattern of work is common in EMS. It may be even more stressful for many dual-income families, who often miss time shared with their children and each other. The need for continuing education also contributes to already strained schedules. Evening meals that could be restful times, for example, even for those who dine by themselves, are too often replaced with high-caffeine beverages and high-fat fast food, all consumed on the run. A healthier diet and lifestyle can help Emergency Medical Responders combat the stressors that are an unavoidable part of the job.

Both short-term and long-term stressors are occupational hazards for Emergency Medical Responders. Fortunately, research in the past 15 years has found ways to help reduce both kinds of stress. The old saying "work hard, play hard" may not be a particularly useful expression. In fact, it may actually cause more difficulties by trying to solve a complex problem with too simple a solution.

Signs and Symptoms of Stress

The way you handle stress can affect both your emotional health and the way you respond to emergencies. Emergency Medical Responders have a duty to confront the psychological effects of the work they do. Ignoring stress does not make it go away. Instead, it may crop up in unexpected forms, such as insomnia, fatigue, heart disease, alcohol use, increased incidence of illnesses, or other disruptive responses. You may find yourself doing less well at work and in your relationships with others. Those who do not find ways to cope with stress can become depressed, suffer physical disorders, experience burnout, and may even have to leave the field permanently.

Recognize the signs and symptoms of stress. They include irritability with family, friends, and coworkers; inability to concentrate; changes in daily activities, such as difficulty sleeping or nightmares, loss of appetite, and loss of interest in sexual activity; and anxiety, indecisiveness, guilt, isolation, and loss of interest in work or poor performance. In addition, you might experience constipation, diarrhea, headaches, nausea, and hypertension.

stressor ▶ any emotional or physical demand that causes stress.

burnout ▶ an extreme emotional state characterized by emotional exhaustion, a diminished sense of personal accomplishment, and cynicism.

IS IT SAFE?

Being safe means being on top of your game at all times. Burnout can cause you to become distracted and complacent, which can cause you to miss an unsafe scene or potential hazard. You must take care of yourself both physically and emotionally to be at your best at all times.

OBJECTIVE

13. Describe common physical, emotional, and psychological responses to stress.

continued

The woman's sobs slowly taper off and, as her bloody hands drop to the ice, Jake sees that she is losing consciousness. Her eyes are shifting groggily from him to the crowd of onlookers and to the small boy who is now being comforted by a teenage girl. Jake wants so badly to help the woman somehow, to apply pressure to stop her bleeding, to hug her, and to tell her that she'll be okay—anything. But hepatitis. Wow, he thinks. He doesn't want to get hepatitis.

As the small mumbling crowd watches, the woman's eyes slowly close and she slumps over onto the red ice.

FIRST ON SCENE

Death and Dying

OBJECTIVE

14. Describe common responses to death and dying and strategies to assist oneself and others in coping with death.

As an Emergency Medical Responder, you will at some time have to deal with a patient who has a terminal illness or injury. Such patients and their families will have many different reactions to the death of their loved one. A basic understanding of what they are going through will help you deal with their stress and your own.

When a patient finds out that he is dying, he will go through several stages, each varying in duration and magnitude. Sometimes those stages are not experienced in the same order given below, and sometimes the stages overlap one another. Whatever the length or order of the stages, they all affect both the patient and his family. The stages include the following:

- *Denial, or "Not me."* The patient denies that he is dying and puts off having to deal with the situation. Often, the patient displays strong disbelief.
- *Anger, or "Why me?"* The patient is angry about the situation. This anger is often vented upon family members or even EMS personnel.
- *Bargaining, or "Okay, but first let me . . ."* The patient feels that making bargains will postpone the inevitable.
- *Depression, or "Okay, but I haven't . . ."* The patient becomes sad and depressed and often mourns things that he has not accomplished. He then may become unwilling to communicate with others.
- *Acceptance, or "Okay, I'm not afraid."* The patient works through all the stages and finally is able to accept death, even though he may not welcome it. Frequently, the patient will reach this stage before family members do, in which case he may find himself comforting them.

Many times a patient's family member or loved one will respond by going through these same stages. Do not neglect their need for information and compassion. Several approaches are appropriate when dealing with situations such as these. Emergency Medical Responders may offer patients and their families the following courtesies:

- *Recognize patient needs.* Treat your patient with respect and do whatever is possible to preserve his dignity and sense of control. Speak directly to the patient and avoid talking about him to family members or friends in his presence. Try to respond to his choices about how to handle the situation. Allow the patient to talk about feelings, even though it may make you uncomfortable. Respect the patient's privacy if he does not want to express personal feelings.
- *Be tolerant.* There may be angry reactions from the patient or his family members. Sometimes they will direct their anger at you, but do not take it personally. The patient and family need a chance to vent, and they will often choose whoever is nearby as a target.
- *Listen empathetically.* That is, try to understand the feelings of the patient or family member. There is seldom anything you can do to fix the situation, but sometimes just listening is very helpful.
- *Do not give false hope or reassurance.* Avoid saying things such as, "Everything will be all right." The family knows things will not be right, and they do not want to try to justify what is happening. A simple "I'm sorry" is sufficient.
- *Offer comfort.* Let both the patient and the family know that you will do everything you can to help or that you will help them to find assistance from other sources if needed. Remember, a gentle tone of voice and possibly a reassuring touch, if appropriate, can be very helpful.

OBJECTIVE

15. Describe strategies for minimizing the affects of stress on the Emergency Medical Responder.

Dealing with Stress

Stress may be caused by a single traumatic event, or it may result from the combined effects of several incidents. It is important to remember that a severe incident can cause different reactions in different people. Stress also may be caused from a combination of factors, including personal problems, such as friends and family members who just do not understand the job. It is frequently necessary for health-care providers to work on holidays, weekends, and during important family events. This can be frustrating to friends and family members, which may cause stress for the provider. It also can be difficult when family and friends do not understand the strong emotions involved in responding to a serious incident.

Ways in which an Emergency Medical Responder can deal with stress include making lifestyle changes and participating in professional counseling.

Lifestyle Changes

It is often difficult to make changes in the habits or the lifestyle you have developed, but it is essential to consider the effects that current conditions have on your well-being. Remember that your health is of primary importance. Look carefully at your life habits and consider making adjustments.

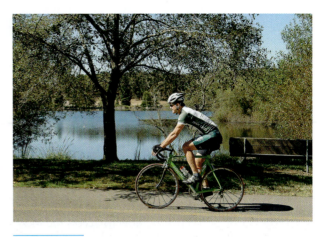

Figure 3.10 • Making lifestyle changes includes exercising regularly.

There are several strategies you can use to help develop your ability to cope with stress (Figure 3.10). They include the following:

- *Develop more healthful and positive dietary habits.* Avoid fatty foods and increase your carbohydrate intake. Also reduce your consumption of alcohol, sugar, and caffeine, which can negatively affect sleep patterns and cause irritability.
- *Exercise regularly.* Properly performed exercise helps reduce stress. It also can help you to deal with the physical aspects of your responsibilities, such as carrying equipment and performing other physically demanding emergency procedures.
- *Devote time to relaxing.* Consider trying relaxation techniques, such as deep-breathing exercises and meditation.
- *Change your work environment or shifts,* if possible, to allow more time to relax with family or friends, or ask for a rotation to a less stressful assignment for a brief time.
- *Seek professional help* from a mental-health professional, a social worker, or a member of the clergy. It is important to develop a healthy perspective about what you do. Being an Emergency Medical Responder is what you do, not who you are.

Critical Incident Stress Management

Critical incident stress management (CISM) is designed to help EMS personnel cope with job-related stress. The **critical incident stress debriefing (CISD)** is one part of it. CISD is a process in which teams of trained peer counselors and mental-health professionals meet with rescuers and health-care providers who have been involved in a major incident. These meetings are usually held within 24 to 72 hours after the incident. The goal is to assist the providers in dealing with the stress related to that incident.

Participation in a CISD is strictly voluntary. No one should ever be forced or coerced to attend. Participants are encouraged to talk about their reactions to the incident. It is *not* a critique. All participants should be made aware that whatever is said during a debriefing will be held in the strictest confidence, both by the participants themselves and the debriefing team. CISDs can be helpful in assisting EMS personnel to better understand their reactions and feelings both during and after an incident. Attendees also will come to understand that other members of the team were very likely experiencing similar reactions.

In the opening discussion, everyone is encouraged to share but not forced to do so. Then the debriefing teams offer suggestions on how to deal with and prevent further stress. It is important to realize that stress after a major incident is both normal and to be expected. The CISD process can be very helpful in speeding up the recovery process.

IS IT SAFE?

Be alert for signs of stress and burnout in those with whom you work. A large part of staying safe is having a partner who is looking out for your safety as well as his or her own. One of the best ways to deal with stress is to talk about it. If you see signs of stress in others, offer to talk to them and help them deal with the stressors that are affecting them.

OBJECTIVE

16. Describe the key components of critical incident stress management (CISM).

critical incident stress management (CISM) ▶ an in-depth, broad plan designed to help rescue personnel cope with the stress resulting from a highly stressful incident.

critical incident stress debriefing (CISD) ▶ a process in which teams of professional and peer counselors provide emotional and psychological support to EMS personnel who are or have been involved in a critical (highly stressful) incident.

CISD

While CISD is a valuable tool in helping to maintain a healthy mind-set, it cannot stand alone. Follow-up care may be needed for some providers, and an ongoing assessment of affected providers should be done to determine if additional personal assistance is indicated. Do not be afraid to speak to your personal physician about any unusual or concerning symptoms, and recognize that even the most experienced health-care providers may need emotional and psychological care at some point in their careers.

Your instructor will inform you of situations in which CISD should be requested and how to access the local system.

WRAP-UP

FIRST ON SCENE

Ten minutes after the woman fell, a group of firefighters and EMTs are walking gingerly across the ice. They are sliding a gurney piled high with equipment bags toward her. Jake explains to the first uniformed rescuer what happened and lowers his voice as he mentions the hepatitis.

The crews, already wearing gloves, quickly put an oxygen mask on the woman, control her bleeding, and secure her to a long yellow board. As they are lifting her onto the gurney, she wakes.

"I think she'll be okay," the EMT at the head of the gurney says to Jake. "It was the right thing to call us."

Jake accompanies them to the edge of the rink and watches the crews take her and the boy out of the arena. He again looks down at his hands. He decides never again to be caught without a pair of exam gloves.

CHAPTER REVIEW

Summary

- It is important for the Emergency Medical Responder to establish a baseline health status prior to beginning work to ensure that he or she is healthy and prepared for the work. Part of this assessment includes ensuring you have received the appropriate immunizations.

- Standard precautions include maintaining a philosophy that all patients are potentially infectious and taking all necessary precautions to minimize the risks of becoming exposed to disease-causing pathogens.

- Proper body substance isolation (BSI) precautions should be taken prior to making contact with all patients. BSI precautions include wearing personal protective equipment such as gloves, eye protection, and protective gowns when necessary.

- Pathogens can enter the body one of four ways: by injection, absorption, inhalation, or ingestion.

- Know your company's specific procedure should you suffer an exposure to a patient's blood or body fluids. At a minimum you must immediately wash the area with warm soap and water and contact your supervisor.

- Exposure to pathogens is just one potential hazard when caring for patients. Emergency scenes are full of other hazards, such as moving traffic, downed power lines, spilled fuel or chemicals, and violent patients. You must always keep personal safety your top priority and utilize appropriately trained resources to help mitigate these hazards.

- Stress is an emotionally disruptive or upsetting condition that occurs in response to adverse external influences. Stressors are those factors that cause stress. As an Emergency Medical Responder you must be aware of the common causes of stress and the typical ways that stress may exhibit itself.

- If not properly managed, stress can become very disruptive. It can cause negative changes in behavior and attitude as well as physical changes that are not healthy for the Emergency Medical Responder.

- You must learn to develop good coping mechanisms for many of the common stressors of the job. Eating a healthy balanced diet, getting regular exercise, and maintaining a balanced work life are all important.

- Critical incident stress management (CISM) can be helpful for many when trying to manage the affects of stress following a critical incident.

Take Action

SLIPPERY WHEN WET

Learning to put on and remove protective gloves is an important skill for all Emergency Medical Responders. One way that you can practice this skill is to don a pair of disposable gloves and spread a generous portion of shaving cream over both gloved hands. The shaving cream is used to simulate blood or other body fluids. Now carefully try to remove the gloves, one at a time, without splattering the shaving cream. The gloves will be difficult to remove when they are wet, but with enough practice you will become skilled at safely removing them.

STRESSED OUT

Most EMS systems around the country have specialized teams of people who are trained to assist EMS personnel who have been exposed to a critical incident. These teams will provide support and assistance for those who were directly involved in the incident and help them understand the reactions that they may be experiencing. Ask your instructor or another EMS professional in your area how to access these resources.

First on Scene Run Review

Recall the events of the "First on Scene" scenario in this chapter and answer the following questions, which are related to the call. Rationales are offered in the Answer Key at the back of the book.

1. Why should Jake ask if he can help?

2. Did Jake do the right thing by not controlling the bleeding? Why or why not?

3. Is there another way that Jake could control the bleeding?

Quick Quiz

To check your understanding of the chapter, answer the following questions. Then compare your answers to those in the Answer Key at the back of the book.

1. Which one of the following statements about exposures and infections is most accurate?
   a. All exposures result from an infection.
   b. All infections result from an exposure.
   c. Infection and exposure are the same thing.
   d. Vaccines help protect against an exposure.

2. Which one of the following is NOT a common pathogen encountered in EMS?
   a. Rabies
   b. HIV
   c. Hepatitis
   d. Tuberculosis

3. Which one of the following types of BSI precautions is most likely going to protect you from an exposure to tuberculosis?
   a. Gloves
   b. Eyeglasses
   c. HEPA mask
   d. Gown

4. You have arrived at a scene of a vehicle collision and there are downed power lines across the road. Which one of the following resources is most appropriate to manage this hazard?
   a. Law enforcement
   b. Fire department
   c. HAZMAT team
   d. Utility company

5. All of the following are common emotional reactions of an Emergency Medical Responder who has faced serious trauma, illness, or death, EXCEPT:
   a. depression.
   b. burnout.
   c. low blood pressure.
   d. insomnia.

6. The best definition of the term *stressor* is anything that:
   a. produces wear and tear on the body's resources.
   b. consumes the attention of the person experiencing stress.
   c. puts pressure on the body.
   d. causes significant behavioral changes.

7. Common causes of stress for Emergency Medical Responders include all of the following EXCEPT:
   a. driving with lights and sirens.
   b. multiple-casualty incidents.
   c. severely injured pediatric patients.
   d. the scene of a violent crime.

8. All of the following are terms used for the stages of death and dying EXCEPT:
   a. denial.
   b. anger.
   c. bargaining.
   d. refusal.

9. Which one of the following would be the best response by an Emergency Medical Responder to family members who are facing the death of a loved one?
   a. Avoid talking directly to the patient.
   b. Do not tolerate angry reactions.
   c. Try your best to understand their feelings.
   d. Tell them everything will be okay.

10. All of the following are common signs and symptoms of stress EXCEPT:
    a. irritability.
    b. difficulty sleeping.
    c. increased appetite.
    d. difficulty concentrating.

11. Which one of the following statements about critical incident stress is MOST accurate?
    a. It is rarely caused by a single incident.
    b. It can be the result of many incidents over a long period of time.
    c. It affects all people the same way.
    d. It can always be avoided with proper preparation.

12. Which one of the following is the BEST definition of critical incident stress management?
    a. It is a broad plan designed to help EMS personnel cope with job-related stress.
    b. It mainly consists of a defusing process.
    c. It is a mandatory process in which all responders must participate.
    d. It focuses on the appropriateness of patient care delivered at the scene.

13. Take body substance isolation (BSI) precautions:
    a. for TB and HBV patients only.
    b. for any ill or injured patient.
    c. only for patients who have a known infection.
    d. only for patients who are bleeding.

14. Which one of the following is the pathogen that most often affects the lungs and can be spread by a patient coughing?
    a. HIV
    b. Hepatitis B
    c. Meningitis
    d. Tuberculosis

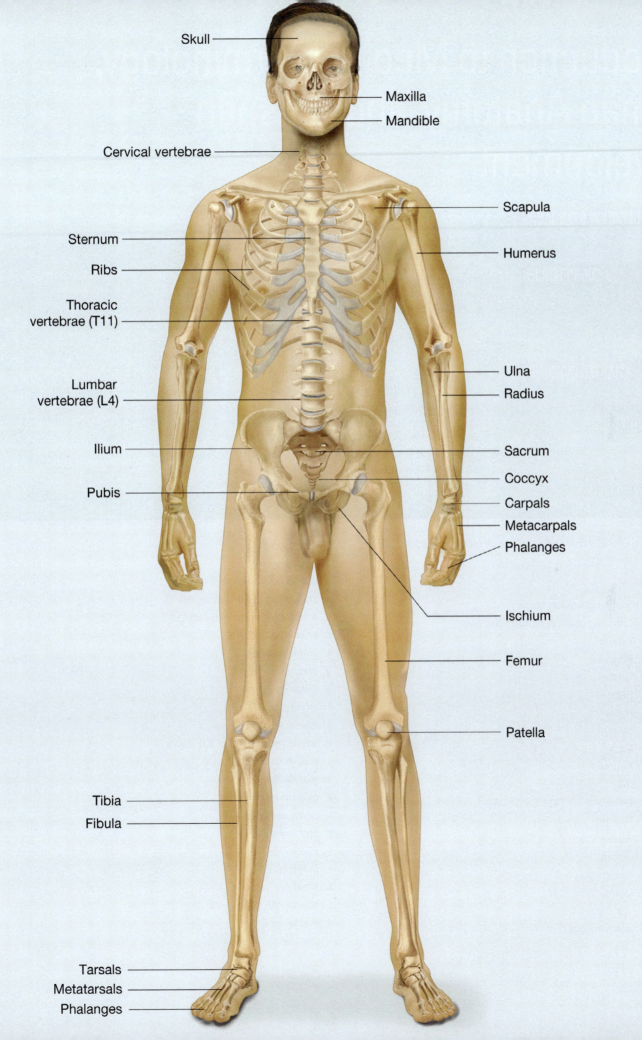

Skull

Maxilla

Mandible

Cervical vertebrae

Scapula

Sternum

Humerus

Ribs

Thoracic
vertebrae (T11)

Lumbar
vertebrae (L4)

Ulna

Radius

Ilium

Sacrum

Coccyx

Pubis

Carpals

Metacarpals

Phalanges

Ischium

Femur

Patella

Tibia

Fibula

Tarsals

Metatarsals

Phalanges

CHAPTER 4

Introduction to Medical Terminology, Human Anatomy, and Lifespan Development

EDUCATION STANDARDS

• Anatomy and Physiology, Medical Terminology, Pathophysiology, Lifespan Development

COMPETENCIES

• Uses simple knowledge of the anatomy and function of the upper airway, heart, vessels, blood, lungs, skin, muscles, and bones as the foundation of emergency care.
• Uses simple medical and anatomical terms.
• Uses simple knowledge of shock and respiratory compromise to respond to life threats.
• Uses simple knowledge of age-related differences to assess and care for patients.

CHAPTER OVERVIEW

As an Emergency Medical Responder, you will not be able to provide the most appropriate care for an ill or injured patient unless you can perform a complete and accurate patient assessment. To do so, you must be familiar with the normal human anatomy. You also must know the language and terms used to describe it. This knowledge will make it possible for you to communicate accurately with other health-care providers about your patient. It also will help you properly document the care that you provide.

This chapter introduces you to the anatomy of the human body, including its major systems and their basic functions. It also introduces you to basic medical terminology and the terms used to describe a patient's position and condition.

OBJECTIVES

Upon successful completion of this chapter, the student should be able to:

COGNITIVE

1. Define the following terms:
   a. Common prefixes and suffixes *(p. 59)*:
      Arterio-
      Brady-
      Cardio-
      Hemo-
      Hyper-
      Hypo-
      Naso-
      Neuro-
      Oro-
      Tachy-
      Thermo-
      Vaso-
      -ectom
      -graphy/graph
      -gram
      -itis
      -ology/ologist
      -osis
      -ostomy
      -otomy
      -scopy/scopic
   b. abdominal cavity *(p. 64)*
   c. abdominal quadrants *(p. 64)*
   d. anatomical position *(p. 60)*
   e. anatomy *(p. 60)*
   f. anterior *(p. 60)*
   g. diaphragm *(p. 64)*
   h. distal *(p. 61)*
   i. inferior *(p. 61)*
   j. lateral *(p. 61)*
   k. lateral recumbent *(p. 61)*
   l. medial *(p. 61)*
   m. midline *(p. 61)*
   n. palpate *(p. 65)*
   o. pelvic cavity *(p. 64)*
   p. physiology *(p. 61)*
   q. posterior *(p. 60)*
   r. prone *(p. 61)*
   s. proximal *(p. 61)*
   t. superior *(p. 61)*
   u. supine *(p. 61)*
   v. thoracic cavity *(p. 63)*

FIRST ON SCENE

"George 14, George 1-4," says the dispatcher, interrupting Stephanie's cell phone call.

"Go ahead for George 14," Stephanie says after snapping the phone shut.

"George 14, respond to Highway 4 between Ottoman and West Carlin for a check on the welfare of Adam 9. He was on a traffic stop about four minutes ago and we can't get a response now."

"Copy." Stephanie puts her cruiser into drive and activates the lights and siren. "George 14 responding from Okalusa Drive and Southwest 14th." She realizes her stomach is tight and growing nauseous as she covers the distance to Scott's location.

He was having radio trouble earlier in the day, so she thinks it's probably nothing. Then again, the department has

been making an increasing number of drug-related arrests now that summer is here, and the lake is attracting visitors at a record pace. She forces herself to focus on the road ahead as she travels along the dusk-lit concrete surface of Highway 4.

Cresting the hill just past the West Carlin exit, she sees a patrol car on the shoulder of the highway, takedown lights still flashing, but nothing else. No other vehicles, no movement, and no police officer. As she pulls up to the empty, idling car her stomach drops. She has to force her hand to stop trembling as she grabs the radio mic. There, sprawled in the dirt on the side of the road and not moving, is State Patrolman Scott Patnode.

Medical Terminology

Every profession has its own language. It consists of a unique set of terms, jargon, and phrases that must be learned by all who participate to ensure clear, concise, and efficient communication among all members. Medical terminology is a very specialized language used by medical professionals. Yet you might be surprised to discover how much of it you already know. Thanks to exposure to vast amounts of media, most of us hear this language every day.

One of the first steps in your journey to becoming an excellent Emergency Medical Responder is to learn the language of medicine. There are college courses devoted to medical terminology. It will be important to study and memorize those terms. Once you begin caring for patients and seeing and hearing how terms are used during patient care, it will become much easier to remember them. Please do search the Internet, because there are hundreds of valuable resources on the Web related to teaching and learning medical terminology.

You might find it interesting to know that there are two categories of medical terms: descriptive, which includes terms that describe shape, size, color and function, and

OBJECTIVE

2. Apply knowledge of basic medical terminology to interpret common medical terms.

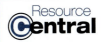

Check out the online medical dictionary to discover new medical terms.

eponyms. Eponyms are terms that honor the person who first discovered or described an anatomical structure or perhaps developed a procedure or instrument. Examples of eponyms include the fallopian tubes, which are named after the 16th-century Italian anatomist Gabriello Fallopio, and the eustachian tubes located in the ear, which are named after another Italian anatomist, Bartolommeo Eustachio. Because eponyms are not very descriptive, there has been a movement in recent years to replace many eponyms with more descriptive terms.

There are three basic parts to most descriptive medical terms. They are the root, the prefix, and the suffix. Here is an example of a medical term with each of the parts identified:

Medical term: **myocarditis**

Prefix: **myo** = muscle

Root: **card** = heart

Suffix: **itis** = inflammation

By using the prefix, root, and suffix of the word *myocarditis* you can determine that the proper definition of the medical term is "inflammation of the heart muscle."

Table 4.1 introduces you to some of the more common medical word roots. It is not essential that you memorize all of the word roots; however, the more of these you

TABLE 4.1 | Common Medical Root Words

ROOT	MEANING	EXAMPLE
Stomato	= mouth	Stomatitis (Inflammation of the lining of the mouth)
Dento	= teeth	Dentist
Glosso/linguo	= tongue	Glossitis, lingual nerve (inflammation of the tongue)
Gingivo	= gums	Gingivitis (inflammation of the gums)
Encephalo	= brain	Encephalitis (inflammation of the brain)
Gastro	= stomach	Gastritis (inflammation of the stomach)
Entero	= intestine	Gastroenteritis (inflammation of the lining of the stomach and intestines)
Colo	= large intestine	Colitis (inflammation of the colon)
Procto	= anus/rectum	Proctitis (inflammation of the rectum)
Hepato	= liver	Hepatitis (inflammation of the liver)
Nephro/rene	= kidney	Nephritis, renal artery (inflammation of the kidney)
Orchido	= testis	Orchiditis (inflammation of the testes)
Oophoro	= ovary	Oophoritis (inflammation of an ovary)
Hystero	= uterus	Hysterectomy (removal of the uterus)
Dermo	= skin	Dermatitis (inflammation of the skin)
Masto/mammo	= breast	Mammography (image of the breast)
Osteo	= bones	Osteoporosis (disease that causes weakening of the bones)
Cardio	= heart	Electrocardiogram (ECG) (electrical tracing of the heart)
Cysto	= bladder	Cystitis (inflammation of the bladder)
Rhino	= nose	Rhinitis (inflammation of the nasal membranes)
Phlebo/veno	= veins	Phlebitis (inflammation of a vein)
Pneumo/pulmo	= lung	Pneumonitis (inflammation of a lung)
Hemo/emia	= blood	Hematoma (localized swelling caused by blood)

TABLE 4.2 | Common Prefixes

Arterio-	= artery	Arteriosclerosis (hardening of the arteries)
Brady-	= slow	Bradycardia (slow heart rate)
Cardio-	= heart	Electrocardiogram (ECG)
Hemo-	= blood	Hematology (the study of the blood)
Hyper-	= over, above, beyond	Hyperglycemia (high blood sugar levels)
Hypo-	= below, under	Hypothermia (low body core temperature)
Naso-	= nose	Nasopharyngeal airway (airway placed in the nose)
Neuro-	= nerve	Neuropathy (disease of the nervous system)
Oro-	= mouth	Oropharyngeal airway (airway placed in the mouth)
Tachy-	= rapid	Tachycardia (rapid heart rate)
Thermo-	= heat	Thermometer (instrument for measuring temperature)
Vaso-	= blood vessel	Vasoconstriction (constriction of the blood vessels)

learn, the more you will understand about your patient's conditions and ailments. An example of a common medical word root is *therm*. This is the root of the word *thermometer*, which you know is the tool used to measure body temperature. You will notice that some words have two roots. This is because some have both a Latin and a Greek origin.

Tables 4.2 and 4.3 provide lists of common prefixes and suffixes along with meanings and an example of each used in a medical term. They are just a small sampling of all the possible prefixes and suffixes that make up the world of medical terminology. You do not have to memorize all of them, but learning even some will ensure a good head start on building your medical vocabulary.

TABLE 4.3 | Common Suffixes

-ectomy	= to cut out, remove	Appendectomy (removal of the appendix)
-graphy/graph	= recording an image	Mammography (x-ray of the soft tissue of the breast)
-gram	= the image (X-ray)	Mammogram
-itis	= inflammation	Tonsillitis (inflammation of the tonsils)
-ology/ologist	= to study, specialize in	Cardiologist (physician who studies the heart)
-osis	= abnormal condition	Cyanosis (bluish coloration of the skin)
-ostomy	= to make an opening	Colostomy (a surgical opening in the colon)
-otomy	= to cut into	Tracheotomy (surgical hole placed in the trachea)
-scopy/scopic	= to look, observe	Colonoscopy (examination of the inner colon)
-emia	= blood	Anemia (deficiency of red blood cells)

Note: The suffixes -graphy, -graph, and -gram are very common and always refer to the recording of a diagnostic image such as an X-ray, CT scan, or MRI scan.

anatomy ▶ the study of body structure.

anatomical position ▶ the standard reference position for the body in the study of anatomy; the body is standing erect, facing the observer, arms are down at the sides, and the palms of the hands are forward.

anterior ▶ the front of the body or body part.

posterior ▶ the back of the body or body part.

Figure 4.1 • Terms of direction.

Positional and Directional Terms

The following are some basic terms that may be used to refer to the human body (Figure 4.1):

- *Anatomical position.* Whenever you describe anything related to human **anatomy** or the location of injuries and their signs and symptoms, it is always assumed that the patient is in what is called the **anatomical position**. In this position, the patient is standing upright, facing forward with arms down at the sides, with the palms of the hands forward. References to all body structures and locations assume that the body is in this position.
- *Right and left.* When referring to the human body, right and left are always described as seen from the patient's perspective. Even though you may think this is simple, it is easy to get confused and make references to your own left and right.
- *Anterior and posterior.* The term **anterior** refers to the front of the body. The term **posterior** refers to the back of the body.

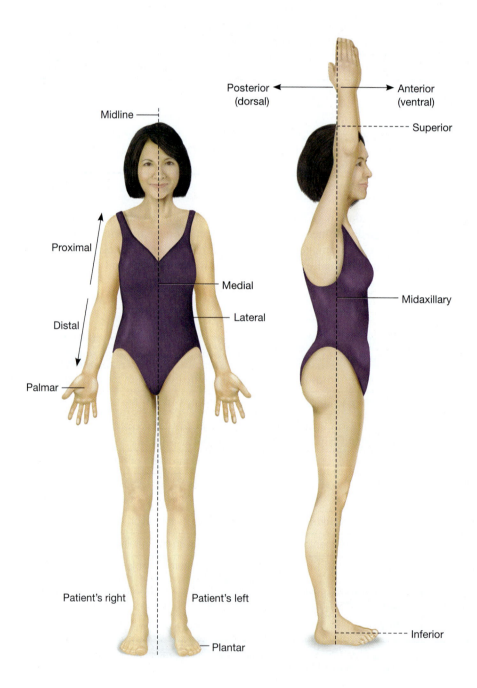

- *Midline.* The **midline** is an imaginary vertical line that divides the body into right and left halves. Anything toward the midline is said to be **medial**. Anything away from the midline is said to be **lateral**. For example, when considering the anatomical position with the palms forward, the thumbs can be described as on the lateral (away from midline) side of the hand, and the little fingers are described as on the medial (near the midline) side of the hand.

There are other directional terms that can be useful. **Superior** means toward the top of the head, as in "the eyes are superior to the nose." **Inferior** means toward the feet, as in "the mouth is inferior to the nose." *Superior* and *inferior* are usually reserved for structures in the head, neck, and torso. Notice that you cannot say something is superior or inferior unless you are comparing at least two points of reference. The heart is not simply superior; it is superior to the stomach. Because you are using the anatomical position for all your references to the body, most medical professionals will understand what you mean when you say a wound is just above the right eye. For this reason, terms such as *superior* and *inferior* may be optional.

Proximal and **distal** are also important terms to learn and use. To use the terms correctly, you must have a point of reference and two structures that can be compared. The two terms are most commonly used to describe anatomy related to the limbs. The point closest to the torso is said to be *proximal*, while the point farthest away is *distal*. It helps to think that the close point is in the proximity of the reference, while the far point is some distance away. Thus the elbow is said to be proximal (closer to the torso) to the wrist and the hand as distal (further from the torso) to the wrist. The knee is proximal to the ankle and the foot as distal to the ankle. Trying to remember all this in an emergency situation can be confusing. Take the opportunity to use the classroom setting to practice the proper use of these terms.

In addition to directional terms, there are specific positional terms with which you should become familiar (Figure 4.2). Positional terms include the following:

- **Supine** means lying face up.
- **Prone** means lying face down.
- *Recovery position*, also referred to as the **lateral recumbent** position, means lying on one's side.
- *Semi-Fowler's position* refers to the patient sitting up at an angle.
- *Trendelenburg position* refers to the patient supine at an angle with feet elevated.

The documentation of the patient's position may be of medical significance and also may become part of the legal record of how a patient was first seen. As with directional terms, positional terms should be learned and practiced so that they become part of your normal vocabulary and documentation.

Most Emergency Medical Responders do not deal with emergencies on a daily basis. Unless you review and use anatomical terms often, you may forget them over time. Be aware that medical and rescue personnel are trained to take your information. They will not be confused if you say *front, back, above,* and *below*. Never let terminology stand in the way of clear communication with EMS providers, physicians, and other medical professionals.

Overview of the Human Body

Human anatomy refers to the structure of the human body. **Physiology** refers to the function of the body and its many systems. Students beginning training in Emergency Medical Responder courses are often a little worried about having to learn anatomy and physiology. Don't be. As an Emergency Medical Responder, you must know basic bodily structures, but not in as much detail as more highly trained medical personnel.

Do not become overly concerned with trying to learn each and every anatomical term. A head is still a head, and feet are still feet. However, you will need to learn some

midline ▶ an imaginary vertical line used to divide the body into right and left halves.

medial ▶ toward the midline of the body.

lateral ▶ to the side, away from the midline of the body.

superior ▶ toward the head (e.g., the chest is superior to the abdomen).

inferior ▶ toward the feet (e.g., the lips are inferior to the nose).

proximal ▶ closer to the torso.

distal ▶ farther away from the torso.

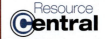

Learn more about anatomical landmarks by viewing an animation.

supine ▶ the patient is lying face up.

prone ▶ the patient is lying face down.

lateral recumbent ▶ the patient is lying on his side.

physiology ▶ the function of the body and its systems.

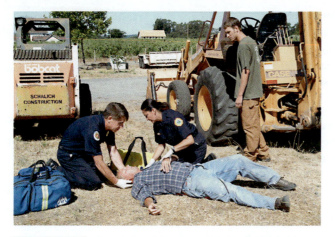

Figure 4.2a • Supine position.

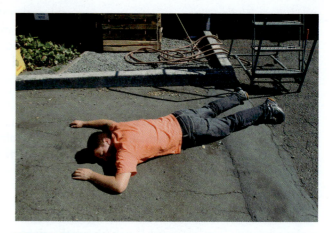

Figure 4.2b • Prone position.

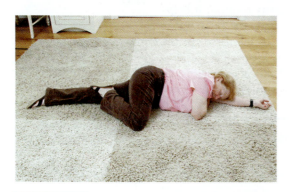

Figure 4.2c • Recovery (lateral recumbent) position.

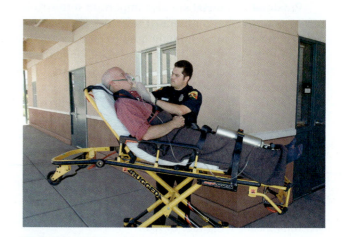

Figure 4.2d • Semi-Fowler's position.

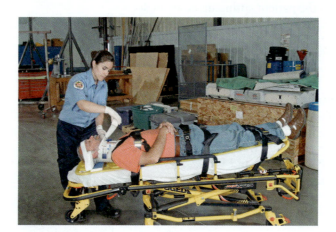

Figure 4.2e • Trendelenburg position.

new terms and make them as much a part of your vocabulary as everyday terms, such as *heart* and *lungs*.

Regions of the Body

To be an Emergency Medical Responder, you must be able to look at a person's body and know the major internal structures and the general location of each (Figure 4.3). Your

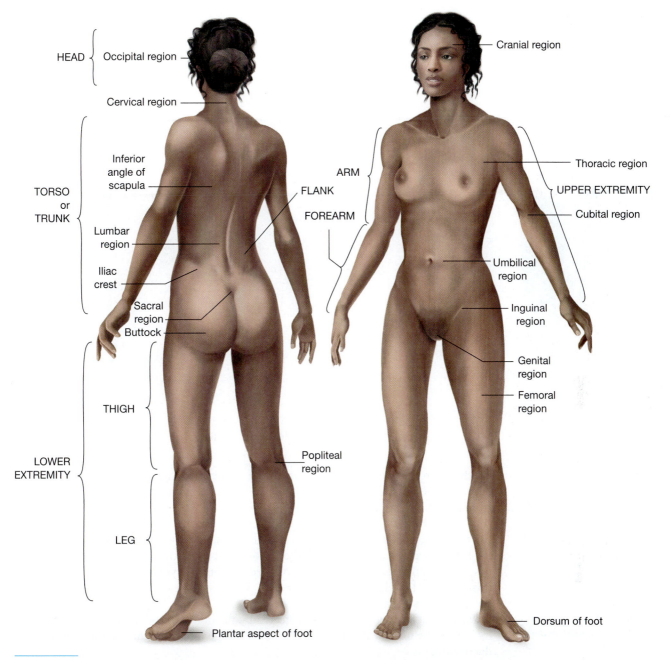

HEAD { Occipital region

Cranial region

Cervical region

TORSO or TRUNK

Inferior angle of scapula

ARM

FLANK

Thoracic region

UPPER EXTREMITY

FOREARM

Cubital region

Lumbar region

Iliac crest

Umbilical region

Sacral region

Inguinal region

Buttock

Genital region

Femoral region

THIGH

LOWER EXTREMITY

Popliteal region

LEG

Dorsum of foot

Plantar aspect of foot

Figure 4.3 • Regions of the body.

concern is not how the body looks dissected or how the body looks on an anatomical wall chart. You must be concerned with living bodies and knowing where things are located as you look from the outside.

Body Cavities

There are four major body cavities—cranial, thoracic, abdominal, and pelvic (Figure 4.4). Housed in these cavities are the major organs (Scan 4.1), blood vessels, and nerves.

- *Cranial cavity.* The *cranial cavity* houses the brain and its specialized membranes. The spinal cord runs out of the cranium and down through the center of the vertebrae of the spine. The bones of the spine protect the spinal cord and its specialized membranes.
- *Thoracic cavity.* The **thoracic cavity**, also known as the chest cavity, is enclosed by the rib cage (Figure 4.5). It holds and protects the lungs, heart, great blood vessels, part of the windpipe (trachea), and part of the esophagus, which is the tube leading from

OBJECTIVES

4. Identify the four major body cavities.

5. Describe the anatomy contained in each of the body cavities.

thoracic cavity ▶ the anterior body cavity that is above (superior to) the diaphragm. Also called *chest cavity*.

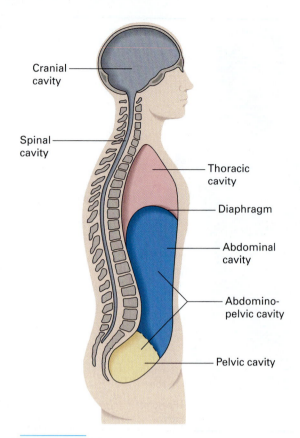

Figure 4.4 • Main body cavities.

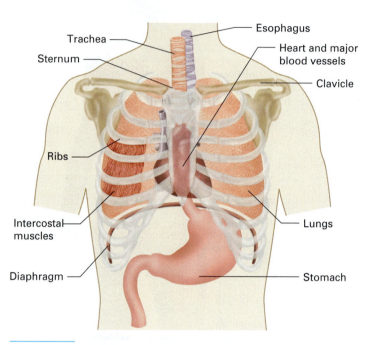

Figure 4.5 • The chest cavity.

diaphragm ▶ the muscular structure that divides the chest cavity from the abdominal cavity.

abdominal cavity ▶ the anterior body cavity that extends from the diaphragm to the pelvic cavity.

pelvic cavity ▶ the anterior body cavity surrounded by the bones of the pelvis.

abdominal quadrants ▶ four divisions of the abdomen used to pinpoint the location of pain or injury: right upper quadrant (RUQ), left upper quadrant (LUQ), right lower quadrant (RLQ), and left lower quadrant (LLQ).

the throat to the stomach. The lower border of the chest cavity is the **diaphragm**, a dome-shaped muscle used in breathing. The diaphragm separates the chest cavity from the abdominal cavity.

- *Abdominal cavity.* The **abdominal cavity** lies between the chest cavity and the pelvic cavity. The stomach, liver, gallbladder, pancreas, spleen, small intestine, and most of the large intestine can be found in the abdominal cavity. Unlike the other body cavities, the abdominal cavity is not surrounded by bones. If you consider the organs in this cavity and the lack of bony protection, it is easy to see why trauma to the abdomen can result in severe injury.
- *Pelvic cavity.* The **pelvic cavity** is protected by the bones of the pelvic girdle. This cavity houses the urinary bladder, portions of the large intestine, and the internal reproductive organs.

Abdominal Quadrants

The abdomen is a large body region that contains many vital organs. The navel, or umbilicus, is the main point of reference when describing the abdomen, which is divided into four **abdominal quadrants** (Figure 4.6). They are:

- *Right upper quadrant (RUQ).* Contains most of the liver, the gallbladder, and part of the small and large intestine.
- *Left upper quadrant (LUQ).* Contains most of the stomach, the spleen, part of the small and large intestine, and part of the liver.
- *Right lower quadrant (RLQ).* Contains the appendix and part of the small and large intestine.
- *Left lower quadrant (LLQ).* Contains part of the small and large intestine.

Some organs are located in more than one quadrant, as you can see from the preceding list. Pelvic organs also are included in these quadrants, with the urinary bladder being assigned to both lower quadrants.

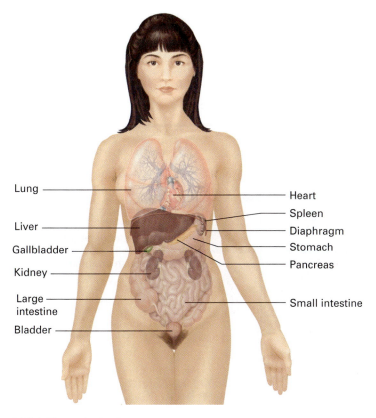

Lung

Liver

Gallbladder

Kidney

Large intestine

Bladder

Heart

Spleen

Diaphragm

Stomach

Pancreas

Small intestine

4.1.1 | The major body organs.

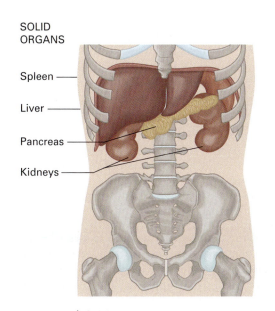

SOLID ORGANS

Spleen

Liver

Pancreas

Kidneys

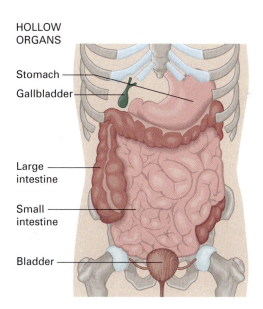

HOLLOW ORGANS

Stomach

Gallbladder

Large intestine

Small intestine

Bladder

4.1.2 | Solid and hollow organs.

When assessing a patient's abdominal area, be sure to **palpate** the soft areas to the rear of the abdomen on each side. These soft areas are located on the flank (posterior), just above (superior to) the pelvic bones. This area contains the kidneys and is susceptible to injury because it is not protected by bone. The kidneys are a special case. They are not contained within the abdominal cavity because they are located behind the membrane that lines the cavity. The location of the kidneys makes them subject to injury from blows to the midback. Any pain or ache in the back may involve the kidneys. Most of the pancreas and the aorta are also located behind the abdominal cavity membrane. The pancreas is mostly in the right upper quadrant, and the aorta lies just in front of the spinal column.

palpate ▶ to examine by feeling with one's hands.

Figure 4.6 • The abdominal quadrants.

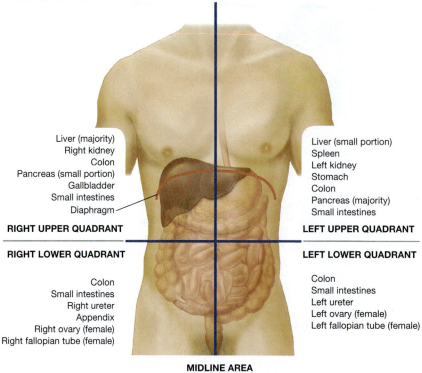

Liver (majority)
Right kidney
Colon
Pancreas (small portion)
Gallbladder
Small intestines
Diaphragm

Liver (small portion)
Spleen
Left kidney
Stomach
Colon
Pancreas (majority)
Small intestines

RIGHT UPPER QUADRANT

LEFT UPPER QUADRANT

RIGHT LOWER QUADRANT

LEFT LOWER QUADRANT

Colon
Small intestines
Right ureter
Appendix
Right ovary (female)
Right fallopian tube (female)

Colon
Small intestines
Left ureter
Left ovary (female)
Left fallopian tube (female)

MIDLINE AREA

Bladder - Uterus (female) - Prostate (male)

FIRST ON SCENE

continued

"Scott!" Stephanie drops to her knees in the dirt next to her colleague, pulls on a pair of gloves, and tears open his bloody uniform shirt. There is a perfectly round hole in his chest just below the right nipple, and dark blood is dripping steadily from the wound. She rolls him up onto his side to check his back, and he moans, grabbing weakly at her arms. There is a large, ragged hole just below his right shoulder blade, and blood is bubbling thickly out onto the ground.

She grabs her portable radio and keys the mic. "Control, George 14, Adam 9 has been shot. I need you to let the responding ambulance know that Adam 9 has an entrance wound just inferior to the right nipple and an exit wound just medial to the right shoulder blade. He is responsive to pain and has noisy breathing. I don't see anything else."

She then drops the radio into the dust, places one hand over each of Scott's wounds, and applies steady pressure.

Body Systems

Now that you have a better understanding of the common terms used to describe the anatomy of the body, it is time to explore the anatomy and *physiology* (essential processes, activities, and functions) of each major body system. Throughout this text, specific anatomy and some basic functions are covered as they apply to illness, injury, and Emergency Medical Responder care.

When body systems are functioning properly, they all support something called perfusion. *Perfusion* is the adequate flow of well-oxygenated blood and nutrients to all body

From the Medical Director

How Things Work

Just as you would not take your car to a mechanic who could not identify the working parts, you cannot fully grasp what is wrong with your patient without understanding his various systems. As with the mechanic, understanding how things work helps you predict how they will fail. In medicine, the parts are anatomy, their function is physiology, and how they fail is called pathophysiology.

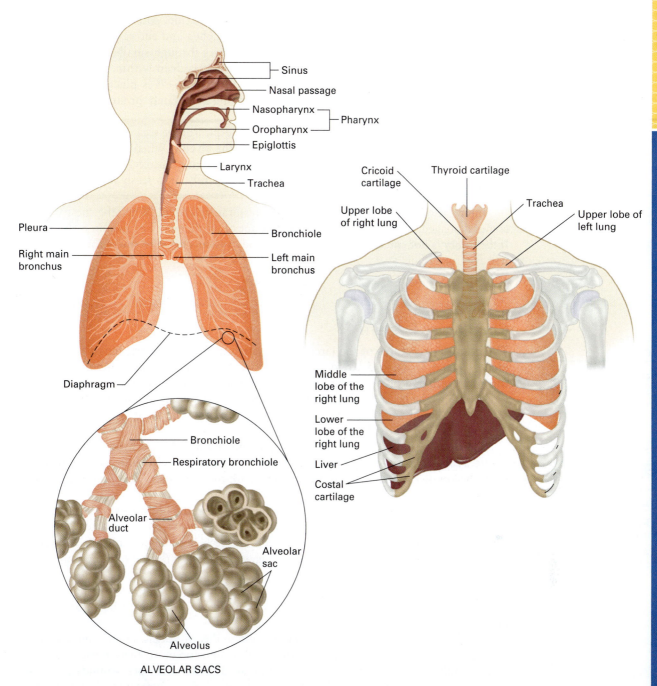

4.2.1 | The respiratory system.

systems, especially the vital organs. When a body system stops functioning properly, or fails completely, it can have an immediate and often life-threatening affect on the rest of the body. The term *pathophysiology* refers to the abnormal function of the body or one of its systems due to disease or injury.

The Respiratory System

The primary structures associated with the respiratory system include the nose (nasopharynx), mouth (oropharynx), trachea, lungs, bronchi, bronchioles, alveoli, and associated muscles related to breathing (Scan 4.2). The respiratory system is primarily

OBJECTIVE

6. Describe the anatomy and physiology of the respiratory system.

responsible for the exchange of oxygen and carbon dioxide. After air enters the body through the nose and mouth, it passes down the trachea and enters the lungs through the right and left bronchus. From there the air passes through smaller passages called bronchioles and eventually ends up at the alveoli. It is deep within the lungs at the alveoli that the exchange of oxygen and carbon dioxide takes place. Perfusion can be adversely affected if the patient is not breathing adequately or stops breathing all together.

There are many diseases that can affect the respiratory system. Many diseases disrupt the delivery of oxygen all the way down to the alveoli. When this happens, blood is allowed to circulate through the lungs without picking up oxygen or dropping off carbon dioxide. Soon, the other body systems that rely on a fresh supply of oxygen begin to fail.

Injury also can affect the function of the respiratory system. When the chest wall becomes damaged, or a lung collapses, the amount of air that can be taken in is decreased. If the injury is not cared for promptly, other body systems begin to starve for oxygen and will eventually fail.

Circulatory System

The primary structures of the circulatory system include the heart, blood vessels, and blood (Scan 4.3). There are two sides to the circulatory system—the arterial system that carries oxygenated blood to the body and the venous system that returns unoxygenated blood back to the heart and lungs. The main job of the circulatory system is to carry well-oxygenated blood and other nutrients to the body's cells, and assist with the removal of wastes and carbon dioxide from the cells.

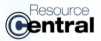
The heart is a hollow, muscular organ that pumps 450 million pints of blood in the average lifetime. Its upper chambers, the atria, receive unoxygenated blood from the venous system. The lower chambers are the ventricles. They pump blood out of the heart.

The right atrium receives unoxygenated blood from the body. It is then moved into the right ventricle, where it pumps the blood to the lungs to receive oxygen. The oxygenated blood then returns to the left atrium before being pumped into the left ventricle. The left ventricle is the largest and strongest chamber of the heart and pumps blood out to the body.

The heart muscle (myocardium) receives its blood supply by way of the coronary arteries. It is when the coronary arteries become blocked that a heart attack can occur.

All three components of the circulatory system (heart, vessels, blood) must be functioning properly to maintain good perfusion. First and foremost, there must be an adequate supply of blood within the system. Damaged tissues and open wounds can cause life-threatening bleeding. Next, the blood vessels must remain intact and functioning normally (constricting and dilating). The function of the blood vessels can be affected by both illness and injury. Last, the heart, which serves as the pump for the whole system, must be functioning normally. It must be pumping at a good rate and with enough force to maintain a good blood pressure. The heart's function can be affected by both illness and injury, thus causing poor perfusion.

Any blood vessel that carries blood away from the heart is called an artery. Arteries have strong muscular walls and are very elastic. They are able to change their diameter depending on the circumstances. The smallest arteries are called *arterioles*.

Any blood vessel that carries blood back to the heart is referred to as a vein. The walls of the veins are not as thick or elastic as those of the arteries. Some veins have valves to prevent the backward flow of blood. The smallest veins are called *venules*.

Cardiovascular System

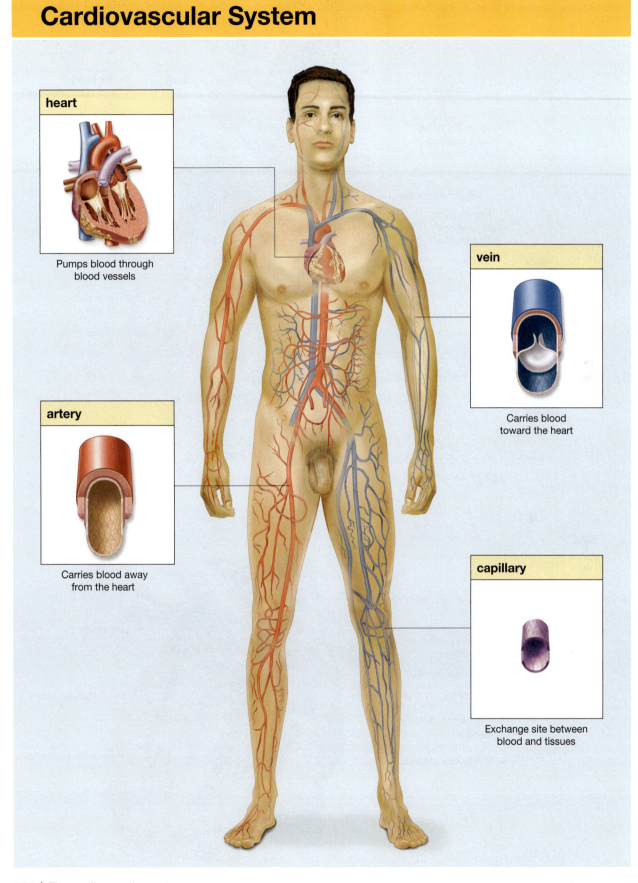

heart

Pumps blood through blood vessels

artery

Carries blood away from the heart

vein

Carries blood toward the heart

capillary

Exchange site between blood and tissues

4.3.1 | The cardiovascular system.

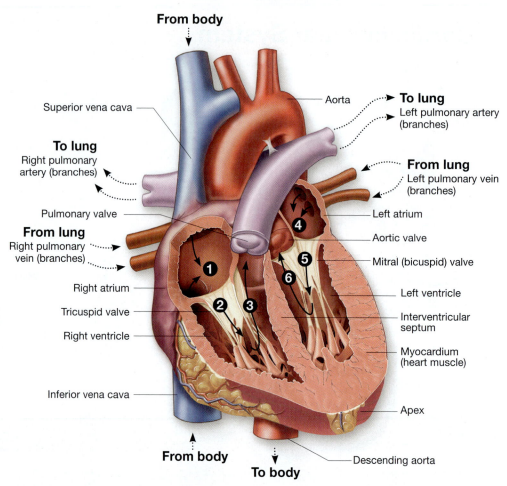

From body

Superior vena cava

Aorta

To lung
Left pulmonary artery
(branches)

To lung
Right pulmonary
artery (branches)

From lung
Left pulmonary vein
(branches)

Pulmonary valve

Left atrium

From lung
Right pulmonary
vein (branches)

Aortic valve

Mitral (bicuspid) valve

Right atrium

Left ventricle

Tricuspid valve

Interventricular
septum

Right ventricle

Myocardium
(heart muscle)

Inferior vena cava

Apex

From body

Descending aorta

To body

4.3.2 | Blood flow through the chambers of the heart.

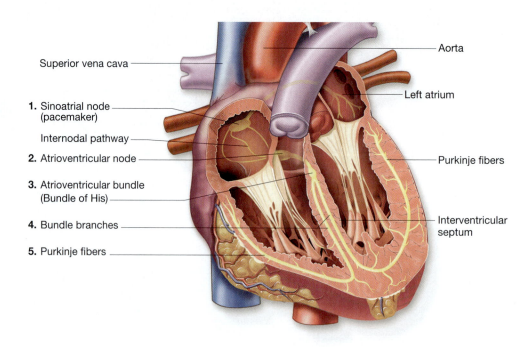

Superior vena cava

Aorta

Left atrium

1. Sinoatrial node
(pacemaker)

Internodal pathway

2. Atrioventricular node

Purkinje fibers

3. Atrioventricular bundle
(Bundle of His)

4. Bundle branches

Interventricular
septum

5. Purkinje fibers

4.3.3 | The cardiac conduction system.

Skeletal System

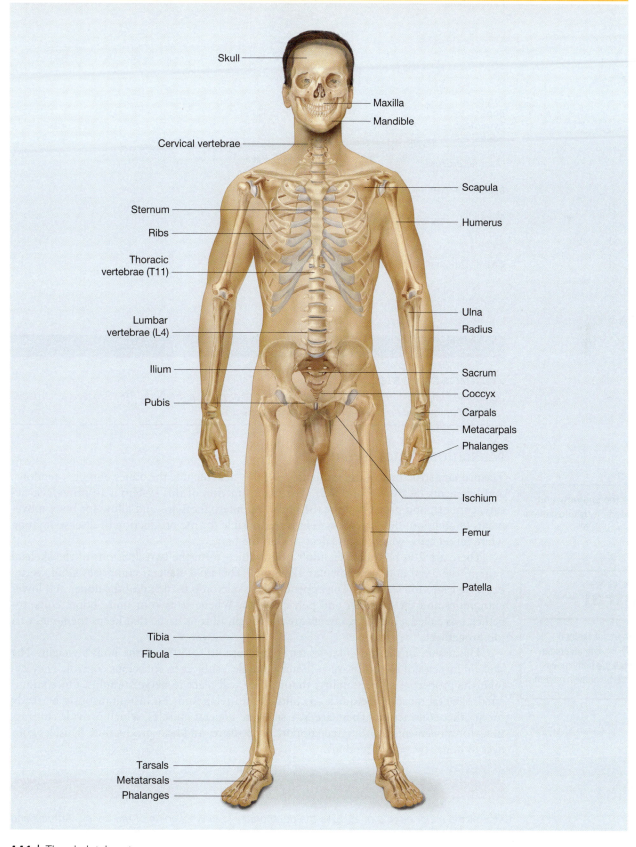

- Skull
- Maxilla
- Mandible
- Cervical vertebrae
- Scapula
- Sternum
- Humerus
- Ribs
- Thoracic vertebrae (T11)
- Lumbar vertebrae (L4)
- Ulna
- Radius
- Ilium
- Sacrum
- Pubis
- Coccyx
- Carpals
- Metacarpals
- Phalanges
- Ischium
- Femur
- Patella
- Tibia
- Fibula
- Tarsals
- Metatarsals
- Phalanges

4.4.1 | The skeletal system.

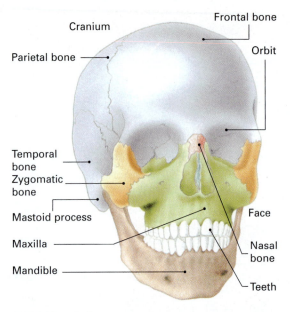

4.4.2 | The skull.

Atherosclerosis

As people age, cholesterol causes narrowing of the arteries in the body. This is called atherosclerosis and is the leading cause of heart attacks and strokes.

OBJECTIVE

8. Describe the anatomy and function of the musculoskeletal system.

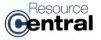

Learn more about skeletal anatomy by viewing an animation, and how the body moves by videos of the body in motion.

Musculoskeletal System

The primary structures of the musculoskeletal system include the bones, muscles, tendons, and ligaments (Scans 4.4 and 4.5). The main function of this system is to provide structure, support, and protection for the body and internal organs and allow for body movement. In addition, the skeletal system is responsible for the production of disease-fighting white blood cells, which occurs deep within the bone.

There are 206 bones in the adult body, which form the two divisions of the skeletal system, the axial and appendicular skeletons. The axial skeletal comprises skull, vertebrae, rib cage, and sternum. The appendicular skeleton is made up of the upper and lower extremities and the shoulder and pelvic girdles. Whenever two or more bones come together, it is called a joint. Ligaments are the tough, fibrous tissue that keeps the bones of a joint together.

The tissues of the muscular system constitute 40%–50% of the body's weight. The skeletal muscles of the body are voluntary muscles, subject to conscious control. They exhibit the properties of excitability; that is, they will react to nerve stimulus. Once stimulated, skeletal muscles are quick to contract and relax and can instantaneously be ready for another contraction. There are 501 separate skeletal muscles, which provide contractions for movement, coordinated support for posture, and heat production. Muscles connect to bones by way of tendons.

▶ **GERIATRIC FOCUS** ◀

One of the major effects of aging is the deterioration and weakening of the bones. Arthritis and osteoporosis are major contributors to this process. Approximately 33% of all falls involving the elderly result in at least one fractured bone, most commonly the hip and/or pelvis.

Muscular System

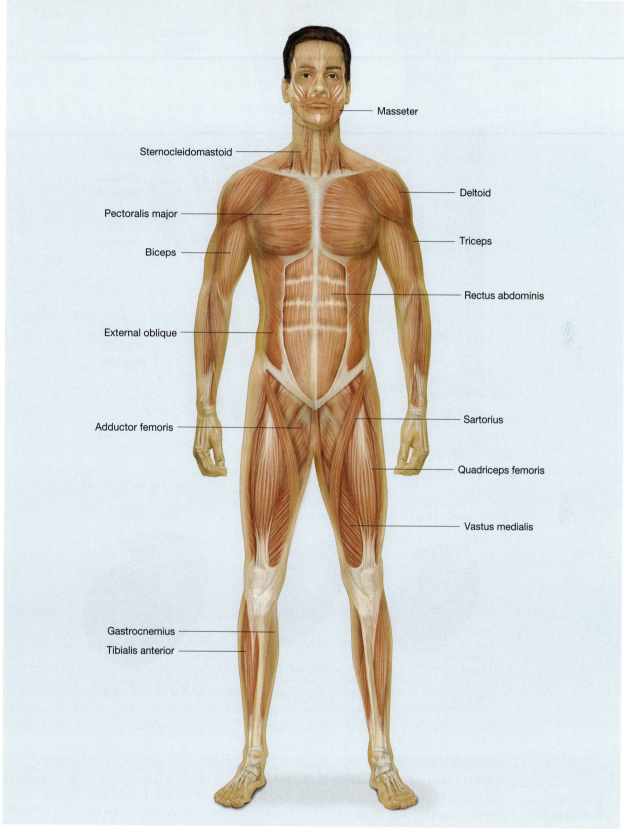

Masseter

Sternocleidomastoid

Deltoid

Pectoralis major

Triceps

Biceps

Rectus abdominis

External oblique

Adductor femoris

Sartorius

Quadriceps femoris

Vastus medialis

Gastrocnemius

Tibialis anterior

4.5.1 | The muscular system.

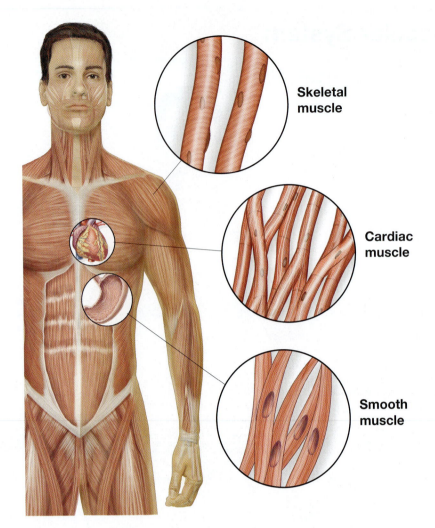

4.5.2 | Three types of muscles.

Skeletal muscle

Cardiac muscle

Smooth muscle

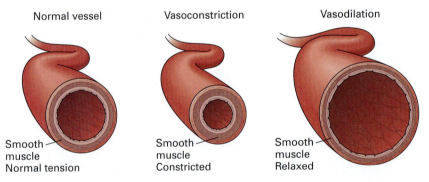

Normal vessel

Vasoconstriction

Vasodilation

Smooth muscle Normal tension

Smooth muscle Constricted

Smooth muscle Relaxed

4.5.3 | Smooth muscle is capable of constricting (getting smaller) and dilating (getting larger).

Nervous System

The primary structures of the nervous system include the brain, spinal cord, and nerves that extend out to all parts of the body (Scan 4.6). Its main function is to control movement, interpret sensations, regulate body activities, and generate memory and thought. Structures within the nervous system may be classified according to divisions: central, peripheral, and autonomic. The central nervous system includes the brain and spinal cord. The sensory (incoming) and motor (outgoing) nerves make up the peripheral nervous

Nervous System

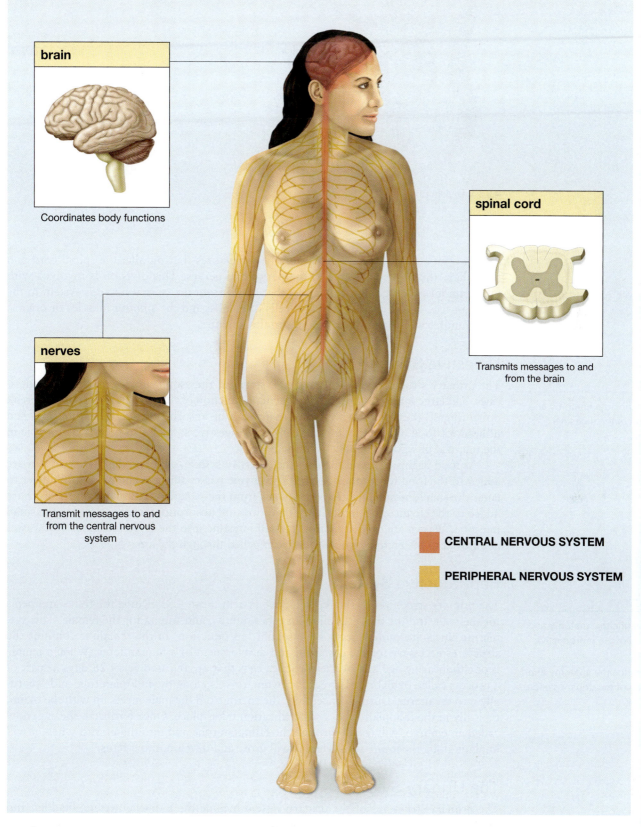

brain

Coordinates body functions

spinal cord

Transmits messages to and from the brain

nerves

Transmit messages to and from the central nervous system

■ CENTRAL NERVOUS SYSTEM

■ PERIPHERAL NERVOUS SYSTEM

4.6.1 | The nervous system.

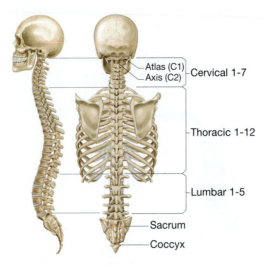

Atlas (C1)
Axis (C2)
Cervical 1-7
Thoracic 1-12
Lumbar 1-5
Sacrum
Coccyx

4.6.2 | Divisions of the spinal column.

system. The autonomic nervous system has structures that parallel the spinal cord and then share the same pathways as the peripheral nerves. This division is involved with motor impulses (outgoing commands) that travel from the central nervous system to the heart muscle, blood vessels, secreting cells of glands, and the smooth muscles of organs. The impulses will stimulate or inhibit certain activities.

Digestive System

The primary structures of the digestive system are the esophagus, stomach, small intestines, and large intestines (Scan 4.7). The main function of this system is to properly break down (digest) the food that we eat so that it can be absorbed through the intestines and utilized for food and energy for our cells. The digestive system also plays a major role in the removal of waste products from the body.

As food begins to travel through the digestive system, acid and digestive enzymes are added to the food to produce chyme. The chyme passes through the pyloric sphincter to enter the small intestine. Digestive enzymes from the pancreas and bile from the liver are added to the chyme. The processes of digestion and absorption are completed in the small intestine. Wastes are carried from the small intestine into the large intestine. The wastes are moved to the rectum, where they are expelled through the anus.

Reproductive System

The primary structures of the reproductive system (Scan 4.8) include the testes and penis for the male and the ovaries, fallopian tubes, uterus, and vagina for the female. This system produces hormones needed for sexual reproduction. In the female it contains the structures necessary for the gestation and development of a human fetus. When a female is of childbearing age, the ovaries produce eggs that are released every 28 days as part of a process called ovulation. The egg, or ovum, travels along the fallopian tube and eventually into the uterus. During conception, the sperm from the male meets up with the ovum, typically in the fallopian tube, and fertilization takes place. Once fertilized, the egg, now called an embryo, will travel through the fallopian tube and into the uterus, where it will implant along the inside wall. Here it will grow and develop into a fetus.

The Urinary System

The primary structures of the urinary system include the kidneys, ureters, bladder, and urethra (Scan 4.9). The main function of this system is to remove chemical wastes from the body and help balance water and salt levels in the blood. This waste is moved from the

Digestive System

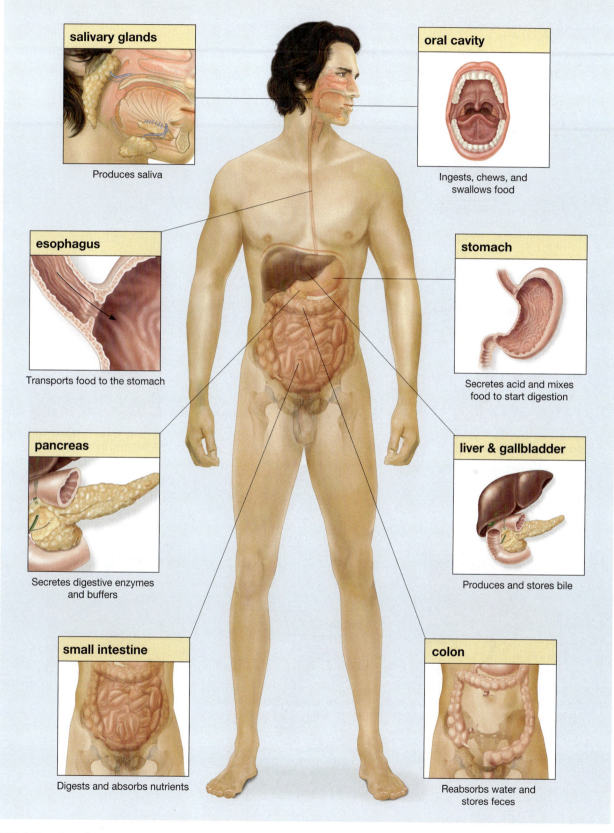

salivary glands

Produces saliva

oral cavity

Ingests, chews, and swallows food

esophagus

Transports food to the stomach

stomach

Secretes acid and mixes food to start digestion

pancreas

Secretes digestive enzymes and buffers

liver & gallbladder

Produces and stores bile

small intestine

Digests and absorbs nutrients

colon

Reabsorbs water and stores feces

4.7.1 | The digestive system.

Male Reproductive System

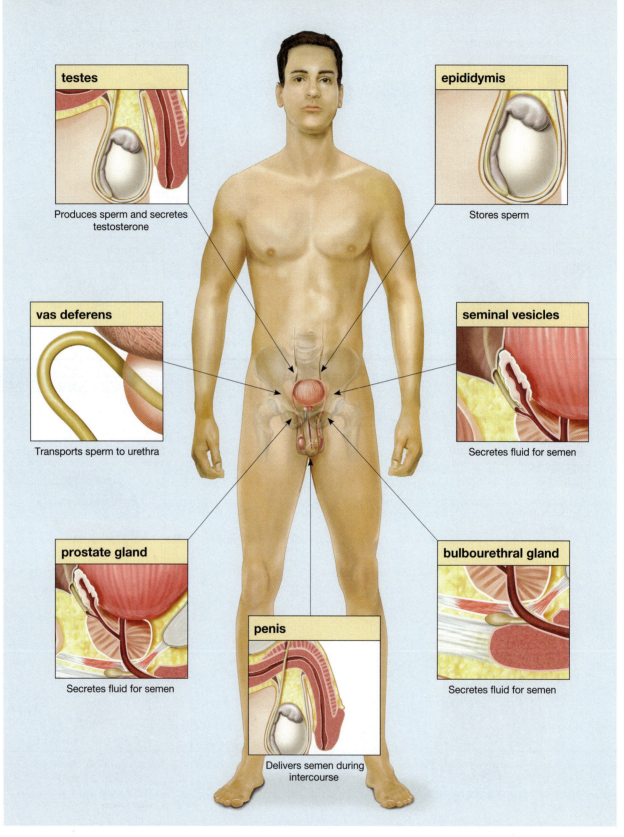

testes

Produces sperm and secretes testosterone

epididymis

Stores sperm

vas deferens

Transports sperm to urethra

seminal vesicles

Secretes fluid for semen

prostate gland

Secretes fluid for semen

penis

Delivers semen during intercourse

bulbourethral gland

Secretes fluid for semen

4.8.1 | The male reproductive system.

Female Reproductive System

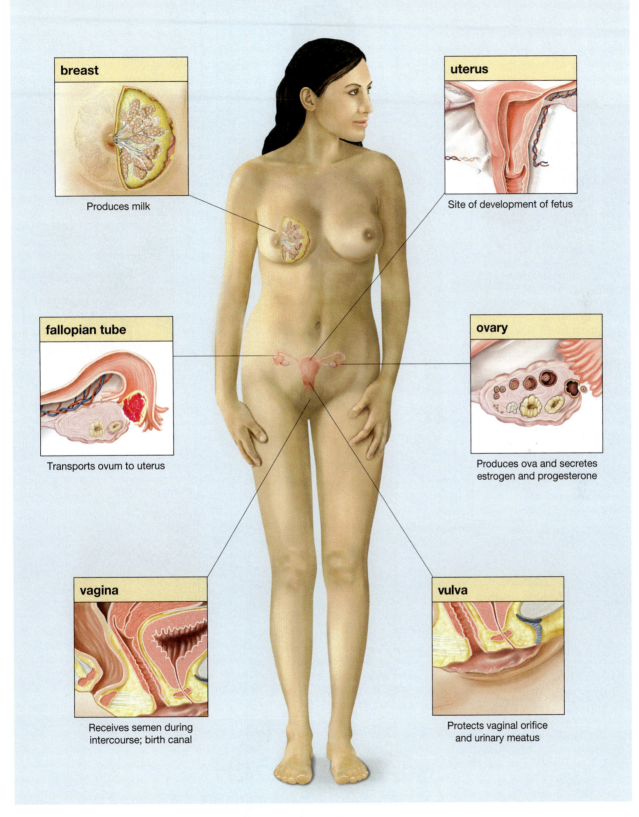

breast

Produces milk

uterus

Site of development of fetus

fallopian tube

Transports ovum to uterus

ovary

Produces ova and secretes estrogen and progesterone

vagina

Receives semen during intercourse; birth canal

vulva

Protects vaginal orifice and urinary meatus

4.8.2 | The female reproductive system.

Urinary System

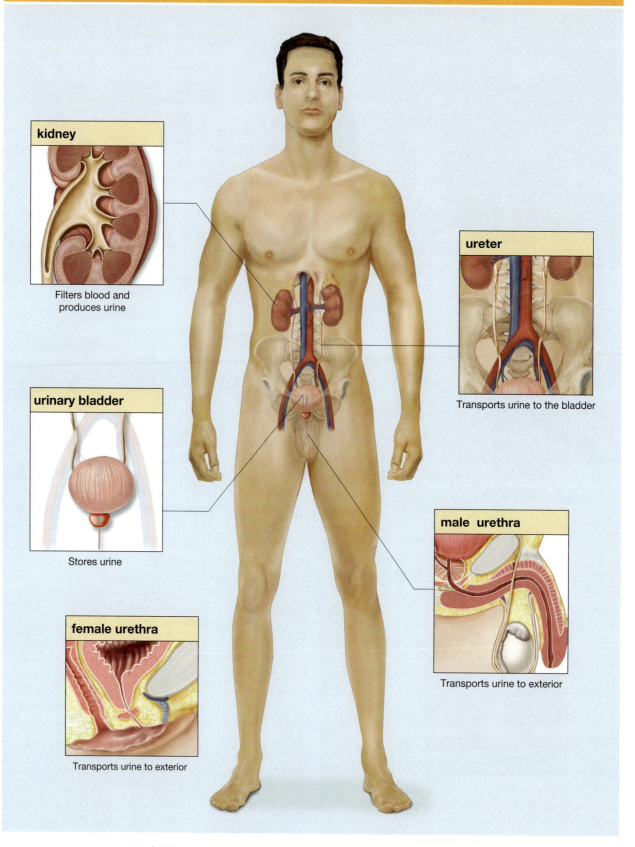

kidney

Filters blood and produces urine

urinary bladder

Stores urine

female urethra

Transports urine to exterior

ureter

Transports urine to the bladder

male urethra

Transports urine to exterior

4.9.1 | The urinary system.

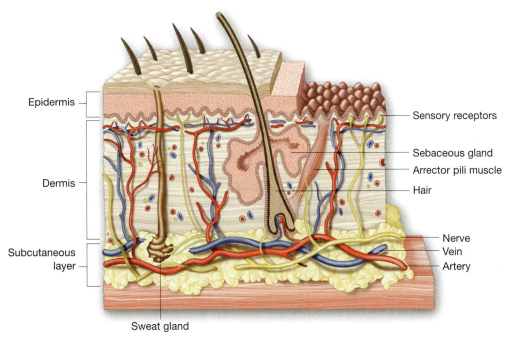

4.10.1 | The anatomy of the skin.

kidneys to the urinary bladder by way of small tubelike structures called ureters. A similar structure called a urethra extends from the bladder to the outside of the body. This allows for the removal of the urine from the body.

Integumentary System

The largest organ of the body is the skin (Scan 4.10). It covers the body's many tissues, organs, and systems. In the adult, the skin covers about 3,000 square inches (1.75 square meters) and weighs about six pounds. It protects the body from heat and cold, as well as from toxins in the environment, such as bacteria and other foreign organisms. It regulates body temperature and senses heat, cold, touch, pain, and pressure. It also regulates body fluids and chemical balance. The skin is actually part of the integumentary system, which includes all the layers of the skin, nails, hair, sweat glands, oil glands, and mammary glands.

▶ GERIATRIC FOCUS ◀

As people age, the skin loses an important component called collagen. The result in the elderly is skin that is very thin and less elastic. This means that it can be easily damaged by simple falls or rough handling.

Endocrine System

The endocrine system is made up of many hormone-producing glands and is responsible for the regulation of many of the processes within the human body (Scan 4.11). Some of the glands that make up the endocrine system include the thyroid, pituitary, adrenal, pancreas, and gonads. Some of the processes that the endocrine system regulates are metabolism, physical size, strength, hair growth, voice pitch, and reproduction. This is accomplished primarily through the production and release of specialized chemicals called hormones.

OBJECTIVE

13. Describe the anatomy and function of the skin.

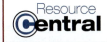

Get more information about both the integumentary and the endocrine systems.

OBJECTIVE

14. Describe the anatomy and function of the endocrine system.

Endocrine System

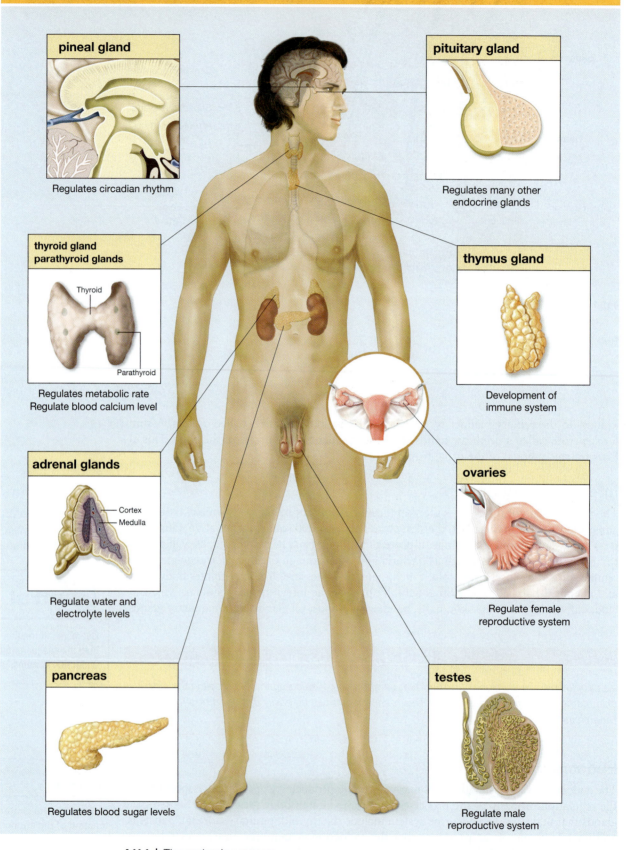

pineal gland

Regulates circadian rhythm

pituitary gland

Regulates many other endocrine glands

thyroid gland parathyroid glands

Thyroid

Parathyroid

Regulates metabolic rate
Regulate blood calcium level

thymus gland

Development of immune system

adrenal glands

Cortex
Medulla

Regulate water and electrolyte levels

ovaries

Regulate female reproductive system

pancreas

Regulates blood sugar levels

testes

Regulate male reproductive system

4.11.1 | The endocrine system.

One of the more common hormones is produced by the pancreas and is called insulin. Insulin is the hormone responsible for the regulation of glucose (sugar) levels in the blood. Another hormone that you may have heard of is called epinephrine. This is produced by the adrenal gland and is responsible for stimulating the nervous system by causing increased heart rate, heart contractions, constriction of the blood vessels, and dilation of the air passages.

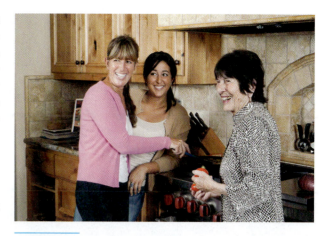

Figure 4.7 • Generations.

Lifespan Development

Throughout its lifespan, the human body undergoes significant change as it grows, develops, ages, and matures (Figure 4.7). These changes occur in three primary areas: biological (the physical body), cognitive (the mind), and psychosocial (how the person interacts with its surroundings). Each phase of development has its unique characteristics that the Emergency Medical Responder must become familiar with to provide the best care possible.

The lifespan development ranges from birth through old age and can be divided into the following phases:

OBJECTIVE

15. Describe the major phases of lifespan development.

- Neonate (birth to 28 days)
- Infant (birth up to 1 year old)
- Toddler (1–3 years old)
- Preschooler (3–6 years old)
- School-age (6–12 years old)
- Adolescent (12–18 years old)
- Early adulthood (18–40 years old)
- Middle adulthood (40–60 years old)
- Late adulthood (60 to the end of life)

In some cases, the specific definition of an infant or child will vary depending on the context in which you are providing care. This is the case in the context of CPR and automated external defibrillator (AED) use. Procedures will change according to the child's physical size more so than the exact age.

The weight used for calculating the size of equipment used and medication doses for children is always given in kilograms. You must learn to estimate the weight of the children you encounter and be able to convert pounds into kilograms.

- 1 kilogram = 2.2 pounds
- 1 pound = 0.45 kilograms

Developmental Characteristics

Because of the different behavioral characteristics of children at different ages, it is useful to become familiar with some broad understandings and expectations for the common stages of child development and how they will affect your assessment of the patient.

Neonates and Infants (Birth up to 1 Year)

When approaching newborns or infants (Figure 4.8), it is important to keep in mind two important ideas: they will not like to be cold, and they do not like to be separated from their parents or primary caregivers. Once infants are crying from discomfort or anxiety, your assessment will surely become much more difficult to perform. A good part of the assessment exam can be done visually, while you are taking the history from the parent or caregiver.

Toddlers (1–3 Years)

The toddler (Figure 4.9) has developed a sense of independence through walking and talking but still is unable to reason well or communicate complex ideas. The toddler does not

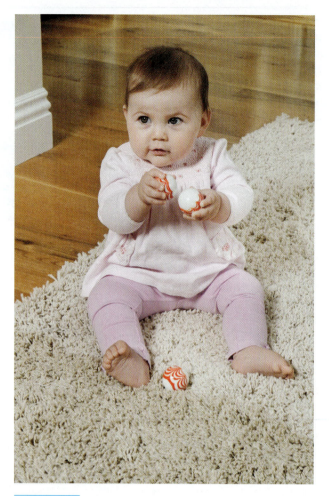

Figure 4.8 • Infant.

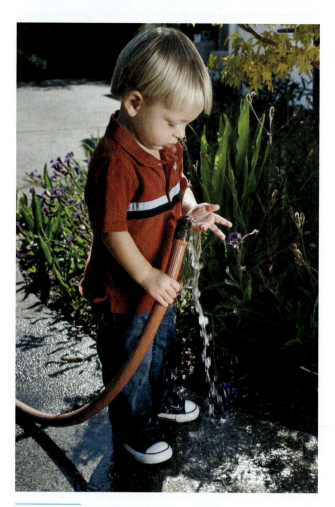

Figure 4.9 • Toddler.

like to be touched by strangers or separated from parents. Like the infant, a good part of the assessment exam can be done visually, while you are taking the history from the parent or caregiver. The alert child will be watching you closely. Even when speaking to the adults, use a calm, quiet voice. This may help to calm the toddler.

When beginning your assessment, listen to heart and lung sounds by pulling up the child's shirt and placing the bell of your stethoscope underneath it, rather than trying to undress the child. Examine the toddler's chest before the head. Use a quiet, confident, soothing voice, and allow the child to hold a toy or favorite object while being examined. When using a stethoscope, it may be helpful to first place it on a parent or favorite stuffed animal to show the child that it does not hurt.

Toddlers may understand injury, illness, or separation from family as punishment, so they need lots of reassurance that they are not to blame and that their parents or caregivers are with them or know where they are.

From the Medical Director

Different Approach

Whenever I approach a child patient, I remember to "get low and go slow." You must gain their confidence even if you know that you may have to cause them some pain as you help them. If there is no clear life-threatening condition, you should first engage the parents. Once the child feels that you are trusted by his parents, he is more likely to trust you as well.

Preschoolers (3–6 Years)

Preschool children (Figure 4.10) have developed concrete thinking skills that allow them to understand and follow instructions. It is important to ask them for their version of how they feel and what happened. Like toddlers, preschoolers may believe they are being punished by an illness or injury for wrong-doing. They are very frightened of potential pain and the sight of blood. They need lots of reassurance and respond well to simple explanations that avoid medical or complicated terminology.

Separation causes them anxiety, so allow the parent or caregiver to hold or sit near the child as you begin your examination. In an effort to build trust, begin your examination with the extremities and then the trunk, followed by the head. The preschooler is typically quite modest, so replace items of clothing after taking them off, or allow the child to help you by pulling up his or her shirt or exposing the area of injury.

School-Aged Children (6–12 Years)

By the time children reach school age (Figure 4.11), they have a basic understanding of the body and its functions, and they usually try to cooperate with the physical exam. They are able to communicate and understand more complex ideas. However, they are very literal, so avoid using confusing language and be aware that they are listening to every word you say, even if you are not talking to them.

School-aged children are aware of and afraid of death and dying as well as pain, deformity, blood, and permanent injury. They benefit from reassurance as well as inclusion in discussions involving their care.

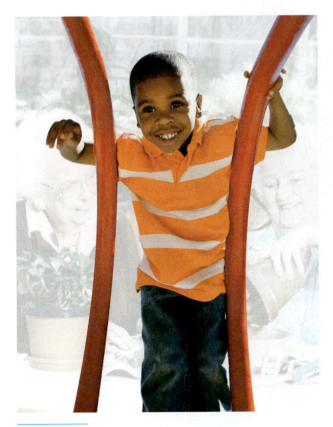

Figure 4.10 • Preschooler.

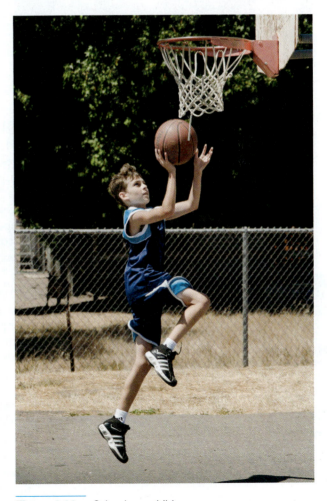

Figure 4.11 • School-age child.

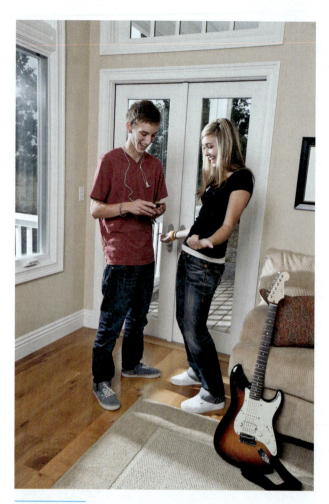

Figure 4.12 • Adolescent.

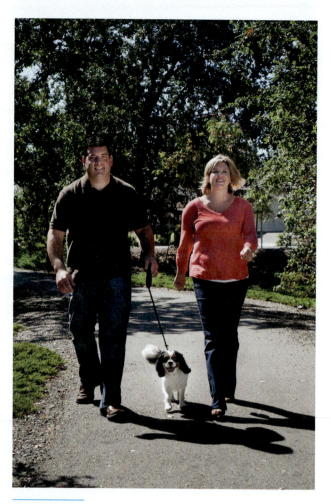

Figure 4.13 • Early adult.

Adolescents (12–18 Years)

The adolescent child (Figure 4.12) has a more thorough understanding of anatomy and physiology and is able to process and express complex ideas. Adolescents are frequent risk takers but poor judges of consequence. They are afraid of disfigurement and permanent injury yet often believe they are immortal or indestructible. They want to be treated as adults, but they may need the same level of support and reassurance as a younger child. Speaking to the adolescent respectfully and non-judgmentally will improve your ability to obtain an accurate history. Protecting adolescents' privacy and modesty may gain their trust. It may be helpful to interview or examine them away from parents or caregivers.

Early Adulthood (18–40 Years Old)

It is during early adulthood (Figure 4.13) when most of us complete our formal education and begin to consider starting families of our own. It is during this time that we are at the peak of health and are traditionally very active. Adults between the ages of 18 and 40 make up a large number of those involved in traumatic injuries and accidents.

Middle Adulthood (40–60) Years

It is during middle adulthood (Figure 4.14) that many develop routines that become well established, and the focus of life often shifts to the rearing of children. It is also the time in life that many physiological changes occur, not the least of which is a noticeable decrease in the ability to see and hear well. It is

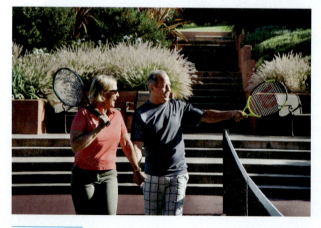

Figure 4.14 • Middle adult.

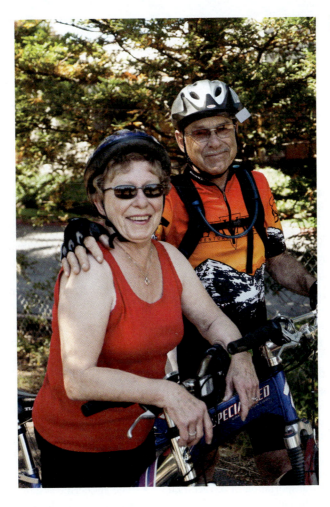

Figure 4.15 • Late adult.

also during this time that people get shorter, hair begins to turn gray, and more permanent wrinkles appear in the skin.

Late Adulthood (60 to the End of Life)

For many, late adulthood (Figure 4.15) represents a period in life when they experience many pronounced changes in the body. Those changes can be greatly influenced by individual lifestyle but can include continued decline in the ability to see, hear, taste, and smell. Mobility can become difficult for some, and the awareness of one's own mortality is ever present. One of the characteristics common to late adulthood is a decrease in the ability to perceive pain. This can make it difficult for the Emergency Medical Responder to accurately assess illness and injury during the patient assessment. It is also common for people in this age group to have overlapping illnesses for which they are taking multiple medications.

WRAP-UP

FIRST ON SCENE

It seems like forever before Stephanie hears sirens approaching. Scott has yet to do anything except flutter his eyelids and groan. Although the direct pressure seems to have stopped most of the bleeding, Scott appears to be struggling more to breathe. Thankfully, she hears vehicle after vehicle rolling to a stop nearby, and the screaming sirens quickly are replaced by a multitude of slamming doors and running feet.

"Okay, we're here now," a woman says and puts her hand on Stephanie's trembling shoulder. She lets go of Scott and stands up. He is immediately surrounded by firefighters and medics, who are tearing open packages and shouting to each other. She takes a few steps back and is caught in the tight embrace of the shift supervisor. "You did real good, kid," he says into her ear. "You did exactly what you were supposed to do."

CHAPTER REVIEW

Summary

- The medical profession has a unique language all its own. To become a valuable participant in this new world, you must learn some of the common word roots, suffixes, and prefixes specific to medical terminology.

- All descriptions relating to illness, injury, and patient care must refer to the patient in the anatomical position. This is a standardized position that is used by all medical professionals and will allow descriptions to be standardized and consistent.

- There are four major body cavities within the human body: the cranial, thoracic, abdominal, and pelvic. These are areas that contain major organs and can hide significant blood loss.

- The cranium contains the brain and soft tissues surrounding the brain. The thorax contains the heart, lungs, and major vessels. The abdomen contains many of the vital organs, such as the liver, spleen, pancreas, gallbladder, and intestines. The pelvic cavity contains the bladder and intestines as well as the uterus, fallopian tubes, and ovaries of the female.

- The respiratory system comprises the upper airway, larynx, trachea, bronchi, bronchioles, and alveoli. It is responsible for the movement of air into and out of the body and the exchange of oxygen and carbon dioxide. The primary muscle of respiration is the diaphragm.

- The cardiovascular system comprises the heart, vessels, and blood. It is responsible for the transportation of oxygen-rich blood and nutrients throughout the body.

- The musculoskeletal system comprises the muscles, bones, and connective tissues such as ligaments and tendons. It provides structure and support for the body and allows mobility. It also provides protection against injury and helps support the immune system.

- The nervous system comprises the brain, spinal cord, and nerves. It is divided into the central nervous system (brain and spinal cord) and the peripheral nervous system (nerves). It allows for the control of all movement and the function of many of the vital systems throughout the body, such as heart rate and breathing rate.

- The digestive system comprises the esophagus, stomach, and intestines. The primary function of the digestive system is to break down the food we eat so that it can be properly metabolized by the cells of the body. It also serves as a means to eliminate solid waste from the body.

- The reproductive system comprises the testes and penis in the male and the ovaries, fallopian tubes, uterus, and vagina in the female. This system is responsible for producing the hormones necessary for reproduction as well as maintaining the structures to support gestation of the fetus in the female.

- The urinary system comprises the kidneys, ureters, bladder and urethra. It is responsible for the filtration and removal of waste from the blood as well as helping to maintain proper water and salt levels in the blood.

- The integumentary system includes all layers of the skin and the structures that support hair/nail growth, sweat glands, and oil ducts. The skin is made up of three layers: the epidermis, dermis, and subcutaneous. The skin helps protect us from harmful pathogens as well as maintain a stable body temperature.

- The endocrine system comprises many hormone-producing glands such as the thyroid, pituitary, adrenal glands and is responsible for the regulation of many of the body's important processes.

- As the human body grows and develops from a newborn infant into an adult, it passes through several developmental stages. There are significant biological, cognitive, and psychosocial changes at each stage of development. The better you understand these changes, the better you will be at assessing your patients and providing the proper care.

Take Action

"WHERE DO I HURT?"

Being able to accurately describe the location of a sign or symptom is an important skill that you must learn to become an effective member of the EMS team. This activity will help you learn to properly describe the anatomical location of a series of random injuries or symptoms. Using a fellow classmate and a roll of masking tape, one of you will place small pieces of tape at various locations on your body. Begin with only two or three pieces of tape and keep them on the anterior side of the body. Next, the person with the tape will stand before the other person in the anatomical position. Using proper anatomical terms, your partner must describe in writing the location of the imaginary injuries or symptoms represented by the tape. To make the activity

more challenging, place the pieces of tape in various locations on the body and have the "patient" lie on the floor in different positions.

VIRTUAL ANATOMY TOUR

This activity will help you learn the location of the various organs in the abdominal cavity. You will need a fellow classmate, and one of you will play the role of patient while the other plays the role of student. With the patient lying supine on the floor, the student carefully palpates the four quadrants of the abdomen while describing the anatomy located in each quadrant. You may refer to your book as necessary until you have memorized the location of all the major organs.

First on Scene Run Review

Recall the events of the "First on Scene" scenario in this chapter and answer the following questions, which are related to the call. Rationales are offered in the Answer Key at the back of the book.

1. Describe the elements of a good scene size-up.

2. What did Stephanie accomplish by placing her hand over the wound?

3. Which organs could be damaged with a gunshot to the chest?

Quick Quiz

To check your understanding of the chapter, answer the following questions. Then compare your answers to those in the Answer Key at the back of the book.

1. Which one of the following best describes the anatomical position?
   a. Standing upright with arms at the sides
   b. Lying supine with arms outstretched and palms up
   c. Standing with hands at the sides and palms forward
   d. Lying prone with arms held straight out, palms down

2. The navel is on the _____ aspect of the body.
   a. posterior
   b. anterior
   c. inferior
   d. superior

3. The spine can be felt (palpated) on the _____ aspect of the body.
   a. posterior
   b. anterior
   c. inferior
   d. superior

4. The imaginary line that bisects the body into two halves (left and right) is known as the:
   a. proximal break.
   b. inferior aspect.
   c. recumbent line.
   d. midline.

5. Any location on the body that is closer to the midline is referred to as:
   a. medial.
   b. recumbent.
   c. lateral.
   d. inferior.

6. The thumb is considered _____ to the palm.
   a. distal
   b. proximal
   c. lateral
   d. medial

7. A bruise that is on the anterior thigh just above the knee could be described as _____ to the knee.
   a. distal
   b. proximal
   c. lateral
   d. medial

8. The chin is _____ to the mouth.
   a. superior
   b. lateral
   c. inferior
   d. medial

9. The nose is _____ to the mouth.
   a. superior
   b. lateral
   c. inferior
   d. medial

10. A patient that is found lying face down is said to be in the _____ position.
    a. recumbent
    b. lateral
    c. supine
    d. prone

11. A patient with a suspected spine injury will likely be placed on a long spine board flat on his back or in a _____ position.
    a. recumbent
    b. lateral
    c. supine
    d. prone

12. The recovery position is also known as the _____ position.
    a. lateral recumbent
    b. lateral
    c. superior
    d. stroke

13. The bladder is located in which body cavity?
    a. Cranial
    b. Thoracic
    c. Abdominal
    d. Pelvic

14. The _____ cavity is also known as the thoracic cavity.
    a. pelvic
    b. chest
    c. abdominal
    d. cranial

15. The _____ separates the thoracic cavity from the abdominal cavity.

   a. pelvic wall
   b. midline
   c. diaphragm
   d. stomach

16. All of the following can be found in the abdominal cavity EXCEPT the:

   a. stomach.
   b. liver.
   c. spleen.
   d. heart.

17. The _____ cavity contains the liver and part of the large intestine.

   a. pelvic
   b. abdominal
   c. thoracic
   d. cranial

18. The _____ is found in the upper left quadrant of the abdomen.

   a. appendix
   b. stomach
   c. kidney
   d. liver

19. An infection of the appendix would most likely cause pain in the _____ quadrant.

   a. upper right
   b. upper left
   c. lower right
   d. lower left

20. The _____ is/are found in an area behind the abdominal cavity.

   a. kidneys
   b. bladder
   c. small intestine
   d. gall bladder

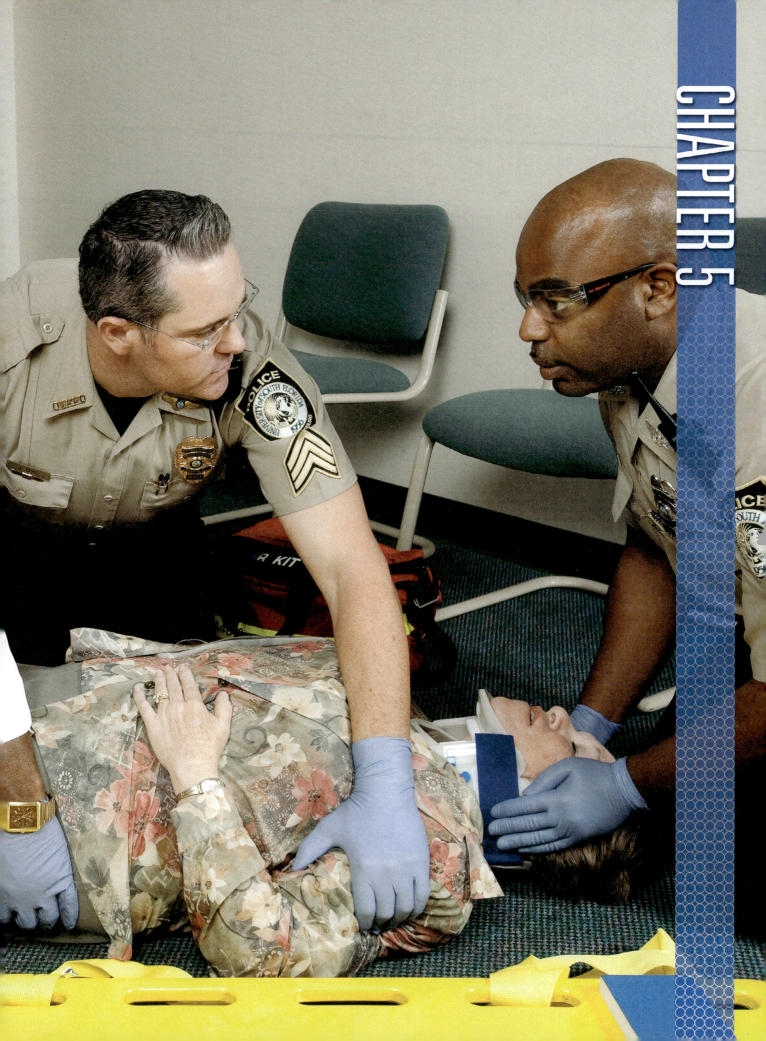

Principles of Lifting, Moving, and Positioning of Patients

CHAPTER OVERVIEW

Many Emergency Medical Responders are injured every year because they attempt to lift or move a patient or piece of equipment improperly. Back injuries are the most common and have the greatest potential to end what could otherwise be a long and rewarding EMS career. One of the most important things that you can do for yourself, your coworkers, and your patients is to learn how to lift and move patients and objects using proper body mechanics.

Just as critical as knowing *how* to move patients properly is knowing *when* they should be moved. There are many factors that you must consider before moving a patient, such as the safety of the scene, the patient's condition, and the number of rescuers available to assist.

This chapter discusses common situations in which an Emergency Medical Responder may be required to move patients. It also will explain some simple lifting and moving techniques utilizing proper body mechanics that will make it possible for you to be a safe and healthy Emergency Medical Responder for many years to come.

OBJECTIVES

Upon successful completion of this chapter, the student should be able to:

COGNITIVE

10. Explain the criteria for utilizing patient restraint. (p. 110)

11. Identify various types of patient restraints. (p. 110)

12. Explain the technique for the proper restraint of a patient. (p. 111)

13. Explain complications associated with restraining a patient. (p. 111)

15. Demonstrate the proper technique for standard moves, urgent moves, and emergent moves.

16. Demonstrate the proper use of equipment used to transport patients.

17. Demonstrate the proper technique for placing a supine patient into the recovery position.

18. Demonstrate the proper technique for log-rolling a patient.

PSYCHOMOTOR

14. Demonstrate the use of proper body mechanics while performing various patient moves.

AFFECTIVE

19. Value the importance of proper body mechanics when participating in simulated patient moves and lifts.

Jesse Daniels had just put a new CD into the stereo when the front right tire on his car exploded, sending ropy pieces of black rubber in all directions. He grabbed the steering wheel with both hands and eased the small car completely off the road and onto the shoulder. He got out, swearing under his breath, and walked around to the front of the car to inspect the damage. The tire wasn't just flat. It was gone. A bare, bent wheel was the only thing that remained.

A man driving a pickup stopped in the roadway next to Jesse's car and shouted through the open passenger window, "Is everything okay?"

"Yeah. I just have to put the spare on," Jesse shouted back, knowing that he was definitely going to be late for his Emergency Medical Responder class at the community college.

"I'll pull over and help!" the man yelled back. Jesse smiled and started to say, "Thanks!" but the man and his pickup truck were suddenly gone in a deafening explosion of twisting metal, rushing air, and spinning chrome wheels. Jesse stumbled back, fell onto the ground, and watched in horror as a speeding semitrailer flashed larger than life just beyond the tips of his tennis shoes for a split second before vanishing with the sound of locked-up tires roaring across the pavement.

Principles of Moving Patients

Body Mechanics

Proper **body mechanics** is the proper and efficient use of your body to facilitate lifting and moving. These are important steps that Emergency Medical Responders must follow to lift efficiently and to prevent injury.

Before you lift or move a patient or an object, it is important to first plan what you will do and how you will do it (Figure 5.1). Estimate the weight of the patient or object and then, if needed, request additional help. It is also important to consider any physical limitations that may make lifting difficult or unsafe for you and those assisting you. Whenever possible, lift with a partner whose strength and height are similar to yours. Clearly communicate with your partner and with the patient when you are ready to lift, and continue to communicate throughout the process. Eye contact is an important component when coordinating a lift. So, to ensure good communications, make sure you and your partner make eye contact before initiating any lift.

When you are ready to lift, follow the rules of proper body mechanics to minimize the chances of injury to yourself, your coworkers, or the patient. They are as follows:

- Position your feet properly. They should be on a firm, level surface and positioned a comfortable width apart. Take extra care if the surface is slippery or unstable. It may be necessary to postpone the move until more help or equipment is on hand.

body mechanics ▶ the use of the body to facilitate lifting and moving to minimize injury.

OBJECTIVES

2. Describe the characteristics of proper body mechanics.

3. Explain the importance of using proper body mechanics.

4. Explain the hazards of not using proper body mechanics when lifting and moving patients.

5. Explain the importance of active communication during patient lifts and moves.

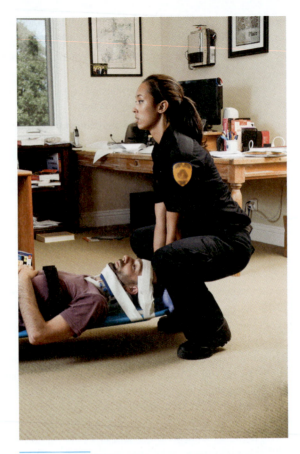

Figure 5.1a • To begin the power lift, keep your back straight and eyes on your partner.

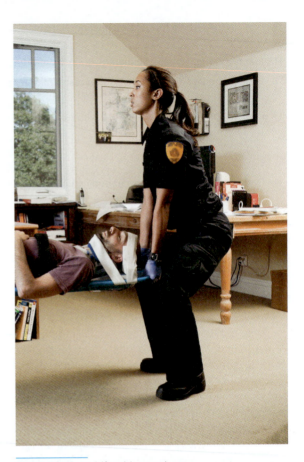

Figure 5.1b • Lift with your legs.

Figure 5.1c • While moving, keep the weight as close to your body as possible.

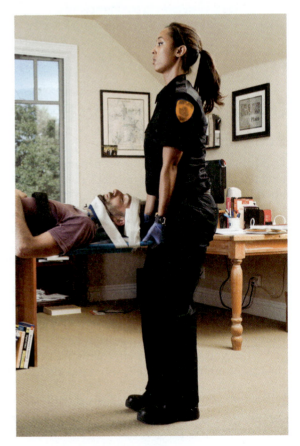

- Lift with your legs. Keep your back as straight as possible and bend at your knees. Try not to bend at the waist any more than you absolutely have to. This technique is known as a **power lift**.
- When lifting an object with one hand, avoid leaning to either side. Bend your knees to grasp the object, and keep your back straight.
- Minimize twisting during a lift. Attempts to turn or twist while you are lifting can result in serious injury.
- Keep the weight as close to your body as possible. The farther the weight is from your body, the greater your chance of injury.
- When carrying a patient on stairways, use a chair or commercial stair chair instead of a wheeled stretcher whenever possible. Keep your back straight, and let your legs do the lifting. If you are walking backward down stairs, ask someone to "spot" you, by walking behind you and placing a hand on your back to help guide and steady you (Figure 5.2).

With the proper technique, moving and lifting patients and objects can be done safely. Use proper body mechanics on every call.

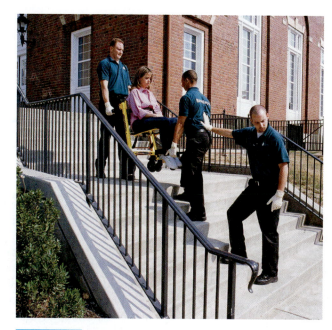

Figure 5.2 • When you use a stair chair, have someone spot you as you walk backward down stairs.

When to Move a Patient

In general, an Emergency Medical Responder should only move a patient when absolutely necessary. Your primary role is to assess the patient, provide basic emergency care, and continue to monitor the patient's condition until more advanced personnel arrive. Emergency situations in which it may be necessary to move a patient include the presence of a dangerous environment where the patient is at risk for further injury; when you cannot adequately assess airway, breathing, and circulation (ABCs) or bleeding; or when you are unable to gain access to other patients who need lifesaving care. You also may be called on to assist other EMS responders in accomplishing *standard* patient moves. Those are the lifting and moving of patients for non-emergent reasons such as comfort or preparation for transport.

Whenever possible, encourage the patient to remain at rest, even when the patient appears to be able to move. Remember that not all signs of an illness or injury show themselves immediately, and sometimes patients do not realize how sick or injured they really are. In addition, some patients may not be straightforward in answering your questions or may even deny or hide the existence of an illness or injury.

Emergency Moves

There are times when a patient must be moved immediately, even if you do not have the appropriate people or equipment to do so. These situations call for an **emergency move**. An emergency move should be considered in the following situations:

- The patient and/or the rescuers are in immediate danger. Situations that involve uncontrolled traffic, fire or threat of fire, possible explosions, impending structural collapse, electrical hazards, toxic gases, and other such dangers may make it necessary to move a patient quickly.
- Lifesaving care cannot be given because of the patient's location or position. The inability to properly assess and care for problems with a patient's airway, breathing, circulation or the inability to properly manage uncontrolled bleeding makes it necessary to move a patient quickly.
- You must move a patient to gain access to other patients who need lifesaving care. This is seen most often in motor-vehicle crashes.

power lift ▶ a technique used to lift a patient who is on a stretcher or cot.

OBJECTIVE

6. Differentiate between a standard move and an emergency move, and state when each should be used.

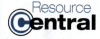

Read additional information on lifting and moving patients.

IS IT SAFE?

Sometimes the best decision is *not* to move the patient. If the patient is too heavy or in an awkward position, or you simply do not have enough people to help, consider a new plan or call for additional help.

emergency move ▶ a patient move that is carried out quickly when the scene is hazardous, care of the patient requires immediate repositioning, or you must reach another patient who needs lifesaving care.

Emergency moves rarely provide any protection for a patient's injuries, and they may even cause the patient tremendous pain. Still, sometimes the need to move a patient to ensure his safety or to provide lifesaving care outweighs the risks associated with moving the patient quickly.

One of the greatest dangers in moving a patient quickly is the possibility of making a spine injury worse. If the patient is on the floor or ground, it is important to make every effort to pull the patient in the direction of the long axis of the body. This is the line that runs down the center of the body from the top of the head and along the spine. By pulling this way, you will provide as much protection to the spine as possible.

Drags

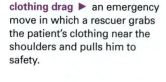

clothing drag ▶ an emergency move in which a rescuer grabs the patient's clothing near the shoulders and pulls him to safety.

One of the most common types of emergency move is the drag. In this type of move, patients are pulled by their clothes, feet, or shoulders or by using a blanket (Scan 5.1). Notice that drags provide little if any protection for the neck and spine.

In most cases, drags are initiated from the shoulders by pulling along the long axis of the body. This causes the remainder of the body to fall into its natural anatomical position, with the spine and all limbs in normal alignment. Avoid dragging a patient sideways, with one arm or one leg, unless absolutely necessary. A sideways drag can cause twisting motions of the spine that may aggravate existing injuries.

When using a drag to move a patient down stairs or down an incline, grab the patient under the shoulders and pull the patient head first as you walk backward. If possible, try to cradle the patient's head in your forearms as you drag.

FIRST ON SCENE

continued

Jesse climbed to his feet and watched the big rig slow to a crawl and pull off onto the shoulder several hundred feet down the highway. The twisted heap that once was a pickup truck sat smoking in the middle of the road just beyond it, the bed curled up over the top of the cab like a huge metal scorpion. Jesse looked back up the highway and saw a car and another semi bearing down on the scene, heading right into the setting sun. He turned and sprinted as fast as he could down the shoulder of the road, past the parked semi, and up to a point where he was even with the wrecked pickup.

"Help me!" Incredibly the man in the pickup was alive and seemed fully conscious. Jesse could clearly see him in

the deformed but still intact cab of the truck. "My legs are...uh...I think they're gone. What do I do?" The man kept looking over at Jesse and then back down into his own lap.

Jesse saw the other vehicles approaching rapidly. He began to yell and wave his arms, trying to get the drivers' attention. The car arrived seconds later, swerved around the wreckage and continued on without braking, throwing up bits of broken glass and metal as it sped by.

"Help me, please!" The man was now screaming over the deafening rumble of a rapidly approaching semi.

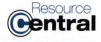

Learn more about proper lifting.

Other Emergency Moves

There are many other techniques that can be used to move a patient quickly. Some require only one rescuer (Scan 5.2), while others require two rescuers. Remember that any emergency move must be justified and should be carried out as quickly as possible.

Standard Moves

standard move ▶ the preferred choice when the situation is not urgent, the patient is stable, and you have adequate time and personnel for a move.

A **standard move** is the preferred choice when the situation is not urgent, the patient is stable, and you have adequate time and personnel for a move. Standard moves should be carried out with the help of other trained personnel or bystanders. Take care to prevent additional injury to the patient, as well as to avoid patient discomfort and pain.

Note: Always pull in the direction of the long axis of patient's body. Do not pull a patient sideways. Avoid bending or twisting the patient's trunk.

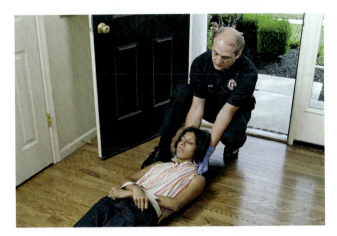

5.1.1 | Clothing drag, or shirt drag.

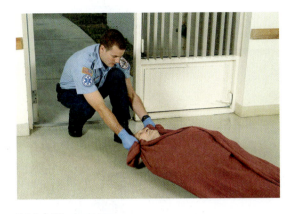

5.1.2 | Blanket drag.

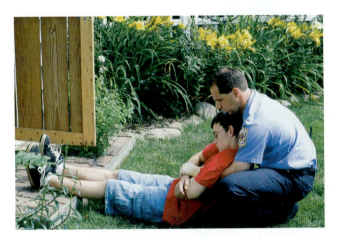

5.1.3 | Shoulder drag.

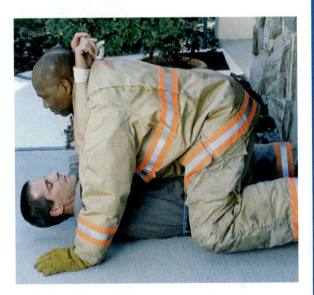

5.1.4 | Firefighter's drag.

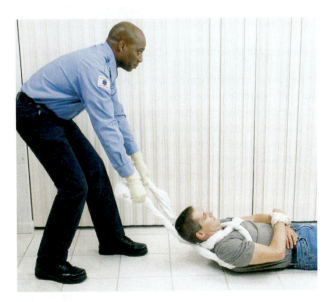

5.1.5 | Strap drag.

Chapter 5 Principles of Lifting, Moving, and Positioning of Patients **97**

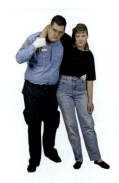

5.2.1 | One-rescuer crutch.

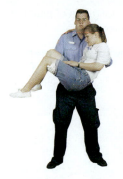

5.2.2 | Cradle carry.

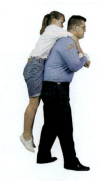

5.2.3 | Pack strap carry.

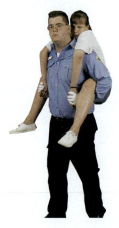

5.2.4 | Piggy back carry.

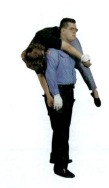

5.2.5 | Firefighter's carry.

firefighter's drag ▶ a move in which the rescuer straddles the supine patient, secures the patient's hands behind the rescuer's neck, and then crawls to safety while dragging the patient underneath him.

blanket drag ▶ a method used to move a patient by placing him on a blanket or sheet and pulling it across the floor or ground.

firefighter's carry ▶ a method used to walk to safety with a patient securely placed over one shoulder.

direct ground lift ▶ a standard lift in which three rescuers move a patient from the ground to a bed or stretcher.

Follow these rules when preparing to use a standard move:

- Complete a primary assessment.
- Choose an appropriate number of rescuers for the specific type of move.
- Take care to avoid compromising a possible neck or spine injury. Avoid moving a patient who has neck pain, numbness, or weakness.
- Consider splinting suspected fractures, depending on the patient's condition.

The following are situations in which a standard move may be appropriate:

- The patient is uncomfortable or his position is aggravating an injury.
- Emergency care requires moving the patient. This is usually seen in cases in which there are no suspected spine injuries. Problems due to extreme heat or cold, such as heat cramps, heat exhaustion, hypothermia, and local cold injuries (frostbite and freezing), are good examples. Reaching a source of water for washing in cases of serious chemical burns also may be a reason to move a patient.
- The patient insists on being moved. If a patient will not listen to the reasons why he should not be moved and tries to move on his own, you may have to assist. Avoid trying to restrain the patient. Sometimes a patient becomes so upset that stress worsens his condition. If this type of patient can be moved, and the move is short, you may have to make the move to keep him calm and relieve his stress.

Direct Ground Lift

The **direct ground lift** is a standard move that can be used to move a patient from the ground or floor to a bed or stretcher. This move is not recommended for use on patients

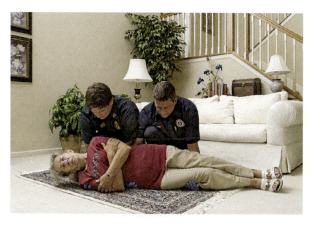

5.3.1 | Position your arms under the patient. Be sure to cradle the head.

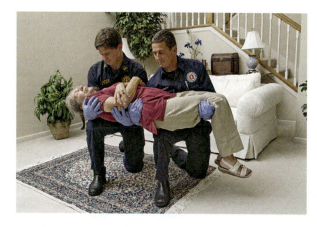

5.3.2 | Lift the patient to your knees and roll toward your chests.

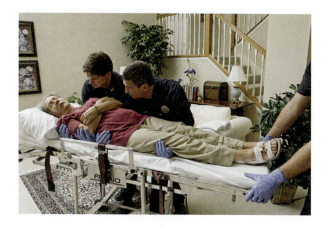

5.3.3 | On signal, move the patient to the carrying device.

with possible neck or spine injuries. Although it can be accomplished by two people, three are recommended for the safety of all involved.

To perform a direct ground lift (Scan 5.3), the patient should be lying face up (supine), and the arms should be placed on the chest. You and your helpers should line up on one side of the patient. One rescuer should be at the patient's head, another at her midsection, and another at the lower legs. Each of you should drop to the knee closest to the patient's feet.

The rescuer at the head should place one arm under the patient's neck and grasp the far shoulder to cradle the head. The other arm should be placed under her back, just above the waist. The rescuer at her midsection should place one arm above and one arm below the buttocks. The rescuer at the patient's lower legs should place one arm under the patient's knees and the other arm under her ankles.

On the signal of the rescuer at the head, everyone should lift the patient up to the level of their knees. Then, on signal, the rescuers should roll the patient toward their chests. Finally, on signal, everyone should stand while holding the patient. The patient can now be moved, reversing the process when it is time to place her in a supine position.

Extremity Lift

An **extremity lift** requires two people (Scan 5.4). This lift is ideal for moving a patient from the ground to a chair or the stretcher. It also can be used to move a patient from a chair to the stretcher. It should not be performed, however, if there is a possibility of head, neck, spine, shoulder, hip, or knee injury or any suspected fractures to the extremities that have not been immobilized.

extremity lift ▶ a move performed by two rescuers, one lifting the patient's arms and one lifting the patient's legs.

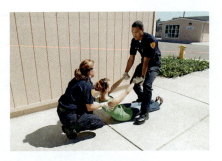

5.4.1 | To get the patient into a sitting position, one rescuer pushes from behind while the other pulls from the wrists.

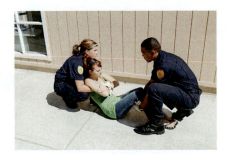

5.4.2 | The rescuer at the head places arms under patient's armpits and grasps patient's wrists. While facing the patient, the rescuer at the feet grasps patient's legs behind the knees.

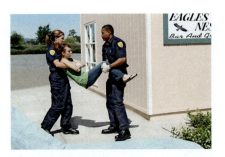

5.4.3 | You can now carry the patient a short distance or place her on a stretcher or chair.

The patient should be placed face up, with knees flexed. You should kneel at the head of the patient, placing your hands under her shoulders. Have your helper stand at the patient's feet and grasp her wrists. Direct your helper to pull the patient into a sitting position, while you push the patient from the shoulders. (Do not have your helper pull the patient by the arms if there are any signs of suspected fractures.) Slip your arms under the patient's armpits and grasp the wrists. Once the patient is in a semi-sitting position, have your helper crouch down and grasp the patient's legs behind the knees.

Direct your helper so that you both stand at the same time. For example, "Ready? Lift on three. One, two, three, lift." Then move as a unit when carrying the patient. Try to walk out of step with your partner to avoid swinging the patient. The rescuer at the head should direct the rescuer at the feet as to when to stop the carry and when to place the patient down in a supine or seated position.

Direct Carry Method

direct carry ▶ a carry performed to move a patient with no suspected spine injury from a bed or from a bed-level position to a stretcher.

The **direct carry** is performed to move a patient with no suspected spine injury from a bed or from a bed-level position to a stretcher (Scan 5.5). First, position the stretcher perpendicular to the bed, with the head end of the stretcher at the foot of the bed. Prepare the stretcher by unbuckling straps and removing other items. Then, two rescuers should stand between the bed and the stretcher, facing the patient. The first rescuer should slide an arm under the patient's neck and cup the shoulder, while the second rescuer slides a hand under the patient's hip and lifts slightly. The first rescuer then slides his other arm under the patient's back, while the second rescuer places his arms underneath the patient's hips and calves. Finally, both rescuers should slide the patient to the edge of the bed, lift/curl him toward their chests, and rotate and place him gently onto the stretcher.

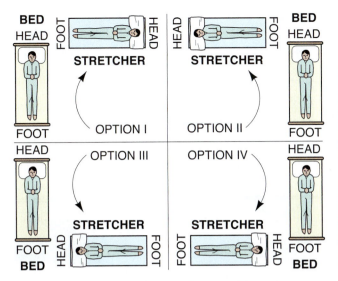

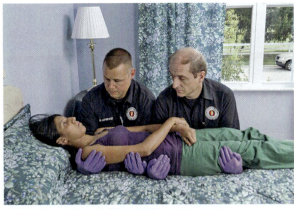

5.5.1 | Stretcher is placed at 90-degree angle to bed, depending on room configuration. Prepare stretcher by lowering rails, unbuckling straps, and removing other items. Both Emergency Medical Responders stand between stretcher and bed, facing patient.

5.5.2 | Position your arms under the patient and slide the patient to the edge of the bed.

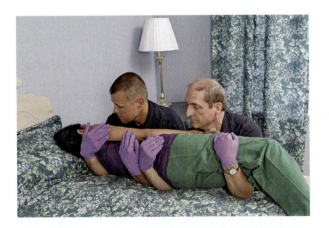

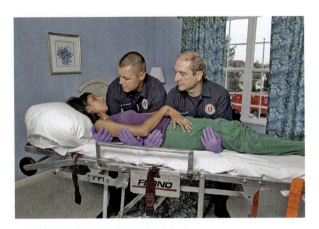

5.5.3 | Lift the patient and curl her toward your chests.

5.5.4 | Rotate and place the patient gently on the carrying device.

Draw Sheet Method

An additional method of moving a patient with no suspected spine injury from a bed to a stretcher is the **draw sheet method**. This method may be performed from the side of the bed or from either the head or the foot of the bed. Select a method that gives you the easiest access to the patient. Figure 5.3 illustrates this move from the side of the bed.

draw sheet move ▶ a method for moving a patient from a bed to a stretcher.

To perform the draw sheet method from the side of the bed, begin by loosening the bottom sheet under the patient and positioning the stretcher next to the bed. Be sure to secure the stretcher so that it does not move while transferring the patient from the bed to the stretcher.

Next, adjust the height of the stretcher to match the level of the bed, lower the rails, and unbuckle the straps. Both rescuers should reach across the stretcher and roll the sheet against the patient. Grasp the sheet firmly at the patient's head, chest, hips, and knees. Finally, draw the patient onto the stretcher, sliding him in one smooth motion.

Several devices have been developed in recent years to make the task of moving patients from stretcher to bed easier and safer. Devices such as slider boards and slide bags

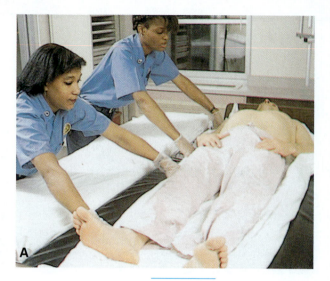
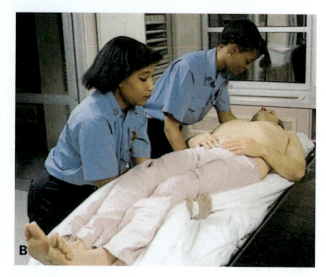

Figure 5.3 • Draw sheet method of moving a patient from a bed to a stretcher.

(Figure 5.4) are in use in many hospitals and nursing care homes. Become familiar with the use of these devices before you attempt to use them the first time.

Equipment for Transporting Patients

OBJECTIVE

7. Identify the common devices used for transporting patients.

EMTs and advanced life support (ALS) personnel will often ask Emergency Medical Responders to assist with preparing the patient for transport and with lifting, moving, and loading patients into the ambulance. To help with those tasks, you must be familiar with the various carrying and "packaging" devices used by EMS personnel. (Many Emergency Medical Responder courses do not include information and practice on immobilization devices. Your instructor will teach you the procedures if you will be expected to perform them in your jurisdiction.)

Typical equipment used for packaging and loading a patient into an ambulance includes a wheeled stretcher. This device has many names depending on the area of the country. Common names include gurney, stretcher, cot, or pram. It is used to transport a patient from the scene of the emergency to the ambulance and from the ambulance to a hospital bed. It is secured in the back of an ambulance by way of a simple locking mechanism. In addition, the head and the foot ends of many stretchers can be elevated to make the patient comfortable or to assist in caring for certain conditions such as difficulty breathing.

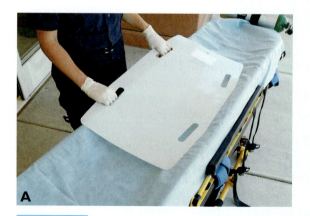

Figure 5.4a • Example of a slider board.

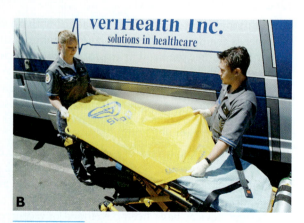

Figure 5.4b • Example of a slide bag.

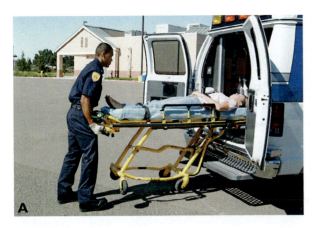

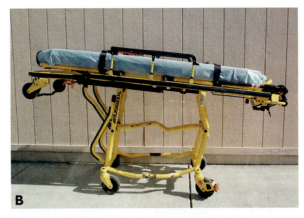

5.6.1 | Single-operator stretcher.

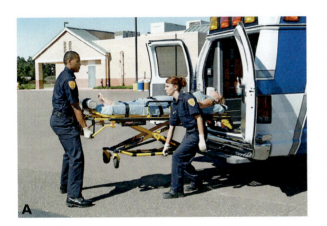

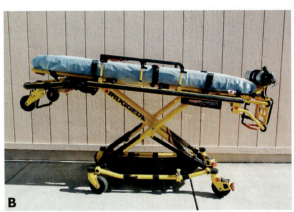

5.6.2 | Dual-operator stretcher.

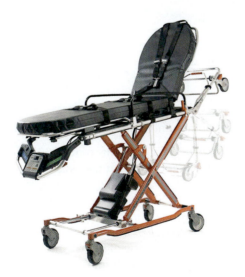

5.6.3 | Electric/pneumatic-lift stretcher. These eliminate the need for heavy lifting.

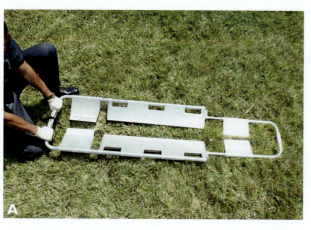
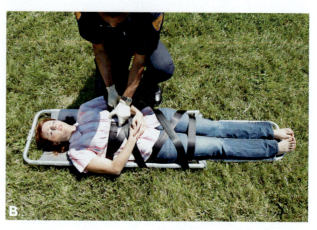

5.7.1 | Scoop stretchers. (A) These stretchers are ideal for moving patients in the position they are found. (B) Once in place, the patient must be properly secured to the device before moving.

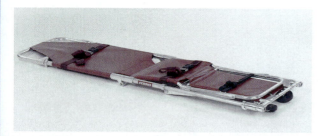

5.7.2 | Portable stretcher. Beneficial for carrying supine medical patients down stairs.

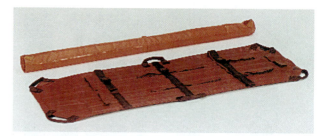

5.7.3 | Flexible stretcher. Used in restricted areas or narrow hallways.

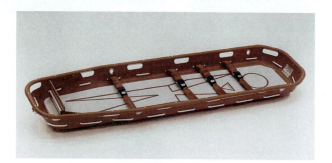

5.7.4 | Basket stretcher. Used in rescue situations and to transport over rough terrain.

There are many brands and types of wheeled stretchers. Some of them are (Scan 5.6):

- *Single-operator stretcher.* This type of stretcher allows a single operator to load the stretcher into the ambulance without the assistance of a second person. The undercarriage is designed to collapse and fold up as the stretcher is pushed into the ambulance.
- *Dual-operator stretcher.* This type of stretcher requires a second person to lift the undercarriage prior to pushing it into the ambulance.
- *Electric/pneumatic-lift stretcher.* This is the newest type of stretcher on the market and is equipped with a pneumatic or electric mechanism that will lift and lower the stretcher at the touch of a button. It minimizes the need for rescuers to lift a stretcher with a patient on it, thereby significantly reducing the risk of back injury.

Other types of equipment used for moving patients include the following (Scans 5.7 and 5.8):

- *Portable stretcher.* This type of stretcher is also known as a folding or flat stretcher. It is much lighter than a standard wheeled stretcher and makes the task of moving a

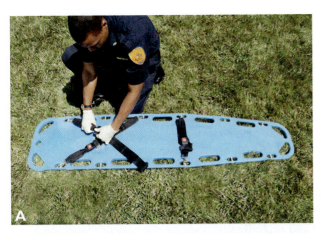
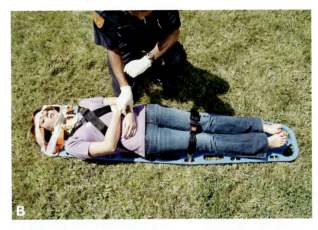

5.8.1 | Long spine board. (A) This backboard is used to immobilize the spine of a supine patient. (B) Long spine board with patient properly secured in place.

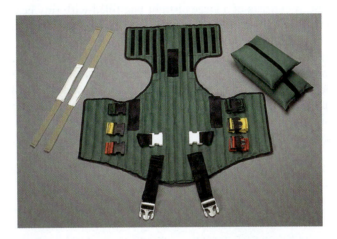

5.8.2 | Vest-type extrication device. This device facilitates the extrication of a seated patient, while stabilizing the patient's head, neck, and spine.

patient down stairs or out of tight spaces much easier. Portable stretchers are typically a combination of canvas and aluminum, and they usually fold or collapse for easy storage.

- *Flexible stretcher.* This stretcher is made of rubberized canvas or other flexible material such as heavy plastic, often with wooden slats sewn into pockets. The flexible stretcher usually has three carrying handles on each side. Because of its flexibility, it can be useful in restricted areas or narrow hallways.
- *Stair chair.* The stair chair helps rescuers move seated medical patients down stairways and through tight places where a traditional stretcher will not fit. Newer brands are made of sturdy folding frames with either canvas or hard plastic seats and are easy to store. They have wheels that allow rescuers to roll them over flat surfaces. Some models have a tractor-tread mechanism that allows them to easily slide down stairways just by tilting them.
- *Basket stretcher.* This device is sometimes referred to as a Stokes basket. It is most commonly used for wilderness or cliff rescue situations.
- *Scoop stretcher.* This device is typically made of hard plastic or aluminum. It is called a scoop stretcher because it splits vertically into two pieces, which can be used to "scoop" the patient up. Newer models are sturdier and more rigid than older ones and provide more support to the spine. However, a scoop stretcher is commonly used for picking up and moving a patient with hip injuries or multiple injuries rather than

IS IT SAFE?

Whenever walking backward down stairs to move a patient, it is best to have a second person walk behind you and act as a spotter. Have your spotter place a hand on your back and talk you down the stairs.

for spine injuries. It is also used for transferring a patient from a bed or the floor to a wheeled stretcher or from the wheeled stretcher to the hospital bed.

- *Spine board.* Spine boards are also known as backboards. The long spine board is used for patients who are found lying down or standing and have a suspected spine injury. Short spine boards are becoming less common as they are being replaced by the vest-type extrication device. Short boards are used primarily for removing patients from vehicles when it is suspected that they have neck or spine injuries. Once secured to the short spine board, the patient may be moved from a sitting position in the vehicle to a supine position on a long spine board. Short boards are difficult to use in late-model cars that have bucket seats because they do not fit the contour of the seat.

- *Vest-type extrication device.* The extrication vest is used to help immobilize and remove patients found in a seated position in a vehicle. It wraps around the patient's torso to stabilize the spine and has an extended section above the vest with side flaps for stabilizing the patient's head and neck. Rescuers secure the patient's head, neck, and torso with straps and padding. The vest has handles that aid in lifting the patient out of the vehicle and onto a long spine board.

- *Full-body immobilization device.* The most common type is the full-body vacuum splint. It consists of a large airtight bag filled with tiny beads. As the patient is placed on the device, it can be molded to fit the shape and contours of the patient's body. Once it is in place, a portable vacuum is activated to remove the air from the bag. The result is a hard cast-like splint that immobilizes the patient.

- *Pedi-board.* Special spinal immobilization boards are made to fit infants and children. The back of a child's head is larger proportionately than an adult's, so boards have a depression in the head end to fit. However, it is still necessary to pad the child's body from the shoulders to the heels to ensure the airway is in a neutral position while secured on the board.

continued

FIRST ON SCENE

Jesse could see the driver of the oncoming semi, immersed in a conversation on his cell phone, simply move the steering wheel to the left, guiding the huge truck onto the grassy center divide of the highway, where it passed the collision scene without so much as downshifting. Once the truck's flatbed trailer cleared the wreckage, it returned to the roadway and continued off into the distance.

"Please, please, help me!" The man, his face contorted with pain and terror, was now screaming at Jesse.

There were more oncoming vehicles, but at the moment they were nothing more than colorful specks on the distant horizon. Jesse ran to the pickup and was able to force the passenger-side door open, breaking it back onto the hinges. He reached over and released the driver's seat belt and found that the bench seat of the truck was covered with blood.

The man fell over onto the passenger side, grabbing for Jesse's arm. Jesse could see that both of his legs were severed, pinched between the truck's displaced engine and the now raised floor of the cab. He quickly glanced down the highway, saw the glint of the sun on a windshield, slid his hands under the man's arms, and began moving backward as fast as he could.

OBJECTIVE

8. Explain the purpose of the "recovery position," and state when it should be used.

recovery position ▶ the position in which a patient with no suspected spine injuries may be placed, usually on the left side. Also called the *lateral recumbent position.*

Patient Positioning

Proper positioning of patients is one of the most important skills an Emergency Medical Responder can learn. Proper positioning is important for many reasons, including patient comfort and proper airway maintenance.

Recovery Position

A patient with no suspected spine injury should be placed on his side to help maintain an open and clear airway. This is especially helpful for unresponsive patients. This position is commonly called the **recovery position** or *lateral recumbent position.* Unless the patient's condition

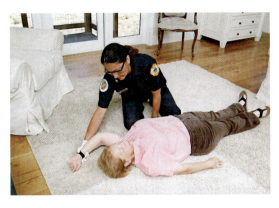

5.9.1 | Move the closest hand of the patient above his head.

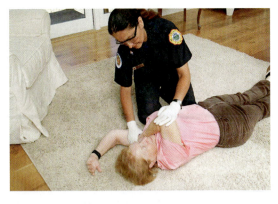

5.9.2 | Move the patient's far hand across to the opposite shoulder, next to the patient's cheek.

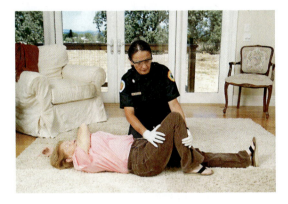

5.9.3 | Bring the patient's far leg to the flexed position.

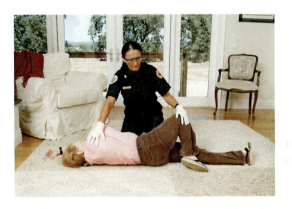

5.9.4 | Using the knee and shoulder, carefully pull the patient onto his side.

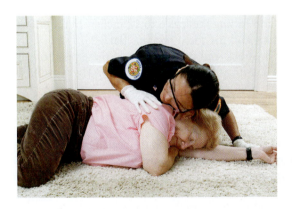

5.9.5 | Adjust the knee and shoulder to stabilize the patient. Then recheck the patient's ABCs.

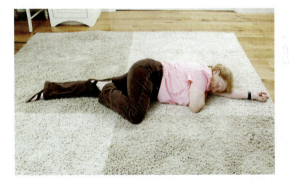

5.9.6 | Once properly positioned, the knee and elbow will support the patient.

suggests otherwise, place the patient on his left side. Because most stretchers secure against the driver's-side wall in ambulances, this positioning will have him face the EMT for the ride to the hospital. Remember that patients with injuries, especially suspected spine injuries, should not be moved until additional EMS resources arrive to evaluate and stabilize them.

To place a patient in the recovery position, perform the following steps (Scan 5.9):

1. Kneel beside the patient on his left side. Raise the patient's left arm straight out above his head.

2. Cross the patient's right arm over his chest, placing his right hand next to his left cheek.

3. Raise the right knee until it is completely flexed.

4. Place your right hand on the patient's right shoulder and your left hand on the patient's flexed right knee. Using the flexed knee as a lever, pull toward you, guiding the patient's torso in a smooth rolling motion onto his side. The patient's head will rest on his left arm.

5. As best as you can, position the patient's right elbow and knee on the floor so that they act like a kickstand, preventing the patient from rolling completely onto his stomach. Place the patient's right hand under the side of his face. The arm will support the patient in this position. The hand will cushion his face and allow the head to angle slightly downward for airway drainage.

Always position yourself appropriately to manage the patient's airway and monitor his mental status. Place the patient in the recovery position at the first sign of a decreased level of responsiveness.

Fowler's and Semi-Fowler's Positions

Many patients with no suspected spine injuries may be placed in either a position of comfort or in specific positions that allow for more effective care of particular conditions. This may include patients with medical complaints such as chest pain, nausea, or difficulty breathing. For example, breathing can often be aided by placing the patient in either a **Fowler's position** (full sitting) or a **semi-Fowler's position** (semi-sitting).

Trendelenburg Position

The **Trendelenburg position** may be used for patients who you suspect may be suffering from shock. The use of this position varies around the country, so you should always follow local protocol. It is achieved by placing the patient in a supine position on a device such as a long backboard or flexible stretcher and raising the foot end of the board or stretcher up approximately 12 to 18 inches. This position keeps the patient's body completely flat while tilting him at a slight head-down angle.

The **shock position** is another option that may be helpful for the patient who you think could be suffering from shock. This position should only be used for patients exhibiting signs of shock but have no evidence of trauma or injury. This position is achieved by placing the patient in a supine position and raising the legs 6 to 12 inches. In the shock position, the patient's legs are bent at the hips and the torso remains flat.

There may be times when a patient is in shock and one or more of these positions is not recommended, such as a patient with a significant head or chest injury. Always follow local protocols when positioning patients.

Log Roll

To move a prone patient to a supine position and ensure stability of the head and spine where a trauma injury is suspected, perform a **log roll**. A log roll is also the most common method for transferring a supine patient onto a long backboard when there is a likelihood of neck or back injury. This move can be done with as few as two rescuers, but three is ideal to minimize twisting of the patient's spine during the procedure. Perform the following steps:

1. One rescuer should kneel at the top of patient's head and hold or stabilize the head and neck in the position found. Notice which way the patient's head is facing, as you will most likely want to roll her in the opposite direction.

2. A second rescuer should kneel at the patient's side opposite the direction the head is facing. Quickly assess the patient's arms to ensure there are no obvious injuries. Raise and extend the patient's arm that is opposite the direction the head is facing. Position that arm straight up above the head. This allows for easy rolling and provides support for the head during the roll. This is especially helpful if you must do the log roll alone.

3. The third rescuer should kneel at the patient's hips.

4. Rescuers should grasp the patient's shoulders, hips, knees, and ankles. If only one rescuer is available to roll the patient, he should grasp the heavy parts of the torso—the shoulders and hips.

OBJECTIVE

9. Describe the following patient positions, and state when each should be used: Fowler's, semi-Fowler's, shock, Trendelenburg.

Fowler's position ▶ a position in which a patient is placed fully upright in a seated position, creating a 90-degree angle.

semi-Fowler's position ▶ semi-seated position in which the patient reclines at a 45-degree angle.

Trendelenburg position ▶ a position in which the patient is placed flat on his back with his legs and feet raised.

shock position ▶ elevation of the feet of a supine patient 6 to 12 inches. Recommended for shock that is not caused by injury.

IS IT SAFE?

The most important person during a log roll is the person at the head. He must think ahead and position his hands in anticipation of the movement of the patient from face down to face up. Positioning the hands incorrectly will result in an awkward hand and body position of the rescuer and may result in excessive movement of the patient's neck.

log roll ▶ a method used to move a patient with a suspected spine injury from the prone position to the supine position.

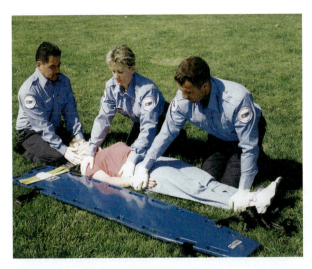

5.10.1 | Manually stabilize the patient's head and neck as you place the board parallel to the patient. Maintain manual stabilization throughout the log roll.

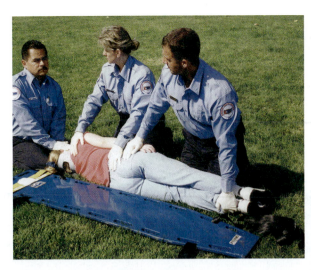

5.10.2 | Kneel at the patient's side opposite the board. Reach across the patient and position your hands. Inspect the patient's back.

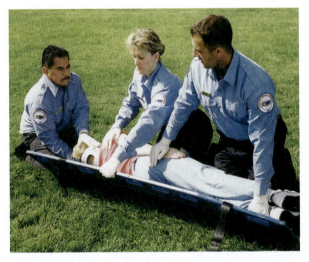

5.10.3 | On command from the rescuer at the head, as a unit roll the patient toward you. Then move the spine board into place.

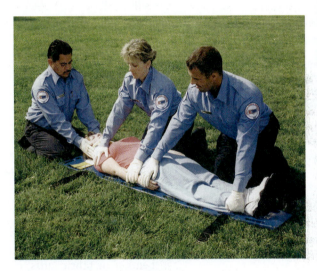

5.10.4 | Lower the patient onto the spine board at the command of the rescuer at the head. Center the patient on the board.

5. The rescuer at the patient's head should signal and give directions: "On three, slowly roll. One, two, three, roll together." All rescuers should slowly roll the patient toward the rescuers in a coordinated move, keeping the spine in a neutral, in-line position. It is important to note that the rescuer holding the head should not initially try to turn the head with the body. Because the head is already facing sideways, allow the body to come into alignment with the head. Once the body and head are aligned, approximately half way through the roll, the rescuer at the head will then move with the body, keeping the head and body aligned until the patient is in the supine position.

Sometimes the patient is already supine but must be placed on a blanket or spine board. If this is the case, perform steps 1–5 above. Without removing your hands, continue with the following (Scan 5.10):

1. The rescuer at the patient's head should continue stabilization of the patient's head and neck until other rescuers position a blanket or long spine board (backboard) behind the patient.

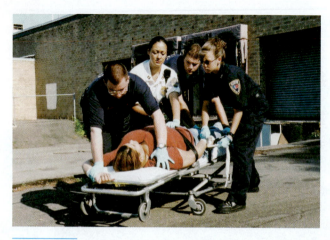

Figure 5.5 • Restraining a patient to a gurney.

restraint ▶ the process of securing a combative patient's body and extremities to prevent injury to himself or others.

2. At a signal from the rescuer at the head, they should slowly roll the patient in a coordinated move onto the blanket or spine board.

3. Finally, they should make sure the patient is positioned on the center of the spine board. If an adjustment is necessary, keep the spine in neutral alignment.

Restraining Patients

It may become necessary to **restrain** a patient when he becomes a danger to himself or others. Patients who are suffering from an illness or injury can suddenly become combative and begin lashing out those around them. Patients suffering from a behavioral problem or psychiatric emergency may also suddenly refuse care and may attempt to leave the scene. Depending on the situation, it may be necessary to restrain the patient to protect yourself or him from further harm (Figure 5.5). In a perfect world, you would leave the job of restraining a patient to law enforcement personnel, but this is not always possible. Whenever possible, be sure to have law enforcement present when attempting to restrain a patient. It is very important to follow local protocol.

Types of Restraints

Patients can either be *physically* or *mechanically* restrained. Physical restraint means holding the patient with your hands or legs so they cannot move, whereas mechanical restraint means applying some sort of device to the patient to restrict his movements. Restraining a patient with your body is not ideal since it does not allow for you to provide medical care. The use of mechanical restraints is a better option for a patient with an altered mental status who is a danger to himself or others (Figure 5.6).

Handcuffs, shackles ("leg irons"), plastic zip-ties, and belly chains (a chain that is wrapped around a person's waist with handcuffs attached) are examples of hard restraints. These devices are used primarily by law enforcement and will rarely be used in medical situations.

Leather or fabric cuffs, cloth straps, rolls of gauze, cravats, sheets, and clothing are examples of soft restraints. You will find these items effective and more suited to properly restraining medical patients without causing further injury.

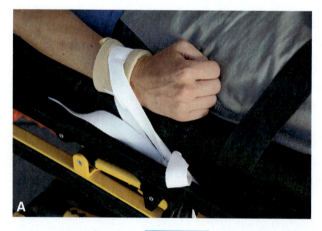

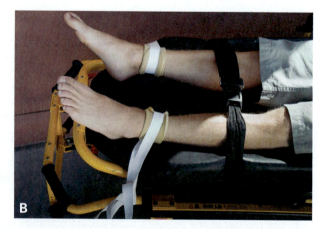

Figure 5.6 • Examples of soft restraints. (A) Restraint of the arm and (B) use of restraints for the legs.

Use Restraint

Physically restraining a patient should be the last resort taken only when it is clear that without doing so the patient may harm himself. Your personal safety is paramount. If you are injured, then the number of patients on the scene is doubled. Use the least amount of restraint necessary to protect the patient from harm, and do not be afraid to stop and evaluate whether your actions are making things better or worse. There is nothing wrong with a tactical retreat and reassessment of the situation. It may be better to wait until additional help arrives.

Patient Restraint

Attempting to restrain a patient is dangerous and can place you, your fellow rescuers, and the patient at risk for injury. Consider all your options before attempting restraint, and always follow local protocol. Follow these guidelines when attempting to restrain a patient:

- Ensure that you have adequate assistance—at least four people, including you.
- Clearly plan the action so that all participants are clear about their responsibilities.
- Stay outside of the patient's range of motion until ready to act.
- Once the plan is clear, act immediately.
- Approach the patient all at once, with each assistant assigned to control a particular limb.
- Talk to the patient calmly during the restraining process.
- Secure all limbs with appropriate restraining equipment.
- DO NOT secure the patient face down.
- Consider administering supplemental oxygen by nonrebreather mask.
- Check the patient's airway, breathing, and circulation often following restraint.
- Clearly document the reason for restraining the patient as well as the procedure and equipment used.
- Ensure that the group uses only the force required to effectively restrain the patient.

Positional Asphyxia

The most serious complication associated with improperly restraining uncooperative or combative patients is called **positional (or *restraint*) asphyxia**. This is where a person is restrained in a position that either blocks the airway (such as with the chin held tightly to the chest) or in a manner that does not allow full expansion of the chest and lungs. Either of these can rapidly lead to death and both are completely avoidable if proper technique is used and the restrained patient is continually assessed.

Restraint Injuries

Another complication, one that is much more common than positional asphyxia, is the injury of the patient, the rescuers, or both during the restraint process. Effective planning and communication among the rescuers and rapid decisive action will go a long way toward preventing injuries while restraining a combative patient. Proper training in the application of restraint devices will also help to prevent injury to the patient once he is restrained.

OBJECTIVE

12. Explain the technique for the proper restraint of a patient.

IS IT SAFE?

It is not always a good idea to attempt to restrain a combative patient. If the patient is armed, too physically strong, potentially under the influence of drugs, or in an unsafe area or you do not have enough assistance, you should maintain your distance and attempt to keep the patient engaged until adequate and appropriate assistance arrives.

OBJECTIVE

13. Explain complications associated with restraining a patient.

positional asphyxia ▶ refers to death resulting from the securing of a person in the prone position, limiting his ability to breathe adequately. Also called *restraint asphyxia*.

WRAP-UP

By the time the emergency crews arrive, summoned by the driver of the semi that had initially hit the pickup, several more cars and big rigs have sped through the collision scene. One even clipped the demolished pickup with a large chrome bumper, sending it skittering off the highway and into a ditch.

Jesse had pulled the injured man onto the side of the road. The semi driver who had hit the pickup comes running up to the scene. Shaken and winded, he offers, "Can I help?" Grateful, Jesse shows him how to hold the man's head in a neutral, in-line position while Jesse applies pressure to the bleeding legs with his jacket.

Later, the paramedic who arrives with the ambulance credits Jesse's quick thinking and actions with ultimately saving the patient's life.

FIRST ON SCENE

Summary

- It is critical to understand and apply proper body mechanics when lifting either patients or objects, since failure to use appropriate techniques can cause career-ending injuries.

- When lifting, always keep the weight as close to your body as possible, avoiding leaning or twisting, and use your leg muscles to lift the weight.

- When two or more responders are preparing to move a patient, eye contact and effective communication are very important to ensure a smooth process and to minimize the risk of injury to them or the patient.

- Although Emergency Medical Responders should ideally provide care for patients where they find them and provide comfort until more advanced help arrives, it is sometimes necessary for the patient to be moved from the immediate area for his own safety or care. The emergency move most appropriate to the situation should be used.

- The recovery position is effective to care for an unresponsive patient's airway when a spine injury is not suspected.

- Patients can be uncooperative or even combative for a wide range of reasons. If a patient needs to be restrained for his own safety, or the safety of others, it is important to only use the force necessary to apply proper restraints.

- Never restrain a patient in the prone position, because this can lead to death from positional asphyxia, a condition where the patient cannot breathe due to the manner in which he has been restrained.

Take Action

INSTANT REPLAY

It is very common for athletes to watch videos of themselves to identify where they could improve their techniques, and Emergency Medical Responders can use the same process for developing better body mechanics. First, obtain a digital video camera and assemble a group of four or more students: one to act as the patient, two to be EMRs, and one to film the exercise.

You should then record yourselves performing the different patient moves detailed in this chapter, immediately reviewing each video and critiquing it from the standpoint of proper body mechanics. Rotate roles so everyone has the opportunity to see and improve their technique. Consider creating a before-and-after compilation highlighting the initial techniques and the revised techniques following the critiquing process.

First on Scene Run Review

Recall the events of the "First on Scene" scenario in this chapter and answer the following questions, which are related to the call. Rationales are offered in the Answer Key at the back of the book.

1. How could Jesse make the scene safe prior to entering?

2. How could Jesse help the driver of the pickup that was hit by the semi-trailer?

3. What would be the proper way to remove the patient from the pickup?

Quick Quiz

To check your understanding of the chapter, answer the following questions. Then compare your answers to those in the Answer Key at the back of the book.

1. *Proper body mechanics* is best defined as:
   a. properly using your body to facilitate a lift or move.
   b. using a minimum of three people for any lift.
   c. contracting the body's muscles to lift and move things.
   d. lifting with your back and not your legs.

2. An Emergency Medical Responder should immediately move a patient EXCEPT when the patient:
   a. has a blocked airway.
   b. is bleeding severely.
   c. has mild shortness of breath.
   d. is in cardiac arrest.

3. When lifting a patient, your feet should be placed:
   a. one in front of the other.
   b. shoulder-width apart.
   c. a comfortable distance apart.
   d. as close together as possible.

4. Good body mechanics means keeping your back _____ and bending at the knees when lifting a patient or large object.

   a. at a 45-degree angle
   b. straight
   c. curved
   d. slightly twisted

5. The load on your back is minimized if you can keep the weight you are carrying:

   a. as close to your body as possible.
   b. at least six inches in front of you.
   c. at least 18 inches in front of you.
   d. as low as possible.

6. What type of move is used when there is no immediate threat to the patient's life?

   a. Emergency
   b. Standard
   c. Rapid
   d. Nonrapid

7. Which one of the following would be the best choice for a stable patient with a suspected spine injury?

   a. One-rescuer assist
   b. Cradle carry
   c. Two-rescuer assist
   d. Shoulder drag

8. Which one of the following patients would best be served by being placed in the recovery position?

   a. A child who is unresponsive following a seizure
   b. An adult in cardiac arrest and in need of CPR
   c. A child who is face down and unresponsive in a pool
   d. An adult victim of a vehicle collision

9. Before restraining a combative patient, the Emergency Medical Responder should obtain _____ approval.

   a. law enforcement
   b. medical direction
   c. ALS
   d. supervisor

10. Which one of the following devices would be best suited to carry a responsive patient with no suspected spine injury down a flight of stairs?

   a. Flexible stretcher
   b. Wheeled stretcher
   c. Scoop stretcher
   d. Stair chair

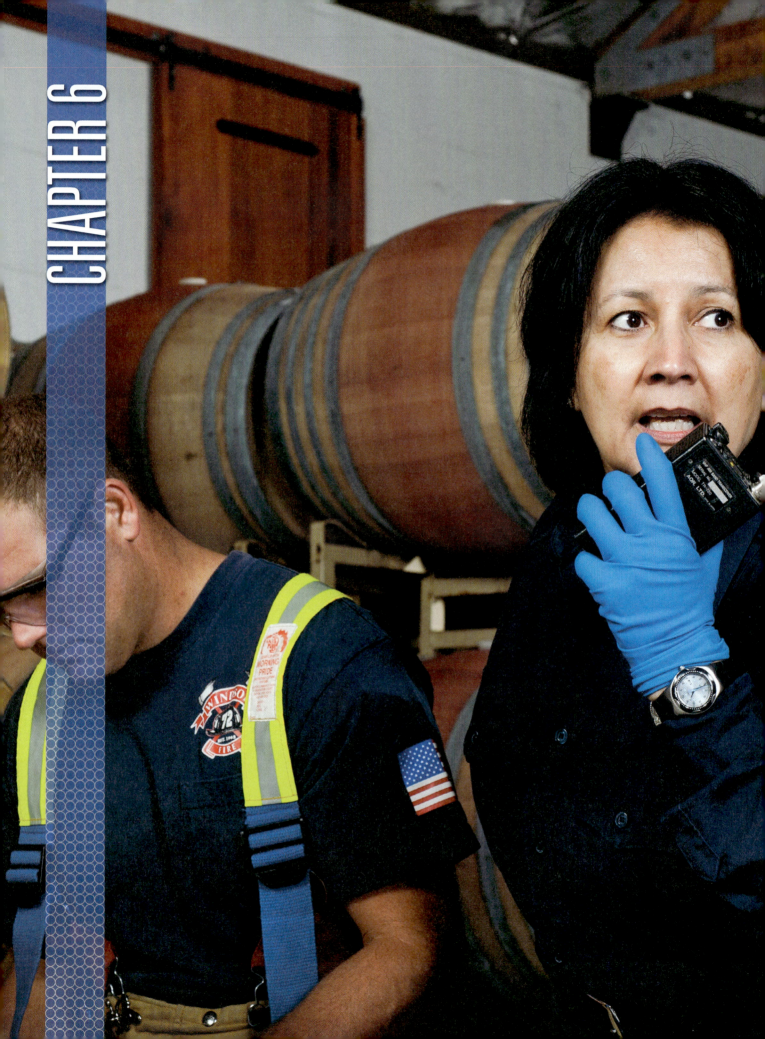

CHAPTER 6

Principles of Effective Communication

EDUCATION STANDARDS
- Preparatory—EMS System Communication, Therapeutic Communication

COMPETENCIES
- Uses simple knowledge of the EMS system, safety/well-being of the Emergency Medical Responder, medical/legal issues at the scene of an emergency while awaiting a higher level of care.

CHAPTER OVERVIEW

The chapter on medical terminology introduced you to the importance of learning the language of medicine. Without a clear understanding of that unique language, it would be very difficult to function in EMS in any meaningful way. Learning the words, phrases, and jargon that are unique to EMS is only half of the equation. You also must be able to communicate your message in a way that others will understand. Not only will you be communicating with other EMS professionals, but you also will be communicating with ill and injured patients of all ages and cultural backgrounds. Your ability to communicate clearly and confidently, and in a manner that all parties understand, will be the key to your success. This chapter will introduce the common elements of effective communication as well as strategies to improve communication with diverse groups. It also will introduce you to some of the communication devices commonly used in EMS today.

OBJECTIVES

Upon successful completion of this chapter, the student should be able to:

COGNITIVE

1. Define the following terms:
   a. base station radio *(p. 121)*
   b. body language *(p. 116)*
   c. communication *(p. 116)*
   d. interpersonal communication *(p. 119)*
   e. message *(p. 117)*
   f. portable radio *(p. 121)*
   g. receiver *(p. 117)*
   h. repeater *(p. 121)*
   i. sender *(p. 117)*
   j. therapeutic communication *(p. 119)*
   k. transfer of care *(p. 120)*
2. State the four types of communication. *(pp. 116)*
3. Describe the components of communication. *(p. 117)*
4. Describe common barriers to effective communication. *(p. 118)*
5. Describe the strategies for effective communication. *(p. 118)*
6. Describe the characteristics of therapeutic communication. *(p. 119)*
7. Describe the elements of an appropriate verbal transfer of care. *(p. 120)*
8. Describe strategies for successful interviewing. *(p. 120)*
9. Describe strategies for successful communication specific to pediatric and geriatric populations. *(p. 120)*
10. Identify common communication devices used in EMS. *(p. 121)*
11. Describe the proper technique for communicating via radio. *(p. 121)*

PSYCHOMOTOR

12. Demonstrate effective communication strategies when dealing with instructional staff, classmates, and simulated patients.
13. Utilize therapeutic communication strategies to establish effective relationships with classmates and simulated patients.
14. Deliver an appropriate verbal transfer of care following a simulated patient encounter.
15. Demonstrate proper technique when communicating via radio.

AFFECTIVE

16. Model sensitivity to cultural/age differences in all communications.

"Dispatch, Engine 86 en route to medical aid at 144 Paradise Way." Kaitlyn sets down the radio receiver as she and her firefighter partner, Nick, head toward their destination.

As they pull up to a modest cabin home, they waste no time grabbing their jump bags and getting to the door. Nick knocks loudly and shouts, "Graham County Fire, you called for assistance?"

Immediately, the door cracks open, and a man peers through, looking agitated. He has on a turban and robe of some sort. "It is my wife, Amilah," he says with a thick accent. "She is bleeding. Please miss, you must help."

The man leads Kaitlyn and Nick into a back room where a woman is sitting on the floor, dressed in traditional Muslim clothing. A moderate-sized blood stain is clearly visible on the carpet beneath her. Kaitlyn quickly kneels at her side, but the man holds Nick back: "No, you stay back!"

Kaitlyn looks up to see Nick's shocked expression, and at that moment, more fire and EMS personnel enter the open door, filling the entryway. The man's eyes open wide and he shouts, "No! All of you get back! Get back from here!"

What Is Communication?

Webster's New College dictionary defines the word *communicate* this way: "to have an interchange of ideas or information, to express oneself effectively." Sounds simple enough, doesn't it? While all may agree on what the word means, things begin to quickly break down when we attempt to make this simple act happen. Take a look at the following example of one person's attempt to communicate:

> "I know that you believe you understand what you think I said, but I am not sure that what you heard is not what I meant."

This probably made perfect sense to the person who said it, but to you and me, it seems to get more confusing each time we read it.

You will be communicating with a wide variety of individuals during the course of a typical emergency call or duty shift. It is extremely important that you understand the characteristics of good **communication** and understand what to do when communication goes bad. Here is a list of just some of the potential individuals and roles that you will likely be expected to communicate with on a regular basis:

communication ▶ the activity of conveying information.

- Patients
- Your partner
- Other EMS personnel
- Fire personnel
- Law enforcement personnel
- Hospital personnel
- Bystanders
- Family members
- Friends of patients

This group represents a wide variety of people, making the task of communicating effectively more challenging.

IS IT SAFE?

Poor, incomplete, or wrong information has been the cause of many unsafe and dangerous situations. When the stakes are high, be sure to use clear and concise communication. Always ask clarifying questions when you don't understand something.

Types of Communication

All communication can be placed into one of four broad categories. They are:

- *Verbal.* Words and sounds that make up the language we speak
- *Nonverbal.* **Body language**, eye contact, and gestures
- *Written.* The use of letters and words to express the language we speak
- *Visual.* Signs, symbols, and designs

OBJECTIVE

2. State the four types of communication.

body language ▶ communication using the movements and attitudes of the body.

First Impressions

I have often said, "I may not look like a doctor, but I play one at work." The truth of the matter is that regardless of how we may want to react to the scene or to the smell, appearance, or behavior of the patient, we must be aware of our patient's perception of us.

Verbal communication can be further broken down into different types, such as interpersonal and therapeutic. As an Emergency Medical Responder you will also use specific tools to facilitate communication, such as radios and computer terminals.

The Communication Process

If I told you that we were going to communicate, what is the first thing that comes to mind? For most of us it is the word *talking*. While talking is clearly a way by which to communicate, it only represents one half of the total equation. The other half of an effective communication model involves listening (Figure 6.1).

There is a lot going on during any communication. There must be a **sender**, the one who is introducing a new thought or concept or initiating the communication process. There is the **message**, which is the thought, concept, or idea being transmitted. There is the **receiver**, the one for whom the message is intended. The model in Figure 6.1 illustrates the many steps that a message must go through, regardless of how simple or complex it is, before the process can be effective. If the message gets blocked or misinterpreted at any one of the steps, the meaning of the message may get lost. When we are dealing with issues related to safety and patient care, poor communication can be dangerous and even deadly.

Transmitting the Message

Now that you know the mechanics of how messages are processed, it will be helpful to have a basic understanding of how most messages are being transmitted. Take a look at Figure 6.2 to see how messages are actually getting across to the receiver.

Research suggests that 55% of communication is delivered by way of body language, which includes gestures, expressions, posture, and many other physical manifestations. About 38% of the message is transmitted by way of the voice—its quality, tone, and inflections, which all express important pieces of the message. Only 7% of any given message is transmitted by the specific words used. So, you can see how this all might work well when you are physically located next to or in front of the person with whom you are communicating. However, a significant amount of the communication in EMS occurs via the radio or a computer screen. Knowing this, you can begin to understand

KEY POINT ▼

Remain aware of what message your body language might be sending. In many situations your body language may be speaking louder than your words.

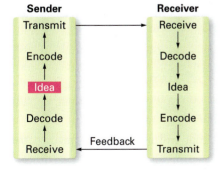

Figure 6.1 • A message must pass through many steps in the communication process.

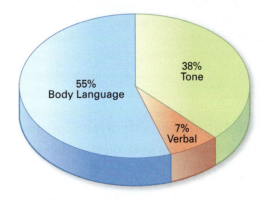

Figure 6.2 • Communication is delivered in many forms.

how not being able to see the person you are communicating with can create many barriers for effective communication.

Barriers to Communication

OBJECTIVE

4. Describe common barriers to effective communication.

There will always be barriers to communication. Dr. Eric Garner is a leading researcher and educator in the area of communication, and he has identified seven barriers to effective communication.

- *Physical.* A physical barrier is any barrier either real or perceived that separates the sender and the receiver. Examples of physical barriers include walls, doors, distance, and territories or zones.
- *Perceptual.* Everyone brings different experiences to the table. People see things differently and have unique perspectives that can differ in so many ways.
- *Emotional.* This can be one of the biggest barriers when dealing with ill and injured patients. It includes fear, mistrust, and suspicion and can be difficult to overcome in the short time we are with our patients.
- *Cultural.* Each year the United States becomes more culturally diverse. Not understanding some of the basic cultural differences that exist can cause significant barriers that will prevent you from delivering the best care possible.
- *Language.* Not being able to communicate with your patient due to language differences can be an overwhelming barrier for many novice EMS personnel. While no one expects you to learn several languages, it will be very beneficial to learn some common words and phrases related to patient care if you live in a culturally diverse environment.
- *Gender.* Simply being a male responding to a female victim of sexual assault or vaginal bleeding can cause barriers the patient is not willing to remove. Gender also can play a role culturally.
- *Interpersonal.* A person's attitudes and beliefs or dislike for the sender/receiver can interfere with the message being communicated.

KEY POINT ▼

There are many factors that can get in the way of effective communication, not the least of which is personal attitude. When you are on duty, you must put all personal problems and interpersonal issues aside and focus on providing the best patient care possible.

As you can see by the list above, there are many reasons why a message might get blocked or misinterpreted. The first step in becoming a better communicator is simply gaining an awareness of the many barriers that can interfere with communication.

OBJECTIVE

5. Describe the strategies for effective communication.

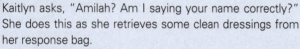

continued

FIRST ON SCENE

Kaitlyn asks, "Amilah? Am I saying your name correctly?" She does this as she retrieves some clean dressings from her response bag.

Amilah nods, looking as if she might faint, and Kaitlyn continues, "Can I check the bleeding to see how I can help you?" Again Amilah nods. Kaitlyn lifts Amilah's dress, gasping at the sight of the blood covering both legs all the way up to her pelvis.

"We are going to need a medic here," Kaitlyn says as she starts to wipe away some of the blood, "I've got a lot of bleeding and no injury I can see."

"No man can see her like this," the husband protests, "It is improper! Disrespectful!"

"Amilah," Kaitlyn says, lowering the woman's skirt to protect her privacy, "I can't help you alone, and you need to get to a doctor right away." Kaitlyn looks into Amilah's scared eyes and touches her shaking hand. She turns to Amilah's husband and pleads, "Amilah has lost a lot of blood, and the EMS personnel behind you must get her to a hospital. Please, please let them pass. We will be as respectful as possible."

Amilah finally speaks, her voice weak, "Makeen, please." Makeen looks seriously at her. He then drops the privacy blanket and allows Nick to move past him.

Strategies for Effective Communication

Resource Central

Learn more about effective communication.

The following are some simple ideas and strategies that will help you become a better communicator:

- Speak clearly and use words and terminology that the receiver will understand. You should not use medical jargon when speaking to a patient, but you should use proper medical terminology when speaking to another medical professional.

- Keep an open mind and resist the urge to be defensive. It is natural to respond defensively when you do not understand or disagree with a message. When this happens, both parties tend to shut down, and any chance of good communication is minimized.
- Become an active listener. Active listening is more than just "paying attention." It means putting your biases aside and making every effort to understand what the other person is saying. Active listening includes using eye contact when appropriate and asking clarifying questions to further define the message.
- Be assertive when appropriate, especially when safety is at stake. Do not passively accept what the other person is saying if you see things differently. Respectfully state your point in a manner that will ensure that you are heard.
- Remain aware of the influence that body language plays in effective communication. Pay attention to your own body language, and ensure that it shows you are listening and attentive to the message.
- Accept the reality of miscommunication. Even the best communicators fail at times. Do not allow yourself to get frustrated, but instead take the miscommunication as a lesson and use it to improve your own communication.

Interpersonal Communication

One of the most important forms of verbal communication is called **interpersonal communication**. Interpersonal communication most often occurs between three or fewer participants who are in close proximity to one another. This is often the case when two or three Emergency Medical Responders are working a shift together or when the communication occurs between caregivers and a patient. A main characteristic of good interpersonal communication is that feedback between the sender and receiver is immediate.

Therapeutic Communication

We are all familiar with the old saying, "Sticks and stones may break my bones, but words will never hurt me." We have also experienced the effects of a verbal attack and know that words can indeed hurt nearly as much as a broken bone. Research has proven beyond a doubt that what you say to your patients can make a big difference in their ability to manage their illness or injury. *"What we say to our patients can relieve pain and anxiety, speed up the healing process, shorten recovery time, and in many cases save a life."**

Therapeutic communication can be defined as the face-to-face communication process that focuses on advancing the physical and emotional well-being of a patient. How you talk to your patients can make a difference in how they respond to the illness or injury and to you.

There are three objectives of therapeutic communication that you must be aware of to maximize the results for both you and the patient.

- *Collecting information.* This is referred to as the patient history. The more information you can gather about the current situation as well as all prior medical history will make it much easier to properly care for the patient.
- *Assessing behavior.* Here you are carefully observing the patients behavior, looking for subtle signs that may offer clues to their condition.
- *Educating.* One of your responsibilities as a patient advocate is to inform and educate patients about their condition. The hope is that with proper education patients will make better decisions regarding their own medical care.

One of the key components of successful therapeutic communication is trust. You will have only a few moments at the beginning of your patient encounter to establish trust. Without trust, the patient may withhold important information about his condition or history, and in the worst case he may refuse care altogether.

---

*Prager, J., and J.S. Acosta. (2002). *The Worst Is Over: What to Say When Every Moment Counts—Verbal First Aid to Calm, Relieve Pain, Promote Healing, and Save Lives.* San Diego: Jodere Group.

IS IT SAFE?

Getting off on the wrong foot with a patient can be dangerous. A patient who thinks you have a bad attitude will often shut down and be reluctant to share important information.

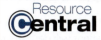

Resource **Central**

Learn about another possible obstacle to effective communication—cultural competence.

interpersonal communication ▶ a form of communication where the participants are dependent on one another and have a shared history.

OBJECTIVE

6. Describe the characteristics of therapeutic communication.

therapeutic communication ▶ the face-to-face communication process that focuses on advancing the physical and emotional well-being of a patient.

Strategies for Successful Interviewing

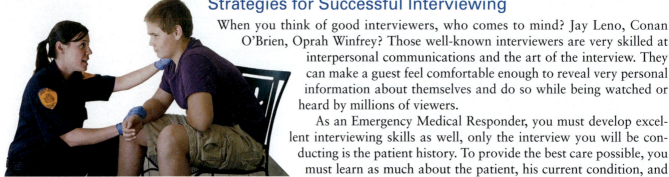

When you think of good interviewers, who comes to mind? Jay Leno, Conan O'Brien, Oprah Winfrey? Those well-known interviewers are very skilled at interpersonal communications and the art of the interview. They can make a guest feel comfortable enough to reveal very personal information about themselves and do so while being watched or heard by millions of viewers.

As an Emergency Medical Responder, you must develop excellent interviewing skills as well, only the interview you will be conducting is the patient history. To provide the best care possible, you must learn as much about the patient, his current condition, and any pertinent prior medical history in a very short period of time.

The following strategies will help you establish a good rapport with your patients and maximize your ability to obtain a good medical history (Figure 6.3):

Figure 6.3 • Positioning yourself at or below eye level with the patient will demonstrate caring and compassion.

OBJECTIVE

8. Describe strategies for successful interviewing.

Read about alternate methods of communication with children.

OBJECTIVE

9. Describe strategies for successful communication specific to pediatric and geriatric populations.

transfer of care ▶ the physical and verbal handing off of care from one health-care provider to another.

- Immediately introduce yourself and your level of training.
- Obtain the patient's name early, and use it frequently during your interview.
- Position yourself at or below the patient's eye level whenever possible.
- Ask one question at a time, and allow the patient ample time to respond.
- Listen carefully to everything the patient tells you.
- Restate the patient's answers when necessary for clarification.

Developing your interviewing skills will take some time. Whenever possible, listen in on others who are interviewing the patient and pay attention to their techniques. Notice what works and what does not work and use these lessons to your advantage.

Your interviewing strategies may need to be modified, depending on the age of your patient (Figure 6.4). For instance, obtaining a thorough medical history from a child may be impossible if the child does not know and trust you. In this instance you will need to rely on parents or other caregivers who know the child's history.

▶ GERIATRIC FOCUS ◀

Obtaining a good history from the geriatric population has its challenges as well. Hearing loss, multiple illnesses, and dementia can make it difficult to get a clear picture of what is going on. Speak slowly, clearly, and loudly enough to be heard. Be extra patient, and allow plenty of time for the patient to process your question and formulate an answer. Resist the desire to jump to conclusions because the patient appears to be confused or is responding slowly.

continued

FIRST ON SCENE

Kaitlyn looks down at Amilah as they load her into the ambulance. She hasn't let go of her hand once, and she makes sure to explain everything the EMTs have done when controlling the bleeding, knowing that Amilah is both fearful and embarrassed by this necessary breech of privacy. "You must go with her," Makeen says to Kaitlyn. "I would feel better knowing that you are there, miss."

"Makeen," Kaitlyn says before the fire crew closes the ambulance door, "I'm going to do everything I can to help her, and I will stay with her until you get to the hospital, all right?"

Makeen nods and runs to his pickup truck parked in the driveway, yelling back, "Thank you, miss."

OBJECTIVE

7. Describe the elements of an appropriate verbal transfer of care.

Transfer of Care

The verbal **transfer of care** happens at the scene when care of the patient is transferred from one care provider, the Emergency Medical Responder, to the next care provider, the ambulance crew. Another verbal transfer of care will occur when the ambulance crew turns care of the patient over to the staff at the hospital. This is a very important component of what is called the continuum of care, and it helps to ensure that the care is consistent and appropriate as the patient moves from care provider to care provider.

The verbal transfer of care may be modified based on the patient's condition. If the patient is critical, the transfer of care may be very short and to the point. Do not be offended if the ambulance crew does not want to take the time for a complete report when the patient is in need of immediate attention.

A good transfer of care should contain all of the following elements, regardless of whether the transfer happens at the scene or at the hospital:

- Patient's name and age
- Chief complaint
- Brief account of the patient's current condition
- Past pertinent medical history
- Vital signs
- Pertinent findings from the physical exam
- Overview of care provided and the patient's response to that care

Keep in mind that you may have to ask for a verbal transfer of care from anyone who may be at the scene before you, such as bystanders, family members, and law enforcement officers. Do not expect them to be able to provide a thorough verbal handoff. You will need to ask specific questions to obtain the information that you need.

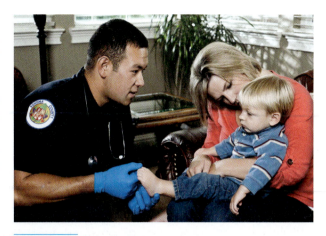

Figure 6.4 • You may have to alter your approach, depending on the age of your patient.

Radio Communications

All EMS systems are connected by a very sophisticated system of hardware and software designed to allow all of the resources in the system to communicate with one another. At the heart of these systems are the radios, pagers, and specific frequencies that connect each and every vehicle and person in the system. This system is set in motion when someone initiates an emergency response by calling 911.

A typical radio system is made up of a combination of transmitters, receivers, **repeaters**, and antennae. Dispatch centers utilize powerful **base station radios** that can transmit over a wide area. When terrain is a factor and hills and mountains obstruct radio signals, specialized mountaintop repeaters are used to capture the signal and redirect it to the appropriate receiver.

EMS personnel often carry both pagers and handheld (portable) radios that allow them to communicate with the dispatch center and each other (Figure 6.5). Pagers are used to notify response personnel of an emergency call, and **portable radios** are used to communicate directly with the dispatch center before, during, and after a call.

The use of radios requires a specific protocol when communicating with others within the system. For instance, you cannot simply push the button and speak any time you feel like it. Doing so might interrupt another person using the same frequency. Instead, you should listen first and begin your transmission when there is a break in the "traffic" on your frequency. The term *radio traffic* is the common jargon for the verbal communication that takes place over a radio.

Imagine that you are "Rescue One" and you want to ask your dispatch center (Central Dispatch) to repeat the address where the emergency call is located. The conversation might go something like this:

RESCUE ONE: Central Dispatch, this is Rescue One with a request.

CENTRAL DISPATCH: Rescue One, Central Dispatch, go ahead with your request.

OBJECTIVES

10. Identify common communication devices used in EMS.

11. Describe the proper technique for communicating via radio.

repeater ▶ a fixed antenna that is used to boost a radio signal.

base station radio ▶ a high-powered two-way radio located at a dispatch center or hospital.

portable radio ▶ a handheld device used to transmit and receive verbal communications.

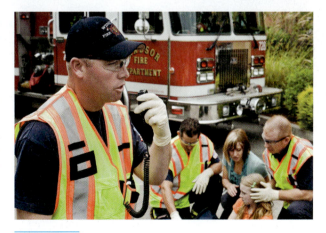

Figure 6.5 • Portable radios are still the most common communication tool used in EMS.

RESCUE ONE: Central Dispatch, Rescue One, can you repeat the address for our call?

CENTRAL DISPATCH: Rescue One, Central Dispatch, you are responding to 2760 Woolsey Road. That's two seven six zero Woolsey Road. Do you copy?

RESCUE ONE: Central Dispatch, Rescue One, confirming two seven six zero Woolsey Road.

CENTRAL DISPATCH: Rescue One, that's affirmative.

Do you see the pattern there? When you wish to contact another resource in the system, it is standard protocol to state the radio identifier (specified name) of the resource you are calling first, in this case Central Dispatch. Follow that with your radio identifier, Rescue One. This is especially important when there are several resources using the same frequency, also known as a channel.

It is normal to be somewhat shy or intimidated by the prospect of having to talk on the radio in the beginning. Not to worry. It quickly becomes second nature, and you will soon learn to enjoy talking with others on the radio.

One way to become more familiar with radio protocol is to listen to a scanner. A scanner is a specialized radio that only receives radio traffic. Most scanners today can be programmed to receive just about any frequency, so you should be able to program it to the frequencies of the EMS system in your area. If you do not want to purchase a scanner, you also can listen to live radio traffic on the Internet. A simple Web search should turn up live radio traffic in your area.

WRAP-UP

FIRST ON SCENE

"That was ridiculous," Nick moans as he and Kaitlyn make their way to the engine, "How could he keep us back when his wife was bleeding like that?"

"It's just cultural, Nick," Kaitlyn says. "You don't mess with people's beliefs. You just try to find a common understanding and then work with it. Makeen just needed to trust us. We're all human."

Nick nods and says, "I guess it's cool how you thought to contact the hospital en route to get a woman doctor and a private room ready for Amilah."

"Communication is key, my friend," Kaitlyn sighs, smiling, "and it saved a life today."

CHAPTER REVIEW

Summary

- Communication is a complex process that involves the interchange of ideas or information. It requires a sender, receiver, and a message.

- There are four types of communication: verbal, nonverbal, written, and visual.

- Some of the more common barriers to effective communication include physical, perceptual, emotional, cultural, language, gender, and interpersonal. All of these factors can interfere with the communication process.

- Some strategies for effective communication include:
  - Speaking slowly and clearly
  - Resisting the urge to be defensive
  - Utilizing active listening techniques
  - Being aware of body language and the messages it sends

- Therapeutic communication is a specific type of communication that focuses on advancing the physical and emotional well-being of a patient. The objectives of therapeutic communication include:
  - Collecting information
  - Assessing behavior
  - Providing education

- Some strategies for successful interviewing include:
  - Immediately introducing yourself and your level of training
  - Obtaining the patient's name early and using it frequently during your interview
  - Positioning yourself at or below the patient's eye level whenever possible
  - Asking one question at a time and allowing the patient ample time to respond

- Listening carefully to everything the patient tells you
- Restating the patient's answers when necessary for clarification

- As an Emergency Medical Responder, your skill of verbal transfer of care or "handoff" is an important one. The elements of an appropriate verbal transfer of care include:
  - Patient's name and age
  - Chief complaint
  - Brief account of the patient's current condition
  - Past pertinent medical history
  - Vital signs
  - Pertinent findings from the physical exam
  - Overview of care provided and the patient's response to that care

- Remember that you may have to modify your communication approach depending on the age of the patient. This is especially true for the very young and the very old.

- The use of technology for the purposes of communication is quite common in EMS. Radios and pagers are a primary source of communication between dispatch centers and field personnel and hospitals. Base station radios are high-powered transmitters that broadcast a signal over a large area. Sometimes repeaters are used to boost the signal when distance and terrain are a factor.

- There is a common protocol for how to communicate with another person or agency using a radio. Each transmission should begin with the identifier (name) of the person or agency you are calling followed by your identifier (name).

Take Action

PRACTICE BY LISTENING

One of the best ways to begin learning proper radio protocol is to listen to live radio traffic. You can do this in a couple of ways. The first is to borrow or purchase a radio scanner. This is a small handheld device that can be programmed to receive local radio traffic from just about any source—fire, police, or EMS. Another way to listen to live radio traffic is to use the Internet. Go to www.radioreference.com. This Web site will allow you to listen in on thousands of different frequencies across the nation. In many instances you will be able to listen in on local police, fire, or EMS frequencies in your area.

First on Scene Run Review

Recall the events of the "First on Scene" scenario in this chapter and answer the following questions, which are related to the call. Rationales are offered in the Answer Key at the back of the book.

1. Did Kaitlyn and Nick check to see if the scene was safe? What would you do differently to ensure that the scene was safe?

2. How would you work with someone who had a different cultural/belief system from your own?

3. What role does communication play in this situation?

Quick Quiz

To check your understanding of the chapter, answer the following questions. Then compare your answers to those in the Answer Key at the back of the book.

1. The word *communicate* is best defined as:
   a. expressing oneself to another.
   b. talking to another person verbally.
   c. an interchange of ideas or information.
   d. understanding what another person is saying.

2. The words and sounds that make up a language is a description of which type of communication?
   a. Verbal
   b. Nonverbal
   c. Written
   d. Visual

3. Nonverbal communication is best characterized by:
   a. written words.
   b. spoken words.
   c. body language.
   d. signs and symbols.

4. All of the following are components of the communication process, EXCEPT:
   a. sender.
   b. receiver.
   c. idea (message).
   d. frequency.

5. Research suggests that the majority of a message is delivered by way of:
   a. body language.
   b. voice (tone).
   c. word use.
   d. eye contact.

6. The distance that exists between two parties that are communicating by radio is an example of which type of barrier?
   a. Perceptual
   b. Language
   c. Physical
   d. Interpersonal

7. What type of communication most often occurs between three or fewer participants who are in close proximity to one another?
   a. Therapeutic
   b. Direct
   c. Visual
   d. Interpersonal

8. All of the following are goals of therapeutic communication, EXCEPT:
   a. pain management.
   b. collecting information.
   c. assessing behavior.
   d. providing education.

9. A good transfer of care should contain all of the following, EXCEPT:
   a. patient's name and age.
   b. patient's address.
   c. chief complaint.
   d. vital signs.

10. Which one of the following is the best example of an appropriate radio call?
    a. Engine 6, this is MedCom. Respond to 1111 Sonoma Ave.
    b. Engine 6, respond to 1111 Sonoma Ave.
    c. This is MedCom, calling Engine 6.
    d. MedCom, come in Engine 6.

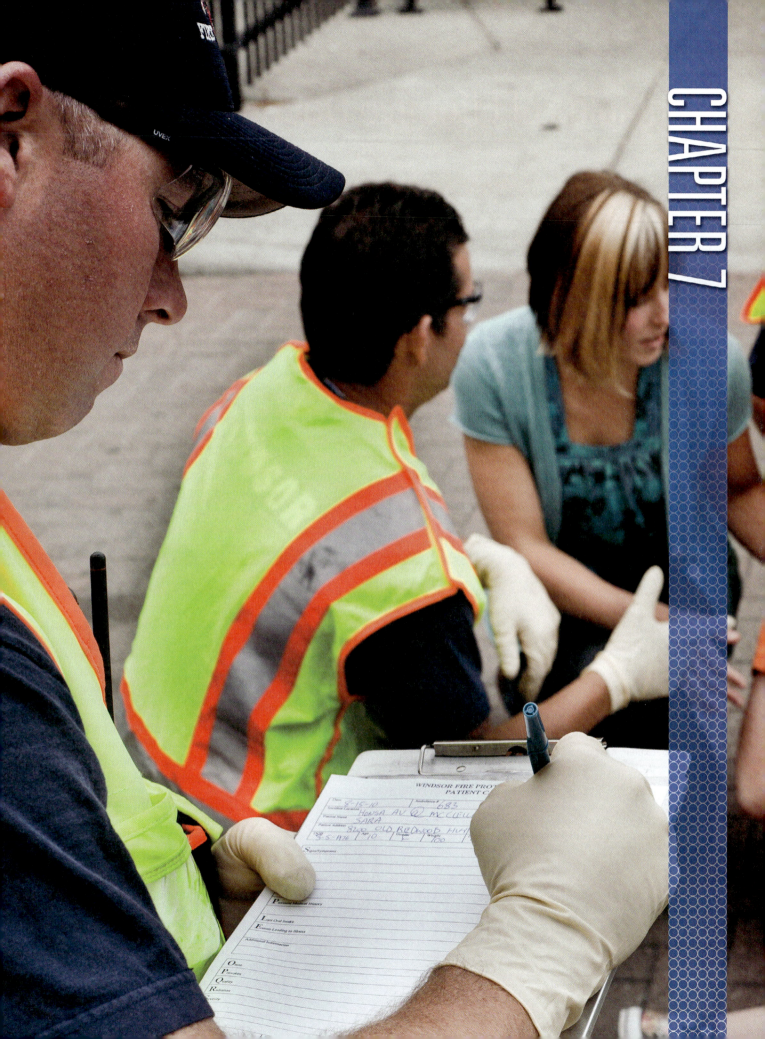

Principles of Effective Documentation

CHAPTER OVERVIEW

Properly documenting the assessment and care of patients is a vitally important part of what you will be doing as an Emergency Medical Responder. Your written reports—usually called run reports or patient care reports (PCRs)—will follow a patient through the health-care system as the only lasting record of the care that you provided and your abilities as an Emergency Medical Responder.

Of course, documentation has many other uses. It is used in the short term by emergency department personnel to get a clear picture of the patient's situation when first encountered by EMS responders, the illness or injuries discovered, and exactly what care was given prior to arrival at the hospital.

Also, documentation can play an important role in minimizing your liability as an Emergency Medical Responder. If someone questions the care you provided to a patient, good clear documentation is going to be the best way to address those concerns in a thorough, accurate way.

As an EMS professional, you should take pride in everything that you do, which includes how effectively you document your assessment and care of each patient.

OBJECTIVES

Upon successful completion of this chapter, the student should be able to:

COGNITIVE

1. Define the following terms:
   a. continuity of care *(p. 127)*
   b. electronic documentation *(p. 130)*
   c. minimum data set *(p. 129)*
   d. patient care report (PCR) *(p. 129)*
2. Explain the purpose(s) of the patient care report. *(p. 127)*
3. Describe the elements of a typical patient care report. *(p. 129)*
4. Describe the minimum data set required for the documentation of patient care. *(p. 130)*
5. Explain the procedure for correcting errors made during documentation. *(p. 130)*
6. List various tools used to document patient care in the field setting. *(p. 130)*

PSYCHOMOTOR

7. Demonstrate the ability to accurately document a simulated patient encounter.
8. Properly correct an error made during documentation.

AFFECTIVE

9. Value the importance of complete and accurate documentation.

Battalion chief Lorenzo Hernandez leans back in his chair and rubs the bridge of his nose before setting his glasses back into place.

"So," he says, seeing that the young firefighter across the desk from him has finished reading the patient care report. "I'll ask you again. At what point during that call did you realize that the patient had stopped breathing, and what exactly did you do about it?"

The other man looks at him pleadingly, glancing from the piece of paper in his hands and back up to the steady gaze of the chief several times before speaking.

"I can't imagine that I didn't start rescue breathing," is all he can say.

"You know what?" Hernandez leans forward and taps his index finger on the desk to accentuate his words. "I believe you, Shane. You're a solid firefighter and a good Emergency Medical Responder, one who would start rescue breathing immediately for a patient who had stopped breathing. But the lawyer representing that patient in his lawsuit against the city knows nothing about you except what you wrote in that PCR. And based on that narrative, you look like a pretty negligent Emergency Medical Responder."

Patient Care Reports

The documentation that you provide is a permanent record of the patient care you performed. When you provide excellent, patient-centered prehospital care, you may be proud of your abilities. However, poor documentation performed after the fact will tarnish the record of what you have done for anyone reviewing the documentation later.

The reporting done by Emergency Medical Responders can take on many names, depending on your region or service. Some call the reports simply "run reports," others **patient care reports** or prehospital care reports (Figure 7.1). Some patient care reports are done by hand, but more and more emergency care services are adopting computerized (or electronic) documentation (Figure 7.2). Regardless of how the reports are completed, there are many reasons for accurate and complete documentation. These include:

- *Continuity of care.* Your report may be referenced at any time during the transport or hospital care of the patient for the vital signs you obtained, medications or treatments you administered, or your observations at the scene.
- *Education.* Your written report may be used as an example for others of proper documentation. If you responded to an unusual or challenging call, it may be used as a basis for training other providers who may encounter similar patients or situations.
- *Administration.* The report will be used for the compiling of statistical analysis on issues that affect your agency or community.
- *Quality assurance.* Reports created by you and others in your agency or organization may be reviewed as part of a structured process to improve the overall quality of the EMS system.
- *Legal.* The report you created is a legal document. It may be called into a civil or criminal court for any number of reasons.

OBJECTIVE

2. Explain the purpose(s) of the patient care report.

KEY POINT ▼

The old saying, "If you didn't document it, you didn't do it" is true when it comes to patient care reports. If the actions that you took and care that you provided are not included in your documentation, the only conclusion a person reading your report can reach is that you simply didn't do it.

continuity of care ▶ refers to how each new provider, who is assuming care for a patient, is properly informed of the patient's progression, so he can watch for trends and continue effective treatments.

From the Medical Director

Patient Care Reports

Your patient care narrative will in most cases be the only means by which your medical director can determine the appropriateness of your care. Often your documentation is passed on to arriving EMS units who will incorporate them into their own reports. While most encounters will be for minor illness and injury, the critical encounter requires detailed documentation. You may find that you only need to provide EMS with "field notes," which are summaries of your care, but you should complete a full patient care report for your service's records. This provides you better protection against liability and further allows your Medical Director to provide optimal feedback.

TRIP #			
MEDIC #			
BEGIN MILES			
END MILES			
CODE___/___		PAGE___/___	
UNITS ON SCENE			

Rural/Metro Ambulance

50 Years of Serving Others

EMERGENCY TRIP SHEET – CONDITION CODES 1 THROUGH 71

BILLING USE ONLY

DAY				
DATE				
RECEIVED				
DISPATCHED				
EN-ROUTE				
ON SCENE				
TO HOSPITAL				
AT HOSPITAL				
IN-SERVICE				

NAME   SEX M F DOB ___/___/___

ADDRESS   RACE

CITY   STATE   ZIP

PHONE ( )   -   PCP DR.

RESPONDED FROM   CITY

TAKEN FROM   ZIP

DESTINATION   REASON

SSN   -   -   MEDICARE #   MEDICAID #

INSURANCE CO   INSURANCE #   GROUP #

RESPONSIBLE PARTY   ADDRESS

CITY   STATE   ZIP   PHONE ( )   -

EMPLOYER

CREW	CERT	STATE #

TIME	ON SCENE (1)	ON SCENE (2)	ON SCENE (3)	EN-ROUTE (1)	EN-ROUTE (2)	AT DESTINATION
BP						
PULSE						
RESP						
EKG						

IV THERAPY
SUCCESSFUL Y N # OF ATTEMPTS _____
ANGIO SIZE _____ ga.
SITE _____
TOTAL FLUID INFUSED _____ cc
BLOOD DRAW Y N INITIALS

INTUBATION INFORMATION
SUCCESSFUL Y N # OF ATTEMPTS _____
TUBE SIZE _____ mm
TIME _____ INITIALS _____

MEDICAL HISTORY

CONDITION CODES

MEDICATIONS

TREATMENTS

TIME	TREATMENT	DOSE	ROUTE	INIT

ALLERGIES

C/C

EVENTS LEADING TO C/C

PERTINENT FINDINGS

ASSESSMENT

TREATMENT

GCS E___ V___ M___ TOTAL =

GCS E___ V___ M___ TOTAL =

HOSPITAL CONTACTED

CPR BEGUN BY   B   P   TIME BEGUN

EMS SIGNATURE

AED USED Y N BY:

RESUSCITATION TERMINATED - TIME

LIFETIME SIGNATURE AUTHORIZATION

I request that payment of authorized Medicare benefits be made on my behalf to Rural/Metro Ambulance for any ambulance service or supplies provided to me by Rural/Metro Ambulance. I authorize any holder of medical information or documentation about me to release to the Health Care Financing Administration and its agents and carriers, as well as to Rural/Metro Ambulance any information or documentation needed to determine these benefits payable for related services or any services provided to me by Rural/Metro Ambulance now or in the future.

Signature _____   Date _____

( ) OSHA REGULATIONS FOLLOWED

Figure 7.1 • Example of a patient care report form.

Elements of the PCR

Standard **patient care reports (PCRs)** used throughout the EMS industry all share several specific sections. These are:

- *Run data.* This section includes information about the call itself, such as the names of the Emergency Medical Responders responding, the organization they work for, the date and time of the incident, and even certification levels of those providing patient care. This section may also include the final outcome of the call, such as a patient's refusal to be treated or the name of the person who assumed patient care from you. Remember, all names, times, and locations recorded on your PCRs must be accurate since continued care, billing, and statistical information will all depend on the information you provide.
- *Patient data.* This section includes all the information about the patient, such as:
  - Name, address, date of birth, sex
  - Nature of the call
  - Detailed notes on the patient's complaint
  - Mechanism of injury and assessment
  - Care administered prior to arrival of Emergency Medical Responders
  - Vital signs
  - SAMPLE history
  - Changes in the patient's condition

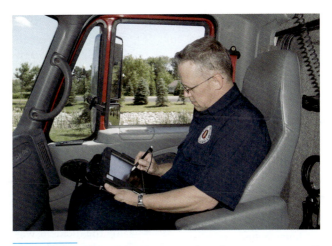

Figure 7.2 • Electronic documentation of an emergency call is becoming more common.

OBJECTIVE

3. Describe the elements of a typical patient care report.

patient care report (PCR) ▶ a document that provides details about a patient's condition, history, and care as well as information about the event that caused the illness or injury.

The information in each of the sections of the report can be entered in various ways:

- *Fill-in.* Data is placed in specifically labeled spaces.
- *Check boxes.* Some patient care reports have boxes that can be checked for information such as patient history, nature of illness, and care provided.
- *Narrative.* Space is provided for you to write your objective "story" documenting the patient's history, assessment, or care information that does not otherwise fit in check boxes or that requires expansion on the details.

The information you write in the narrative should be *objective* rather than *subjective*. Objective information comprises straightforward facts. Subjective information is up for interpretation and may even include descriptions of how people feel about something. The statement, "The patient's right forearm was swollen and angulated," is objective, whereas the statement, "I believe the patient was attempting to perform a dangerous trick on his skateboard," is subjective.

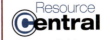

Resource **Central**

Learn more about effectively documenting your patient care experience.

minimum data set ▶ the essential information that must be gathered and documented on every patient care report.

continued

FIRST ON SCENE

Firefighter Shane Lasko closes his eyes and tries to remember the details of the call that occurred nearly eight months earlier. He has been working out of Station Four, covering the eastern edge of the city, a sprawling industrial area known for manufacturing-related trauma calls during the day and fights and overdoses at night. He can remember the fire engine rolling to a stop at the abandoned warehouse. There also was a tan-colored sedan parked haphazardly among toppled garbage cans, the sun glinting off of the haze of cracks on the car's windshield.

He opens his eyes and looks at the on-scene time on the PCR in his hands: 2357.

"Wait a minute." He slides the document back onto the chief's desk and shakes his head wearily. "This call happened at night, and I'm remembering one that happened during the day. I'm getting calls all mixed up. It's just too long ago."

"Shane." Chief Hernandez slides the PCR back into a red folder. "Except for an occasional one that really sticks with you, all of your calls will eventually blend together in your memory. That's why proper documentation and complete, accurate narratives are so critical. You never know when questions will come up about a particular situation long after you've forgotten that it ever even happened."

Figure 7.3 • An example of how to properly document an error in documentation.

The ~~left~~ Jim right pupil was fixed and dilated

IS IT SAFE?

Your documentation will likely become a part of the patient's permanent medical record. It will inform other health-care providers how the patient first presented at the scene. It also will inform them of the care you provided. This is very important to ensure a consistent and safe patient care.

electronic documentation ▶ refers to technology such as computers, PDAs, and cellular phones and their use to document patient condition and care.

Minimum Data Set

In an effort to standardize the information collected from EMS calls around the nation, the U.S. Department of Transportation (DOT) has defined what it calls a **minimum data set**. Regardless of how much information any single agency collects on each call, the data must include all items on the minimum data set. The minimum data set includes:

- Time the incident was reported to 911
- Time of dispatch
- Time of arrival at the patient's location
- Time the patient was transported from the incident location
- Time the patient arrived at the destination (hospital, aid station, etc.)
- Time the patient care was transferred to more advanced providers
- Patient's chief complaint
- Patient's vital signs
- Patient's demographics (age, gender, race, weight)

Correcting Errors

There may be times when you write something incorrectly while completing a patient care report, such as writing that the patient's heart rate was 97 instead of 79. In this case you would cross out the incorrect item with a *single* line, initial it, and write the correct number beside or above it (Figure 7.3). Never completely cover the incorrect information, because it may appear that you are attempting to hide something.

Methods of Documentation

An increasing number of EMS agencies and organizations are moving toward **electronic documentation**, but not all services are going down the same path. It is important for Emergency Medical Responders to have a general understanding of the different patient care documentation tools (Figure 7.4). They include:

- *Paper forms.* These traditional PCR forms are filled out by hand.
- *Computer-scan forms.* These PCR forms are completed by hand, but they use a fill-in-the-bubble format so they can be scanned into a computer for easy information management and statistics gathering.

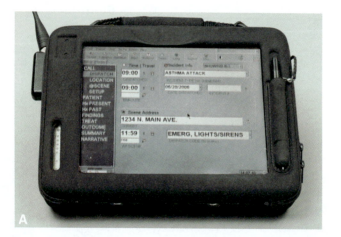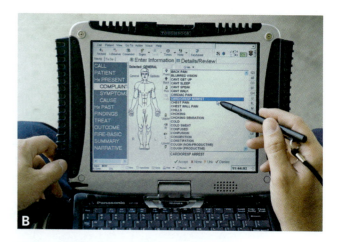

Figure 7.4 • Two types of electronic tablets used for documenting patient care.

- *PDAs or handheld computers.* Specialized software allows emergency care professionals to enter PCR information into small handheld computers. The information can then be downloaded to other computer devices at the hospital, base, or main office.
- *Laptop computers.* Software available for laptop or tablet-type computers allows responders to complete a PCR on the computer and either print it from a docking station or even send it wirelessly to a hospital or central database.
- *Data-enabled cellular devices.* Some advanced cellular data devices can operate PCR applications that allow responders to complete and send documentation quickly and easily from their cellular phones.

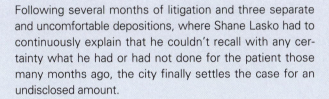

WRAP-UP

FIRST ON SCENE

Following several months of litigation and three separate and uncomfortable depositions, where Shane Lasko had to continuously explain that he couldn't recall with any certainty what he had or had not done for the patient those many months ago, the city finally settles the case for an undisclosed amount.

Shane has since gained a reputation for completing the most clear and concise patient care reports in the entire department and for keeping meticulous records about each and every call that he participates in.

CHAPTER REVIEW

Summary

- Patient care documentation is important for several reasons, from continuity of medical care to legal proceedings in the months and years following an incident. It becomes a permanent part of a patient's medical record and can even be used by EMS organizations to improve the overall quality of local emergency services.

- Patient care reports (PCRs) are usually broken into two main categories (run data and patient data) and are completed using a combination of fill-ins, check boxes, and narrative areas.

- Each PCR has a minimum data set, which is the absolute minimum information that must be documented for each emergency response as defined by the U.S. Department of Transportation.

- Documentation errors should be corrected without trying to obscure the erroneous information, because this could lead to speculation about dishonesty. It is better to put a single line through the mistake, enter the correct information above or beside it, and initial the change.

- Patient care documentation can now be completed in numerous ways: via traditional paper-based forms, high-tech hand-held computers, and data-enabled cellular devices. Even with the technological advancements in documentation, Emergency Medical Responders still need to ensure accuracy and avoid subjectivity when documenting what happened on each response.

Take Action

PLEASE CORRECT ME

You will need several blank PCRs and a partner for this activity. Each person should complete a blank PCR form for an imagined emergency scenario while intentionally making as many documentation mistakes as possible. Leave some areas blank, put incorrect information in other areas, and generally do a less-than-thorough job of completing the form.

Once you are both finished, exchange PCRs and attempt to find as many mistakes and inaccuracies as possible. Rewrite the narrative in a way that would be acceptable.

Do the activity again with two new blank PCR forms, but this time make your errors less obvious and more difficult to find. You will find that it is not as easy as you might think to make intentional errors on the PCRs!

Understand that looking at someone else's PCR with a critical eye will help you to become more critical of your own documentation, which will make you better at completing PCRs.

First on Scene Run Review

Recall the events of the "First on Scene" scenario in this chapter and answer the following questions, which are related to the call. Then decide why is it important for proper documentation on all PCRs. Rationales are offered in the Answer Key at the back of the book.

1. Could you add more info to the PCR after you turn in the report?

2. How would you go about adding information or correcting an error discovered in your documentation?

Quick Quiz

To check your understanding of the chapter, answer the following questions. Then compare your answers to those in the Answer Key at the back of the book.

1. Patient care reports are used for all of the following, EXCEPT:
   a. billing.
   b. press releases.
   c. quality improvement.
   d. lawsuits.

2. Continuity of care is best described as:
   a. ensuring that the same care provider is responsible for treating a patient until admission to the hospital.
   b. ensuring that once a particular treatment is started it is not stopped.
   c. the process where each new care provider is properly updated about the patient's progression.
   d. the proper documentation of the care provided to a patient.

3. You are writing the patient's history on a PCR and inadvertently document an incorrect medication. You should:

   a. discard the document and begin again.

   b. completely mark out the incorrect medication name with your pen so no one will be able to see it and become confused.

   c. not worry about it, since Emergency Medical Responders do not administer medications.

   d. correct the error with a single, initialed line.

4. "The patient complained of chest pain, but I believe that he was just trying to avoid getting a speeding ticket," is an example of a(n) _____ statement.

   a. subjective

   b. pertinent

   c. objective

   d. erroneous

5. Which one of the following would NOT be included in a standard Emergency Medical Responder patient care report?

   a. The exact location where the patient was initially contacted

   b. That the patient was suffering from a heart attack

   c. The names of the ambulance personnel who assumed care of the patient

   d. The cause of the injury

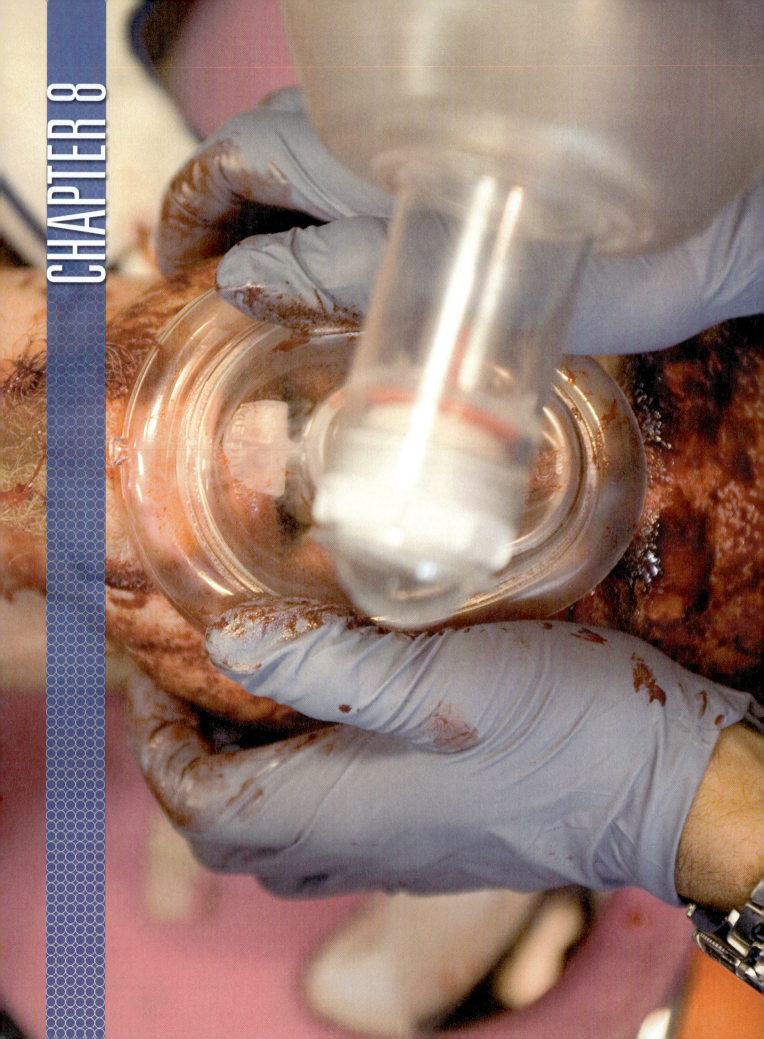

CHAPTER 8

Airway Management and Ventilation

EDUCATION STANDARDS • Airway Management—Airway Management, Respiration, and Artificial Ventilation

COMPETENCIES • Applies knowledge (fundamental depth, foundational breadth) of anatomy and physiology to ensure a patent airway, adequate mechanical ventilation, and respiration while awaiting EMS response for patients of all ages.

CHAPTER OVERVIEW Breathing is life. Each hour of every day the human body takes approximately 900 breaths. When everything is functioning properly, the air we breathe enters the body through the mouth and nose and travels deep into the lungs. Blood that circulates through the lungs picks up the oxygen and drops off carbon dioxide. The heart then pumps the freshly oxygenated blood to the rest of the body. This continuous process is a simple one that we do not usually think about—until we cannot do it.

This chapter explains the process of breathing and the importance of an open and clear airway. It also discusses how to recognize and provide emergency care for patients who are not breathing adequately or who may not be breathing at all.

OBJECTIVES

Upon successful completion of this chapter, the student should be able to:

COGNITIVE

1. Review the anatomy and physiology of the respiratory system. (See Chapter 4.)
2. Define the following terms:
   a. abdominal thrusts *(p. 152)*
   b. accessory muscles *(p. 140)*
   c. agonal respirations *(p. 140)*
   d. apnea *(p. 137)*
   e. bag-mask device *(p. 154)*
   f. biological death *(p. 138)*
   g. cardiac arrest *(p. 137)*
   h. chest thrust *(p. 152)*
   i. clinical death *(p. 138)*
   j. cyanosis *(p. 138)*
   k. diaphragm *(p. 138)*
   l. dyspnea *(p. 140)*
   m. epiglottis *(p. 138)*
   n. exhalation *(p. 149)*
   o. gag reflex *(p. 154)*
   p. gastric distention *(p. 145)*
   q. head-tilt/chin-lift maneuver *(p. 141)*
   r. hypoxia *(p. 137)*
   s. inhalation *(p. 138)*
   t. inspiration *(p. 138)*
   u. jaw-thrust maneuver *(p. 141)*
   v. laryngectomy *(p. 147)*
   w. larynx *(p. 138)*
   x. nasopharyngeal airway (NPA) *(p. 154)*
   y. oropharyngeal airway (OPA) *(p. 154)*
   z. patent airway *(p. 140)*
   aa. pharynx *(p. 138)*
   bb. pocket face mask *(p. 143)*
   cc. positive pressure ventilation *(p. 141)*
   dd. pulmonary resuscitation *(p. 141)*
   ee. rescue breathing *(p. 141)*
   ff. respiration *(p. 136)*
   gg. respiratory arrest *(p. 137)*
   hh. respiratory compromise *(p. 136)*
   ii. respiratory distress *(p. 136)*
   jj. stoma *(p. 145)*
   kk. tidal volume *(p. 140)*
   ll. trachea *(p. 138)*
   mm. ventilation *(p. 141)*
3. State the oxygen concentration of room air. *(p. 141)*
4. Describe the common causes of respiratory compromise. *(p. 137)*
5. Differentiate between clinical and biological death. *(p. 137)*
6. Describe the signs of a patent airway. *(p. 140)*

7. Describe the signs and symptoms of adequate and inadequate breathing. *(p. 140)*

8. Explain the appropriate steps for rescue breathing with a barrier device. *(p. 143)*

9. Describe common causes of airway obstruction. *(p. 148)*

10. Differentiate between anatomical and mechanical airway obstruction. *(p. 148)*

11. Describe the signs and symptoms of a partial and a complete airway obstruction. *(p. 149)*

12. Describe the care for a patient with a partial and complete airway obstruction (adult, child, infant). *(p. 150)*

13. Describe the management of a patient's airway when there is a suspected spine injury. *(p. 142)*

14. Explain the indications and contraindication for the insertion of an oropharyngeal airway. *(p. 155)*

15. Explain the indications and contraindications for the insertion of a nasopharyngeal airway. *(p. 158)*

16. Explain the benefits, indications, and contraindications of positive pressure ventilation. *(p. 141)*

17. Describe the signs of adequate versus inadequate ventilations. *(p. 144)*

18. Explain the indications for oral and nasal suctioning. *(p. 162)*

19. Differentiate between manual, electric, and oxygen-powered suction devices. *(p. 162)*

20. Differentiate the airway management of a pediatric, adult, and geriatric patients. *(p. 145)*

PSYCHOMOTOR

21. Demonstrate the proper use of the head-tilt, chin-lift maneuver.

22. Demonstrate the proper use of the jaw-thrust maneuver with and without a pocket mask.

23. Demonstrate the proper use of an oropharyngeal airway (OPA).

24. Demonstrate the proper use of a nasopharyngeal airway (NPA).

25. Demonstrate the proper technique for oral suctioning using both a battery-powered and hand-operated suction device.

26. Demonstrate the proper technique for nasal suctioning using both a battery-powered and hand-operated suction device.

27. Demonstrate the proper use of a bag mask device (adult, child, infant).

28. Demonstrate the proper technique for providing positive pressure ventilations for a patient with inadequate respirations (adult, child, infant).

29. Demonstrate the proper technique for caring for a foreign body airway obstruction (adult, child, infant).

AFFECTIVE

30. Value the priority of airway management in the overall assessment and care of the patient.

31. Explain the rationale for using a barrier device when ventilating a patient.

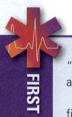

FIRST ON SCENE

"Lindsey!" The neighbor's voice is full of panic. "Lindsey, are you home?"

Lindsey Perez, full-time mother and part-time volunteer firefighter, had been dozing in the backyard with a paperback novel shielding her eyes from the sun. "Yeah, Kayla, I'm back here," she says, lifting the book up and squinting toward the back fence and her neighbor's red face.

"Lindsey. Quick. It's Camille!" the neighbor stammers. "She fell off the pool slide onto the cement, and she's not moving."

Lindsey jumps up from her lounge chair and races to the gate separating the two backyards. Hunter, Kayla's

husband and Camille's stepfather, is kneeling over the motionless girl protectively.

"Nobody move her!" he says, probably louder than he intended. "I think her neck might be hurt."

Lindsey looks past Hunter and sees the girl lying awkwardly semiprone on the concrete with her chin propped against her chest.

"Kayla, I need you to call 911 right now." Lindsey kneels next to the girl. "And Hunter, we need to gently roll her over."

respiration ▶ the act of breathing; the exchange of oxygen and carbon dioxide that takes place in the lungs.

respiratory compromise ▶ a general term used to describe when a patient is not breathing adequately.

respiratory distress ▶ refers to breathing that becomes difficult or labored.

Breathing

Why We Breathe

To maintain life, we breathe. The act of breathing is called **respiration**, during which oxygen is brought into the body. The body's cells, tissues, and organs need oxygen for life, and all life requires energy. The body uses oxygen to produce the energy needed to contract muscles, send nerve impulses, digest food, and build new tissues. In addition, the breathing process removes carbon dioxide from cells and gives it off as waste. This process also is called respiration.

CPR

When you deliver chest compressions during CPR, blood is pumped from the heart to the brain and, just as important, to the arteries supplying the heart. When starting CPR, you do not need to give oxygen yet because there is a large reserve of oxygen in the blood that can be extracted simply by providing high-quality chest compressions.

The process of breathing maintains a constant exchange of carbon dioxide and oxygen. If breathing is not adequate or if it stops, carbon dioxide accumulates in the body's cells and becomes a deadly poison. A patient who is not breathing adequately is said to be experiencing **respiratory compromise**. An early sign of respiratory compromise is **respiratory distress**. Respiratory distress is usually obvious because the patient is clearly having trouble breathing. If not managed properly, respiratory compromise can lead to a condition in which the cells begin to starve for oxygen. This is called **hypoxia**. If adequate breathing is not restored quickly, the patient may stop breathing altogether. This is known as **respiratory arrest**.

There are many causes of respiratory compromise, including medical conditions such as asthma, bronchitis, heart attack, and severe allergic reactions. There are also other factors that can cause difficulty breathing, such as exposure to toxic substances or inhalation of super-heated air.

By regulating the levels of carbon dioxide in the blood and tissues, the respiratory system plays a key role in keeping a normal acid–base balance. This is measured using a pH scale. A low pH indicates too much acid and may be caused by a buildup of carbon dioxide, as may be seen in a patient suffering from hypoxia. Cells live and function within a narrow range of pH. If breathing is not adequate or if it fails, this balancing function stops. If the blood pH level goes too far one way or the other on the scale, cells stop functioning and die. The brain is also very sensitive to improper levels of pH balance. Without proper pH, brain functions quickly cease, including the ones that control breathing.

The absence of breathing is called **apnea**, and once apnea sets in, the heart will soon stop as well. This is known as **cardiac arrest**. The heart requires a continuous supply of oxygen to function. The moment both heartbeat and respirations stop, a condition called **clinical death** occurs. Over the next four to six minutes, oxygen is depleted and cells begin to die. This is the period when it is most critical for the patient to receive CPR. If the patient's cells do not receive oxygen within 10 minutes, irreversible death may occur. The organ affected first, and the most critical one, is the brain. Biological death occurs during this 4- to 6-minutes time frame (Figure 8.1). **Biological death** occurs when too many brain cells die. Clinical death can be reversed; biological death cannot.

How We Breathe

Breathing is automatic. Even though you can temporarily control depth and rate, that control is short term and is soon taken over by involuntary orders from the respiratory centers of the brain. If you try to hold your breath, these centers will urge you to breathe and then take over and force you to breathe. If you try to breathe slow, shallow breaths while running, those brain centers will automatically adjust the rate and depth of breathing to suit the needs of your body. Asleep, or even unresponsive, if there is no damage to these respiratory centers and the heart continues to circulate oxygenated blood to the brain, breathing will be an involuntary, automatic function. The needs of your cells, not your will, are the determining factors in the control of breathing.

The lungs are elastic and expandable. This expansion is limited by the size of the chest cavity and the pressure within the cavity pushing back on the lungs. To inhale, the size of the chest cavity must increase and the pressure

OBJECTIVE

4. Describe the common causes of respiratory compromise.

hypoxia ▶ a condition in which there is an insufficient level of oxygen in the blood and tissues.

respiratory arrest ▶ the absence of breathing.

apnea ▶ the absence of breaths.

cardiac arrest ▶ the absence of a heartbeat.

OBJECTIVE

5. Differentiate between clinical and biological death.

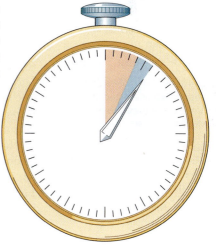

☐ Clinical death—the moment breathing and heartbeat stop

☐ Biological death—within 4–6 minutes

Figure 8.1 • Without oxygen, brain cells begin to die within 10 minutes. Cell death may begin in as little as four minutes.

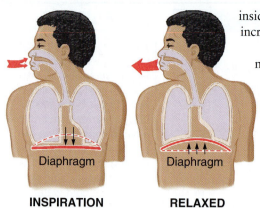

Diaphragm

Diaphragm

INSPIRATION

RELAXED

Figure 8.2 • The respiratory cycle.

inside the cavity must decrease. A simple law governs respiration: as volume increases, pressure decreases.

The volume of the chest cavity is increased by muscle contraction. This may sound backward because contractions usually make things smaller. However, as the muscles between the ribs contract, they pull the front of the ribs up and out. The primary muscle of breathing is the **diaphragm**. When the diaphragm contracts, it moves downward. Both actions result in an increase in the size and volume of the chest cavity.

With each **inhalation**, or breath taken in, the volume of the chest cavity increases, causing a decrease in the pressure within the lungs. (Figure 8.2 illustrates the breathing process.) When this occurs, the lungs expand automatically. As the lungs expand, the volume inside each lung increases. This means that the pressure inside each lung will decrease. As you know, air moves from high pressure to low pressure. (A punctured automobile tire demonstrates this principle.) So, when the pressure inside the lungs becomes less than the pressure in the atmosphere, air rushes into the lungs. It moves from high pressure (atmosphere) to low pressure (lungs). It will continue to do so until the pressure in the lungs equals the pressure in the atmosphere.

For exhaling (or breathing out), the process is reversed. The diaphragm muscle and the muscles between the ribs relax, which reduces the volume in the chest cavity. As the cavity gets smaller, pressure builds in the lungs until it becomes greater than the pressure in the atmosphere, when we must exhale. Air flows from high pressure (full lungs) to low pressure (atmosphere).

Respiratory System Anatomy

Several important parts of the respiratory system have been discussed: the respiratory centers in the brain and the muscles of respiration, including the diaphragm and those between the ribs. Other major structures of the respiratory system include the upper and lower airways (Figure 8.3):

- *Nose.* The nose is the primary path for air to enter and leave the system.
- *Mouth.* The mouth is the secondary path for air to enter and leave the system.
- *Throat.* An air and food passage, the throat is called the oral **pharynx**.
- *Epiglottis.* A leaf-shaped structure, the **epiglottis** covers the larynx when we swallow, which prevents food and fluids from entering the trachea.
- *Trachea.* The trachea is an air passage to the lungs. It is located below the larynx and is commonly called the windpipe.
- *Larynx.* An air passage at the top of the trachea, the larynx is known as the voice box (the structure that contains the vocal cords).
- *Bronchial tree.* The bronchial tree is formed by tubes that branch from the trachea and take air to the lungs. Its two main branches are the right and left main stem bronchi, one for each lung. They branch into secondary bronchi in the lobes of the lungs. The secondary bronchi then branch into still smaller bronchioles, and eventually into alveoli, the microscopic air sacs where the exchange of gases actually takes place.
- *Lungs.* The lungs are elastic organs containing the bronchi, bronchioles, terminal bronchioles, and the alveoli.
- *Alveoli.* These are the small air sacs at the end of the terminal bronchioles where blood cells replenish their oxygen supply and release their accumulated carbon dioxide.

Respiratory Cycle

When the breathing muscles (the diaphragm and those between the ribs) contract and enlarge the chest cavity, air flows through the mouth and nose, into the throat, past the epiglottis, and into the trachea. Air then flows into the left and right main stem bronchi and then through the smaller bronchioles to the clusters of alveoli. The alveoli are

clinical death ▶ the moment when breathing and heart actions stop.

biological death ▶ occurs approximately four to six minutes after onset of clinical death and results when there is an excessive amount of brain cell death.

diaphragm ▶ the dome-shaped muscle that separates the chest and abdominal cavities. It is the major muscle used in breathing.

inhalation ▶ the process of breathing in. See *inspiration*.

inspiration ▶ refers to the process of breathing in, or inhaling. Opposite: *expiration*.

cyanosis ▶ bluish discoloration of the skin and mucous membranes; a sign that body tissues are not receiving enough oxygen.

pharynx ▶ the throat.

epiglottis ▶ a flap of cartilage and other tissues located above the larynx. It helps close off the airway when a person swallows.

larynx ▶ the section of the airway between the throat and the trachea that contains the vocal cords. Also called *voice box*.

trachea ▶ the windpipe.

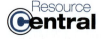

Review your lung anatomy by labeling the lungs.

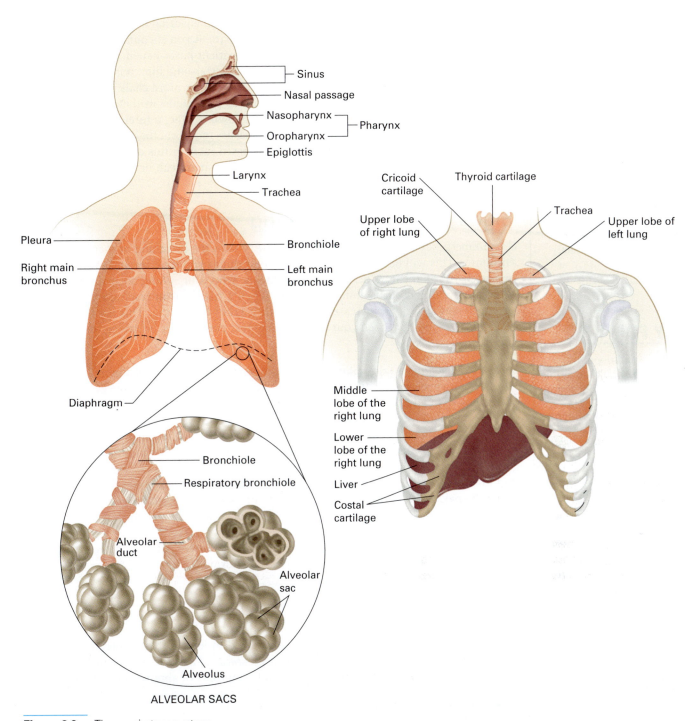

Figure 8.3 • The respiratory system.

Labels in figure:
Sinus
Nasal passage
Nasopharynx
Oropharynx
Pharynx
Epiglottis
Larynx
Trachea
Pleura
Bronchiole
Right main bronchus
Left main bronchus
Diaphragm

Cricoid cartilage
Thyroid cartilage
Trachea
Upper lobe of right lung
Upper lobe of left lung
Middle lobe of the right lung
Lower lobe of the right lung
Liver
Costal cartilage

Bronchiole
Respiratory bronchiole
Alveolar duct
Alveolar sac
Alveolus
ALVEOLAR SACS

surrounded by tiny blood vessels called *capillaries*. It is here in the alveoli that oxygen and carbon dioxide exchange takes place. Oxygen travels through the walls of the alveoli and into the blood, which delivers it to the cells. Carbon dioxide travels from the blood through the alveoli walls, where it is eliminated when we exhale. When working properly, this process of gas exchange is called respiration.

An Open and Clear Airway

Before a breath can be taken, there must be an open and clear path into the lungs. This path is commonly called the airway, and it consists of the passages that make up the nose (nasopharynx), mouth (oropharynx), throat (pharynx), and trachea. When an airway is

KEY POINT ▼

A patent airway is free of all obstructions and allows for the movement of air both in an out of the lungs without difficulty. Noisy breathing is always a sign of a partial airway obstruction.

patent airway ▶ an airway that is open and clear.

Listen to a variety of breath sounds.

tidal volume ▶ the amount of air being moved in and out of the lungs with each breath.

dyspnea ▶ difficult or labored breathing.

accessory muscles ▶ muscles of the neck, chest, and abdomen that can assist during respiratory difficulty.

agonal respirations ▶ an abnormal breathing pattern characterized by slow, shallow breaths that typically occur following cardiac arrest.

open and clear it is said to be patent. Assessing for and ensuring a **patent airway** will be one of the very first steps in the assessment of any patient you encounter.

In most situations it will be obvious that the patient has a patent airway because he will be awake, sitting up, and talking normally to those around him. It is when the patient is unresponsive that assessing the airway can become a bit more challenging. An airway can become blocked by anything small enough to get caught in the airway. Common causes of airway obstruction include the patient's own tongue, a foreign object such as a piece of food or a small toy, and swelling of the tissues that form the airway. How to manage an airway that has become blocked is discussed later in this chapter. For now, just know that without a patent airway there is no way a patient can breathe adequately.

Signs of Normal Breathing

As an Emergency Medical Responder, you must assess the breathing of every patient you encounter. This will become one of the very first things you look for and evaluate as you approach your patient. When observing someone who is breathing normally, the process of breathing in and out is almost invisible. When a patient is in respiratory distress, the most obvious sign is an increase in the work it takes to breathe. This is called *work of breathing*. As you approach your patient, you must evaluate his breathing for the following characteristics:

- Look for adequate **tidal volume**. This is amount of air being moved in and out of the lungs with each breath. Tidal volume can be assessed by observing the even and effortless rise and fall of the chest with each breath.
- Listen for air entering and leaving the nose and mouth. The sounds should be quiet like a soft breeze (no gurgling, gasping, wheezing, or other unusual sounds).
- If the patient is unresponsive, you may feel for air moving into and out of the nose and mouth.
- Observe skin color. Although every person's skin is a different color, the skin should not be pale or cyanotic (tinted blue). Look for these signs, especially around the lips and eyes and in the nail beds, where it will be obvious if the patient is not breathing adequately.
- Observe the patient's level of responsiveness. A responsive patient who is not having difficulty breathing is almost always breathing normally.

Signs of Abnormal Breathing

A patient who is unable to breathe normally is said to have difficulty breathing or be in respiratory distress. This is sometimes called *shortness of breath*, and the medical term is **dyspnea**. The following are common signs and symptoms of abnormal breathing:

- Increased work of breathing
- Absent or shallow rise and fall of the chest
- Little or no air heard or felt at the nose or mouth
- Noisy breathing or gasping sounds
- Breathing that is irregular, too rapid, or too slow
- Breathing that is too deep or labored, especially in infants and children
- Use of **accessory muscles** in the chest, abdomen, and around the neck
- Nostrils that flare when breathing, especially in children
- Skin that is pale or cyanotic (tinted blue)
- Sitting or leaning forward in a tripod position in an effort to make breathing easier

Another form of abnormal breathing that is common during cardiac arrest is called **agonal respirations**. Agonal respirations are characterized by slow, sporadic gasps of air from an unresponsive patient. Those gasping breaths should not be mistaken for normal breathing.

Rescue Breathing

Rescue breathing may be necessary when a patient is not breathing normally or has stopped breathing altogether. When you perform rescue breathing, you are breathing for the patient. This is also referred to as **positive pressure ventilation** or just simply **ventilation**. Rescue breaths are indicated when a patient, either responsive or unresponsive, is unable to breathe in and out with an adequate rate and volume to sustain life. On the other hand, rescue breaths are not appropriate for a responsive or unresponsive patient who is breathing with a normal rate and volume.

Because you provide air that has already been in your lungs to the patient, you might wonder if you are providing enough oxygen. The atmosphere contains about 21% oxygen. The air exhaled from your lungs can contain up to 16% oxygen. This is more than enough oxygen to keep most patients biologically alive until they can receive supplemental oxygen.

OBJECTIVE

16. Explain the benefits, indications, and contraindications of positive pressure ventilation.

rescue breathing ▶ the act of providing positive pressure ventilations for a patient who has inadequate respirations.

OBJECTIVE

3. State the oxygen concentration of room air.

continued

FIRST ON SCENE

"I don't think we should move her," Hunter says, grabbing Lindsey's wrists as she touches the unresponsive girl's shoulder. "Shouldn't we wait for the ambulance?"

"Hunter, she has no airway right now. She's not breathing." Lindsey easily shakes her arms from Hunter's grasp.

"Now unless we get her airway open, she's not going to last until the ambulance gets here."

Kayla screams from the back door of the house, one hand over the telephone receiver. "Do what she says!"

Opening the Airway

Before a patient can breathe normally or before you can provide rescue breaths, the patient must have an open and clear airway. You must ensure that the nose, mouth, and back of the throat are clear of any obstructions. In an unresponsive patient, the muscles begin to relax, and the tongue can drop into the back of the throat and obstruct the airway. The simple act of tilting the head and lifting the chin could relieve this problem. If a patient is responsive and showing signs of obstruction, such as choking (panicked appearance and hands at the throat), the problem is not likely to be the tongue. Immediately begin the steps for choke saving that will be discussed later in this chapter.

Repositioning the Head

In an unresponsive patient, simply repositioning the head may be enough to open the airway. If the patient is lying down with his head on several pillows or up against some object with head flexed forward, tilt the head back slightly by removing pillows or by repositioning the patient so that his head is not flexed forward. You may place one flat pillow beneath the patient's shoulders to help maintain the airway. Note that patients under the influence of alcohol or drugs often have trouble holding a head position that will keep the airway open.

There are two methods of opening the airway. The first is the **head-tilt/chin-lift maneuver,** and it is used for ill or injured patients with no suspected spine injury. The second is the **jaw-thrust maneuver,** which is used for patients who you suspect may have an injury to the spine.

Head-Tilt/Chin-Lift Maneuver

To perform the head-tilt/chin-lift maneuver, place one hand on the patient's forehead and two fingers of your other hand on the bony part of the patient's chin. Gently tilt the head back while lifting the chin. Be careful not to compress the soft tissues under the jaw. Lift up the patient's chin so the lower teeth are almost touching the upper teeth (Figure 8.4).

positive pressure ventilation ▶ the process of using external pressure to force air into a patient's lungs, such as with mouth-to-mask or bag-mask ventilations.

ventilation ▶ the supplying of air to the lungs. See *pulmonary resuscitation.*

pulmonary resuscitation ▶ a technique by which breaths are provided to a patient in an attempt to artificially maintain normal lung function. Also called rescue breathing or artificial ventilation.

head-tilt/chin-lift maneuver ▶ technique used to open the airway of a patient with no suspected neck or spine injury.

jaw-thrust maneuver ▶ technique used to open the airway of a trauma patient with possible neck or spine injury.

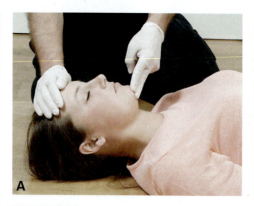

IS IT SAFE?

It is important to carefully consider the potential for spine injury before opening the patient's airway. For example, the absence of an obvious mechanism of injury does not automatically rule out spine injury. A patient found unresponsive in an alley could have been assaulted and therefore may have a neck or back injury. When in doubt, always take appropriate spinal precautions.

OBJECTIVE

13. Describe the management of a patient's airway when there is a suspected spine injury.

KEY POINT ▼

It is important to understand that if you are caring for a patient who has been injured and you are unable to effectively open the airway using the jaw-thrust maneuver, you must use the head-tilt/chin-lift maneuver instead. An open airway is always your first priority.

IS IT SAFE?

The Occupational Safety and Health Administration (OSHA) and the Centers for Disease Control and Prevention (CDC) guidelines state that EMS personnel can reduce the risk of contracting infectious diseases by using pocket face masks with one-way valves and HEPA filter inserts when ventilating patients. Always have one on hand. Also wear protective gloves during assessment and care of all patients.

Figure 8.4 • Use the head-tilt/chin-lift maneuver to open the airway if there are no spine injuries. (A) First, position your hands. (B) Then, tilt the patient's head back as far as it will comfortably go.

This maneuver will lift the tongue away from the back of the throat and allow air to flow freely as the patient breathes. It also will move the neck, which you do not want to do if the patient has a possible spine injury. In such cases, use the jaw-thrust maneuver.

Jaw-Thrust Maneuver

The jaw-thrust maneuver is the recommended method for opening the airway of patients with possible neck or spine injuries (Figure 8.5). Position yourself at the top of the patient's head. Reach forward and place the index and middle fingers of each hand on either side at the angles of the jaw. You may press your thumbs against the cheekbones for leverage. Lift the jaw forward. Do not tilt or rotate the patient's head.

This method also can be used in conjunction with a **pocket face mask** when assisted ventilations are required.

Barrier Devices

All Emergency Medical Responders should use barrier devices, such as pocket face masks or face shields, when providing rescue breaths. When you perform rescue breathing, you can come into direct contact with the patient's body fluids, such as respiratory secretions,

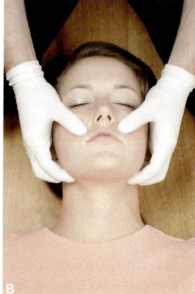

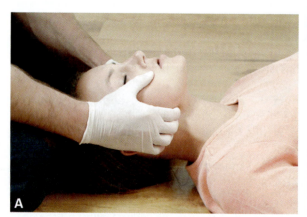

Figure 8.5 • Use the jaw-thrust maneuver if there are possible neck or spine injuries. (A) Side view and (B) front view of the Emergency Medical Responder's hand position.

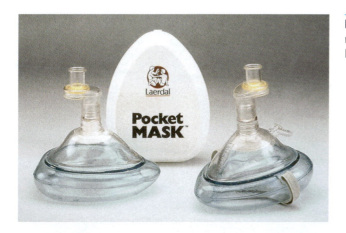

Figure 8.6 • Pocket face mask with one-way valve and HEPA filter.

pocket face mask ▶ a device used to help provide ventilations. It has a chimney with a one-way valve and HEPA filter. Some have an inlet for supplemental oxygen.

KEY POINT ▼

The mouth-to-mouth and mouth-to-nose procedures are no longer accepted as safe practices for Emergency Medical Responders. Laypeople learn these methods because they do not normally carry barrier devices. Even so, it is still common for all rescuers to learn how to deliver mouth-to-mouth and mouth-to-nose techniques because of the possibility of being in situations where there are no protective devices or where there are more patients than devices at the scene. Those who advocate rescue breathing without protective devices state that it is the rescuer's decision to provide ventilation without adequate rescuer protection.

KEY POINT ▼

It is common for patients who are not breathing to vomit during the resuscitation effort. If you carry a suction device and are trained in its use, it is highly recommended that you have it out and available for use whenever you are providing rescue breaths for a patient. Always follow local protocols.

OBJECTIVE

8. Explain the appropriate steps for rescue breathing with a barrier device.

saliva droplets, blood, or vomit. Take all steps necessary to ensure protection from infectious diseases. Always protect yourself.

One example of a barrier device is the pocket face mask. Pocket face masks are available in many sizes and should fit the patient and seal easily to the facial contours of the adult, child, or infant. Pocket face masks are typically made of durable plastic and have a replaceable one-way valve and filter. Some variations have an oxygen inlet to allow for the administration of supplemental oxygen.

Another example of a barrier device is the face shield, which is a durable plastic sheet with a built-in filter. When folded and stowed, it is small enough to be attached to a key ring; unfolded, it is large enough to cover the patient's lower face and act as a barrier to help prevent direct contact with body fluids.

Mouth-to-Mask Ventilation

The mouth-to-mask technique of providing rescue breaths is the recommended method when there is only a single rescuer present. It is quick to set up and relatively easy to facilitate. A pocket face mask allows you to provide ventilations without having to make direct skin-to-skin contact. The mask should have a one-way valve in the stem to minimize the chances of the rescuer breathing in exhaled air from the patient. The pocket face mask that you use should also come with the disposable filter called a *high-efficiency particulate air (HEPA) filter* (Figure 8.6). It snaps inside the pocket face mask and traps air droplets and secretions that may contain dangerous pathogens.

The pocket face mask is made of soft plastic material that can be folded and carried in your pocket. It is available with or without an oxygen inlet. You provide mouth-to-mask ventilations through a chimney on the mask (Figure 8.7). If the mask has a second port for oxygen, you can simultaneously ventilate the patient with air from your lungs and with additional oxygen from an oxygen source.

Another advantage of the pocket face mask is that it allows you to use both hands to maintain a proper head-tilt or jaw-thrust and still hold the mask firmly in place. It is relatively easy to keep a good seal between the face mask and a patient's face with this device. The pocket face mask also can be used with or without an airway adjunct (discussed later in the chapter).

To provide mouth-to-mask ventilations, make sure you are wearing appropriate PPE, and then follow these steps:

1. Kneel beside the patient and confirm unresponsiveness.

2. Open the airway, using the most appropriate maneuver.

3. Firmly hold the mask in place while keeping the airway open. To accomplish this, place both thumbs and index fingers on the cone of the mask to form a C around both sides. Apply even pressure on both sides of the mask.

4. Take a normal breath and breathe slowly into the one-way valve, delivering each breath over one second. Air will enter the airway through the patient's nose and slightly open mouth. Watch for the patient's chest to rise. Remember that there is no

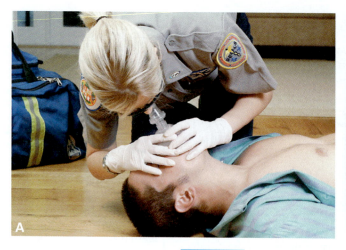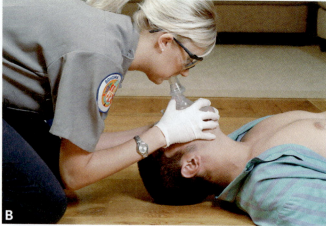

Figure 8.7 • Deliver ventilations using (A) the lateral position or (B) the cephalic position.

need to remove your mouth to allow the patient to exhale. The patient's exhaled air will escape through separate vents in the one-way valve. If air does not enter on the initial breath, reposition the patient's head and try again. If air still does not enter, perform the steps for clearing an obstructed airway (explained later in the chapter).

5. If the initial breath is successful, but the patient does not begin breathing adequately on his own, begin CPR.

An alternative method for ventilating with a pocket mask is to kneel at the top of the patient's head. Place both thumbs and index fingers on the cone of the mask to form a C around both sides. Place the third, fourth, and fifth fingers of each hand under the jaw to form an E on both sides of the patient's jaw. Apply even pressure on both sides of the mask while maintaining a head tilt.

The best indication that you are providing good ventilations is obvious chest rise and fall with each ventilation. If you find that your efforts to ventilate the patient are *not* adequate, you must make adjustments, such as increasing the volume, changing the rate of ventilations, or adjusting the seal between the mask and the patient's face. It is not unusual to see the patient's skin color improve with good ventilations.

Mouth-to-Shield Ventilation

To provide mouth-to-shield ventilations, make sure you are wearing appropriate PPE, and then follow these steps:

1. Kneel beside the patient and confirm unresponsiveness.

2. Open the airway, using the most appropriate maneuver.

3. Place the barrier over the mouth. Keep the airway open as you pinch the nose closed.

4. Open your mouth wide and take a normal breath.

5. Place your mouth over the face shield opening. Make a tight seal by pressing your lips against it.

6. Exhale slowly into the patient's mouth until you see the chest rise. If this first attempt to provide a breath fails, reposition the patient's head and try again.

7. Break contact with the face shield to allow the patient to exhale. Quickly take in another breath and ventilate the patient again. You will give two initial breaths.

8. If the patient does not begin breathing adequately on his own, begin CPR.

Continue CPR until the patient begins to breathe on his own, someone with more training takes over, or until you are too exhausted to continue. You must recheck for the presence of a pulse every two minutes.

If you are following the correct procedures and the patient's airway is not obstructed, you should be able to feel resistance to your ventilations as the patient's lungs expand, see the chest rise and fall, hear air leaving the patient's airway as the chest falls, and feel air leaving the patient's mouth as the lungs deflate. Constantly monitor the patient to determine if he has begun to breathe unassisted. Verify the presence of a pulse every two minutes.

The most common problems with the mouth-to-barrier technique are:

- Failure to form a tight seal over the face shield opening and the patient's mouth (often caused by failing to open your mouth wide enough to make an effective seal, as well as pushing too hard in an effort to form a tight seal)
- Failure to pinch the nose completely closed
- Failure to tilt the head back far enough to open the airway
- Failure to open the patient's mouth wide enough to receive ventilations
- Failure to deliver enough air during a ventilation.
- Providing breaths too quickly
- Failure to clear the airway of obstructions.

Two additional problems—air in the patient's stomach and vomiting—are covered later in this chapter.

Mouth-to-Nose Ventilation

Patients may have injuries to the mouth and jaw, missing teeth or dentures, or airway obstructions that will make airway techniques ineffective. For those patients, use the mouth-to-nose technique. (Depending on the location of the obstruction, mouth-to-nose ventilation may not work if mouth-to-barrier ventilation has failed, but it should be tried.)

Follow these guidelines when performing mouth-to-nose ventilations:

1. Use your hand to seal the mouth shut. Do not pinch the nose.
2. Seal your mouth around the patient's nose.
3. Deliver ventilations through the nose.
4. Break contact with the nose and open the mouth slightly to allow the patient to exhale. Keep your hand on the patient's forehead to keep the airway open.

Like mouth-to-mouth ventilation, mouth-to-nose ventilation exposes the rescuer to potentially infectious body fluids.

Special Patients

Among your patients will be infants and children, elderly patients, patients with a **stoma** (surgical hole in the neck for breathing), and trauma victims (some with possible neck and spine injuries).

Infants and Children

The airways of infants (birth to one year) and children (one year to the onset of puberty) have several physical characteristics that are different from adults. In the infant and child:

- The mouth and nose are much smaller and more easily obstructed.
- The tongue takes up more space in the mouth and throat.
- The trachea (windpipe) is smaller and more easily obstructed by swelling. It also is softer and more flexible and can become obstructed by tilting the head back too far (hyperextension).
- The chest muscles are not as well developed, causing the infant and child to depend more on the diaphragm for breathing.
- The chest cavity and lung volumes are smaller, so **gastric distention** (air getting into the stomach) occurs more commonly.

You must recognize and aggressively care for airway and respiratory problems in infants and children. Respiratory distress can quickly lead to cardiac arrest in these patients.

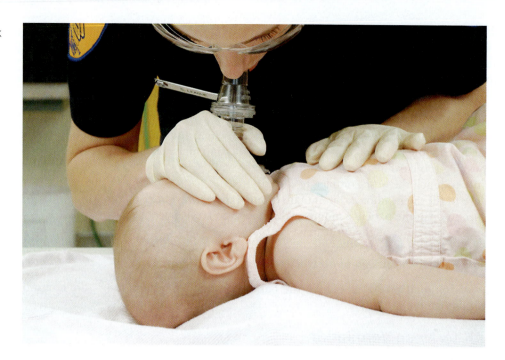

Figure 8.8 • Mouth-to-mask ventilation of an infant.

When assisting ventilations for an infant (Figure 8.8) or small child who has a pulse but is not breathing normally, make sure you take appropriate BSI precautions. Then perform the following steps:

1. Kneel or stand beside the patient and confirm unresponsiveness.
2. Open the airway using the most appropriate maneuver.
3. Using an appropriate barrier device, give one breath every three to five seconds or 12 to 20 breaths per minute. If air does not enter on the initial breath, reposition the head and try again. If air still does not enter, begin CPR.
4. Assist ventilations with gentle but adequate breaths. The volume of breath for the infant or child is determined by ventilating until you see the chest rise. Watch for the chest to rise with each breath.

Note: If there is no reason to suspect spine injury, it is helpful to place a folded towel or similar object under an infant's shoulders to help maintain an open airway.

KEY POINT ▼

Some guidelines allow adult masks to be inverted for use on children.

Terminally Ill Patients

Many terminally ill patients choose to spend their remaining time at home with family and friends. Many others enter a hospice program, which supports and advises the patient and family or makes arrangements with doctors for advance directives such as DNR orders. For guidelines on how to care for hospice or DNR patients, check your jurisdiction for training programs and follow your local protocols.

▶ GERIATRIC FOCUS ◀

Elderly patients may require special care because of changes in their bodies that are normal for aging. First, the lungs may have lost some elasticity, and the rib cage may be more rigid and difficult for you to expand when assisting ventilations. The jaw joints and neck may be stiff and arthritic, which can make it difficult to open the airway, but you will be able to get sufficient air in the patient with the usual maneuvers. With the mouth-to-mask technique, air will still enter the nose, even if the mouth is not open, but your ventilations may have to be a little more forceful. Patients who have lost their teeth and do not use dentures have receding chins and sunken cheeks that make it difficult to seal a mask to the face. Always be aware of resistance to your ventilations and the rise and fall of the patient's chest.

Second, realize that the elderly patient's bones may be more brittle than the bones of younger patients. If elderly patients have fallen, they are more likely to suffer spine injury. When such injuries are possible or when you are in doubt, use the jaw-thrust maneuver to open the airway.

Finally, you may be faced with family members who say such things as, "He's so old. Let him die in peace." Keep in mind that you are charged with the responsibility of assisting all patients who need care, unless direct orders stating otherwise have been given to you by a physician or family member. Any time there is conflict in care priorities, contact medical direction.

Stomas

Some people have had a surgical procedure called a **laryngectomy** to remove part or all of the larynx (voice box). An opening called a stoma is made from outside the neck to the trachea (windpipe) to create an adequate airway for breathing. These patients breathe through that opening (Figure 8.9), not through the nose or the mouth.

Because the patient no longer takes air into the lungs by way of the nose and mouth, you will have to use the mouth-to-mask-to-stoma technique to assist ventilations. Always look to see if there is a stoma. If so, ventilate the patient through the stoma. Currently, there is no specific mask for ventilating these patients, but an infant-size mask often fits, allowing you to establish a seal around the stoma. You also may assist ventilations with a protective face shield or by attaching a bag-valve resuscitator directly to the patient's stoma tube if one is in place in the stoma opening. Follow the protocols of your jurisdiction. Remember, direct contact increases the risk of infection.

When ventilating a stoma patient, take appropriate BSI precautions. Then perform the following steps:

1. Keep the patient's head in a neutral or normal position. Do not tilt the head.
2. Ensure that the stoma is free and clear of any obstructions such as mucus or vomit. Do not remove the breathing tube if one is in place.
3. Use the same procedures as you would for mouth-to-barrier resuscitation, *except:*
   - Do not pinch the patient's nose closed.
   - Place the mask or face shield on the neck over the stoma.

If the chest does not rise, the patient may be a partial neck breather. This means that the patient takes in and expels some air through the mouth and nose. In such cases, you will have to pinch the nose closed, seal the mouth with the palm of your hand, and ventilate through the stoma.

laryngectomy ▶ the total or partial removal of the larynx.

Crash Victims

Opening the airway and assisting ventilations are easier for you to perform when the patient is lying down. This means that a crash victim who is not breathing but who is still in his vehicle must be repositioned. There is always a risk of causing further spine injury if you move the patient, but you must be realistic. If you wait for other EMS personnel to arrive, or if you take time to put on a rigid cervical collar and secure the patient to a spine board, the patient will likely not survive due to a lack of oxygen to the brain. Airway and breathing are always the first priorities of patient care.

Without risking your own safety, take appropriate BSI precautions and reach the victim as quickly as possible. Look, listen, and feel for breathing before moving him. If the patient is breathing, the airway is open and you do not have

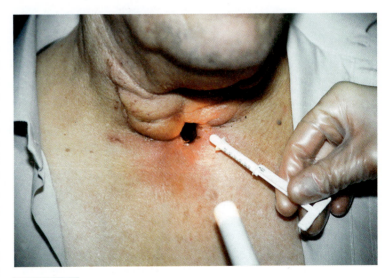

Figure 8.9 • A typical neck stoma.
(© Shout Pictures/Custom Medical Stock Photo)

to move him. If you believe the mechanism of injury may have caused damage to the spine or neck and the patient is not breathing, stabilize the head and open the airway with the jaw-thrust maneuver. Then check again for breathing. If the patient is breathing, keep the airway open while maintaining the head and neck in a neutral position. Monitor breathing until assistance arrives. If the patient is not breathing and his position does not allow you to maintain an airway while you assist ventilations, you will have to reposition him.

Your instructor will show you methods to practice so you can reposition a patient with maximum head stabilization and as little spinal movement as possible.

Air in the Stomach and Vomiting

A common problem with rescue breathing is air in the stomach. It can be caused by overinflating the lungs or breathing too quickly. Remember to carefully watch the chest rise as you ventilate. It will only rise so far. Do not keep ventilating when it stops rising. When the chest rises completely, allow the patient to exhale. Forcing more air than the lungs can hold during ventilation can cause or worsen inflation of the stomach. Air in the stomach will cause the abdomen to distend (get larger). This condition is called *gastric distention*.

Watch for gastric distention when you ventilate a patient. Excessive gastric distention will reduce the ability for the lungs to expand normally. Reduced lung capacity restricts ventilations and reduces oxygen flow to the body. Gastric distention also can cause extra pressure in the stomach, which can result in the patient vomiting.

Do not worry about slight bulging, but you will have to make adjustments if you notice extensive bulging. In cases of air in the stomach where you see a noticeable bulge, reduce the force of your ventilations and do the following:

- Reposition the patient's head to ensure an open airway.
- Be prepared for vomiting. If the patient begins to vomit, turn the patient (not just the head) to one side so the vomit will flow out of the airway and not back into it. (Vomit can obstruct the airway and damage the lungs.) Have suction equipment on hand if you carry it on your unit.
- Do not push on the stomach to release the air. This may cause vomiting, which can block the airway or enter the lungs. Even if the patient is on his side when he vomits, the vomit will not simply flow out. With your gloved hand, clear his mouth with gauze and finger sweeps, or use suctioning equipment.

Airway Obstruction

Causes of Airway Obstruction

OBJECTIVES

9. Describe common causes of airway obstruction.

10. Differentiate between anatomical and mechanical airway obstruction.

The airway is divided into the upper and lower airway. The dividing line is the larynx or vocal cords. Lower airway obstructions are difficult to manage and often require advanced training. You will be able to assess and manage most upper airway obstructions. Many factors can cause the airway to become partially or completely obstructed, including a foreign object lodged in the airway or excess saliva or blood accumulating in the mouth.

The following are examples of upper airway obstructions that you may be able to relieve (Figure 8.10):

- *Obstruction by the tongue (anatomical obstruction).* This is one of the most common causes of airway obstruction in unresponsive patients and is caused when the tongue falls back in the throat and blocks the airway.
- *Foreign objects (mechanical obstruction).* Objects and other matter, such as pieces of food, ice, toys, dentures, vomit, and liquids pooling in the back of the throat, can block the airway.

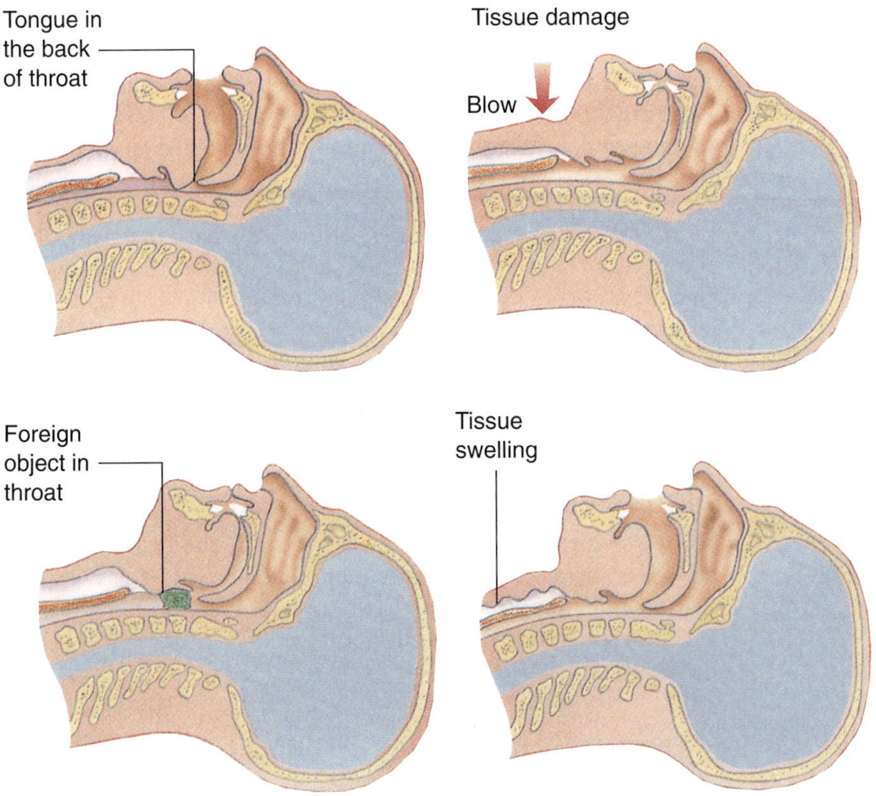

Tongue in the back of throat

Tissue damage

Blow

Foreign object in throat

Tissue swelling

Figure 8.10 • Possible causes of airway obstruction.

The following obstructions may be impossible for you to relieve, but you must still attempt to assist ventilations:

- *Tissue damage.* Tissue damage can be caused by punctures to the neck, crush wounds to the neck and face, upper-airway burns from breathing super-heated air (from a fire or explosion), poisons, and severe blows to the neck. The tissues of the throat and windpipe become swollen and make it difficult for air to flow through the airway.
- *Allergic reactions.* The tissues of the oral pharynx, tongue, and/or the epiglottis become swollen in response to the patient's exposure to something he is allergic to, such as a bee sting or a certain food.
- *Infections.* The tissues of the throat and trachea can become infected and swollen and can produce airway obstruction.

Signs of Partial Airway Obstruction

A patient who is having difficulty breathing may have only a partial obstruction and may still be able to move some air. The signs of partial airway obstruction include the following:

- Noisy breathing, such as the following:
  - *Snoring* is usually caused by the tongue partially or intermittently obstructing the back of the throat.
  - *Gurgling* is usually caused by fluids or blood in the airway or by a foreign object in the trachea.
  - *Crowing* is usually caused by spasms of the larynx (voice box).
  - *Wheezing* is usually due to swelling or spasms along the lower airway caused by asthma, but it does not always mean there is an airway problem. Wheezing may sound serious but is not usually associated with airway obstruction. It is more common during exhalation.

OBJECTIVE

11. Describe the signs and symptoms of a partial and a complete airway obstruction.

exhalation ▶ the process of breathing out.

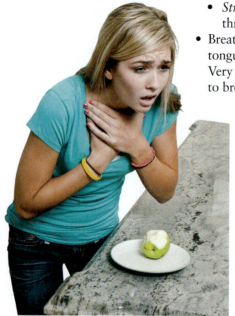

- *Stridor* is a high-pitched harsh sound usually caused by swollen tissue in the throat or larynx (voice box) and typically heard when the patient inhales.
- Breathing is present, but skin is pale or blue at the lips, earlobes, fingernail beds, or tongue. The usual presentation in a responsive patient is fear, panic, or agitation. Very few things invoke terror in a person like a threatened airway or the inability to breathe.

If a responsive patient is experiencing a partial airway obstruction, encourage him to cough. A forceful cough indicates that he has enough air exchange, and coughing may dislodge and expel foreign materials. Do not interfere with the patient's own efforts to clear the airway.

If the patient has poor air exchange and cannot cough or only coughs weakly, begin care as if there is a complete airway obstruction. (Care steps follow later in the chapter.)

Signs of Complete Airway Obstruction

When the airway is completely obstructed, the responsive patient will be unable to speak, breathe, or cough. The patient often will grasp his neck and open his mouth, which is the universal sign of choking (Figure 8.11). The unresponsive patient will not have any of the typical chest movements or the other signs of good air exchange.

Figure 8.11 • Universal sign of choking.

KEY POINT ▼

Do not practice abdominal or chest thrusts on your classmates or any other person. Although important to learn, manual thrusts can be dangerous when performed on a responsive, healthy person. Practice only on the mannequins that are provided by your instructor.

OBJECTIVE

12. Describe the care for a patient with a partial and complete airway obstruction (adult, child, infant).

Clearing a Foreign Body Airway Obstruction

Responsive Adult or Child Patient

Ongoing research conducted by the American Heart Association suggests that the use of **abdominal thrusts** is still the most effective method for clearing the airway of an adult or child who is choking. A slightly different technique is used to clear the airway of an infant.

Abdominal thrusts are achieved by having the rescuer stand behind the patient, place one fist just above the navel, grasp that fist with the other hand, and provide inward and upward thrusts. These thrusts push up on the diaphragm muscle, creating pressure inside the chest cavity and forcing air out of the lungs. As the air is forced out of the lungs, it pushes the foreign object out ahead of it.

Perform the following steps for removal of a foreign body airway obstruction for a responsive adult or child patient (Scan 8.1):

1. Determine that there is complete obstruction or a partial obstruction with poor air exchange. Ask, "Are you choking?" or "Can you speak?" Look and listen for signs of complete obstruction or poor air exchange. Tell the patient you will help.
2. Position yourself behind the patient, and with the index finger of one hand, locate the navel.
3. Make a fist with the other hand and place it against the abdomen thumb side in, just above the navel.
4. Grasp the fist with the first hand and give up to five abdominal thrusts in rapid succession. Watch and listen for evidence that the object has been removed. The patient will begin to cough or speak if the object is removed.

Unresponsive Adult or Child

The following guidelines for the care of an unresponsive patient apply to adults and children (from the age of one year and up). When you suspect a patient may be suffering from an airway obstruction, move swiftly to clear the airway. For unresponsive patients, act quickly to determine if you are able to provide adequate ventilations. Because the tongue is the most common cause of airway obstruction for those patients, make certain to open the airway using the most appropriate maneuver, *prior* to attempting ventilation. Once you have confirmed that you are unable to ventilate, begin CPR. (The specific techniques for performing CPR are explained in Chapter 10.)

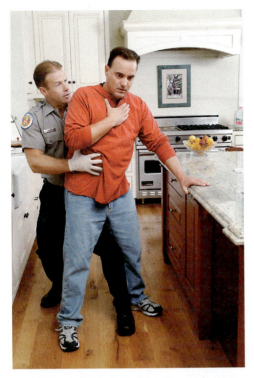

8.1.1 | Stand behind the patient. Place one leg between the patient's legs to obtain a stable stance.

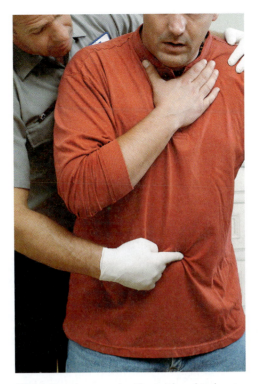

8.1.2 | Reach around with one hand to locate the patient's navel.

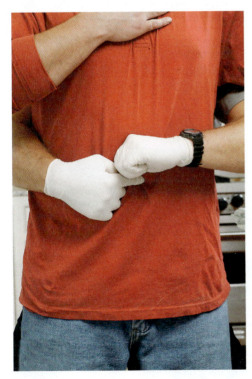

8.1.3 | With the other hand, make a fist and place it just above the patient's navel.

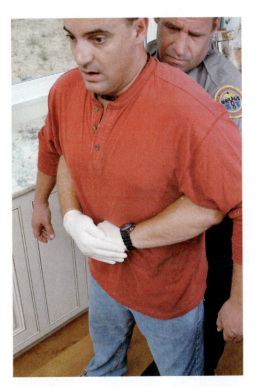

8.1.4 | Grasp your fist with the first hand and pull in and up with swift, firm thrusts.

abdominal thrusts ▶ manual thrusts delivered to create pressure that can help expel an airway obstruction in an adult or child. Also known as *Heimlich maneuver.*

chest thrusts ▶ manual thrusts delivered to create pressure that can help expel an airway obstruction in an infant or in pregnant or obese patients.

KEY POINT ▼

If the unresponsive patient is very large or if you are small, you can deliver effective manual thrusts if you straddle the legs of the supine patient.

KEY POINT ▼

Do not use abdominal thrusts on patients younger than one year of age.

Perform these steps when caring for an unresponsive patient with an airway obstruction:

1. Take the appropriate BSI precautions.
2. With the patient lying face up (supine), tap and shout to assess responsiveness.
3. If unresponsive, direct someone to activate 911.
4. Begin CPR with chest compressions.
5. After each set of 30 compressions, open the airway and check for evidence of a foreign object and remove it if it is visible.
6. Attempt two rescue breaths. If breaths do not go in, continue CPR with chest compressions.

Responsive Infant

The steps for caring for an infant (younger than one year of age) are slightly different from those used for adults and children. For the responsive infant, a combination of **chest thrusts** and back slaps are used to remove the foreign object.

Perform these steps when caring for a responsive infant with an airway obstruction:

1. Take appropriate BSI precautions.
2. Pick up the infant and support him between the forearms of both arms. Support the infant's head as you place him facedown on your forearm. Use your thigh to support your forearm. Remember to keep the infant's head lower than the trunk.
3. Rapidly deliver five back blows between the shoulder blades (Figure 8.12). If this fails to expel the object, proceed to Step 4.
4. While supporting the infant between your arms, turn him over onto his back, again keeping the head lower than the trunk. Remember to support the infant's neck. Use your thigh to support your forearm.
5. Locate the compression site and deliver five chest thrusts with the tips of two or three fingers along the midline of the breastbone (Figure 8.13).

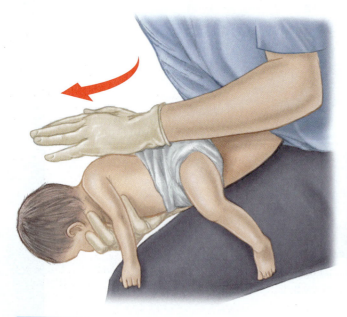

Figure 8.12 • Place the infant over your arm with the head lower than the body and provide 5 back blows.

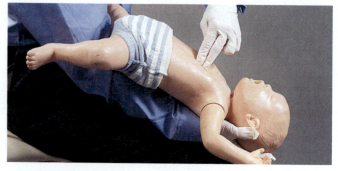

Figure 8.13 • Chest thrusts on an infant.

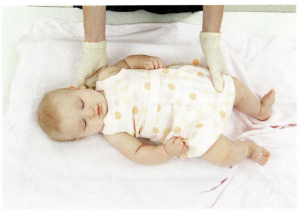

8.2.1 | Place the infant supine on a firm surface.

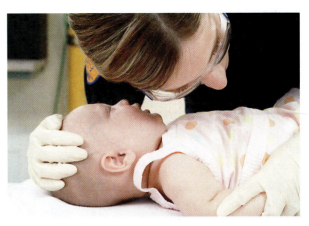

8.2.2 | Assess breathing for no more than 10 seconds.

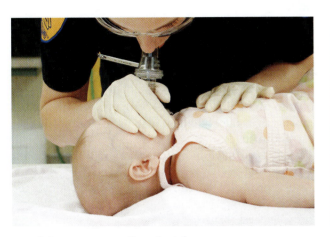

8.2.3 | Attempt to ventilate the infant.

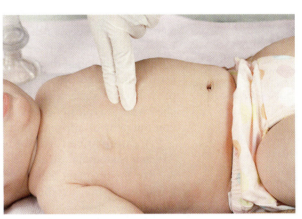

8.2.4 | If unable to ventilate, start CPR beginning with chest compressions.

6. Continue with this sequence of back slaps and chest thrusts until the object is expelled or the infant loses responsiveness.

7. If the infant becomes unresponsive before you can expel the object, begin CPR.

Unresponsive Infant

Perform these steps when caring for an unresponsive infant with an airway obstruction (Scan 8.2):

1. Take the appropriate BSI precautions.

2. With the infant lying face up (supine), tap and shout to assess responsiveness.

3. If the infant is unresponsive, direct someone to activate 911. Then begin CPR with chest compressions.

4. After each set of 30 compressions, open the airway and check for evidence of a foreign object. Remove it if it is visible.

5. Attempt two rescue breaths. If breaths do not go in, continue CPR with chest compressions.

KEY POINT ▼

Back slaps are recommended for conscious infants who have complete airway obstructions. Do not use this procedure on children or adults.

KEY POINT ▼

Chest thrusts must be used for infants, obese patients, and women in the later stages of pregnancy.

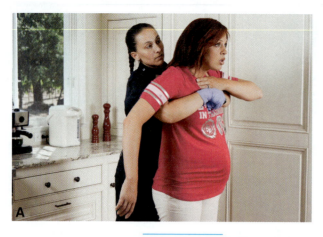 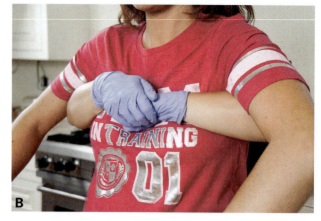

Figure 8.14 • (A) Chest thrust to a pregnant patient. (B) Place the fist of one hand on the sternum and grasp firmly with the other hand.

Obese and Pregnant Patients

Some choking patients present specific challenges that must be overcome if you are going to have any chance of clearing the airway. For example, a patient's large size may prevent you from getting your arms completely around him, making it impossible to provide adequate abdominal thrusts. Providing abdominal thrusts to a pregnant woman can cause serious injury to the developing fetus. For these two responsive patients, attempt to provide chest thrusts as an alternative to abdominal thrusts. For the obese patient, the chest area is typically smaller in diameter than the abdomen, making it more likely that you can provide adequate and successful thrusts.

An alternative for the obese patient is to have him stand against a sturdy wall. Attempt abdominal thrusts from the front.

For the pregnant patient, chest thrusts provide a suitable alternative and eliminate the possibility of injuring the developing fetus (Figure 8.14).

Perform the following steps to provide chest thrusts:

1. Determine that there is complete obstruction or a partial obstruction with poor air exchange. Ask, "Are you choking?" or "Can you speak?" Tell the patient you will help.
2. Position yourself behind the patient and place the thumb side of one fist on the center of the breastbone.
3. Grasp the fist with the other hand and give up to five chest thrusts in rapid succession. Watch and listen for evidence that the object has been removed. If it has, the patient will begin to cough or speak.
4. If the patient's airway remains obstructed, repeat the thrusts until the airway is cleared or until the patient loses responsiveness.
5. If the patient becomes unresponsive before you are able to clear the airway obstruction, direct someone to call 911 and begin CPR.

gag reflex ▶ a retching action, hacking, or vomiting that is induced when something touches a certain level of the patient's throat.

oropharyngeal airway (OPA) ▶ a curved breathing tube inserted into the patient's mouth. It will hold the base of the tongue forward. Also called *oral airway*.

nasopharyngeal airway (NPA) ▶ a flexible tube that is lubricated and then inserted into a patient's nose to the level of the nasopharynx (back of the throat) to provide an open airway. Also called *nasal airway*.

bag-mask device ▶ an aid for pulmonary resuscitation; made up of a face mask, self-refilling bag, and valves that control the one-way flow of air. Also referred to as a *bag-valve mask (BVM)*.

continued

Finger Sweeps

A finger sweep is the technique of using your finger to sweep through the patient's mouth in an attempt to remove a foreign object. It is important to know that you should only perform finger sweeps if you can see an object in the patient's mouth (Figure 8.15). Be careful not to accidentally force the object back down the patient's throat in your attempt to sweep it out.

In most cases, a responsive patient has a **gag reflex**. Probing the mouth with your finger may stimulate the gag reflex and cause vomiting. If this occurs, the patient may inhale the vomit, resulting in the potential for serious illness later. Therefore, only attempt finger sweeps on unresponsive patients and only when you can actually see the object you are going after.

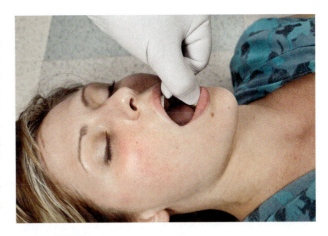

Figure 8.15 • Open the mouth with the crossed-finger technique.

Aids to Airway Management

The use of basic airway adjuncts can help the Emergency Medical Responder provide more effective airway management. There are a variety of such devices in use in EMS systems across the United States. Some of them are used by both EMTs and Paramedics with more advanced training and are not within the scope of the typical Emergency Medical Responder training course. Three types of equipment are commonly used by Emergency Medical Responders: the **oropharyngeal airway (OPA)**, the **nasopharyngeal airway (NPA)**, and the **bag-mask device**. As you learn to use these devices, it is important to understand that they are only adjuncts or aids that assist you in managing a patient's airway and breathing status.

The OPA and NPA help the Emergency Medical Responder maintain an open airway for the patient, allowing more effective ventilations to be delivered to the patient. With less risk of being exposed to the patient's body fluids, the bag-mask device allows the Emergency Medical Responder to deliver better ventilations for those patients who are not breathing adequately on their own. The OPA and NPA are often used together with the bag-mask device to provide the best possible ventilations.

One disadvantage of all adjunct equipment is that it can delay the beginning of resuscitation if it is not readily available. Your pocket face mask and airway adjuncts should always be handy. Never delay the start of ventilations or CPR while you try to find, retrieve, or set up airway adjunct equipment.

Oropharyngeal Airways

Oro- refers to the mouth. *Pharyngeo-* refers to the throat. An oropharyngeal airway (OPA) is a device, usually made of plastic, that can be inserted into a patient's mouth. It has a flange that rests against the patient's lips. The lower portion curves back into the throat and rests against the patient's tongue, restricting its movement and minimizing the chance that it will block the airway. Once a patient's airway is opened manually—by using the

From the Medical Director

Aids to Resuscitation

Either the oropharyngeal or nasopharyngeal airway should be used whenever you perform positive-pressure ventilation. When choosing which airway to use, you can safely assume that the patient who is totally unresponsive and not breathing will tolerate the insertion of an oropharyngeal airway. The patient who is breathing abnormally will more than likely have a gag reflex, which will prohibit the insertion of an oropharyngeal airway. In this case, opt for a nasopharyngeal airway first rather than risk having the patient vomit.

KEY POINT ▼

Do not use the finger-sweep technique on responsive patients or on unresponsive patients who have a gag reflex.

KEY POINT ▼

Finger sweeps can dislodge dentures. If this happens, remove them from the patient's mouth. Do not attempt to replace them.

KEY POINT ▼

Some jurisdictions and agencies do not require or allow Emergency Medical Responders to use special equipment called "airway adjuncts" for airway management or resuscitation. This part of the chapter is provided for those who must learn such skills to meet the requirements of their EMS agency or system. These skills must be learned and practiced on mannequins under your instructor's supervision.

OBJECTIVE

14. Explain the indications and contraindication for the insertion of an oropharyngeal airway.

head-tilt/chin-lift or jaw-thrust maneuver—an OPA may be inserted to help keep the tongue off the back of the throat.

OPAs should only be used in unresponsive patients who do *not* have a gag reflex. These devices can stimulate a patient's normal gag reflex, causing him to vomit. If the unresponsive patient vomits, he can aspirate or breathe the vomit back into his airway and lungs, causing a blockage and possibly a serious infection. If the patient is responsive, even if disoriented or confused, or unresponsive with a gag reflex, do not insert an OPA. Do not continue to insert or leave the airway in the patient's mouth if you meet any resistance or if the patient begins to gag as you insert it.

You may already see that the rules for deciding whether or not to use an OPA may seem contradictory. You are not supposed to use an OPA on a patient with a gag reflex, yet you will not know if the patient has one unless you attempt to insert the OPA first. To resolve this dilemma, you must be very focused as you insert the OPA in your patient. Expect that he may have a gag reflex, and at the first indication that he does, remove the airway.

If you carry a suction unit and are trained to use it, have it ready for any patient who is unresponsive and may need an airway. You do not want to be caught unprepared when your patient vomits.

Measuring the Oropharyngeal Airway

There are numerous sizes of OPAs, designed to fit infants, children, and adults (Figure 8.16). To use this device effectively, you must be able to select the correct size for the patient. Before inserting an airway, hold the device against the patient's face and measure to see if it extends from the center of the mouth to the angle of the lower jaw. The airway also may be sized by holding it at the corner of the patient's mouth and seeing if it will extend to the tip of the earlobe on the same side of the face. You may not find the exact size airway for all patients. If this is the case, choose the airway that is slightly larger rather than one that is slightly smaller.

An airway that is the wrong size has the potential to cause more harm than good. If the airway is too long, it might extend too far into the throat and block the airway. If the device is too short, it will not restrict the movement of the tongue as it should, thus allowing the tongue to block the airway.

Inserting the Oropharyngeal Airway

To insert an OPA, you should (Scan 8.3):

1. Take the appropriate BSI precautions.
2. With the patient on his back, manually open the airway using the head-tilt/chin-lift or jaw-thrust maneuver.
3. Select the appropriate-size airway by measuring from the middle of the mouth to the angle of the jaw or from the corner of the mouth to the earlobe.
4. Insert the airway by positioning it so that its tip is pointing toward the roof of the patient's mouth.
5. Insert the airway and slide it along the roof of the mouth, being certain not to push the tongue back into the throat as you insert the airway.
6. Once the airway is about halfway in, rotate it 180 degrees so that the tip is positioned at the base of the tongue. Allow the flange to rest against the outside of the lips.
7. Monitor the airway constantly. Check to see that the flange of the airway is against the patient's lips. If the airway is too long, it will keep slipping out of the mouth and the flange will not rest on the lips. If the airway is too short, the patient's mouth may remain slightly open in an awkward position.

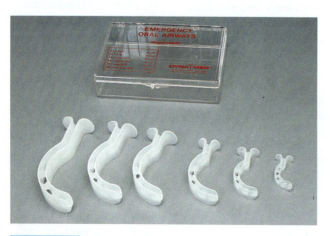

Figure 8.16 • Various sizes of oropharyngeal airways (OPAs).

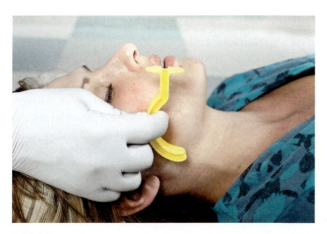

8.3.1 | Properly measure the airway prior to insertion.

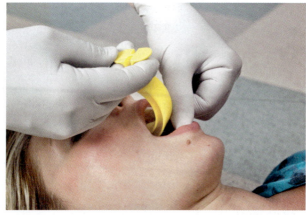

8.3.2 | Insert the airway with the tip pointing to the roof of the patient's mouth. When halfway in, rotate 180 degrees.

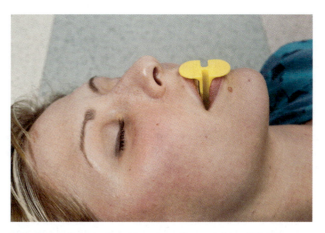

8.3.3 | The flange should rest on the outside of the lips and never any further than the teeth.

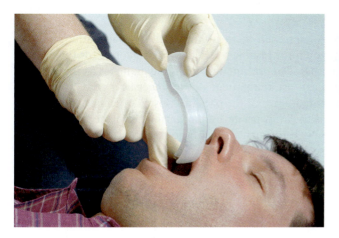

8.3.4a | **Alternative insertion method:** 90 degrees into position. Insert the airway sideways and rotate 90 degrees.

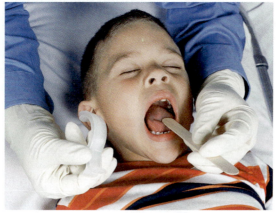

8.3.4b | **Alternative insertion method:** Insertion of an oropharyngeal airway into a child, using a tongue depressor.

Warning: Never practice the use of airways on anyone. Mannequins should be used for developing airway skills.

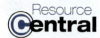
KEY POINT ▼

The OPA is an adjunct. It does not maintain an open airway position by itself. You must still manually maintain the appropriate head position at all times.

OBJECTIVE

15. Explain the indications and contraindications for the insertion of a nasopharyngeal airway.

IS IT SAFE?

Remember that the main contraindication for the use of an NPA is the presence of facial trauma. Inserting an NPA in a patient with a facial fracture could result in the NPA being inserted into the cranial cavity. Carefully consider the mechanism of injury, and assess your patient for signs of facial injury prior to insertion.

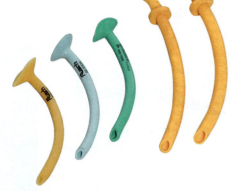

Figure 8.17 • Various types of nasopharyngeal airways (NPAs).

8. Ventilate the patient with the most appropriate technique.

9. Continue to closely monitor the patient's airway. If the patient becomes responsive, he may attempt to remove, displace, or cough up the airway. You must be ready to assist or remove it for him.

An alternative method for inserting an OPA is to insert it sideways into the mouth until it is approximately halfway in. Then simply rotate it 90 degrees. Just as with the first method, make certain that the tip of the airway is positioned at the base of the tongue. This method is less likely to cause trauma to the roof of the patient's mouth during insertion. As with all other skills, follow both your instructor's preference and local protocols.

Infants and Children

To minimize injury to the roof of the mouth of the infant or child while inserting an OPA, the following method is recommended:

1. Use a tongue blade to gently place downward pressure on the tongue.

2. Insert the OPA with the tip pointing toward the tongue and throat, in the same position it will be in after insertion, rather than upside down.

The OPA is inserted in this way because the infant's or child's mouth is smaller than an adult's and the upper portion of the oral cavity is more easily injured. Rotating the airway can damage the soft palate or the uvula.

Nasopharyngeal Airways

The nasopharyngeal airway (NPA) is a soft, flexible tube that is inserted into the nose to create a clear and open path for air. It is the preferred choice when the patient is not totally unresponsive or has a gag reflex. NPAs are the next choice of airway adjunct (after OPAs) because they are less likely to stimulate a gag reflex and therefore do not have to be removed if the patient becomes responsive.

An NPA is easy to insert because you do not have to reposition the patient's head or pry open the mouth. If there is any injury to the mouth, teeth, or oral cavity, the NPA will still provide an open airway for the patient. The only precaution is for patients with possible skull or facial fractures. If there is any indication of head or facial injury, do not insert the NPA. If a facial or skull fracture exists, inserting the NPA may cause it to enter the cranial cavity through the unseen fracture. This could cause direct damage to the brain.

Measuring the Nasopharyngeal Airway

There are numerous sizes of NPAs designed to fit infants, children, and adults (Figure 8.17). To use an NPA effectively, you must be able to select the correct size for the patient. Begin by selecting an airway that is approximately the same diameter as the patient's nostril opening. You also can use the patient's little finger as a guide. (The little finger is often the approximate size of the patient's nostril opening.) Next, make sure that the tube length is appropriate by measuring from the tip of the patient's nose to the earlobe. If the airway is not the correct size, do not use it on the patient. Instead, select another airway and re-measure to check correct size before inserting.

Inserting the Nasopharyngeal Airway

Perform the following steps to insert an NPA (Scan 8.4):

1. Take the appropriate BSI precautions.

2. Select the largest diameter NPA that will fit into the patient's nostril without force. Then measure the length from the tip of the patient's nose to the earlobe.

3. Use a water-based lubricant on the outside of the tube before you insert it. Do not use petroleum jelly or any other non-water-based lubricant.

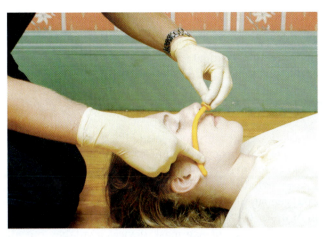

8.4.1 | Measure the NPA from the tip of the nose to the earlobe, or to the angle of the jaw.

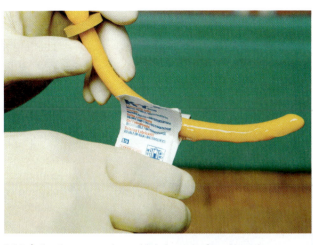

8.4.2 | Apply a water-based lubricant before insertion.

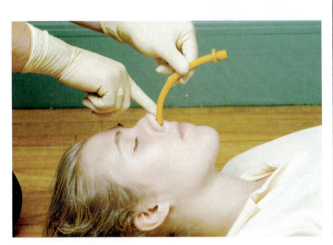

8.4.3 | Gently insert the airway, advancing it until the flange rests against the nostril.

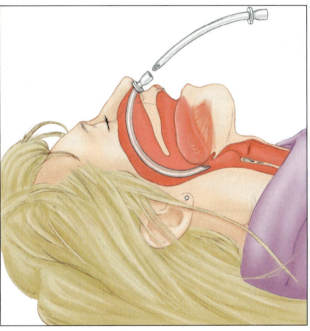

8.4.4 | Nasopharyngeal airway, properly inserted.

4. Keep the patient's head in a neutral position while you gently push the tip of the nose upward. Insert the airway straight back through the nostril. If the airway has a beveled (angled) end, that end should point toward the septum (the midline of the nose). Gently advance the airway until the flange rests firmly against the patient's nostril. Never force the airway. If the airway will not advance into the nostril easily, remove it and try it in the other nostril. If the airway will not advance into the other nostril, make another attempt with an airway that is slightly smaller in diameter.

▶ GERIATRIC FOCUS ◀

Elderly patients are prone to nosebleeds for two reasons. First, they have thin, easily damaged mucosa. Second, many of them are on "blood thinners," such as Coumadin. Take this into consideration when placing an NPA. Ensure that the airway is adequately lubricated and avoid forcing it past any obstruction. Frequently, a rotational maneuver is very successful when inserting an NPA in the elderly.

KEY POINT ▼

Most NPAs are made with the bevel facing to the left; therefore, they are meant to fit into the right nostril. Before inserting the NPA into the left nostril, use a pair of scissors to carefully snip the end of the airway to change the bevel from the left to the right. Then lubricate and insert. It is not recommended to insert an NPA against its natural curvature because it is likely to rotate on its own after being inserted.

Bag-Mask Ventilation

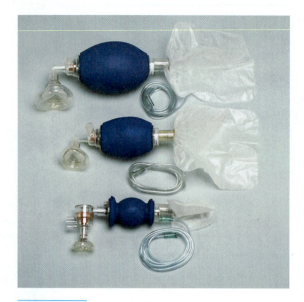

Figure 8.18 • Disposable bag-mask devices.

The bag-mask device is one of the most commonly used devices for ventilating a nonbreathing patient. Some EMS systems also use the bag-mask device to ventilate patients with inadequate respirations (e.g., in drug overdose). The bag-mask device is available in sizes for infants, children, and adults. It also acts as an effective infection-control barrier between you and your patient.

The bag-mask device delivers room air (21% oxygen) to the patient when it is squeezed through the unit to the patient's lungs. (In contrast, a pocket face mask will deliver between 10% and 16% oxygen from your exhaled air.) The bag-mask device can be connected to an oxygen supply source to enrich room air and deliver a concentration of up to 100% oxygen.

There are many brands of bag-mask devices available, but all have the same basic parts: a self-refilling bag, valves that control the one-way flow of air, and a face mask. There is a standard 15/22 mm fitting, so a variety of respiratory equipment and face masks can be used with it. The bag-mask device must be made of material that can be easily cleaned and sterilized. Many EMS systems now use disposable units (Figure 8.18).

The principle behind the operation of the bag-mask device is simple. When you squeeze the bag, air is delivered to the patient through a one-way valve. When you release the bag, fresh air enters the bag from the rear while the exhaled air from the patient flows out near the mask. The exhaled air does not go back into the bag.

There are times when the bag-mask device will not deliver air to the patient's lungs. Sometimes the problem occurs because the patient has an airway obstruction that must be cleared. More often, the problem is caused by an improper seal between the patient's face and mask. If this occurs, you should reposition your fingers and check placement of the mask.

KEY POINT ▼

Most EMS systems recommend that an OPA or NPA should be inserted before attempting to ventilate the patient with a bag-mask device.

Resource Central

Get more information about the equipment needed for bag-mask ventilation.

Also, learn more about performing effective bag-mask ventilations with two rescuers.

▶ GERIATRIC FOCUS ◀

Because the elderly often have recessed chins due to loss of teeth, two hands are frequently required to maintain the mask-to-face seal. Therefore, two rescuers are required to perform bag-mask ventilation.

Two-Rescuer Bag-Mask Ventilation

For the best possible results, the bag-mask device should be used with two rescuers. One rescuer can use two hands to maintain a good mask seal, while the second rescuer squeezes the bag. Note also that for trauma patients who must have their airway opened by the jaw-thrust maneuver, the two-rescuer method is more effective. The rescuer holding the mask in place can more easily perform the jaw-thrust while the other rescuer provides effective ventilations.

Perform the following steps to provide ventilations using the two-rescuer bag-mask technique (Scan 8.5):

1. Take the appropriate BSI precautions.

From the Medical Director

Bag-Mask Technique
When using a bag-mask device, the bag should be squeezed only until the rise of the chest is seen. The bag should be squeezed over one second to avoid over inflation of the lungs and increased gastric distention.

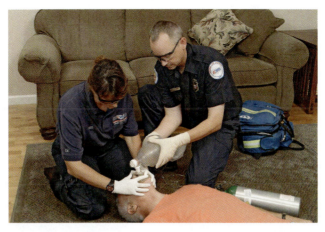

8.5.1 | Proper technique for using the bag-mask device with two rescuers.

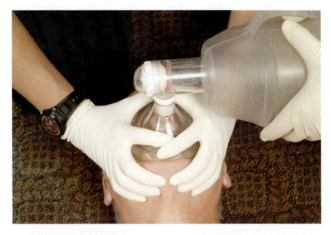

8.5.2 | Proper hand position for bag-mask ventilation with two rescuers.

2. Ensure an open airway, and position yourself at the patient's head. Clear the airway if necessary.

3. Insert an appropriate airway adjunct.

4. Rescuer 1 should kneel at the top of the patient's head, holding the mask firmly in place with both hands.

5. Rescuer 2 should kneel beside the patient's head and connect the bag to the mask (if not already done). He should then squeeze the bag once every five seconds for an adult (once every three seconds for a child or an infant). Ensure adequate rise and fall of the chest each time the bag is squeezed.

The bag-mask device also can be used effectively during two-rescuer CPR by a skilled operator. The ventilator squeezes the bag and provides two back-to-back ventilations following each cycle of compressions.

One-Rescuer Bag-Mask Ventilation

For a single rescuer alone, the bag-mask device can be difficult to operate. This is especially true if you have small hands or do not use a bag-mask device on a regular basis. The most difficult part is maintaining an adequate mask-to-face seal with one hand. If you are assigned a bag-mask device for use in the field, practice using it in the classroom until your technique is well developed.

KEY POINT ▼

In some instances as a single rescuer, it may be more effective to provide assisted ventilations using the mouth-to-mask technique than attempting to use a bag-mask device by yourself.

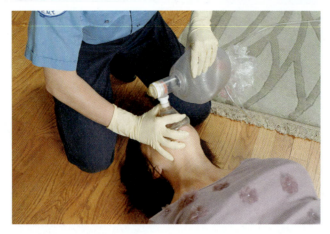

8.6.1 | Proper technique for using the bag-mask device with one rescuer.

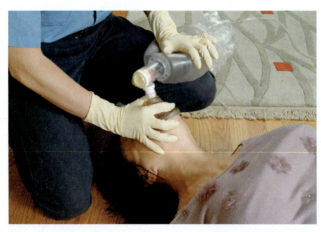

8.6.2 | An alternative is to press the bag against your leg.

KEY POINT ▼

Some EMS systems have decided that one-rescuer bag-mask ventilation skills are poorly maintained and thus have selected the pocket face mask as the preferred ventilation-assist device for Emergency Medical Responders.

OBJECTIVES

18. Explain the indications for oral and nasal suctioning.

19. Differentiate between manual, electric, and oxygen-powered suction devices.

Perform the following steps to ventilate a patient using the bag-mask device as a single rescuer (Scan 8.6):

1. Take the appropriate BSI precautions.
2. Ensure an open airway, and position yourself at the patient's head. Clear the airway if necessary.
3. Insert an appropriate airway adjunct.
4. Use the correct mask size for the patient. Place the apex, or top, of the triangular mask over the bridge of the nose. Rest the base of the mask between the patient's lower lip and the projection of the chin.
5. With one hand, hold the mask firmly in position.
6. With your other hand, squeeze the bag at the appropriate rate, delivering each breath over approximately one second. Observe for adequate rise and fall of the patient's chest.

Suction Systems

To clear blood, mucus, and other body fluids from a patient's airway, an Emergency Medical Responder usually will position the patient on his side (recovery position) or use finger sweeps appropriately. However, a suction device can assist in keeping a patient's

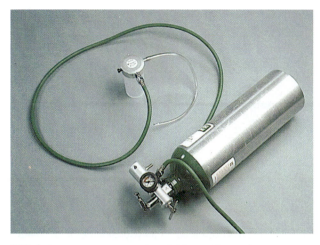

8.7.1 | An oxygen-powered portable suction unit.

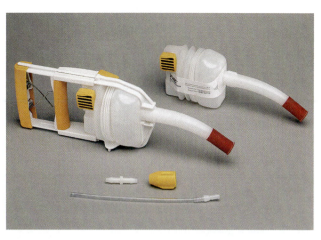

8.7.2 | Manually operated suction device (V-VAC).

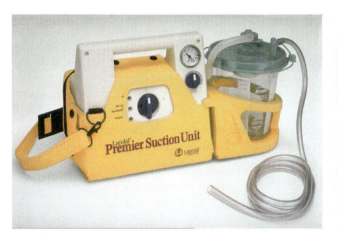

8.7.3 | Battery-powered portable suction unit.

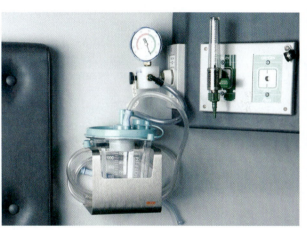

8.7.4 | Mounted suction unit installed in an ambulance patient compartment.

airway clear. There are several types of portable suction units available, including manually powered, oxygen or air powered, and electrically powered units (Scan 8.7).

All types of suction units must have thick-walled, nonkinking, wide-bore tubing; a nonbreakable collection container (bottle); and sterile, disposable, semirigid but flexible or rigid suction tips. The longer, flexible suction tips are usually called *catheters*. Rigid suction tips are sometimes referred to as *tonsil suction tips*.

General Guidelines for Suctioning

- Always use appropriate BSI precautions, including a mouth and eye shield, because the potential for being sprayed with body fluids such as vomit, blood, and saliva are high.
- Keep your suctioning time to a minimum. Remember that while you are suctioning, you are not ventilating. Also, suction removes valuable oxygen along with dangerous fluids. One suggested guideline is to suction for no more than 15 seconds for adults, 10 seconds for children, and 5 seconds for infants.
- If there is a copious amount of fluid in the patient's airway, it may be helpful to roll him onto his side and then suction. You may need to suction, ventilate, and then suction again in a continuous sequence as long as necessary.
- Measure the suction catheter before inserting it into the patient's mouth as you would for an OPA. Prior to inserting into the nose, measure the catheter as you would for an NPA.
- Activate the suction unit only after it is completely inserted and as you withdraw the catheter.

KEY POINT ▼

A manually powered suction unit may have a rubber bulb or a hand- or foot-operated device to produce the vacuum. Follow manufacturer guidelines for operating the device.

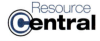

Learn more about safe suctioning techniques.

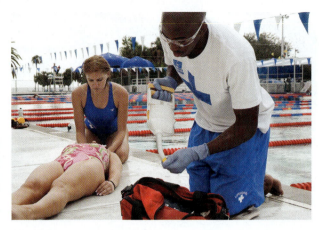

8.8.1 | Prepare suction unit.

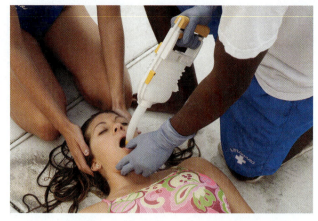

8.8.2 | Insert the device as far as you can see, and initiate suction.

- Twist and turn the tip of the catheter as you are removing it from the mouth, nose, or stoma.
- When suctioning the mouth, concentrate on the back corners of the mouth, where most fluids tend to accumulate. *Do not* place the tip directly over the back of the tongue, because this will likely stimulate the gag reflex.

Suctioning Techniques

There are many variations to the techniques used to suction the mouth, nose, or stoma. However, you *must* follow your own local protocols. In general, you will follow these steps (Scan 8.8):

1. Before suctioning any patient, be sure to take the appropriate BSI precautions.
2. Attach the catheter and activate the unit to ensure that there is suction.
3. Position yourself at the patient's head. If possible, turn the patient onto his side. Follow guidelines for protection of the spine.
4. Measure the catheter prior to insertion.
5. Open the patient's mouth and clear obvious matter and fluid from the oral cavity by letting the mouth drain or by using finger sweeps with a gloved hand.
6. Insert the tip of the catheter to the appropriate depth. Usually, the tip is inserted to the base of the tongue. If you are using a rigid catheter, place the convex (curved-out) side against the roof of the mouth with the tip at the base of the tongue.
7. Apply suction *only* when the tip or catheter is in place at the back of the mouth or base of the tongue and as you begin to withdraw it. Twist and turn it from side to side and sweep the mouth. This twisting action prevents the end of the catheter from grabbing the soft tissue inside the mouth.
8. Remain alert for signs of a gag reflex and vomiting.

WRAP-UP

FIRST ON SCENE

A few minutes later, just as Camille is beginning to blink her eyes and look around, a team of firefighter Emergency Medical Responders appears in the backyard, followed closely by an ambulance crew. The ambulance crew performs an initial assessment and begins oxygen therapy, while the firefighters help secure the girl to a long spine board, move her to the wheeled stretcher, and get her into the ambulance.

"She has good sensation and motor function in her extremities," one of the EMTs says to Lindsey. "I think she probably just got a good bump on the head. It could have been a lot worse."

"Tell me about it," Lindsey says and waves reassuringly at Hunter and Kayla as they get into their car to follow the ambulance.

Summary

- Receiving an adequate supply of oxygen is essential to life. There are many conditions, such as asthma, bronchitis, drowning, and choking, that can disrupt this essential process and cause what we call respiratory compromise.

- Clinical death occurs the moment that both breathing and heartbeats stop. Biological (irreversible) death occurs approximately four to six minutes following clinical death.

- A patent airway is one that is clear and open and allows for the effortless flow of air in and out of the lungs. The air that we breathe contains approximately 21% oxygen and is more than adequate for our daily needs.

- When something disrupts the normal breathing process, breathing becomes inadequate and the patient is at risk of becoming hypoxic. Signs of inadequate breathing include increased work of breathing and shallow, rapid, noisy, or gasping breathing.

- To assist a patient who is not breathing adequately or not at all, you must provide rescue breaths using an appropriate barrier device. Using a firm seal with the mask, you will breathe once every five to six seconds for adults and once every three to five seconds for children and infants.

- There are many causes of airway obstruction, with some of the most common being the patient's own tongue, blood, saliva (anatomical obstructions), and foreign objects such as food or small objects (mechanical obstructions).

- A responsive patient with a complete obstruction is unable to breathe, cough, or speak and will usually look panicked. You must provide immediate care for the removal of the obstruction.

- The preferred method for opening the airway of an unresponsive patient who is uninjured is the head-tilt/chin-lift maneuver. The preferred method for an unresponsive patient with a suspected neck or spine injury is the jaw-thrust maneuver.

- It is important to understand that if you are working with a patient with a suspected neck or spine injury and you are unable to open the airway using the jaw-thrust, you must attempt the head-tilt/chin-lift maneuver.

- Unresponsive patients with no gag reflex should receive an OPA. The OPA helps keep the tongue from falling to the back of the throat and thus blocking the airway.

- For patients with a gag reflex or those who are somewhat responsive, the NPA may be the best choice as an airway adjunct.

- When a patient is not breathing adequately or not at all, you must provide positive pressure ventilations or rescue breaths for your patient.

- The best sign that you are providing good rescue breaths is good chest rise and fall with each breath.

- To minimize the flow of air into the stomach during rescue breaths, you should provide slow, even breaths, and do not overinflate the chest.

- If the patient's airway becomes obstructed with fluid such as saliva, blood, or vomit, it will be necessary to suction the mouth and/or nose to remove this fluid and clear the airway.

Take Action

OPENING THE AIRWAY

Certainly you will have the opportunity to practice opening the airway of a mannequin as well as practice giving rescue breaths using a barrier device. But what you may not realize is that practicing those skills on a mannequin is often very different than on a real person. For this "Take Action," practice two specific skills using a real live person.

The first two skills are the head-tilt/chin-lift and the jaw-thrust maneuvers. First, you must locate a suitable person to serve as your patient. This is best if it is someone you know well, perhaps even a family member. Begin by explaining clearly what it is you want to do with him and then ask him to lie down on the floor flat on his back. Kneeling at the side of his head, practice the head-tilt/chin lift by placing one hand on the forehead and two fingers of the other hand on the bony part of the chin. Now gently tilt the head as far back as it will comfortably go. Remind your patient to just relax and allow you to do the work. The first thing you will notice is that a real patient's head is significantly heavier than that of the mannequin. It is good to get this experience before you are forced into the real situation.

Next, kneel at the top of the patient's head and practice the jaw-thrust maneuver. Remind your patient to relax and let you do the work. Begin by placing your thumbs directly on the cheekbones of your patient. Next, grasp the corners of the jaw with the index and middle finger of each hand. Using your thumbs as counter pressure, pull forward on the corners of the jaw and move the lower jaw upward, creating an exaggerated underbite. By lifting the jaw up, you will bring the tongue with it and keep the tongue from blocking the back of the throat.

Note: Do not practice manual thrusts on a real person, only on mannequins. Even though obstructed airway procedures do not require extremely forceful thrusts, they can cause discomfort or injury. Therefore, although you can practice positioning on people of different sizes, perform the complete maneuver only on mannequins.

First on Scene Run Review

Recall the events of the "First on Scene" scenario in this chapter and answer the following questions, which are related to the call. Rationales are offered in the Answer Key at the back of the book.

1. Did Kayla make the right decision to roll Camille onto her back? What are some reasons you would want to roll someone quickly?

2. What was likely causing the obstruction of Camille's airway?

3. What is your priority when a patient has an obstructed airway as well as a possible neck injury? How do you manage both?

Quick Quiz

To check your understanding of the chapter, answer the following questions. Then compare your answers to those in the Answer Key at the back of the book.

1. Rescue breathing is:
   a. any effort to restart normal heart rhythms.
   b. any effort to revive or restore normal breathing.
   c. the use of mechanical devices to restart breathing.
   d. the ability to restore normal heart rhythm and breathing.

2. When performing the head-tilt/chin-lift maneuver on an adult, tilt the head:
   a. as far back as possible.
   b. into the sniffing position.
   c. to get the tongue to close the epiglottis.
   d. so that upper and lower teeth are touching.

3. The recommended method for opening the airway of a patient with a possible neck or spine injury is the _____ maneuver.
   a. jaw-thrust
   b. mouth-to-nose
   c. abdominal thrust
   d. head-tilt/chin-lift

4. Clinical death occurs when the patient's:
   a. brain cells begin to die.
   b. breathing has stopped for four minutes.
   c. pulse has been absent for five minutes.
   d. heart beat and breathing have stopped.

5. A pocket face mask allows the rescuer to provide ventilations WITHOUT:
   a. having to hold the mask firmly in place.
   b. delivering his own breaths to the patient.
   c. direct contact with the patient's mouth and nose.
   d. worrying about keeping the head and spine in-line.

6. During rescue breathing, you should check for adequate breathing by:
   a. looking for chest rise and fall.
   b. listening for airflow from the mouth and nose.
   c. observing skin color, such as paleness or cyanosis.
   d. looking for chest rise and fall, listening for airflow, and observing skin color.

7. If an infant becomes unresponsive before you can clear an airway obstruction, you should first:
   a. place the infant facedown and lift her chest with your hands.
   b. place her on a firm surface and begin chest compressions.
   c. hold her face up and deliver chest thrusts.
   d. turn her facedown and deliver back slaps.

8. For suctioning a patient, the appropriate BSI precautions include:
   a. pocket face mask.
   b. oropharyngeal airway.
   c. eye and face protection.
   d. folded towel under his shoulders.

9. Which one of the following improves ventilations delivered by way of a bag-mask device?
   a. Inserting an oropharyngeal airway
   b. Applying suction for four to six minutes
   c. Alternating chest thrusts and squeezing the bag
   d. Combining finger sweeps with a mouth-to-mouth technique

10. Which one of the following is recommended for clearing an airway obstruction in an unresponsive 10-month-old baby?
    a. Abdominal thrusts
    b. Chest thrusts
    c. Back slaps and finger sweeps
    d. Abdominal thrusts and finger sweeps

11. The primary muscle of respiration is the:
    a. trachea.
    b. esophagus.
    c. diaphragm.
    d. pharynx.

12. The _____ prevents food and other material from entering the trachea.
    a. tongue
    b. alveoli
    c. pharynx
    d. epiglottis

13. Deep within the lungs, the _____ are the tiny balloon-like structures where gas exchanges take place.

   a. alveoli
   b. bronchioles
   c. trachea
   d. epiglottis

14. All of the following are signs of inadequate breathing EXCEPT:

   a. poor chest rise.
   b. pale or bluish skin color.
   c. use of accessory muscles.
   d. good chest rise and fall.

15. When caring for an unresponsive medical patient, tilting the head back improves the airway by:

   a. lifting the tongue from the back of the throat.
   b. shifting the epiglottis from front to back.
   c. allowing fluids to flow more easily.
   d. opening the mouth.

16. An airway stoma is found on the:

   a. chest.
   b. arm.
   c. neck.
   d. cheek.

17. Noisy breathing is a sign of _____ airway obstruction.

   a. bilateral
   b. complete
   c. adequate
   d. partial

18. You have just made two attempts to ventilate an unresponsive child with an airway obstruction. Your next step is to:

   a. begin chest compressions.
   b. continue to ventilate.
   c. perform five chest thrusts.
   d. provide back slaps.

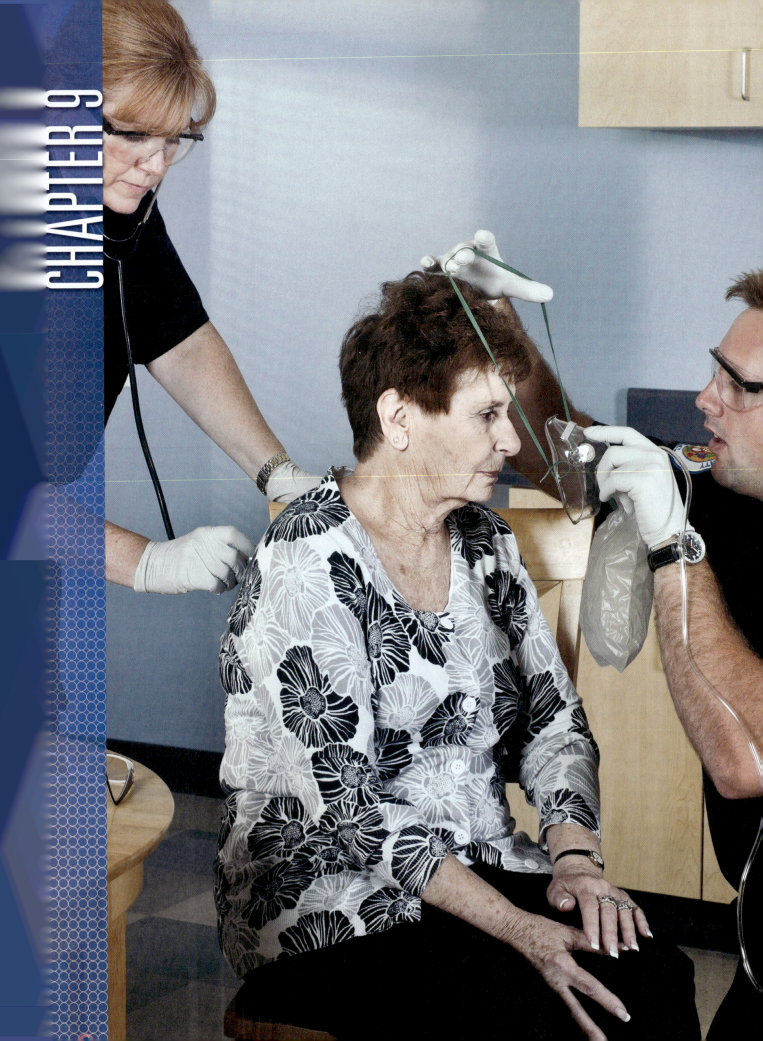

Oxygen Therapy

EDUCATION STANDARDS
- Airway Management—Airway Management, Respiration, and Artificial Ventilation

COMPETENCIES
- Applies knowledge (fundamental depth, foundational breadth) of anatomy and physiology to ensure a patent airway, adequate mechanical ventilation, and respiration while awaiting EMS response for patients of all ages.

CHAPTER OVERVIEW

As you have already learned, a constant supply of oxygen to the body's cells is essential to maintain healthy and properly functioning body systems. When a person becomes ill or injured, the normal flow of oxygen into and throughout the body can become disrupted. In these instances it may be helpful to provide supplemental oxygen to help overcome this deficiency.

This chapter will provide an overview of the proper equipment and techniques necessary to provide your patients with supplemental oxygen. It is important to point out that oxygen is a drug and that not all EMS systems authorize Emergency Medical Responders to administer oxygen. Your instructor will inform you as to the protocols for oxygen administration in your area.

OBJECTIVES

Upon successful completion of this chapter, the student should be able to:

COGNITIVE

1. Define the following terms:
   a. humidifier *(p. 171)*
   b. hydrostatic test *(p. 173)*
   c. liter flow *(p. 174)*
   d. nasal cannula *(p. 175)*
   e. nonrebreather mask *(p. 176)*
   f. O ring *(p. 175)*
   g. oxygen concentration *(p. 170)*
   h. oxygen supply tubing *(p. 179)*
   i. pin index system *(p. 174)*
   j. pressure gauge *(p. 172)*
   k. pressure regulator *(p. 172)*
   l. reservoir bag *(p. 176)*
   m. supplemental oxygen *(p. 170)*
2. Explain the benefits of supplemental oxygen. *(p. 170)*
3. Explain the indications of supplemental oxygen. *(p. 170)*
4. Explain the potential hazards of working with high-pressure cylinders. *(p. 171)*
5. Explain the safe practices when working with high-pressure cylinders. *(p. 173)*
6. Differentiate between the common sizes of oxygen cylinders used in EMS. *(p. 171)*
7. Describe the purpose and functions of an oxygen regulator. *(p. 174)*
8. Explain the indications for the use of a nasal cannula. *(p. 175)*
9. Explain the indications for the use of a nonrebreather mask. *(p. 176)*

PSYCHOMOTOR

10. Demonstrate the proper use of a nonrebreather mask.
11. Demonstrate the proper use of a nasal cannula.
12. Demonstrate the ability to add supplemental oxygen to a pocket mask and/or bag-mask device.
13. Demonstrate the proper technique for attaching a regulator to a cylinder.
14. Demonstrate the ability to identify and troubleshoot a leaky oxygen cylinder/regulator.

AFFECTIVE

15. Recognize the value that supplemental oxygen might offer for most ill and injured patients.

"Emergency Medical Responders," Lawee calls out as she makes her way through the open doorway of an aging townhome. "Someone called us for help?"

"In here!" It is a young women's voice from down the hallway.

Lawee and Matt bring their equipment into the kitchen, where a young woman is kneeling next to an older woman who is hunched over in her wheelchair.

"She's having trouble breathing! I've never seen Grandma this bad before. Mom's gonna kill me if something happens to Grandma. Please help us."

"What's her name?" Lawee asks as she reaches for her oxygen equipment. Lawee notices the discolored and dirty cannula on the woman's face and the oxygen canister lying down beside the wheelchair. The woman is clearly in distress. She is gasping for air as she stares at Lawee through eyes that look unfocused and scared.

"It's Joanne," the young girl answers. "Her name is Joanne. My name is Becky. Please, can you help her?"

Importance of Oxygen

OBJECTIVES

2. Explain the benefits of supplemental oxygen.

3. Explain the indications of supplemental oxygen.

The air in our environment contains approximately 21% oxygen. This concentration of oxygen is more than adequate when all body systems are working properly. When a patient becomes suddenly ill or injured, the normal flow of oxygen throughout the body can be diminished or disrupted.

A patient may need oxygen for many reasons, including respiratory or cardiac compromise, cardiac arrest, shock, major blood loss, injury to the lungs or the chest, airway obstruction, or stroke, just to name a few. The most common indications that a patient may be in need of supplemental oxygen are abnormal signs and symptoms, a significant mechanism of injury, or an increased level of distress:

- *Abnormal signs and symptoms.* These include abnormal vital signs, significant pain, or any complaint that is out of the ordinary.
- *Significant mechanism of injury.* Any person who has suffered a significant injury, regardless if there is an open wound or not, may have sustained damage to the circulatory system resulting in a disruption in normal blood flow to all the vital organs.
- *Increased level of distress.* This refers to anyone who appears to be in significant distress as indicated by difficulty breathing or significant pain.

IS IT SAFE?

It is important to understand that oxygen is a drug. If misused, it can be harmful to some patients. Always follow local protocols when providing supplemental oxygen.

supplemental oxygen ▶ a supply of 100% oxygen for use with ill or injured patients.

oxygen concentration ▶ the amount of oxygen being delivered to a patient.

Many ill or injured patients may benefit from supplemental oxygen. **Supplemental oxygen** is a source of 100% oxygen. It is typically stored in metal or composite cylinders that are available in a wide variety of shapes and sizes. The term **oxygen concentration** refers to the actual percentage of oxygen being delivered to the patient. It is dependent on the delivery device being used and how much room air is being mixed with the oxygen supply. Supplemental oxygen usually is mixed with room air, which is 21% oxygen.

From the Medical Director

Use of Oxygen

Recent research has brought into question the value of supplemental oxygen administration by Emergency Medical Responders as well as other EMS providers. It appears that for some conditions such as cardiac arrest and chest pain, too much oxygen can actually be harmful. Too much oxygen can result in poor neurologic outcomes for those who survive cardiac arrest and larger heart attacks. However, the use of oxygen is deeply engrained into medical practice, and it may take time to fully determine when it is most appropriate to administer or withhold oxygen. Always follow your Medical Director's advice.

So, the actual oxygen concentration available to the patient is somewhere between 21% and 100%.

The air we exhale contains approximately 16% oxygen. Providing rescue breaths without supplemental oxygen provides the patient with only the minimum oxygen required for short-term survival. By providing supplemental oxygen, you will be able to greatly increase the oxygen concentration delivered to your patient.

Many patients may benefit from supplemental oxygen. However, too much oxygen may be harmful to some patients. Be sure to consult with your instructor and local protocols to confirm the standard of care for providing oxygen in your system, area, or region.

Hazards of Oxygen

There are certain hazards associated with oxygen administration, including the following:

- Oxygen used in emergency care is stored under pressure (2,000 pounds per square inch [psi] or greater). If the tank is punctured or if a valve breaks off, the supply tank and the valve can become projectiles, injuring anyone nearby.
- Oxygen supports combustion and causes fire to burn more rapidly.
- Oxygen and oil do not mix. When they come into contact with one another, there can be a severe reaction, which may cause an explosion.

Oxygen Therapy Equipment

A typical oxygen-delivery system includes an oxygen source (oxygen cylinder), a *regulator*, and a delivery device (Figure 9.1). Occasionally a **humidifier** will be added to provide moisture to the oxygen if the patient will be on the system for more than 30 minutes. (Some EMS systems will not allow the use of humidifiers because of improper storage and potential contamination.)

Oxygen Cylinders

When providing oxygen in the field, the standard source of oxygen is a seamless steel or aluminum cylinder filled with pressurized oxygen. The maximum service pressure is equal to

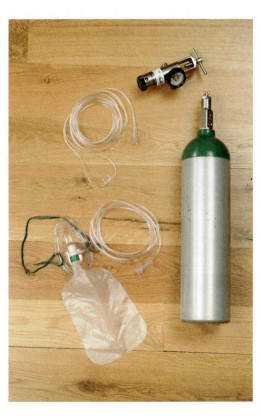

Figure 9.1 • An oxygen-delivery system.

KEY POINT ▼

Oxygen is considered a medication and must be prescribed by a physician. All EMS systems and agencies have a physician responsible for medical oversight who authorizes the use of oxygen for the EMS personnel within their system.

KEY POINT ▼

Patients with a history of chronic lung problems have what is known as a "hypoxic drive." That is, they have become used to the lower levels of oxygen in their lungs and blood. Prolonged use of high-concentration oxygen can lower their drive to breathe, causing respiratory arrest in some patients. This is *not* common in the prehospital setting and is rarely a concern for the Emergency Medical Responder. Never withhold supplemental oxygen from someone in respiratory distress.

OBJECTIVE

4. Explain the potential hazards of working with high-pressure cylinders.

humidifier ▶ a device used to increase the moisture content of supplemental oxygen.

IS IT SAFE?

Oxygen is stored under very high pressure. You must always lay the oxygen cylinder on its side to prevent it from falling over and becoming damaged.

OBJECTIVE

6. Differentiate between the common sizes of oxygen cylinders used in EMS.

Figure 9.2 • Various-size portable oxygen cylinders.

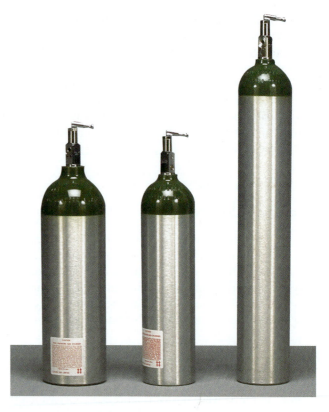

2,000 to 2,200 psi. Cylinders come in various sizes, identified by letters. The smaller sizes that are practical for the Emergency Medical Responder include (Figure 9.2):

- Jumbo D cylinder, which contains about 640 liters of oxygen
- D cylinder, which contains about 425 liters of oxygen
- E cylinder, which contains about 680 liters of oxygen

Part of your duty as an Emergency Medical Responder is to make certain that the oxygen cylinders are full and ready to use before they are needed for patient care. In most cases, you will use a **pressure gauge** to determine the pressure remaining in the tank. The pressure gauge is located directly on the **pressure regulator** and will display the actual pressure inside the tank. A cylinder is considered full at 2,000 psi, half full at 1,000 psi, and one quarter full at 500 psi.

The length of time that you can use an oxygen cylinder depends on the pressure in the cylinder and the flow rate being delivered to the patient. The method of calculating cylinder duration is shown in Table 9.1.

pressure gauge ▶ the device on a regulator that displays the pressure inside a cylinder.

pressure regulator ▶ the device used to lower the delivery pressure of oxygen from a cylinder.

KEY POINT ▼

You cannot tell if an oxygen cylinder is full, partially full, or empty by lifting or moving the cylinder. You must always check the pressure in the cylinder by using the pressure gauge.

TABLE 9.1	Duration of Flow Formula
SIMPLE FORMULA	

$$\frac{\text{Gauge pressure in psi} - \text{residual pressure} \times \text{constant}}{\text{Flow rate in liters/minute}} = \text{Safe duration of flow in minutes}$$

Residual Pressure = 200 psi Cylinder Constant

D = 0.16	G = 2.41
E = 0.28	H = 3.14
M = 1.56	K = 3.14

Determine the life of a D cylinder that has a pressure of 2,000 psi and a flow rate of 10 LPM.

$$\frac{(2,000 - 200) \times 0.16}{10} = \frac{288}{10} = 28.8 \text{ minutes}$$

Most EMS agencies keep a supply of full oxygen cylinders on hand. When a cylinder gets below a predetermined pressure, it should be replaced with a full tank or refilled depending on the procedure where you are working. Many agencies consider 500 psi to be the minimum service pressure for an oxygen cylinder. Oxygen cylinders should never be allowed to go completely empty. If they do, moisture can accumulate inside the tank and cause oxidation or rust to develop. For this reason, never allow the pressure in an oxygen cylinder to fall below 200 psi.

continued

"It looks like her tank is empty," says Matt. "I'm going to transfer her to our tank and switch to a nonrebreather, if that's good with you?"

"Sounds like a plan. You do that while I try to get a respiratory rate," says Lawee.

Joanne's breathing is very labored. They can hear wheezing without a stethoscope. Her skin is cool and almost translucent looking. She is sitting in the tripod position, unable to speak but a few words at a time.

"Becky," Lawee says as she jots down Joanne's respiratory rate. "You said your grandma is on oxygen all the time,

but when we got here, her tank was empty. Do you have any idea how long she has been going without oxygen?"

"No," Becky admits sheepishly. "My brother and I have had to take care of her since we had to cut down on the caretaker's hours. I don't even know how to turn on the oxygen or who to call to order it."

"Okay, Joanne," Matt says to the patient, as the reassuring hiss of oxygen fills the reservoir bag of the nonrebreather mask. "Just breathe as normally as you can. The oxygen is going to help you breathe easier. You are going to be fine, Joanne. We have an ambulance on the way"

Oxygen System Safety

While all oxygen systems are designed with safety in mind, there are several tips that you should be aware of when working with them. The following are some general guidelines to keep in mind with working with high-pressure cylinders:

- Never allow smoking around oxygen equipment.
- Never use oxygen equipment around open flames or sparks.
- Never use grease or oil on devices that will be attached to an oxygen cylinder. Do not handle those devices when your hands are greasy.
- Never put tape on the cylinder outlet or use tape to mark or label any oxygen cylinder or oxygen-delivery equipment. The oxygen can react with the adhesive left behind and produce a fire.
- Never store a cylinder near high heat or in a closed vehicle that is parked in the sun.
- Always keep portable oxygen cylinders lying flat. If you must stand a tank upright, keep your hand on the tank to prevent it from falling over.
- Always use the pressure gauges and regulators that are intended for use with oxygen and the equipment you are using.
- Always ensure that the O ring is in good condition and free of cracks or divots. This will help prevent dangerous leaks.
- Tighten all valves and connections hand-tight only.
- Open and close all valves slowly.
- Always store reserve oxygen cylinders in a cool, ventilated room as approved by your EMS system.
- Always have oxygen cylinders hydrostatically tested. This should be done every five years for steel tanks (three years for aluminum cylinders). The date for retesting should be stamped on the top of the cylinder near the valve.

The U.S. DOT requires that all compressed gas cylinders be inspected and pressure tested at specific intervals. The cylinders used in EMS that contain medical-grade oxygen must be tested every five years. That test is commonly referred to as a **hydrostatic test**. It is used to confirm that no leaks exist. For that test, a visual inspection of the tank must be performed first. Then the tank is filled with water and pressurized to five-thirds the service

OBJECTIVE

5. Explain the safe practices when working with high-pressure cylinders.

KEY POINT ▼

Some oxygen cylinders have met rigorous inspection and testing standards and are allowed to go up to 10 years between test dates. Stamped into the crown of those cylinders immediately following the hydrostatic test date is a five-pointed star.

hydrostatic test ▶ the process of testing high-pressure cylinders.

pressure, or approximately 3,360 psi. The most recent hydrostatic test date must be stamped into the crown of the cylinder and easily readable.

Oxygen Regulators

OBJECTIVE

7. Describe the purpose and functions of an oxygen regulator.

As you know, the pressure in a full oxygen cylinder is approximately 2,000 psi. This is much too high of a pressure to be used directly from the cylinder. A specialized regulator, sometimes called a pressure regulator or oxygen regulator, must be connected to the oxygen cylinder before it may be used to efficiently deliver oxygen to a patient (Figure 9.3).

All oxygen regulators have a minimum of three functions:

- *Reduce tank pressure.* The first function of a regulator is to reduce the pressure of the oxygen leaving the tank to allow for efficient delivery to the patient. It can reduce the pressure from 2,000 psi to between 30 and 70 psi.
- *Display tank pressure.* The second function of the regulator is to display the pressure contained inside the cylinder. It does so by way of a high-pressure gauge. The gauge displays the actual (unregulated) pressure remaining inside the tank. It also lets you know how much oxygen you have left in the tank.
- *Control the delivery of oxygen.* The third function of most regulators is the **liter flow** valve, sometimes called the *flow meter*. The liter flow valve is an adjustable dial on the regulator that allows you to select a specific flow of oxygen to the patient in liters per minute (LPM). An oxygen delivery device, such as a mask, can be connected to the liter flow valve. Then, when it is placed on the patient, it can deliver supplemental oxygen.

liter flow ▶ the measure of the flow of oxygen being delivered through a mask or cannula.

Connecting the Regulator

On portable oxygen cylinders, a yoke assembly is used to secure the pressure regulator to the cylinder valve assembly. The yoke has pins that must mate with the corresponding holes found in the valve assembly. This is called a **pin index system** (Figure 9.4). The position of the pins varies for different gases to prevent an oxygen-delivery system from being connected to a cylinder containing another gas. There are three pins on the regula-

pin index system ▶ the safety system used to ensure that the proper regulator is used for a specific gas, such as oxygen.

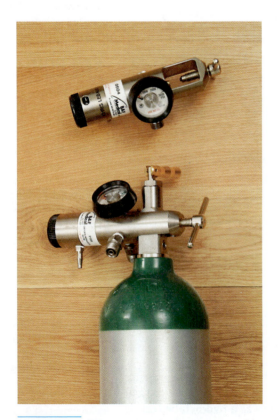

Figure 9.3 • Pressure regulators, one on and one off the tank.

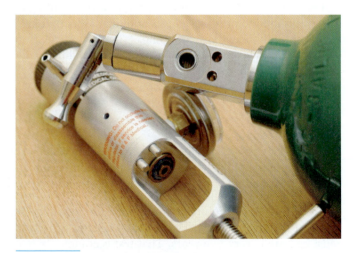

Figure 9.4 • The PIN safety system.

tor that must be matched to three holes on the tank valve. The largest pin is the oxygen port. This pin is the pathway through which oxygen flows from the cylinder to the regulator. Before placing the regulator onto the tank, you must ensure the presence of an O ring. The **O ring** sits over the oxygen port and serves as a gasket and ensures an airtight seal between the regulator and the tank valve.

Before connecting the pressure regulator to an oxygen-supply cylinder, open the cylinder valve slightly for just a second to clear dirt and dust out of the delivery port. This is called "cracking" the cylinder valve.

Humidifiers

A humidifier is an unbreakable container of sterile water that can be placed in-line between the flow valve and the oxygen-delivery device. As the oxygen from the cylinder passes through the water, it picks up moisture from the water. In turn, the oxygen becomes more comfortable for the patient to breathe. Non-humidified oxygen delivered to a patient over a long period of time (usually more than 20 minutes) will dry out the mucous membranes in the airway and lungs.

For the short period of time in which the patient receives oxygen in the field, this is not usually a problem. A problem does arise, though, when humidifiers are not used appropriately. Too often, the task of changing them between patients is overlooked, or the device is opened but not used, which allows it to become contaminated over time. Because of this infection risk and the fact that they are not required for short transports, many EMS systems no longer use humidifiers.

Oxygen-Delivery Devices

You will encounter two types of patients who may need supplemental oxygen: those who are breathing on their own and those who are breathing inadequately or not at all. There are two types of devices that help deliver oxygen to patients who are breathing on their own. The nasal cannula and the nonrebreather mask are the main oxygen-delivery devices used for the field administration of oxygen to breathing patients (Table 9.2).

Nasal Cannula

The **nasal cannula** delivers oxygen into the patient's nostrils by way of two small plastic prongs (Figure 9.5). Its efficiency is greatly reduced by nasal injuries, colds, and other types of nasal airway obstruction. A nasal cannula has an effective flow rate of between 1 and 6 LPM. Those flow rates will provide the patient with an increased oxygen concentration between 25% and 45%. The approximate relationship of oxygen concentration to LPM flow is:

25% oxygen with 1 LPM

29% oxygen with 2 LPM

33% oxygen with 3 LPM

37% oxygen with 4 LPM

41% oxygen with 5 LPM

45% oxygen with 6 LPM

O ring ▶ the gasket used to seal a regulator to the oxygen cylinder.

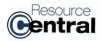

Read more about oxygen humidifiers and about oxygen-delivery devices.

OBJECTIVE

8. Explain the indications for the use of a nasal cannula.

nasal cannula ▶ a device used to deliver low concentrations of supplemental oxygen to a breathing patient.

KEY POINT ▼

Never withhold the concentration of oxygen that is appropriate for the patient. If you are in doubt as to how much oxygen to deliver, contact medical direction for advice.

TABLE 9.2 | Oxygen-Delivery Devices

	FLOW RATE	% OXYGEN DELIVERED	SPECIAL USE
Nasal cannula	1 to 6 LPM	25% to 45%	Most medical patients in mild to moderate distress
Nonrebreather mask	Start with 10 LPM; practical high is 15 LPM	80% to 95%	Most trauma and medical patients in moderate to severe distress

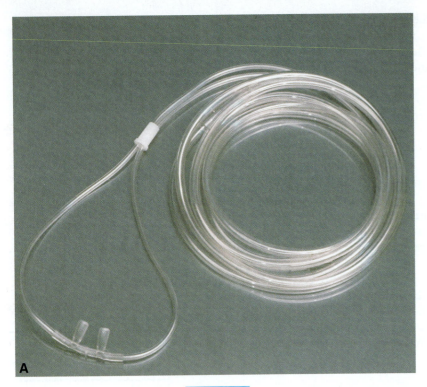
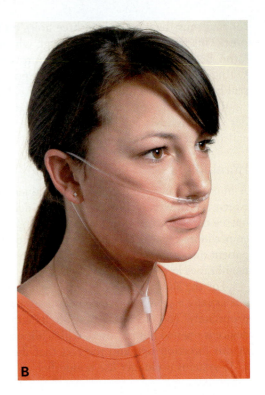

Figure 9.5 • (A) Example of a nasal cannula and (B) a nasal cannula properly placed on the face of the patient.

OBJECTIVE

9. Explain the indications for the use of a nonrebreather mask.

KEY POINT ▼

It is important to understand that the proper use of a nonrebreather mask is not dependent on any particular flow rate. The best way to determine proper flow rate is to choose a rate that allows the reservoir bag to deflate slightly when the patient takes a breath in and to completely reinflate before the next breath.

nonrebreather mask ▶ a device use to deliver high concentrations of supplemental oxygen.

reservoir bag ▶ a device attached to an oxygen-delivery device that temporarily stores oxygen.

For every 1 LPM increase in oxygen flow, you deliver a 4% increase in the concentration of oxygen. At 4 LPM and above, the patient's breathing patterns may prevent the delivery of the stated percentages. At 5 LPM, drying of the nasal membranes is likely. After 6 LPM, the device does not deliver any higher concentration of oxygen and may be uncomfortable for most patients.

Nonrebreather Mask

A **nonrebreather mask** is used when the patient requires a higher concentration of oxygen than the nasal cannula can deliver. The nonrebreather mask consists of a face mask, a one-way valve, and a **reservoir bag.** The reservoir bag must remain full and will ensure that the patient receives the highest concentration of oxygen possible.

It is important that you inflate the reservoir bag *before* placing the mask on the patient's face (Figure 9.6). A full reservoir bag will ensure that the patient will receive a supply of 100% oxygen directly from the reservoir with each breath. This is done by using your finger to cover the one-way valve inside the mask between the mask and the reservoir. Care must be taken to ensure a proper seal with the patient's face. The reservoir must not deflate by more than one-third when the patient takes his deepest breath. You can maintain the volume in the bag by adjusting the oxygen flow. The patient's exhaled air does not return to the reservoir; instead, it is vented through the one-way flaps or portholes on the mask. The minimum flow rate when using this mask is 8 LPM, but a higher flow (12 to 15 LPM) may be required.

Venturi Mask

Another common type of oxygen mask is called the Venturi mask. The key to the Venturi mask is its adjustable "jets" that allow the user to more accurately determine the specific oxygen concentration delivered to the patient. Venturi masks are more commonly seen and used in the hospital setting.

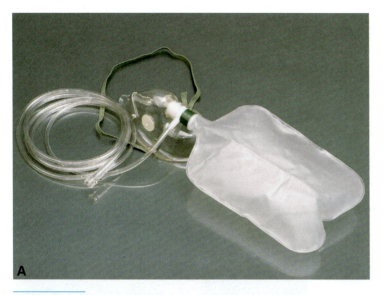

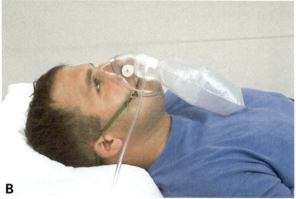

Figure 9.6 • (A) Example of a nonrebreather mask and (B) a nonrebreather properly placed on the face of a patient.

Blow-by Delivery

Another technique for the delivery of supplemental oxygen to a breathing patient is called the blow-by method. It can be used for any patient who will not tolerate having a traditional mask or cannula placed on his face. With the blow-by technique, you can use a nonrebreather mask set to 15 liters and simply have the patient hold the mask as close to the face as comfortable. This technique is especially good for small children who are typically frightened by a mask or cannula.

Be sure that the mask is held as close to the face as possible to ensure that a good supply of oxygen reaches the patient.

Administering Oxygen

Scans 9.1 and 9.2 will take you step-by-step through the process of preparing the oxygen-delivery system and administering oxygen.

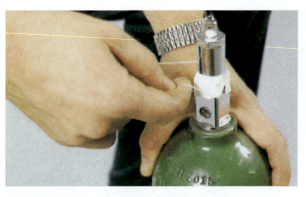

9.1.1 | Remove the plastic wrapper or cap protecting the cylinder outlet.

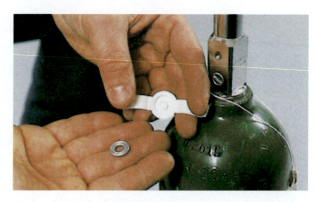

9.1.2 | Keep the plastic washer that is used in some setups.

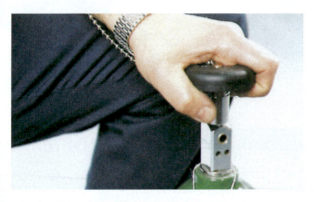

9.1.3 | "Crack" the main valve for one second.

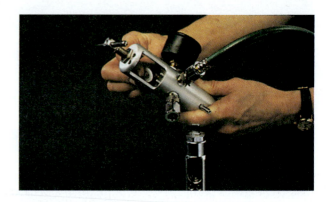

9.1.4 | Place cylinder valve gasket on regulator oxygen port.

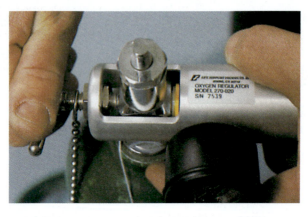

9.1.5 | Tighten T-screw hand-tight. Do not overtighten because this can crush or crack the washer, thus causing a leak.

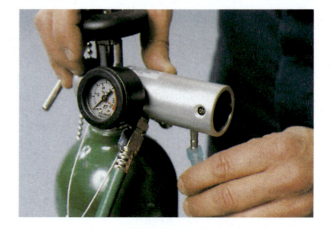

9.1.6 | Attach tubing and delivery device.

Administration of Oxygen to a Nonbreathing Patient

There are three devices commonly used in the EMS setting to provide high-concentration oxygen while providing rescue breaths for a nonbreathing patient. They are the pocket mask with oxygen inlet, the bag-mask device, and the demand-valve device. When using these devices, an appropriate airway adjunct should be inserted, if you are allowed and trained to do so. Always follow local protocol.

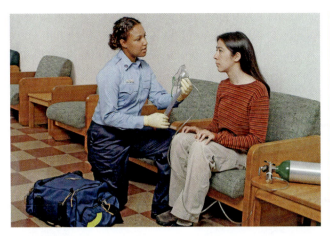

9.2.1 | Explain the need for oxygen therapy.

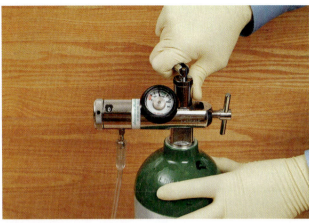

9.2.2 | Open the main valve.

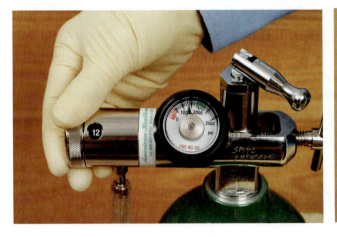

9.2.3 | Attach the delivery device and adjust flow meter.

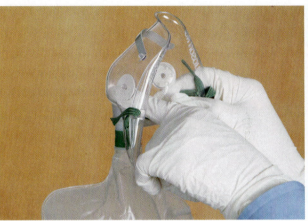

9.2.4 | Be sure to fill the reservoir bag prior to placing it on the patient by turning on the flow and placing your finger over the valve in the mask.

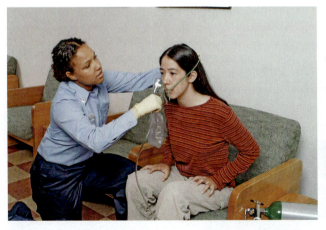

9.2.5 | Position the oxygen-delivery device on the patient.

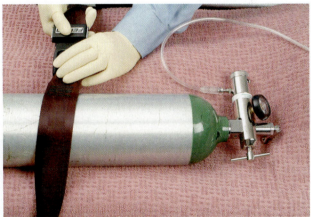

9.2.6 | Secure the cylinder during transfer.

Pocket Mask with Oxygen Inlet

The pocket face mask connected to an oxygen supply can deliver higher concentrations of oxygen than a pocket mask alone. Using **oxygen supply tubing**, connect one end to the liter flow valve of the regulator and the other end to the oxygen inlet on the pocket mask (Figure 9.7). Turn on the liter flow to 10 LPM and use the mask as you normally would to provide rescue breaths.

oxygen supply tubing ▶ the tubing used to connect a delivery device to an oxygen source.

Chapter 9 Oxygen Therapy **179**

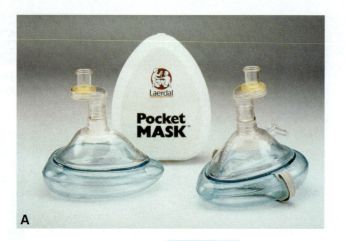

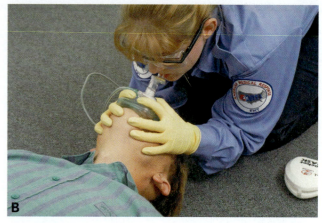

Figure 9.7 • (A) One mask without and one with an oxygen inlet. (B) Rescuer delivering her own breath through the mask's chimney plus oxygen through the inlet.
(Photo courtesy of Laerdal Medical Corporation)

Bag-Mask Device

Most bag-mask devices are capable of accepting supplemental oxygen. When available, attach the bag-mask to an oxygen source and adjust the flow to no less than 15 LPM. Many bag-mask devices have an oxygen reservoir (long tube or bag) to increase the oxygen concentration delivered to the patient. Used without a reservoir, it will deliver approximately 50% oxygen. Used with a reservoir, it will deliver an oxygen concentration up to 100%.

Maintain an open airway, hold a tight mask-to-face seal, squeeze the bag to deliver oxygen, and release the bag to allow for a passive exhalation (Figure 9.8). There is no need to remove the mask when the patient exhales. The bag mask also can be used to assist the breathing efforts of a patient who has inadequate respirations (as in a drug overdose).

The bag mask works best when used by two rescuers. The first rescuer obtains a tight mask-to-face seal and keeps the airway open. The second rescuer squeezes the bag to achieve good chest rise and fall.

> ▶ **GERIATRIC FOCUS** ◀

Many geriatric patients have dentures. When dentures are securely in place, they provide necessary support for the lips, making a mask seal much easier. When dentures are loose or missing, making a good mask seal can be much more challenging.

Figure 9.8 • Bag-mask device connected to an oxygen supply.
(Photo courtesy of Laerdal Medical Corporation)

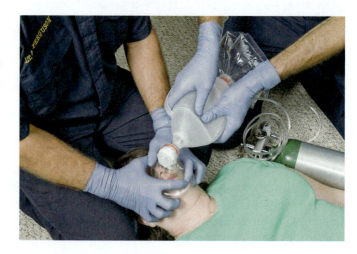

Demand-Valve Device

Extreme caution should be used when ventilating a patient with a demand-valve device. It is very easy to overinflate the lungs, which inhibits blood flow to the heart in cardiac arrest. It can easily cause air to enter the stomach, resulting in gastric distention and vomiting.

Demand-Valve Device

A demand-valve device delivers oxygen through a specialized regulator. That regulator can deliver 100% oxygen "on demand" when the patient inhales. The Emergency Medical Responder also can activate the regulator by pressing a trigger. Standard features of the demand-valve device include a peak flow rate of 40 LPM, an inspiratory pressure-relief valve that opens at approximately 60 cm of water pressure, and a trigger that enables the rescuer to use both hands to maintain a mask seal while activating the device.

To operate a demand valve, place an appropriate-size mask on the demand valve. Follow the same procedures for placing and sealing the mask as you would for the bag-mask device. Then press the trigger to deliver oxygen until the patient's chest rises. Release the trigger after the chest inflates and allow for passive exhalation. Repeat this step as often as necessary for the specific patient. If the chest does not rise, reposition the head or reopen the airway, check for obstructions, reposition the mask, check for a seal, and try again.

Monitor your patient carefully whenever you are providing assisted ventilations. High pressure caused by forcing air or oxygen into a patient's airway can cause air to enter the esophagus and fill the stomach. Air distends the stomach, which presses into the lung cavity and reduces expansion of the lungs. To avoid or correct this problem, carefully maintain a patent airway and mask-to-face seal, and ensure good chest rise and fall with each breath. Do not continue to provide ventilations after chest rise; allow passive exhalation after each breath.

If you suspect neck injury, have an assistant manually stabilize the patient's head or use your knees to prevent head movement. Bring the jaw to the mask without tilting the head or neck and trigger the mask to ventilate the patient.

General Guidelines for Oxygen Therapy

Many patients may benefit from supplemental oxygen. However, there are some patients where too much oxygen may be harmful. Be sure to consult with your instructor and local protocols to confirm the standard of care for providing oxygen in your system, area, or region.

Examples of situations where a patient may benefit from supplemental oxygen include:

- Apnea(not breathing)
- Heart failure
- Shock

It is always important to explain to your patient what you are doing when providing care. Attempting to place a cannula or mask on his face without explaining what you are doing can frighten him. Once frightened, he may have a hard time feeling comfortable with you or the care you are attempting to provide.

Before placing the device on the patient's face, explain that you would like to provide him with oxygen and that it will help him feel better. Show him the device and explain how it works and how it will fit on his face. Then gently place the device on his face and confirm that he is comfortable with it. Adjust it as necessary to make it comfortable. Remind him to breathe as normally as possible.

KEY POINT ▼

Bag-mask and demand-valve devices are not recommended when performing one-rescuer CPR. The preferred device for one-rescuer CPR is a pocket mask with supplemental oxygen.

KEY POINT ▼

The demand valve is recommended for use on adult patients only. Due to the difficulty in controlling the flow through the regulator, there is a risk of overinflating a pediatric patient, causing gastric distention.

IS IT SAFE?

Always use caution when providing positive pressure ventilations. It is possible to overinflate the patient's lungs and cause distention of the stomach. Watch carefully for proper rise and fall of the chest with each ventilation.

If your patient is anxious and seems reluctant to accept the device, provide extra reassurance. In the case of a mask, allow him to hold the device and place it himself. This will allow him to remove the device if he feels the need. Sometimes the mask can make a patient feel claustrophobic. Monitor the patient closely and provide reassurance as necessary if his breathing does not improve.

WRAP-UP

"Joanne's respiratory rate has gone from 32 to 24, and it's a little easier for her to breathe now," Lawee reports to the arriving medics. The patient's coloring has slowly returned to her cheeks, and she is sitting up a little straighter.

"Grandma," Becky says as the medics prepare to transfer the patient from her wheelchair. "Calm down, okay? These people are going to help."

Joanne looks worried and reaches out for her granddaughter. "Don't worry, Joanne," Lawee tells her as the medics connect the oxygen mask to their own bottle. "The oxygen will help your breathing."

"Thank you," Joanne mutters softly.

"No problem," Lawee says, as she looks at Matt and smiles, "though oxygen was the real hero here."

CHAPTER REVIEW

Summary

- A constant supply of oxygen is essential to keep all of the vital body systems functioning properly. Sometimes an illness or injury can disrupt the normal flow of oxygen into the body. In those situations, most ill or injured patients will benefit from supplemental oxygen.

- Oxygen is stored and transported in portable containers called cylinders. The oxygen contained in these cylinders is stored under very high pressure (2,000 psi) and can pose a risk to those working around them if not handled properly.

- When working with high-pressure cylinders, it is important to keep the cylinders lying flat on the ground to minimize the chance they could fall over and be damaged. All valves should be opened and closed slowly, and all cylinders should be stored in a cool environment and away from sources of flame or heat.

- There are many different sizes of oxygen cylinders, but the most commonly used cylinders in EMS are the D, Jumbo D, and the E cylinders.

- A pressure regulator is used to reduce the pressure of the oxygen coming out of the cylinder, which makes it usable for patients. In addition to reducing the pressure, the regulator has a pressure gauge that displays how much pressure is in the tank as well as a liter flow valve that allows for regulation of the flow of oxygen to the patient.

- There are two devices commonly used to provide supplemental oxygen for the breathing patient: the nasal cannula and the nonrebreather mask. The cannula can deliver oxygen concentrations up to 44%. The nonrebreather mask is capable of delivering oxygen concentrations up to approximately 90%.

- The amount of supplemental oxygen provided to a patient will be determined based on such things as mechanism of injury, signs and symptoms, and level of distress.

- When a patient is not breathing adequately on his own, you must provide positive pressure ventilations. This can be performed by using a pocket mask, bag mask, or a demand-valve device.

Take Action

IN-SERVICE OR OUT?

One very important safety precaution that often gets overlooked is the check of the hydrostatic test date of each oxygen cylinder. Your agency or training institution probably has oxygen cylinders for patient care or training. Take some time to inspect each cylinder. Then, specifically look for the hydrostatic test date stamped on the top side of the cylinder. Since this test must occur every five years, and a typical cylinder can last for decades, you may find a cylinder with multiple test stamps. Locate the most current date and determine if the cylinder is expired. Should you find a cylinder that is out of date, be sure to let your instructor, supervisor, or equipment officer know immediately.

First on Scene Run Review

Recall the events of the "First on Scene" scenario in this chapter and answer the following questions, which are related to the call. Rationales are offered in the Answer Key at the back of the book.

1. What kind of questions would you ask Becky about her grandma?

2. What kind of respiratory history would Joanne likely have to be on home oxygen?

3. What information should Lawee give the arriving medic?

Quick Quiz

To check your understanding of the chapter, answer the following questions. Then compare your answers to those in the Answer Key at the back of the book.

1. Supplemental oxygen can be helpful to ill or injured patients by:
   a. reducing the concentration of available oxygen.
   b. increasing the concentration of available oxygen.
   c. helping eliminate carbon dioxide.
   d. increasing the concentration of carbon dioxide.

2. Which one of the following best describes the oxygen consumption of a normally functioning human being?
   a. The body requires a constant supply of oxygen at 79%.
   b. The human body needs a minimum of 10% oxygen to survive.
   c. The body exhales an average of 21% carbon dioxide with each breath.
   d. The average exhalation contains an oxygen concentration of between 10% and 16%.

3. All of the following are reasons a patient might need supplemental oxygen EXCEPT a(n):

   a. significant mechanism of injury.
   b. upset over the breakup of a boyfriend.
   c. suspected heart attack.
   d. difficulty breathing.

4. Which one of the following best defines the term *oxygen concentration*?

   a. Available amount of air to the patient
   b. Amount of oxygen remaining in one exhalation
   c. Ratio between oxygen and carbon dioxide
   d. Concentration of oxygen available to the patient

5. The pressure gauge of a full oxygen cylinder will display approximately _____ psi.

   a. 500
   b. 1,000
   c. 1,500
   d. 2,000

6. A typical oxygen regulator will NOT:

   a. display tank pressure.
   b. display ambient air pressure.
   c. control liter flow.
   d. regulate tank pressure.

7. You are caring for a patient complaining of mild shortness of breath and have her on a nasal cannula at 6 liters per minute. What oxygen concentration are you delivering to the patient?

   a. 25%
   b. 29%
   c. 33%
   d. 45%

8. You are caring for a victim of a motor vehicle crash and have placed her on a nonrebreather mask. Which one of the following best describes how you know the liter flow has been adjusted properly?

   a. The patient is able to speak in complete sentences.
   b. The reservoir bag completely deflates with each breath.
   c. You see no movement of the reservoir bag with each breath.
   d. The reservoir bag refills completely between breaths.

9. You are caring for a patient who was ejected from a vehicle that rolled over. She is alert and responsive. Her respirations are 20 times per minute with good tidal volume and unlabored. Which device is most appropriate to deliver oxygen to this patient?

   a. Nasal cannula
   b. Demand valve
   c. Bag-mask device
   d. Nonrebreather mask

10. In reference to the patient in the previous question: The primary reason you decided to provide supplemental oxygen is due to:

    a. the patient's level of distress.
    b. abnormal vital signs.
    c. the mechanism of injury.
    d. the respiratory rate.

11. You are a single rescuer caring for the victim of a cardiac arrest. Your equipment bag along with a supply of oxygen is within reach. Which one of the following is the most appropriate choice for beginning rescue breaths on this patient?

    a. Pocket mask with supplemental oxygen
    b. Bag mask without supplemental oxygen
    c. Mouth-to-mouth
    d. Waiting for another rescuer before beginning rescue breaths

12. The proper placement of a(n) _____ will help ensure an air-tight fit between the regulator and the tank valve.

    a. cannula
    b. Venturi
    c. O ring
    d. demand valve

13. You are caring for a 12-year-old patient who is having severe difficulty breathing. His respirations are 28 times per minute and shallow. The best choice for oxygen therapy for this patient is a:

    a. demand valve.
    b. nasal cannula.
    c. bag mask.
    d. nonrebreather mask.

14. Which one of the devices listed below is recommended for adult patients only and can be used to provide rescue breaths for a nonbreathing patient?

    a. Bag mask
    b. Demand valve
    c. Venturi mask
    d. Pocket mask

15. One of the most common consequences of overinflating a patient during rescue breaths is:

    a. a ruptured lung.
    b. inadequate chest rise.
    c. gastric distention.
    d. a weak mask seal.

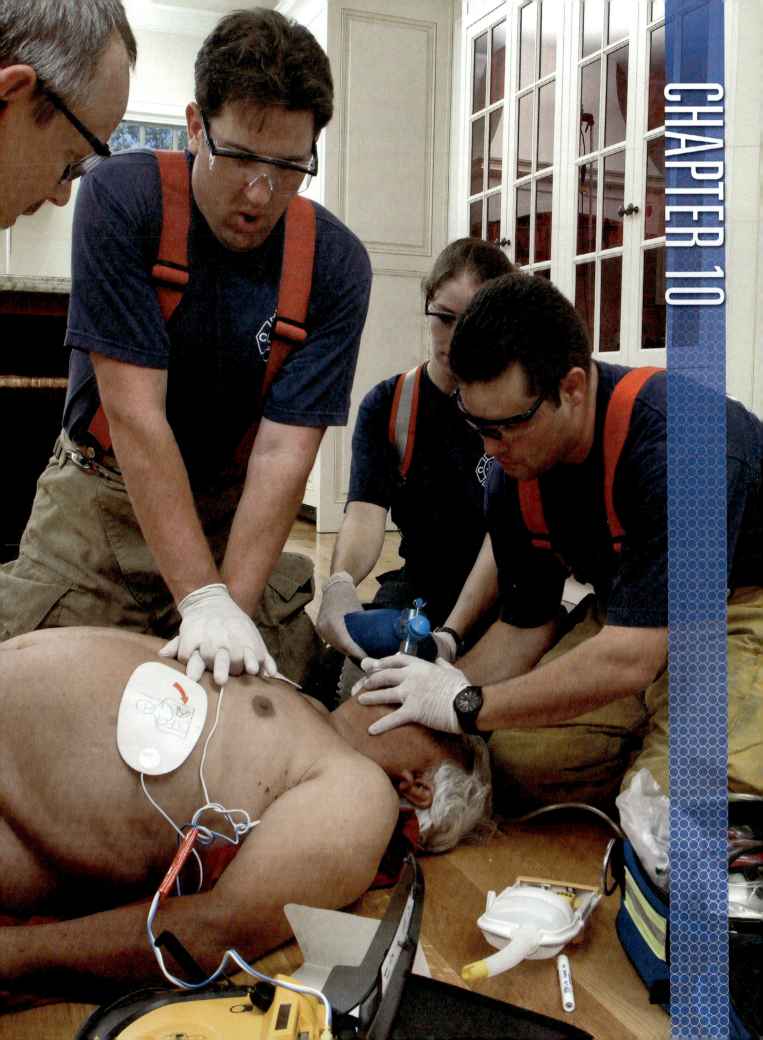

CHAPTER 10

Resuscitation and the Use of the Automated External Defibrillator

• Shock and Resuscitation

• Uses assessment information to recognize shock, respiratory failure or arrest, and cardiac arrest based on assessment findings and manages the emergency while awaiting additional emergency response.

CHAPTER OVERVIEW

Research and statistics from the American Heart Association show that there are approximately 800,000 deaths each year due to cardiovascular disease. Approximately one-third of those people die from sudden cardiac arrest.

Over the years, the techniques of CPR have been refined to increase its effectiveness. It is important to make a point of practicing your CPR skills often and keeping up to date with the latest research findings.

This chapter presents the latest guidelines for CPR as well as the use of the automated external defibrillator.

From the Medical Director

An Epidemic

To gain a better impression of the number who die from cardiac arrest, imagine a fully loaded 757 jetliner crashing. Now imagine three fully loaded 757 jetliners crashing every day, 365 days a year. Would that cause the public to question the safety of air travel? It most certainly would. That is the number of people who are victims of cardiac arrest each year. Yet, little attention is paid to this epidemic. Your efforts as part of the healthcare system can begin to address this issue and make a difference in people's lives.

OBJECTIVES

Upon successful completion of this chapter, the student should be able to:

COGNITIVE

1. Review cardiovascular and respiratory anatomy and physiology in Chapter 4.

2. Define the following terms:

   a. advanced life support (ALS) *(p. 188)*

   b. asystole *(p. 205)*

   c. automated external defibrillator (AED) *(p. 188)*

   d. basic life support (BLS) *(p. 209)*

   e. cardiac arrest *(p. 187)*

   f. cardiopulmonary resuscitation (CPR) *(p. 188)*

   g. chain of survival *(p. 187)*

   h. chest compressions *(p. 188)*

   i. defibrillation *(p. 188)*

   j. fibrillation *(p. 205)*

   k. pediatric patient *(p. 188)*

   l. ventricular fibrillation *(p. 205)*

   m. ventricular tachycardia *(p. 205)*

3. Explain the most common causes of cardiac arrest for adult and pediatric patients. *(p. 188)*

4. Explain the components of the adult "chain of survival." *(p. 187)*

5. Describe the signs of cardiac arrest. *(p. 188)*

6. Explain the steps for performing single-rescuer CPR on an adult, child, and infant. *(p. 190)*

7. Explain the steps for performing two-rescuer CPR on an adult, child, and infant. *(p. 195)*

8. Explain the purpose of an automated external defibrillator (AED). *(p. 205)*

9. Describe the indications and contraindications for the use of an AED. *(p. 208)*

10. Explain the importance of minimizing interruptions during CPR. *(p. 195)*

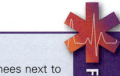
PSYCHOMOTOR

11. Demonstrate the proper technique for performing single-rescuer CPR on a simulated patient in cardiac arrest.

12. Demonstrate the proper technique for performing two-rescuer CPR on a simulated patient in cardiac arrest.

13. Demonstrate the proper use of an AED on a simulated patient in cardiac arrest.

AFFECTIVE

14. Value the importance of prompt assessment and action for patients of cardiac arrest.

15. Demonstrate an understanding of the needs of family members of a victim of cardiac arrest.

"What do you think, Chris?" Kim Jerika, security manager for Western Legends Hotel and Casino, is examining a CCTV video screen closely. "Chris?" She turns to see why the hotel's lead security agent hasn't answered her.

Chris sits several feet from her, both hands on his chest and face ghostly pale. "What's wrong, Chris? Chris?"

She stands quickly, sending her chair crashing into a metal rack of DVD cases. Chris looks up at her, his bulging eyes reflecting the wall of video monitors next to him. He tries to speak several times and then collapses into a heap onto the floor.

"Chris!" Kim screams and drops to her knees next to him, shaking his shoulders. "Are you okay?" There is no response and his eyes, partially hidden behind half-closed lids, stare vacantly at her.

"Okay," Kim says to herself. "Okay, calm down. First thing's first." Kim searches her memory for the procedures that she learned in last spring's Emergency Medical Responder course. She takes a deep breath, rolls Chris onto his back, and checks for any signs of breathing.

The Chain of Survival

Chapter 1 describes the chain of human resources and services in the EMS system. If each link in the chain works quickly and efficiently, the EMS system can provide effective pre-hospital emergency care. The American Heart Association's adult **chain of survival** is another linked system of patient-care events that specifically addresses patients in cardiac arrest (Figure 10.1). For a patient to have the best chance of survival following a **cardiac arrest**, each link in the chain of survival must be strong. The links are:

- Immediate recognition of cardiac arrest and *activation of emergency response system*.
- *Early CPR with an emphasis on chest compressions*. The sooner that chest compressions can be initiated, the sooner circulation can be restored to the patient's brain and vital organs.

OBJECTIVE

4. Explain the components of the adult "chain of survival."

chain of survival ▶ the idea that the survival of the patient in cardiac arrest depends on the linkage of early access, early CPR, early defibrillation, and early advanced life support.

cardiac arrest ▶ when the heart stops beating. Also, the ineffective circulation caused by erratic muscle activity in the lower chambers of the heart (ventricular fibrillation).

AHA ECC Adult Chain of Survival

The links in the new AHA ECC Adult Chain of Survival are as follows:

1. **Immediate recognition of cardiac arrest and activation of the emergency response system**
2. **Early CPR with an emphasis on chest compressions**
3. **Rapid defibrillation**
4. **Effective advanced life support**
5. **Integrated post-cardiac arrest care**

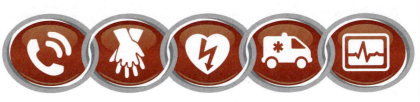

Figure 10.1 • The American Heart Association's Adult Chain of Survival.
Reprinted with permission. 2010 American Heart Association Guidelines for Cardiopulmonary Resuscitation and Emergency Cardiovascular Care, Part 4: CPR Overview. *Circulation.* 2010; 122 [suppl 3]: S676–S684. Copyright 2010 American Heart Association, Inc.

KEY POINT ▼

In some areas, the ABCs of emergency care have one more letter— *D*, which stands for defibrillation.

- *Rapid defibrillation.* **Defibrillation** is the application of an electric shock to a patient's heart in an attempt to convert a lethal rhythm into a normal one. The time from cardiac arrest to defibrillation is an essential factor in the survival rate of out-of-hospital cardiac-arrest patients. The shorter the time between collapse and defibrillation, the better.
- *Effective advanced life support.* **Advanced life support (ALS)** is the care provided by more highly trained EMS personnel such as Advanced Emergency Medical Technicians (AEMTs) and Paramedics. In addition to defibrillators, they provide other interventions, such as advanced airways, intravenous access for fluids, and medications.
- *Integrated post-cardiac arrest care.* A more formal and organized approach to post-cardiac arrest care includes neurologic support and therapeutic hypothermia.

Each link in the chain of survival is essential to improving patient survival. In recent years, defibrillator technology has improved to the point that an **automated external defibrillator (AED)** can be operated with minimal training. Today, AEDs can be found in many public areas such as airports, shopping malls, stadiums, and other public gathering places.

If Emergency Medical Responders in your jurisdiction are permitted to use AEDs, your instructor or Medical Director will provide the appropriate training.

Circulation and CPR

At the center of the circulatory system is the heart. When the heart beats, it acts as a pump. Blood from the body flows into the heart and is sent to the lungs. In the lungs, the blood releases carbon dioxide gathered while circulating through the body and exchanges it for oxygen. This oxygen-rich blood is then returned back to the heart, where it is pumped back out to the body.

There are many things that can affect the proper function of the heart, including injury due to trauma and heart attack. In adults, one of the most common causes of cardiac arrest is a heart attack. In **pediatric patients** the cause of cardiac arrest is most commonly caused by an underlying respiratory problem such as choking or respiratory arrest.

When everything is working properly, the circulatory system keeps oxygenated blood moving to all parts of the body (Figure 10.2). As blood flows through the body, it also gathers nutrients from the small intestines, picks up secretions from special glands, and gives up wastes to the kidneys. This constant exchange is important for proper functioning of the vital organs—and for life.

When the heart stops beating, a person is said to be in cardiac arrest. The signs of cardiac arrest are unresponsiveness, no breathing, and no pulse.

Cardiopulmonary Resuscitation

Cardiopulmonary resuscitation (CPR) is an emergency procedure that involves the application of both external chest compressions and ventilations when heart and lung actions stop. (*Cardio-* refers to the heart, and *pulmonary* refers to the lungs. Resuscitation means to revive.)

During CPR, you must:

- Perform chest compressions to circulate the patient's blood.
- Ensure and maintain an open airway.
- Breathe (ventilate) for the patient.

CPR—How It Works

During the period between clinical death and biological death, irreversible brain damage begins. By performing CPR early, you can circulate oxygenated blood to the brain and help to delay the onset of biological death.

CPR is a series of specific steps that must be performed in a certain manner. CPR begins with the patient lying on his back on a firm surface. You will compress the patient's chest straight down between the nipples. This squeezing of the heart causes an increase in pressure in the chest (thoracic) cavity and forces blood out of the heart and into the arteries to circulate to all parts of the body (Figure 10.3). When compression is relaxed and

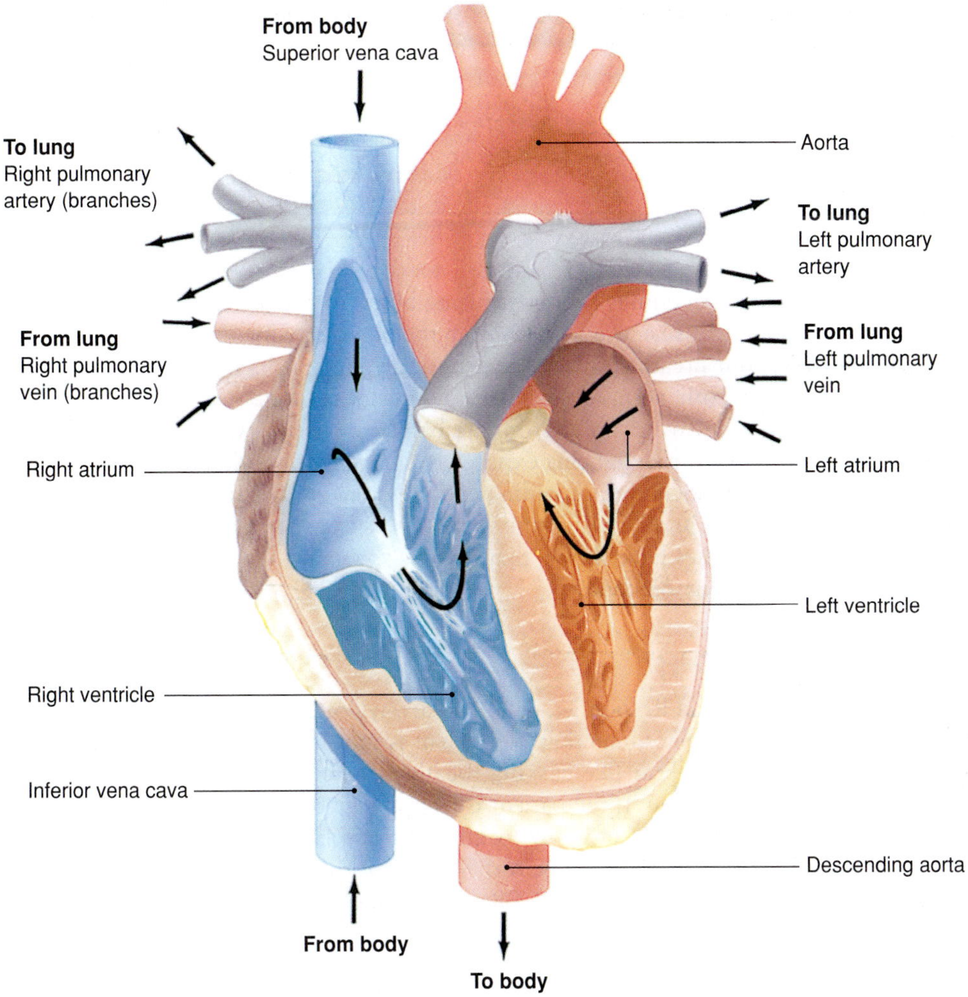

From body
Superior vena cava

To lung
Right pulmonary
artery (branches)

From lung
Right pulmonary
vein (branches)

Right atrium

Right ventricle

Inferior vena cava

From body

Aorta

To lung
Left pulmonary
artery

From lung
Left pulmonary
vein

Left atrium

Left ventricle

Descending aorta

To body

Figure 10.2 • The heart acts as a pump circulating blood to the lungs and the rest of the body.

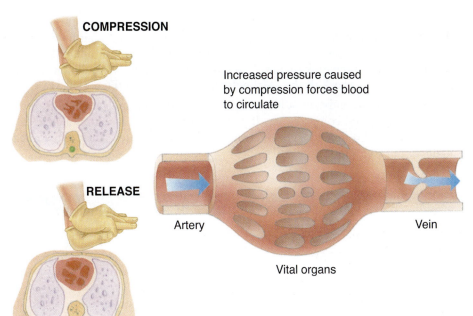

COMPRESSION

RELEASE

Increased pressure caused by compression forces blood to circulate

Artery

Vein

Vital organs

Figure 10.3 • During CPR, pressure in the chest cavity increases with compression, which forces blood into circulation.

Oxygen and CPR

There is oxygen remaining in the blood even after the heart stops beating. The blood in the veins contains oxygen, which can be delivered to the heart and brain simply by providing quality chest compressions.

pressure is released, a vacuum is created, causing blood to flow back into the heart. One-way valves in the patient's heart and veins keep the blood moving in the proper direction.

During CPR, your breaths provide oxygen to the patient's blood, which is then circulated to the brain and other vital organs with each compression.

There may be times when no appropriate barrier device is available and the rescuer does not want to take the risk of being exposed to the patient's bodily fluids. According to the American Heart Association, providing compressions only is significantly better than providing no assistance at all, and it minimizes the risk of the rescuer coming in contact with bodily fluids. Studies have shown that there is some air movement in and out of the lungs with each chest compression.

When to Begin CPR

As an Emergency Medical Responder, you must always perform a primary assessment on your patient. You must determine that the patient is unresponsive and not breathing. He may have breaths that appear like gasping breaths. These gasping breaths are not to be considered normal breathing. If the patient is unresponsive, and not breathing, you must then confirm the absence of a pulse by locating the carotid pulse point in the neck and checking for no more than 10 seconds. If the patient is unresponsive, not breathing, and does not have a pulse, you must begin CPR with chest compressions.

Perform these steps when assessing a patient and performing CPR:

1. Form a general impression of the patient as you approach. Does the patient appear awake or does he appear unresponsive? Start with a gentle tap on the shoulder and shout, "Are you okay?"

2. If the patient is unresponsive, send someone to call 911 and position him on his back on a firm surface.

3. Look for the absence of breathing (no chest rise and fall) or gasping breaths, which are not considered adequate.

4. Assess circulation by feeling for a pulse for at least 5 seconds, but no more than 10 seconds. To assess for a pulse in an adult or child (one year and older), check the carotid pulse in the neck (Figure 10.4). To assess the pulse of an infant (younger than one year), check the brachial pulse in the upper arm (Figure 10.5).

5. If you are alone and cannot locate a pulse, activate 911 and get an AED, if available. Next, begin chest compressions. If you are alone and the patient is a child or an infant, begin CPR immediately and continue for two minutes. Then, if not already done, call 911 and get the AED.

When to Begin CPR

While the steps to determine a patient's responsiveness, breathing, and circulation appear to be made in a particular order, the reality is that all three functions are performed simultaneously. This limits delays in starting CPR, if it is indicated. Another concern many people have is, "What if I start CPR on someone who is not in cardiac arrest?" Studies have shown that CPR is unlikely to stop a patient's heart from beating.

IS IT SAFE?

The American Heart Association strongly suggests the use of appropriate barrier devices when performing CPR on any patient. If you do not have an appropriate barrier device, you may perform compression-only CPR. The act of compressing the chest moves some air in and out of the lungs and is more beneficial than not doing CPR at all.

OBJECTIVE

6. Explain the steps for performing single-rescuer CPR on an adult, child, and infant.

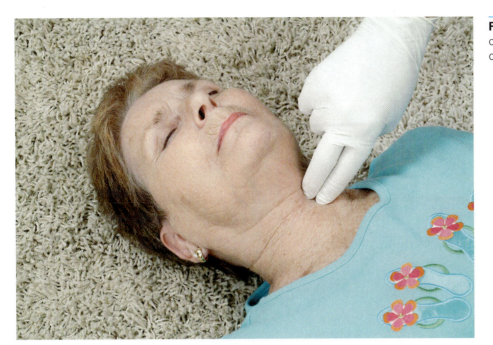

Figure 10.4 • Use the carotid pulse for an adult and a child.

▶ GERIATRIC FOCUS ◀

One of the consequences of aging is that the bowels become less efficient, making constipation a common problem among the elderly. This can be dangerous to those patients who have heart conditions. When they bear down during a difficult bowel movement, the pressure changes inside the chest and abdominal cavity, which can cause a slowing of the heart and dangerous changes in the heart rhythm. This is one of the reasons why many elderly are found unresponsive in the bathroom.

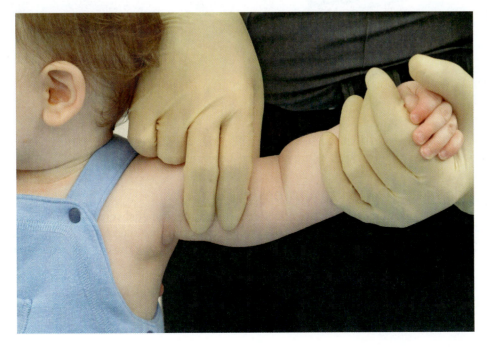

Figure 10.5 • Feel for a brachial pulse for an infant.

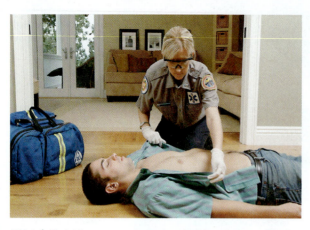

10.1.1 | Quickly move or remove clothing that may be covering the patient's chest.

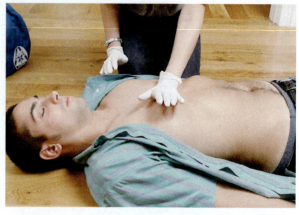

10.1.2 | Then place the heel of one hand on the center of the patient's bare chest, on the lower half of the sternum, along the axis of the sternum.

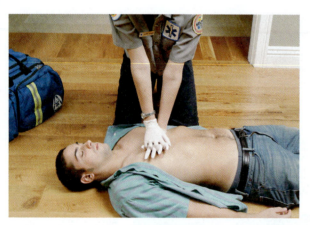

10.1.3 | Put your other hand on top of the first. Either extend or interlace your fingers to keep them off the patient's chest.

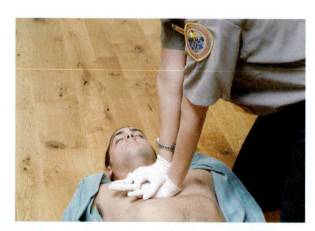

10.1.4 | Make sure your elbows are locked and your shoulders are directly over your hands.

Note: From here on the discussion will center on adult and child CPR, unless otherwise noted. (Infant CPR is addressed later in this chapter.)

Locating the CPR Compression Site

External chest compressions are not effective unless they are delivered to a specific site on the patient's chest (Scan 10.1). If you apply compressions to the wrong site, you may injure the patient or provide ineffective CPR. Steps for locating the compression site on an adult patient are as follows:

1. After determining that the patient needs CPR, place the patient face up on a firm surface, such as the ground or floor. This is necessary for CPR to be effective.

2. Kneel at the patient's side near his shoulder.

KEY POINT ▼

Do not practice CPR on a person with a normal heartbeat, because it can cause serious problems. Practice only on mannequins. Finding the CPR compression site may be practiced on people as well as on mannequins.

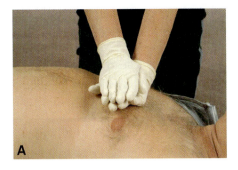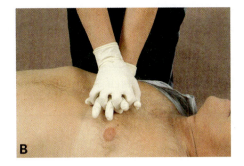

Figure 10.6 • Hand positions at the CPR compression site: (A) extending fingers; (B) intertwining fingers.

3. Quickly move or remove clothing that may be covering the patient's chest.

4. Place the heel of one hand on the center of the patient's bare chest, right between the nipples. This will result in hand placement on the lower half of the sternum.

5. Put your other hand on top of the first. Either extend or interlace your fingers to keep them off the patient's chest.

External Chest Compressions

The correct technique for external chest compressions is as follows:

1. Keep the heels of both hands parallel to each other, one on top of the other, with the fingers of both hands pointing away from you.

2. Keep your fingers off the chest, either extended or interlaced (Figure 10.6). For some it may be easier to do compressions by grasping the wrist of the hand placed at the compression site. Practice different positions until you find one that is comfortable for you.

3. Keep your elbows straight and locked. Do not bend your elbows when delivering or releasing compressions.

4. Position your shoulders over your hands (Figure 10.7). Keep both of your knees on the ground about shoulder width apart.

5. Deliver compressions straight down, and apply enough force to the adult patient to depress the sternum at least two inches. For a child, compress the chest about two inches with the heel of one hand (Figure 10.8). CPR will be effective for the

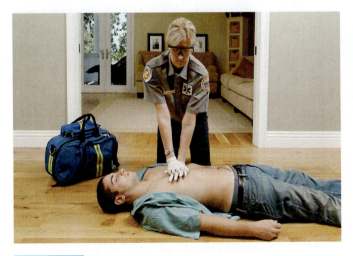

Figure 10.7 • Position your shoulders directly over the compression site.

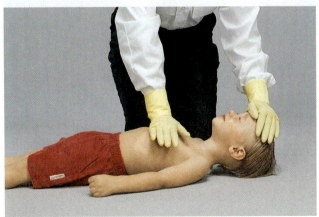

Figure 10.8 • For child chest compression, use the heel of one hand.

patient and less tiring for you if you bend from the hips in a smooth up-and-down motion. Perform chest compressions hard and fast at a rate of at least 100 per minute.

6. Release pressure on the chest completely to allow the patient's heart to refill.

7. You will provide sets of 30 compressions and pause briefly to provide two breaths.

▶ GERIATRIC FOCUS ◀

A youthful skeleton has lots of flexibility and strength not seen in the geriatric skeleton. For this reason, the ability to provide proper chest compressions can be a challenge. It may require significantly more effort to achieve the desired two inches of compression during the first several compressions. In addition, the dry bones of the elderly will be much more brittle and you will likely hear the sound of breaking bones during your first several compressions (crepitus). This is rarely the actual sound of bones breaking but instead the sound of cartilage breaking. This is an expected and necessary outcome of good chest compressions. When you hear the sound of crepitus, double-check your hand position and adjust if necessary. Then continue with chest compressions.

Providing Ventilations During CPR

Follow these guidelines when providing ventilations during CPR:

- After each set of 30 compressions, provide two breaths, one right after the other. Allow the chest to deflate between breaths.
- Deliver each breath slowly over one second.

Do not over-ventilate the patient. If you force too much air into the patient's lungs, the excess air will begin to fill the stomach and may eventually cause the stomach to distend (gastric distention). Provide breaths until you see the chest rise. Then stop and allow the chest to fall.

To provide effective mouth-to-mask ventilations, you may position yourself either at the top of the patient's head or at the patient's side (Figure 10.9). The top of the patient's head is preferred for patients with a pulse but no respirations and for two-rescuer CPR. The lateral position is preferred for one-rescuer CPR. Practice both positions on a mannequin. Remember that good CPR delays the onset of biological death and increases the patient's chances for survival.

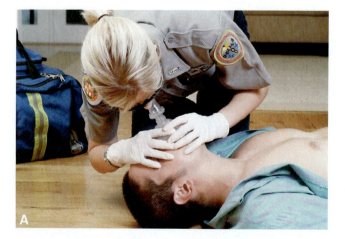
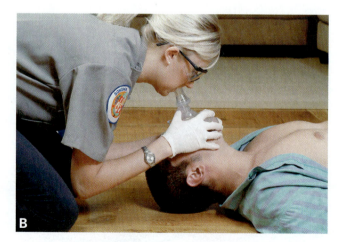

Figure 10.9 • Deliver ventilations from (A) the side the patient's head or (B) from the top of the patient's head.

Due to the loss of calcium in the bones of the elderly, the ribs can become much less flexible and therefore allow far less chest wall movement during breathing. As you check for breathing or provide ventilations, you might not see as much chest rise and fall as on a younger patient. Observe the abdomen for signs of movement, when you assess breathing or provide ventilations. You may see a rise and fall of the abdomen much like you normally would of the chest. Of course, a lack of movement is never good, and you must consider the possibility of a total airway obstruction and provide care accordingly.

Rates and Ratios of Compressions and Ventilations

Effective CPR depends on the correct rate and ratio of compressions and ventilations. For effective CPR, you must:

- Deliver compressions at a rate of at least 100 per minute.
- Provide ventilations at a ratio of two breaths for every 30 compressions. Deliver each breath over one second.
- Once you have begun CPR, avoid interrupting compressions for longer than 10 seconds. Interrupt compressions only for ventilations or for moving the patient.

The rate for chest compressions refers to the speed rather than the number of compressions the rescuer delivers in one minute. Because rescuers must interrupt chest compressions to deliver breaths, the actual number of compressions will be less than 100 per minute. To be sure that you provide compressions at the proper rate of at least 100 per minute, count out loud as you deliver compressions. Deliver two ventilations, each over a period of one second. Quickly relocate the CPR compression site, and continue the next set of compressions.

Effective CPR

You will be performing CPR correctly if:

- Your hands are in the center of the chest over the lower half of the sternum.
- You are compressing the chest at least two inches hard and fast at a rate of at least 100 per minute.
- You see the chest rise and fall during ventilations.
- You interrupt compressions as little as possible.

If you are performing CPR correctly, you may notice the patient's skin color improve, but this does not always occur. Sometimes the patient may try to swallow, gasp, or move his limbs. Those actions do not necessarily mean that he is recovering. However, such movements are signs of life and do mean that you should stop CPR and check for the return of breathing and pulse.

If the patient regains a pulse but is not breathing, stop compressions and continue with ventilations only. Rescue breaths should be delivered at a rate of one breath every five to six seconds or about 10 to 12 breaths per minute. If there is no pulse, continue CPR. Patients will usually require defibrillation and possibly other special medical procedures before they regain heart function. CPR only delays the onset of biological death until special medical procedures can be provided.

OBJECTIVE

10. Explain the importance of minimizing interruptions during CPR.

Adult and Child CPR

The following is a step-by-step procedure for performing one- and two-rescuer CPR. The procedures follow the American Heart Association (AHA) recommendations. The extensive research done by the AHA has found them to be most efficient in saving the lives of

OBJECTIVE

7. Explain the steps for performing two-rescuer CPR on an adult, child, and infant.

TABLE 10.1 | Summary of CPR Techniques

PROCEDURE	ADULT	CHILD	INFANT
Compressions			
Method	Heels of two hands	Heel of one or two hands	Two fingers or two thumbs with hands encircling chest
Depth	At least 2 inches (5 cm)	1/3 the diameter of the chest, or about 2 inches (5 cm)	1/3 the diameter of the chest, or about 1½ inches (4 cm)
Rate	At least 100/minute		
Ventilations (patient with a pulse)			
Method	Barrier device		
Rate	One breath every 5 to 6 seconds	One breath every 3 to 5 seconds	One breath every 3 to 5 seconds
Ratio of Compressions to Breaths			
One rescuer	30:2	30:2	30:2
Two rescuers	30:2	15:2	15:2
Counts			
	1, 2, 3, 4, 5 . . . 30 and breathe, breathe		

patients in cardiac arrest. Also, remember that the following steps are a part of the primary assessment. (See Table 10.1 for a summary of CPR techniques.)

One-Rescuer CPR

To perform one-rescuer CPR on an adult or child (Scan 10.2):

1. Position the patient face up on a hard surface and check for responsiveness. Gently tap the patient's shoulder and ask, "Are you okay?"

2. Check for breathing. If breathing is absent or the patient is only gasping, call out for help. If you are alone with an unresponsive adult patient, call 911 immediately and get a defibrillator, if available. If you are alone with an unresponsive child, provide five cycles of compressions and ventilations (approximately two minutes), then call 911.

3. Check for a pulse for at least 5 seconds, but no more than 10 seconds.

4. If no pulse, begin compressions.

5. Deliver 30 chest compressions. Keep your arms straight, elbows locked, and shoulders directly over the compression site.
   - Compress the adult patient's chest at least two inches. Compressions on a child should be about two inches.
   - Deliver compressions hard and fast at a rate of at least 100 per minute.
   - Release pressure completely to allow the heart to refill.

6. After 30 compressions, open the airway by using the head-tilt/chin-lift maneuver or, if you suspect a spine injury, by using the jaw-thrust maneuver. Provide two slow breaths, one right after the other. Allow the chest to fall between breaths. Watch for chest rise and fall with each breath.

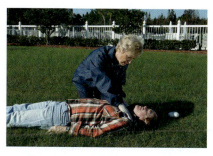

10.2.1 | Establish unresponsiveness and activate EMS. Position the patient and yourself.

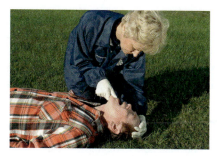

10.2.2 | Look for signs of breathing. If not breathing or only gasping call 911 and check for a pulse.

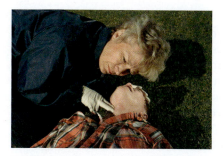

10.2.3 | Check for a pulse for at least 5 seconds but no more than 10 seconds.

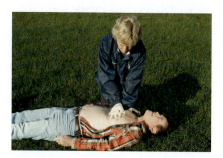

10.2.4 | If no pulse, begin chest compressions.

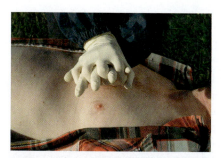

10.2.5 | Provide 30 compressions at a depth of two inches and a rate of at least 100 per minute.

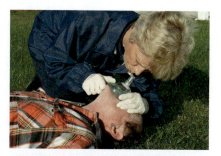

10.2.6 | After 30 compressions, open the airway and provide two ventilations. Each breath should be delivered over one second. Look for chest rise and fall.

7. Continue CPR. Deliver 30 compressions followed by two ventilations.

8. If the patient has a carotid pulse, but no respirations, provide one breath every five to six seconds or 10 to 12 breaths per minute.

9. Do not interrupt CPR for any longer than 10 seconds or longer than is absolutely necessary. If the patient regains a pulse and/or breathing, stop CPR.

Health-care providers, such as Emergency Medical Responders, who have a duty to perform CPR, should also be trained, equipped, and authorized to use an automated external defibrillator (AED).

"Sydney, do you copy?" Kim grabs the portable radio after confirming that Chris is not breathing and doesn't have a pulse.

"Yeah, go ahead," comes a reply with a strong Australian accent.

"I need you to get an ambulance here and bring an AED to the security office right now! Chris is in cardiac arrest!"

She then drops the radio onto the floor next to her, and begins chest compressions.

As Kim counts out loud, she focuses on the hallway monitor to see when Sydney is coming with the AED. Also, because the compressions are making Chris's head bob slowly from side to side, and she doesn't like how his unseeing eyes kept meeting hers.

IS IT SAFE?

Doing CPR as a single rescuer can be very tiring. The more tired you become, the less effective you will be. It is recommended that you change places with another rescuer after every five cycles of 30 compressions and two ventilations. This will minimize the chances of becoming overly tired during the resuscitation effort. It also will provide the best possible CPR for the patient.

KEY POINT ▼

Each rescuer should use his own barrier device with one-way valve and HEPA filter insert to perform two-rescuer CPR safely.

Two-Rescuer CPR

All EMS personnel should learn and remain proficient in both one- and two-rescuer CPR techniques. CPR that is performed by two trained rescuers is more efficient and less tiring for both rescuers (Figure 10.10). Two-rescuer CPR minimizes the transition time between ventilations and compressions and therefore maximizes the effectiveness of both. When performing two-rescuer CPR on a child, the compression-ventilation ratio changes to 15:2.

Use of an AED is also more efficient with two rescuers. One rescuer can begin to set up the AED and attach the electrodes to the patient, while the other rescuer begins a primary assessment of the patient. If you arrive on scene and find that an AED is being used, ensure that the individuals are performing the steps properly and taking the necessary safety precautions. Offer to assist them and support their actions. You also may need to relieve or guide someone who is unsure of the procedure.

Changing from One- to Two-Rescuer CPR

When you assess a patient who has collapsed, your first action is to assess for unresponsiveness. Tap the patient and shout, "Are you okay?" and look for signs of normal breathing. If there is no response and no signs of normal breathing, direct someone to activate the EMS system (or phone the appropriate emergency number). If you are alone, leave the patient long enough to call for help. Then return and continue your assessment. If the patient is a child, provide two minutes of rescue support before calling 911.

In many situations, a bystander may start one-rescuer CPR before Emergency Medical Responders arrive. Upon arrival, assess the patient's pulse before taking over and performing two-rescuer CPR with your partner.

If you arrive as a lone Emergency Medical Responder and determine that a bystander's CPR techniques are inadequate or incorrect, take over one-rescuer CPR. If the bystander is CPR-trained but has no barrier device and is reluctant to ventilate a stranger, perform the ventilations yourself with your own pocket face mask. Have the bystander take over chest compression. Monitor his effectiveness.

If a member of the EMS system is performing CPR when you arrive, begin two-rescuer CPR. To help make a smooth transition from one-rescuer to two-rescuer CPR, follow these steps:

1. If upon arriving on scene you see a rescuer performing CPR, identify yourself. Then, if not already done, activate the EMS system.

2. While the first rescuer is delivering two breaths, get in position next to the patient's chest.

3. After the two breaths, resume chest compressions. The first rescuer should then resume ventilations, providing two ventilations after every 30 of your compressions.

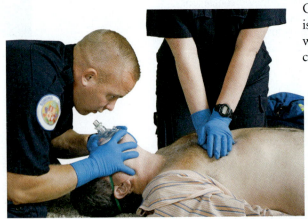

Figure 10.10 • Compressions should be paused to allow for two breaths to be given.

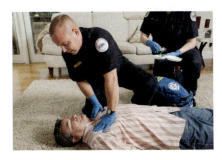

10.3.1 | The first rescuer positions the patient, determines unresponsiveness, and looks for signs of breathing.

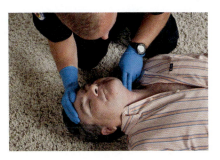

10.3.2 | If there are no signs of breathing, send someone to call 911 and get an AED. Then assess for a pulse for no more than 10 seconds.

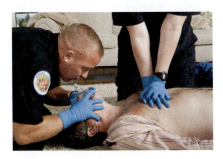

10.3.3 | If no pulse, the second rescuer locates the compression site and begins compressions. Deliver 30 compressions at a rate of at least 100 per minute.

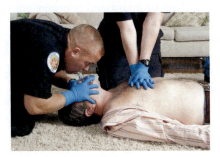

10.3.4 | After each set of 30 compressions the first rescuer provides two slow breaths. The second rescuer should pause compressions to allow for adequate ventilations.

4. Provide compressions at the rate of at least 100 per minute with a pause after every 30 compressions to allow for two ventilations.

5. After two minutes or approximately five cycles of 30 compressions and two ventilations, both you and the other rescuer may change positions.

If the Emergency Medical Responder who arrives on scene to see CPR being performed is equipped with an AED, he should immediately set it up, turn it on, and attach electrodes in preparation for early defibrillation. Do this without interrupting the CPR that is in progress. Stop CPR only when the AED begins to analyze.

Compressions and Ventilations

During two-rescuer CPR, deliver 30 compressions at a rate of at least 100 compressions per minute. After every 30 compressions, deliver two ventilations. The compressor will count aloud so that both rescuers will be able to establish and maintain the correct rate. By hearing the count, the ventilator will be prepared to provide a breath after every 30 compressions while the compressor pauses to allow for adequate ventilation.

CPR Procedure

The complete sequence for two-rescuer CPR is illustrated in Scan 10.3. Your instructor will demonstrate how to ventilate a patient in both positions—top and lateral—using the barrier devices and oxygen-delivery equipment that your jurisdiction requires.

Changing Positions

Regardless of whether or not you or your partner appear tired, it is crucial to rotate positions every two minutes. This prevents fatigue and encourages you to keep your weight off the chest. In addition, ventilations are improved when a new rescuer assumes the role.

Changing Positions

To minimize the effects of fatigue and ensure good chest compressions, rescuers should change positions after ever set of five cycles (approximately two minutes). At the end of 30 compressions, the ventilator will provide two ventilations. Then the rescuers will quickly change positions.

Activating the EMS System

With pediatric patients, it is recommended that the lone Emergency Medical Responder provide two minutes of rescue support before activating EMS. You may be able to carry the child or infant and continue emergency care while calling EMS.

Infant and Neonatal CPR

For purposes of field resuscitation, infant and neonate patients are defined as follows:

- *Infant.* An infant is a baby from birth through one year of age.
- *Neonate.* A neonate is an infant that is less than one month of age.

Positioning the Infant

Just as you do for adults and children, place the infant patient face up on a hard, flat surface. Be aware that when an infant is on his back, his large head can cause the neck to flex forward, potentially closing the airway. To help ensure an open airway, maintain the head in a neutral position. It may be necessary to provide support under the shoulders with a folded blanket or towel (Figure 10.11).

Opening the Airway

For the infant with no spine injury, use the head-tilt/chin-lift maneuver. Tilt the head gently back to a neutral or slightly extended position with one hand. A slight head tilt is often all that is needed. Place your fingers under the bony part of the chin and lift to finish the technique of opening the airway. Be careful not to compress the soft tissues of the neck, because this may obstruct the airway. In cases of suspected spine injury, use the jaw-thrust maneuver.

Assessing Breathing

Assess for signs of breathing. Look for the rise and fall of the chest and abdomen. If there is no breathing, check for the presence of a pulse.

Figure 10.11 • To help manage the airway of an infant, place a folded towel or similar material beneath the shoulders.

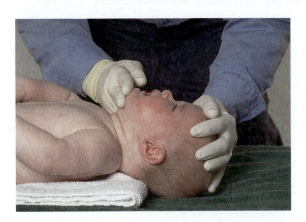

Checking for a Pulse

Follow these steps when assessing for a pulse in an infant:

1. Feel for a pulse at the brachial artery for no less than 5 seconds but no more than 10 seconds.

2. The brachial pulse point is located on the medial side of the arm between the elbow and armpit.

Infant CPR Techniques

Ventilations

If your assessment finds that the infant patient has a good pulse but is not breathing adequately or not at all, provide rescue breaths (ventilations). With the airway open and using an appropriate barrier device, provide ventilations at a ratio of one breath every three to five seconds. The correct volume for each ventilation is the volume that causes the chest to rise. Be careful not to overinflate the lungs, which can cause air to enter the stomach (gastric distention) and, eventually, vomiting.

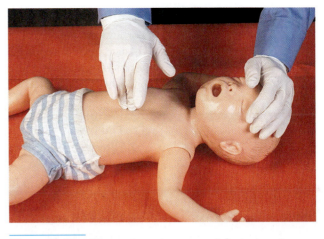

Figure 10.12 • For compressions on an infant, place two fingers on the center of the chest, one finger-width below the nipple line.

You may find it easier to seal your mouth over the infant's mouth and nose. If the patient is a very large infant, seal your mouth over the patient's mouth and pinch the nostrils closed. If you do not see chest rise after repositioning the airway, begin chest compressions.

External Chest Compressions

For infant CPR, external chest compressions and artificial ventilation can easily be performed by a single rescuer or shared between two trained rescuers, depending on available resources.

In infant CPR, apply compressions to the lower half of the breastbone (sternum). Place two fingers on the sternum, one finger-width below the imaginary nipple line (Figure 10.12). Compress the infant's sternum one-third the anterior-posterior diameter of the chest or about one and one-half inches. Compress at a rate of at least 100 per minute.

If possible, maintain an open airway with one hand while compressing the chest with two fingers of the other hand. Provide two rescue breaths after each set of 30 compressions. Watch carefully for the rise and fall of the infant's chest.

When there are two rescuers, the preferred method for chest compressions for the infant is the two-thumbs encircling-hands technique. One rescuer (the compressor) places both thumbs side-by-side over the lower half of the infant's sternum or about one finger-width below the nipple line (Figure 10.13). For very small infants or newborns, you may place one thumb on top of the other. The other rescuer provides ventilations.

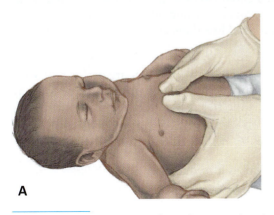
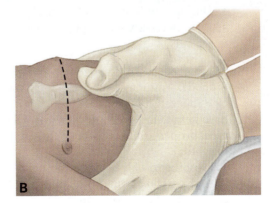

Figure 10.13 • (A) For an infant, place two thumbs side-by-side on the center of the chest just below the nipple line. (B) For newborns (neonate), place two thumbs one on top of the other on the center of the chest just below the nipple line.

Infant CPR Rates and Ratios

For infant CPR, deliver compressions at the rate of at least 100 per minute. For a single rescuer, perform compressions and ventilations at a ratio of 30:2. For two rescuers, perform compressions and ventilations at a ratio of 15:2.

The following steps outline key points for infant CPR:

1. Determine unresponsiveness by gently tapping the bottom of the infant's feet and shouting, "Are you all right?" If no response, then . . .

2. Direct someone to call EMS. If you are alone, provide two minutes of CPR before calling EMS.

3. Position the infant in a supine (face up) position on a flat, hard surface. You may support small infants on your forearm.

4. Check for signs of breathing. If there is no breathing or only gasping breaths, check for a pulse.

5. Determine the presence of a brachial pulse. If there is a pulse but no respirations, provide ventilations at a rate of one breath every three to five seconds. If there is no pulse, or a heart rate of less than 60 per minute, begin compressions.

6. Provide chest compressions. Place two fingers in the center of the chest, one finger-width below the nipple line. Compress at a rate of at least 100 per minute, and provide ventilations at a 30:2 ratio.

Caring for the Neonate

Since neonatal cardiac arrest is almost always due to inadequate breathing or asphyxia, an ABC sequence is recommended. You must first ensure an open and clear airway, provide rescue breaths as appropriate and begin chest compressions. A 3:1 compression-ventilation ratio should be used for most neonatal patients. A 15:2 compression/ventilation ratio (two rescuers) should be considered when the cause of cardiac arrest is cardiac in nature.

Ensuring Effective CPR for All Patients

Unless the proper techniques are performed (Scan 10.4), CPR will not be as effective and the patient has a smaller chance of recovery. For effective CPR for all patients, be sure to remember these important points:

- Place the patient face up (supine) on a hard surface.
- Compress smoothly and to the proper depth. Relax pressure completely between compressions to allow the heart to refill.
- Use the correct rates and ratios.
- Use an appropriate barrier device, place it securely over the face, and ensure a good seal.
- During ventilations, watch the chest for adequate rise and fall.
- Limit necessary interruptions such as pulse and breathing checks to no more than 10 seconds.

In some cases, damage to the chest may occur even when you are performing CPR properly. You may hear a cracking sound while performing compressions, which may be a separation of the cartilage that connects the ribs to the sternum. If you think you have heard ribs crack, do not stop CPR. Check the position of your hands, reposition them properly, and resume CPR. A fractured rib will heal. But stopping CPR will result in death.

Another problem occurs when too much air is forced into the patient's lungs. The excess air overflows out of the lungs and enters the stomach by way of the esophagus. This can result in gastric distention. Do not try to force excess air out of the stomach. To do so might cause the patient to vomit, which could lead to an airway obstruction. In some cases, the patient may *aspirate* (inhale) stomach contents, and if you try to provide breaths, you will force the vomit into the lungs.

IS IT SAFE?

Providing proper chest compressions on an adult will likely result in the separation of the cartilage where the ribs meet the sternum. During the first few compressions, you are likely to feel and hear a popping sound, much like the popping of knuckles. Do not stop CPR. Instead, reconfirm proper hand position and continue to provide good compressions. This is a normal side effect of good chest compressions.

ONE RESCUER	FUNCTIONS	TWO RESCUERS
	• Establish unresponsiveness • Look for signs of breathing • If no response, call 911	
	• Check pulse . . . (5–10 seconds) If no pulse . . . • Begin chest compressions	
	DELIVER COMPRESSIONS **Adult** 30 compressions At least two inches At least 100/minute **Child** 30 compressions About two inches At least 100/minute	
	• After each set of 30 compressions, deliver two breaths	
	COMPRESSION/VENTILATION RATIOS **One Rescuer** Adult/Child 30:2 **Two Rescuers** Child Only 15:2	

To avoid or reduce the amount of air forced into the stomach, always look for the patient's chest to rise as you deliver ventilations. Adjust the size of your breaths so that you see the chest rise, and then allow the patient to passively exhale. If you see the stomach begin to bulge, reposition the patient's head and adjust your ventilations.

If the patient vomits, stop CPR. Take time to clear the patient's airway as best you can by repositioning the patient for drainage and by using your gloved fingers to sweep the mouth. After clearing the airway, resume CPR.

Special CPR Situations

Moving the Patient

Usually, there are only two reasons for an Emergency Medical Responder to move a patient who is receiving CPR: transport and immediate danger at the scene. Most of the time, the patient is moved after the EMTs assume responsibility for care. In preparation for transport when the EMTs arrive, place the cardiac-arrest patient on a long spine board when available. This will allow for easy transfer to the stretcher and provide a firm surface when doing compressions.

Trauma

Many factors complicate CPR when dealing with a victim of trauma. Severe injuries to the patient's face may interfere with your attempts to provide ventilations. Crushing injuries to the patient's chest may lessen the effectiveness of chest compressions. Head, neck, and spine injuries may require that you handle the patient in a special manner.

Many rescuers are unsure about starting CPR on trauma patients. When rescuers find obvious indications of spine injuries, they may feel it is more important to immobilize the spine before they start CPR. If rescuers find a patient with a crushed chest, they may be afraid of causing internal injuries if they perform chest compressions. Patient injuries should not prevent you from starting CPR. If you delay or do not start CPR, the patient will die.

Moving the trauma patient into proper position is a major problem. One concern is spine injury, but CPR is not effective if the patient is in a seated position. Nor is CPR likely to be effective if the patient is on a soft surface, such as a car seat. Patients must be moved to hard surfaces and placed on their backs. While doing so, take into account the possibility of neck and spine injury, and use your hands and arms to initially control and stabilize the head and neck whenever you have to move a patient.

When moving an adult, cradle the head and shoulders in your forearms and attempt to move the patient so that his head stays in line with his body. When moving an infant or a child, always use one hand to support the head and neck of the patient. Again, for CPR to be effective, the patient must be lying face up on a hard surface.

If you must move the patient after starting CPR because of the dangers at the scene, then do so. Try not to interrupt CPR for more than 10 seconds during a move. The total move may have to be done in several stages if conditions allow. Even if your patient has possible neck and spine injuries, start CPR as soon as possible. Do not delay CPR to fully stabilize the neck and spine with a collar and immobilization devices. Use the jaw-thrust maneuver for ventilations to reduce the chances of causing greater injury to the patient.

Hypothermia

Patients who are victims of hypothermia may have vital signs that are very difficult to assess. You should take extra time—at least a full minute—when assessing both pulse and breathing. No attempt should be made to rewarm the patient in the field. Resuscitation attempts should continue until the patient can be rewarmed by the receiving facility. In most cases, a patient is not considered dead until the core body temperature has been raised and he remains unresponsive to resuscitation efforts.

Stopping CPR

When caring for a patient in cardiac arrest, your duties are twofold: to have someone activate EMS and to start CPR immediately. Only a Medical Director or a physician at the scene who has accepted responsibility for the patient may order you not to begin CPR. You also may choose not to begin CPR, if there are obvious signs of prolonged death, such as the presence of muscle rigidity (rigor mortis) and pooling of blood (lividity).

Bystanders and members of the patient's family may tell you that the patient would not want to be resuscitated. You are not to obey such requests without seeing proper documentation.

Even though the patient may have a terminal illness or may be very old, you will still need to provide CPR unless there is a written advance directive present. Quickly let the family know that you understand their feelings, but your duty as an Emergency Medical Responder is to begin CPR. If the family does not have an advance directive for the patient, you must begin CPR.

The longer a patient is in cardiac arrest before CPR is started, the less likely CPR will be effective. However, there are documented cases of adults in cardiac arrest for over 10 minutes who have been resuscitated with no major brain damage. Once you have started CPR, continue to provide CPR until:

- The patient regains a pulse. Then provide ventilations only.
- Spontaneous pulse and breathing begin.
- Equally or more highly trained members of the EMS system can continue in your place.
- You turn over responsibility for patient care to a physician.
- You are exhausted and no longer able to continue.

Automated External Defibrillation

EMS personnel and laypeople are now being trained in the use of a device called an *automated external defibrillator (AED)*. AEDs can assess a heart's rhythm, determine if defibrillation is necessary, and deliver an electrical shock when needed. Almost all jurisdictions have approved and adopted the use of AEDs.

OBJECTIVE

8. Explain the purpose of an automated external defibrillator (AED).

External Defibrillation

Defibrillators are designed to deliver an electrical shock that will stimulate the heart to begin beating normally. The shock does not start a heart that has stopped completely, but it will give the fibrillating heart a chance to spontaneously reestablish an effective rhythm on its own. The entire process is called *defibrillation*.

There are many kinds of defibrillators available today. The two basic kinds are manual defibrillators and automated external defibrillators (AEDs). Manual defibrillators are carried by most ALS providers. They require the rescuer to interpret the patient's heart rhythm and then decide whether the patient should receive a shock. The skills needed to accomplish those tasks require significant training beyond the level of most Emergency Medical Responders and EMTs.

The other type of defibrillator, the AED (Figure 10.14), can be fully automated or semi-automated. The fully automated AED assesses the patient's heart rhythm, advises that a shock is necessary, and delivers the shock without any input from the rescuer. Semi-automated defibrillators analyze the patient's rhythm and simply advise the rescuer if a shock is needed. It is then up to the rescuer to push a button to deliver the shock. For safety reasons, the semi-automated AED is the recommended choice for Emergency Medical Responders.

AEDs are capable of recognizing two very specific abnormal heart rhythms: ventricular fibrillation and ventricular tachycardia. The term **fibrillation** refers to a disorganized electrical activity within the heart that renders the heart incapable of pumping blood. The most common cause of fibrillation is a heart attack. Fibrillation results in a disorganized quivering of the heart muscle much like a spasm or seizure (Figure 10.15).

The most common type of fibrillation affects the lower half (ventricles) of the heart and is called **ventricular fibrillation (VF)**. When a person's heart goes into VF, the brain and other vital organs no longer receive an adequate supply of oxygenated blood and the patient becomes unresponsive. VF does not produce blood flow or a pulse, so the patient will be found unresponsive with no pulse and no breathing. The sooner that VF can be defibrillated, the better the patient's chances are for survival.

AEDs also can recognize the abnormal heart rhythm called **ventricular tachycardia**, or V-tach for short. V-tach is a rapid rhythm that originates in the ventricles and rarely produces a pulse. It does not pump blood very efficiently. Less than 10% of the prehospital cardiac-arrest cases have this problem. Defibrillation may help some of these patients.

In situations where there is no electrical activity within the heart, a condition called **asystole** or sometimes "flat line," AEDs will not be effective.

fibrillation ▶ a disorganized electrical activity within the heart that renders the heart incapable of pumping blood.

ventricular fibrillation (VF) ▶ disorganized electrical activity, causing ineffective contractions of the lower heart chambers (ventricles).

ventricular tachycardia ▶ the abnormally rapid contraction of the heart's lower chambers, resulting in very poor circulation. Also called *V-tach.*

asystole ▶ no electrical activity in the heart; cardiac arrest. Also called *flatline.*

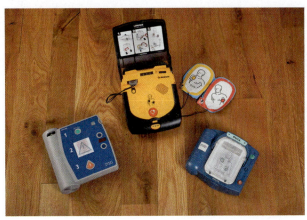

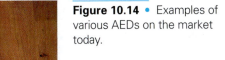
Figure 10.14 • Examples of various AEDs on the market today.

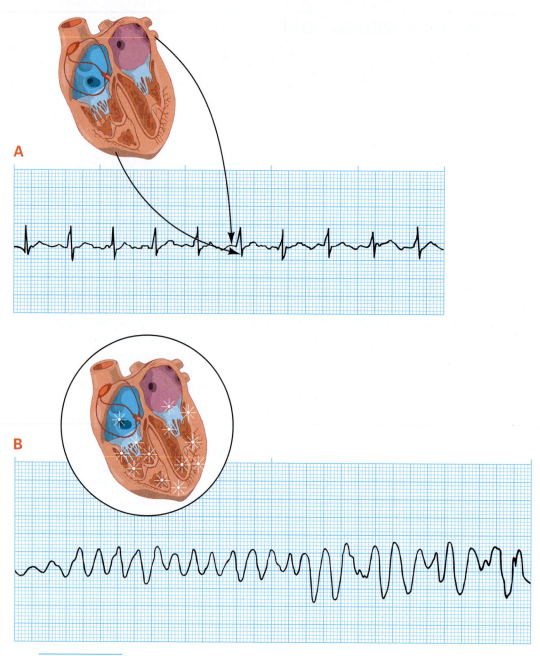

Figure 10.15 • (A) A normal heart rhythm as scene on an EKG monitor. (B) Ventricular fibrillation as seen on an EKG monitor.

continued

Kim's arms and lower back are just beginning to ache, when Sydney turns the corner at the end of the hall and sprints to the locked office door. The sound of footfalls grows louder until they slide to a halt just outside and she hears her fumbling with a set of keys, find the right one, and push the door open.

Fluorescent lights flood the small office, making Kim squint and causing Chris to look hideously pale. "Quick!" Kim shouts. "Get the AED on him!"

Sydney pops the cover open, glancing at the large, cartoon-like directions as he turns the unit on and pulls the electrode pads out. She then grabs Chris's shirt and tears it open, sending small plastic buttons skittering in all directions.

Kim stretches her back, panting, as Sydney yanks the paper backing from each electrode and places each one on Chris's lifeless body.

EMS and Defibrillation

Time is one of the most critical elements in the effort to save the life of a victim of cardiac arrest. Minimizing the time between collapse and the initiation of CPR, between CPR and the delivery of the first AED shock, and between defibrillation and the arrival of more advanced care is the goal of a strong chain of survival. The time between collapse and defibrillation can be divided into four segments:

- *EMS access time.* This is the time from patient collapse until the EMS system is alerted.
- *Dispatch time.* This is the time from the call to the EMS dispatcher to the alert of the personnel who will respond and defibrillate.
- *Response time.* This is the time it takes for the rescuer or crew to reach the patient.
- *Shock time.* This is the time it takes from reaching the patient until the first shock is delivered.

The goal of every EMS system is to reduce the time of each of those four segments. In particular, having rescuers with defibrillators available 24 hours a day shortens the time from dispatch to the arrival of the defibrillator. If the patient can receive the first shock within three to five minutes of collapse, survival is more likely.

Using AEDs

A defibrillator must be ready for use at any given moment. Make certain that you follow manufacturer guidelines to ensure that the defibrillators you use are in working order and prepared for use. Always carry fully charged spare batteries.

Basic Warnings

Emergency Medical Responders may be trained to use either fully automated or semi-automated defibrillators. The Medical Director for your EMS system may have approved one or both of these devices. Whichever your system uses, you are responsible for noting certain warnings when working with AEDs:

- Follow the same precautions that you would for operating any electrical device.
- Only place the AED on a patient who is in cardiac arrest.
- Do not place defibrillator patches over a patient's medication patch or implanted pacemaker. With gloved hands, remove the medication patch and wipe the chest dry.
- Make certain that no one is touching the patient during the "analyze" or "shock" phases.
- Do not attempt to assess or shock a patient who is moving or when the defibrillator or its leads are being moved.
- Do not attempt to defibrillate a patient who is lying in a puddle of water.
- Your Medical Director may have specific guidelines for defibrillating infants younger than one. Follow your local protocols.

> **▶ GERIATRIC FOCUS ◀**
>
> *It is not uncommon for an elderly patient to have an implanted pacemaker/defibrillator. This will be seen as a small round or rectangle object beneath the skin, just below the clavicle or high in the abdomen. Do not place the AED pads directly over such a device.*

Protocols for the use of AEDs for trauma patients vary by state and jurisdiction. Follow your EMS system's protocols and carefully assess the patient and mechanism of injury or the nature of the illness. If you are not certain as to what you are to do, contact medical direction.

KEY POINT ▼

American Heart Association guidelines suggest that all health-care providers should be trained and equipped to provide defibrillation at the earliest possible moment for victims of sudden cardiac arrest.

KEY POINT ▼

Some patients with specific heart conditions may have a small automated defibrillator surgically implanted inside their chest or abdomen. These devices are very much like external AEDs only much smaller. You might not know that this was in place unless the patient or a family member tells you it is there. Your care of a patient in cardiac arrest will not change with the presence of an internal defibrillator.

IS IT SAFE?

Make certain that no one is touching the patient when a shock is delivered. Before pressing the shock button, check the patient from head to toe to be sure.

OBJECTIVE

9. Describe the indications and contraindications for the use of an AED.

IS IT SAFE?

The American Heart Association has indicated that it is safe and appropriate to use an AED on a patient who is lying on a wet surface. It is, however, important to ensure that they are *not* lying in a puddle of standing water. If this is the case, simply drag the patient out of the puddle and continue your care. Also, it is important that the surface of the patient's chest where the pads are to be placed is dry.

American Heart Association guidelines also indicate that metal surfaces pose no shock hazard to either the patient or the rescuer.

When to Place an AED

The use of a defibrillator must follow specific procedures of care and assessment. You must determine if the patient is indeed a candidate for the placement of an AED. To be a candidate, the patient must:

- Be unresponsive
- Have no carotid pulse
- Have no normal respirations

All of the criteria must be met before you can place an AED on a patient who is in suspected cardiac arrest.

Perform a primary assessment to confirm that the patient is indeed in cardiac arrest. If you are first on the scene and have confirmed the patient meets all of the criteria, begin CPR and place the AED as soon as possible. If you do not have an AED, continue CPR.

If you arrive on scene with an AED and someone else is providing CPR, your job will be to prepare and attach the defibrillator. Make certain that both of you are clear of the patient before delivering a shock.

If a cardiac arrest is witnessed, you should begin CPR immediately and place an AED just as soon as it is available. In the event of an unwitnessed cardiac arrest, some medical directors may recommend performing CPR for approximately two minutes before attempting to defibrillate. This will provide circulation to the heart muscle, which may increase the chances of successful defibrillation in some patients.

Attaching the Defibrillator

The procedure for attaching the AED to a patient is the same for both semi-automated and fully automated AEDs. While the first rescuer performs CPR, the rescuer operating the AED should perform the following steps:

1. Bare the patient's chest. If the patient's chest is wet, quickly wipe it dry. Make certain the patient is not lying in a puddle of standing water. Ground that is wet with no standing water is safe for defibrillation.

2. Place electrodes on the patient's bare, dry chest, one at a time. It may be necessary to shave the chest, because hair can prevent the electrodes from sticking properly. Place one pad on the patient's upper right chest below the collarbone (clavicle) and next to the breastbone (sternum). Place the second pad on the patient's left side just below the nipple line. Most pads and devices have illustrations on them showing the correct placement of the pads (Figure 10.16).

Figure 10.16 • Correct placement of AED electrode pads.

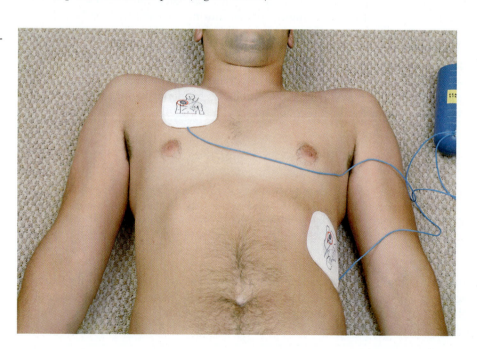

3. Finally, ensure that the electrodes are firmly plugged into the device. Some electrodes come connected and others need to be plugged in after the pads have been placed. Follow the specific directions for your device.

AEDs will not function properly unless the pads fully adhere to the patient's chest and the cables are tightly inserted into the device. If either of these problems exist, the "No contact" or "Check electrodes" prompt will sound or appear on the AED.

Operating the Fully Automatic AED

The following describes the operational procedures for a typical fully automatic AED. There are many models available. You must be familiar with the one that you will use. Follow the manufacturer's operating instructions for the specific AED you will be using.

Once turned on and attached to the patient, the latest models of fully automatic AEDs will assess the patient's heart rhythm, determine if a shock is indicated, charge to a pre-set energy level, and deliver the shock to the patient—all without further input from the rescuer. Many of the AEDs have voice and text prompts that advise the rescuer with messages such as "Shock advised. Do not touch the patient," "Charging. Stand clear," and "Stop CPR. Check breathing and pulse." Should this voice system fail, the rescuer is expected to know what to do and how to ensure personal safety.

To operate a fully automated external defibrillator, you should:

1. Assess the patient to confirm that he is in cardiac arrest.
2. Have your partner or someone trained in **basic life support (BLS)** begin CPR while you set up the AED. If you are alone, make sure that EMS has been called and immediately attach the AED.
3. Turn on the AED and attach the electrodes. Once the electrodes are in place, the AED will begin to analyze the patient's rhythm. Make sure no one is touching the patient.
4. Depending on the patient's rhythm, the AED will deliver one shock.
5. Following the shock, immediately begin CPR. (The most current AEDs are programmed to pause for two minutes after each shock to allow for CPR.)
6. After two minutes, the AED will advise you to stop CPR. It will then re-analyze the heart rhythm and, if indicated, deliver another shock. This sequence of one shock and two minutes of CPR should continue until more advanced care providers arrive.

If at any time the patient goes into a rhythm that is not shockable, the AED will advise you to check the patient and begin CPR as appropriate.

If the patient does have a pulse, leave the defibrillator attached. Maintain an open airway, monitor pulse and breathing, and continue supportive procedures until more advanced EMS personnel arrive and take over patient care.

Operating the Semi-Automated Defibrillator

The following is an example of the operational procedure for a semi-automatic AED. There are several semi-automatic models currently available. Follow the instructions given in the manufacturer's manual for your specific model, and always follow your EMS system's protocols for the AED you use.

Once turned on and applied to the patient, semi-automatic AEDs will analyze the rhythm and advise if a shock is necessary. Some models require the rescuer to push a button to begin the analysis sequence. In either case, the AED will automatically charge to a preset energy level. At this point, it is necessary for the rescuer to push a button to deliver the shock (Scan 10.5).

The same assessment and safety procedures that apply to the fully automatic AEDs also apply to the operation of the semi-automatic AEDs. Some older models may not have a voice synthesizer. Regardless of the model, they all require the rescuer to push a button to deliver the shock.

IS IT SAFE?

The fully automated AED is not recommended for use by Emergency Medical Responders since it will deliver a shock without any input from the operator. If you find yourself on the scene where a fully automated AED is in use, listen carefully to the device for voice prompts prior to the delivery of a shock. Be certain that no one is touching the patient when the device delivers a shock.

basic life support (BLS) ► externally supporting the circulation and respiration of a patient in respiratory or cardiac arrest through CPR.

KEY POINT ▼

The AED sequence presented here is a typical protocol that is programmed into many AEDs from the factory. Each EMS system has its own protocols for the use of AEDs, and may differ from what is presented here. Some jurisdictions may require Emergency Medical Responders to give a different number of shocks before transporting or continuing CPR, while others may require rescuers to perform CPR for two full minutes or perform some other step before preparing and attaching the defibrillator. Always know and follow local protocols before attempting to use an AED.

KEY POINT ▼

Always follow the manufacturer's manual and your EMS system's guidelines for the defibrillator you use.

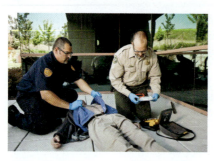

10.5.1 | Once you have confirmed the patient is unresponsive and has no pulse, turn on the AED and bare the patient's chest.

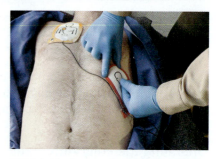

10.5.2 | Place the pads and connect the cable to the device (if not already connected).

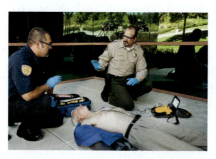

10.5.3 | When prompted, clear the patient and press the shock button.

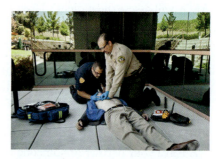

10.5.4 | After delivery of the shock, immediately begin chest compressions.

To operate a semi-automatic AED, you should:

1. Assess the patient to confirm that he is in cardiac arrest.

2. Have your partner or someone else trained in basic life support begin CPR while you set up the AED. If you are alone, make sure that EMS has been called and immediately attach the AED.

3. Turn on the AED and attach the electrodes. Once the electrodes are in place, the AED will begin to analyze the patient's rhythm. If necessary, push the "Analyze" button. Make certain that no one is touching the patient.

4. If a shockable rhythm is detected, the AED will advise so and charge to the appropriate energy level. When needed, the AED will prompt you to push the Shock button.

5. After you push the Shock button, the AED will deliver one shock.

6. Following the shock, immediately begin CPR. (The most current AEDs are programmed to pause for two minutes after each shock to allow you to perform CPR.)

7. After two minutes, the AED will advise you to stop CPR. It will then re-analyze the heart rhythm and, if indicated, advise the rescuer to deliver another shock. This sequence of one shock and two minutes of CPR should continue until more highly trained providers arrive.

Potential Problems

Most of the problems with AED operations can be easily corrected. Most problems involve the poor attachment of the pads or cables. Making certain that the pads are in full contact with the patient's chest and that the cables are tightly connected to the device usually is all that is needed.

Make sure the patient's chest is dry and free of anything that can prevent the pad from adhering well, such as hair or medication patches that occupy the pad placement sites. With gloved hands, remove any medication patches and wipe off any medication remaining on the patient's chest. If you have to shave the pad placement areas of the patient's chest, use a disposable safety razor provided in the AED kit for this purpose.

Most AEDs are programmed to run self-diagnostic checks every 24 hours. Should one of the self-checks detect a failure of any of the AED's internal systems, an error message or audible alarm will sound alerting the rescuer to the failure. It is important to know the error messages that can be displayed by your specific device. Some errors are only advisory in nature and allow continued use of the device, while others indicate a failure of a major system, rendering the AED inoperable. Become familiar with all error messages and alarms.

Quality Assurance

To be effective, a prehospital AED program requires ongoing evaluation to identify and correct any problems. This process of assessment and quality assurance should focus on specific situations that involve standard operating procedures, physician-directed standing orders, care delivered by the rescuers, performance of the equipment, routine maintenance, and effectiveness of training programs. Changes in any aspect of the program must be the result of Medical Director evaluation and orders.

Some AEDs have a voice-recording device built in that will provide an audible record of the resuscitation and defibrillation incident. All AEDs have an internal recording device that can capture a digital recording of the patient's heart rhythm, including shocks delivered. This information can be downloaded onto a computer so that the Medical Director can evaluate the event. Evaluation is an important part of any AED program and serves to improve and ensure quality patient care.

Be certain to carefully document all incidents involving the use of an AED. Your notes should include the time you arrived on scene, your assessment findings, how many shocks you delivered, and the patient's response following each shock.

Part of your equipment inspection and assessment should include the operation of your AED recording devices. Follow the manufacturer's instructions and your EMS system's recommendations to correct any problems before the unit is put into service. In addition, it is important to ensure that the AED kit includes the necessary supplies at all times, such as an extra battery, an extra set of electrode pads (adult and pediatric), razors, and towels.

WRAP-UP

FIRST ON SCENE

The afternoon crowd in the casino is sparse (mostly retirees whose RVs are parked haphazardly in the adjoining lot), so not many people notice as the ambulance crew pulls their gurney through the main doors and walk quickly to the bank of elevators. Once on the third floor, they meet a woman with an Australian accent who directs them down a long, doorless hallway to the facility's CCTV room. A woman in a disheveled business suit is sitting cross-legged on the floor next to an older man in the recovery position.

"It worked," she says with a huge, tired smile. The patient is breathing steadily and slowly running his fingers over the foam pads stuck to his chest.

"You're a very lucky man," one of the EMTs says as she places an oxygen mask on the patient's face. "It looks like this young lady over here saved your life."

Chris looks over at Kim, who is now blushing, and smiles weakly as he pats her hand. "Thank you," he mouths, the hissing oxygen louder than his quiet words.

Summary

- Like the chain of EMS resources, the chain of survival is also a linked system of patient-care events. These events include immediate recognition and activation of EMS, early CPR, rapid defibrillation, effective advanced life support (ALS), and integrated post-cardiac arrest care.

- The survival of the brain is dependent on the activities of breathing and circulation. When the heart stops beating, a patient is in cardiac arrest and cannot circulate oxygenated blood to the brain. The major signs of cardiac arrest are unresponsiveness, no breathing, and no pulse.

- If a patient is unresponsive, check for signs of breathing. If the patient is not breathing or has only gasping breaths, call 911 and check a pulse. If the patient has no pulse, begin chest compressions immediately.

- If you are alone and caring for a pediatric patient, provide two minutes of CPR before leaving the child to activate EMS.

- To provide proper CPR, you will place the patient in a supine position on a hard surface. If the patient is unresponsive, check for signs of breathing. If he is not breathing or showing only gasping breaths, begin compressions:
  - For an adult, provide compressions at a rate of at least 100 per minute and a depth of two inches.
  - For a child (age one to onset of puberty), provide compressions at a rate of at least 100 per minute and compress the chest about two inches.

- For an infant (up to one year of age), provide compressions at a rate of at least 100 per minute and compress the chest one-third the depth of the infant's chest or about one and one-half inches.

  After 30 compressions, provide two rescue breaths over one second each and begin compressions again. Do not stop CPR for more than 10 seconds other than to move the patient because of danger on scene. Continue CPR until the patient regains a pulse and/or breathing or until you are relieved by an equally or more highly trained person, care for the patient is accepted by a physician, or until you can no longer continue because of exhaustion.

- Automated external defibrillators (AEDs) are lifesaving units used by Emergency Medical Responders and available in many public areas. AEDs are electrical devices that can convert certain lethal heart rhythms to a normal cardiac rhythm and must be used with caution and according to specific protocols.

- The general steps for the use of a typical AED are as follows: Confirm that the patient is unresponsive and has no breathing or pulse. Turn on the AED, expose the patient's chest, and securely attach the pads. Wipe dry or shave hair, if necessary. Follow the AED's prompts to defibrillate and check breathing and pulse. Follow AED prompts to check a pulse or start CPR if there is no pulse.

Take Action

LOCAL RESOURCES

As more and more people become trained, AEDs are becoming more available. It is quite common to find AEDs available for public access in airports, shopping malls, amusement parks, and any place that attracts the public in large numbers. In fact, there are probably several businesses in your own town or city that have an AED and personnel trained in its use.

For this activity, identify at least three public locations that have AEDs available. You will have to make some calls or talk to people who work in different locations. You may wish to contact the following agencies and locations to ask if they have AEDs available in the event of a cardiac arrest. Also ask which employees are trained in their use.

- *Large shopping malls.* Often it is the security staff that carries the AED and is trained in its use.
- *Large employers.* Many large employers have employee volunteers who are trained to respond to medical emergencies.
- *Police agencies.* Some jurisdictions have all police vehicles equipped with AEDs.
- *Public venues.* such as fairgrounds, race tracks, zoos, and amusement parks.

First on Scene Run Review

Recall the events of the "First on Scene" scenario in this chapter and answer the following questions, which are related to the call. Rationales are offered in the Answer Key at the back of the book.

1. Did Kim respond appropriately following Chris's collapse to the floor? What should you look for when determining if your patient is breathing?

2. Was it the correct decision for Sydney to put the AED on Chris? What are the criteria for someone who gets an AED?

3. What information should you give the EMTs when they arrive?

Quick Quiz

To check your understanding of the chapter, answer the following questions. Then compare your answers to those in the Answer Key at the back of the book.

1. The appropriate rate of compressions during CPR is _____ per minute.
   a. 80 to 100
   b. no faster than 80
   c. at least 100
   d. no faster than 120

2. You are caring for an adult patient who was found unresponsive. You observe only gasping respirations. What is the most appropriate next step?
   a. Open the airway and give a breath.
   b. Call 911 and get an AED.
   c. Begin chest compressions.
   d. Attach the AED.

3. The recommended location for assessing for the presence of a pulse on a child is at the _____ artery.
   a. brachial
   b. carotid
   c. radial
   d. femoral

4. What is the recommended rate of compressions for infant CPR?
   a. At least 100 per minute
   b. As fast as possible
   c. 80 to 100 per minute
   d. 60 to 80 per minute

5. What is the recommended ratio of chest compressions to ventilations for an adult patient in cardiac arrest?
   a. 30 to 2
   b. 15 to 2
   c. 5 to 1
   d. 3 to 1

6. You are caring for an adult victim of sudden cardiac arrest. To give this patient the best chance for survival, you should provide immediate:
   a. CPR and no defibrillation.
   b. defibrillation without CPR.
   c. CPR with defibrillation within 10 minutes.
   d. CPR with defibrillation within three minutes.

7. Which one of the following is the best reason to provide rescue breathing to a nonbreathing patient?
   a. It is an effective way to provide oxygen to the patient.
   b. It can clear a blocked airway with little effort.
   c. It can defibrillate the heart if done quickly enough.
   d. It helps to circulate blood to the brain and lungs.

8. You are caring for a child who has a good pulse but is not breathing on her own. You should provide rescue breaths for this patient once every _____ seconds.
   a. three to five
   b. five to six
   c. six to seven
   d. 10 seconds

9. Which one of the following statements best describes the appropriate ventilation volume for a nonbreathing child?
   a. Twice that of an infant
   b. The weight minus the age
   c. Enough to cause the chest to rise
   d. Exactly half the volume of an adult

10. After assessing responsiveness, you must check for the presence of normal breathing. Do this by:
    a. shaking the patient.
    b. looking for chest rise.
    c. observing pupil response.
    d. sweeping the mouth for obstructions.

11. You are caring for an unresponsive adult patient who is not breathing but has a pulse. You should:
    a. provide finger sweeps.
    b. begin chest compressions.
    c. give five back blows.
    d. provide rescue breaths every five to six seconds.

12. You are alone when you discover and remove a four-year-old child from a public pool. When should you call 911?
    a. After providing two minutes of CPR
    b. Immediately after removing him from the pool
    c. After 10 minutes of CPR with no response
    d. After rescue breaths but before compressions

13. Which one of the following represents the most appropriate hand location for chest compressions on an adult?
    a. At the lower half of sternum
    b. At the top of the sternum
    c. Over the left side of the chest
    d. On the very bottom of the sternum

14. You are caring for an infant who is unresponsive and not breathing. Your initial attempt to deliver a rescue breath is not successful. Which one of the following is most likely the cause?
    a. The child has asthma and cannot breathe.
    b. The airway is likely blocked by an airway spasm.
    c. The child is choking on a foreign object.
    d. You probably did not open the airway properly.

15. You are at a Little League baseball game and see a parent collapse onto the ground. You are the first person to the woman. What is the first thing you should do?
    a. Place her in the recovery position.
    b. Send someone to call 911.
    c. Check for responsiveness.
    d. Give two slow breaths.

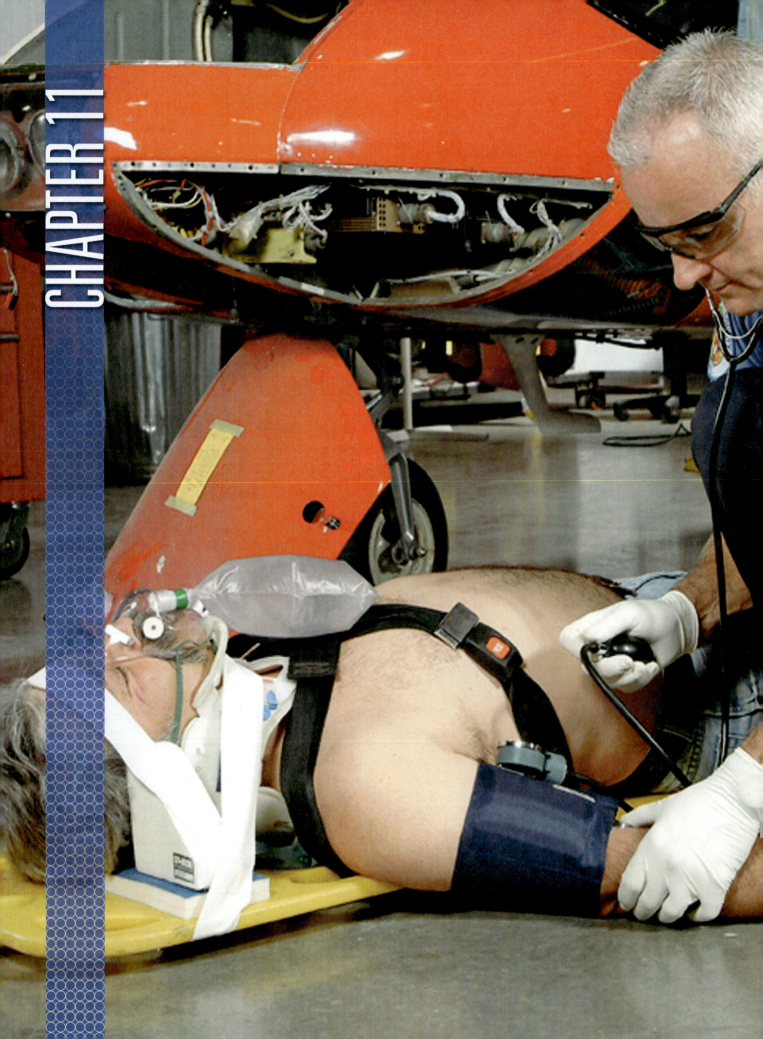

CHAPTER 11

Obtaining a Medical History and Vital Signs

EDUCATION STANDARDS
- Assessment—Secondary Assessment, History Taking

COMPETENCIES
- Use scene information and simple patient assessment findings to identify and manage immediate life threats and injuries within the scope of practice of the Emergency Medical Responder.

CHAPTER OVERVIEW

Two of the most powerful skills that you must develop to properly care for ill or injured patients are asking good questions and accurately assessing a patient's vital signs. Together, they make up much of the assessment for each and every patient you encounter. Obtaining a good medical history requires that you become comfortable asking very personal questions related to a patient's medical condition. You must learn the appropriate questions to ask for the current situation as well as the ones that will provide insight into pertinent past medical history.

In addition to developing your interviewing skills, you must learn the skills necessary to properly obtain complete and accurate vital signs for each patient you encounter. Obtaining vital signs requires several isolated skills that will enhance your ability to see, touch, and hear what is going on with your patient. This chapter introduces you to basic principles and offers many tips that will assist you in developing your proficiency with obtaining a medical history and vital signs.

OBJECTIVES

Upon successful completion of this chapter, the student should be able to:

COGNITIVE

1. Define the key terms introduced in this chapter:
   a. auscultation *(p. 228)*
   b. baseline vital signs *(p. 222)*
   c. blood pressure *(p. 227)*
   d. capillary refill *(p. 226)*
   e. chief complaint *(p. 217)*
   f. cyanotic *(p. 232)*
   g. diaphoretic *(p. 232)*
   h. diastolic *(p. 227)*
   i. medical history *(p. 216)*
   j. mental status *(p. 221)*
   k. OPQRST *(p. 219)*
   l. palpation *(p. 228)*
   m. pulse *(p. 224)*
   n. respiration *(p. 222)*
   o. SAMPLE history tool *(p. 218)*
   p. sign *(p. 217)*
   q. stethoscope *(p. 228)*
   r. symptom *(p. 217)*
   s. systolic *(p. 227)*
   t. trending *(p. 222)*
   u. vital signs *(p. 221)*
   v. work of breathing *(p. 223)*

2. Explain the importance of a thorough medical history. *(p. 216)*

3. Differentiate between a sign and a symptom. *(p. 216)*

4. Describe the components of the SAMPLE history tool. *(p. 218)*

5. Describe the components of the OPQRST assessment tool. *(p. 219)*

6. Explain the role that monitoring vital signs plays in the overall assessment and care of the patient. *(p. 222)*

7. State the characteristics that are obtained and measured when assessing respirations, pulse, blood pressure, skin signs, and pupils. *(p. 221)*

8. Describe the methods used to assess each of the five vital signs. *(p. 221)*

9. Differentiate the techniques used to assess a pulse in an infant, child, and adult patient. *(p. 225)*

...mal and abnormal vital sign values for the ...ult patient. *(p. 224)*

...the ability to properly obtain and accurately ...ocument vital signs.

AFFECTIVE

12. Demonstrate a caring and compassionate attitude with classmates and simulated patient.

"Call an ambulance, Hernandez, I'm on my way over!" Kate Terrance, a newly certified Emergency Medical Responder, slams the phone down and ducks under her desk to grab the first aid bag. As she dashes down the entryway of the quiet, empty lodge, she begins to run the coming scenario through her mind. It will take EMS a good 15 minutes to reach the hotel on this side of the lake, so she knows she will have time to prepare a sturdy set of vitals.

"There you are, Kate!" The young hotel employee seems shaken. "I called for an ambulance, but they said it is 20 minutes or so away."

"I figured as much," Kate replies. She eyes the man lying on a poolside chaise. His breathing is quick and watery sounding, and his skin is pale and glistening. Although his clothes are completely dry, Kate thinks he might have nearly drowned. "Hello, sir, my name is Kate, and I'm a trained Emergency Medical Responder. What seems to be the problem?"

The man starts saying something in Spanish, but it is interrupted by gasps of breath. "Hernandez," Kate says, pulling out her vitals kit, "I need your help with this one, kid."

Obtaining a Medical History

2. Explain the importance of a thorough medical history.

medical history ▶ previous medical conditions and events for a patient.

3. Differentiate between a sign and a symptom.

It is safe to say that a good patient assessment is likely to result in good patient care. A good patient assessment includes knowing how to ask questions and discover information that is not immediately obvious. All of the information that you gather about the patient's current and previous medical conditions is referred to as the patient's **medical history**.

Much of what you learn about your patient during the assessment comes from what the patient tells you (Figure 11.1). When the patient is unresponsive and there is no one at the scene who can answer your questions, you are at a great disadvantage, and so is your patient.

The first thing you must know about obtaining a patient history is the difference between a sign and a symptom. **Signs** are something you can see and observe about your patient. Think of signs much like those along the road that are telling you to stop or yield, or, worse yet, that you are going the wrong way! If you are alert and paying attention, those signs tell you a lot about what is going on around you. The same applies to patient care. A sign can be pale skin or a rapid pulse or an open wound to the chest. All signs are obvious if you are alert and properly trained on how to look for them.

Symptoms are very different and much more difficult to discover. A **symptom** is something the patient feels and may complain about. Symptoms are most commonly discovered through asking questions about what they are experiencing at the time. Symptoms can be obvious or very subtle. One of the most common symptoms that a patient can experience is pain. Another common symptom is nausea. Certainly you have experienced both of these symptoms on more than one occasion and for various reasons. Table 11.1 shows common examples of both signs and symptoms.

Your assessment must be focused on gathering and documenting as many pertinent signs and symptoms as possible to ensure that your care, and the care that others provide after you, is appropriate.

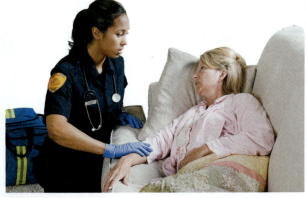

Figure 11.1 • Get down at eye level with your patient and make good eye contact as you begin your medical history.

TABLE 11.1 | Common Signs and Symptoms

SIGNS	SYMPTOMS
Blood pressure	Pain
Pulse	Nausea
Respirations	Shortness of breath
Skin color, temperature, moisture	Chest pressure
Bleeding	Headache
Pupils	Dizziness
Bruising	Blurred vision
Unresponsive	Fatigue
Disoriented	Cough
Deformity	Anxiety

Interviewing Your Patient

In most situations an alert patient is your best source of information. Nearly every patient encounter with an alert patient will begin with questioning them about what they are feeling or what happened that made them call for assistance. This is referred to as the patient's **chief complaint**. Whenever appropriate, it is best to direct your questions to the patient. In the case of a very young child, it is usually more appropriate to interview a parent, guardian, or caregiver. If the patient is unresponsive, you must look to other sources for this information. Family members, bystanders, and first responders should all be questioned as appropriate to gather as much information about the patient as possible.

Ask questions slowly and clearly, using a caring tone of voice. Allow plenty of time for the patient to process and respond to your question before asking another one. Repeat or rephrase the question if necessary. Listen carefully to what the patient is telling you, and document important details as necessary. There is little that frustrates patients more than when the Emergency Medical Responder does not listen and they must repeat answers they have already given.

The level of cooperation and quality of answers that you receive can be greatly influenced by the rapport you establish early on. This also can be influenced by others on the scene. A simple sequence can be used for most situations and will work well for quickly establishing a good rapport with your patient. Read the following dialogue and see if you can identify the five components of the sequence:

> EMERGENCY MEDICAL RESPONDER: "Hello, my name is Chris. I'm with the fire department, would you mind if I ask you some questions?"
>
> PATIENT: "Hi Chris. Uh, no, I don't mind.
>
> EMERGENCY MEDICAL RESPONDER: "What is your name?"
>
> PATIENT: "Jordan."
>
> EMERGENCY MEDICAL RESPONDER: "How old are you, Jordan?"
>
> PATIENT: "I'm 48."
>
> EMERGENCY MEDICAL RESPONDER: "Jordan, you look like you are in quite a bit of discomfort. Can you tell me what you are feeling right now?"
>
> PATIENT: "I was out back cutting down weeds with the mower when I suddenly felt tightness in my chest."

sign ▶ something that can be observed or measured when assessing a patient.

symptom ▶ something that the patient complains of or describes during the secondary assessment.

chief complaint ▶ the main medical complaint as described by the patient.

KEY POINT ▼

Being a good interviewer means being a good listener. There is nothing more frustrating for a patient than having to answer the same question over and over.

Building Rapport

I have found that treating patients as equals improves communication. Talk to them as you would someone you are meeting for the first time at work. Be respectful and avoid the use of medical jargon. Ask clear questions and do not interrupt the patient. Simple courtesy often results in obtaining the most accurate history.

Did you identify the five components of the sequence? Here they are:

- *Introduction.* "Hello, my name is Chris. I'm with the fire department." This tells the patient the role that you play in the team and is just good courtesy.
- *Consent.* "Would you mind if I ask you some questions?" Obtaining consent to care for the patient is not only good manners but is also a legal requirement.
- *Patient's name.* "What is your name?" Using a patient's name frequently is one of the most effective ways to establish a rapport and gain the confidence of your patient.
- *Patient's age.* While it is often easy to guess a patient's age, it is just as easy to ask and get the actual age.
- *Chief complaint.* "Jordan, you look like you are in quite a bit of discomfort. Can you tell me what you are feeling right now?" Obtaining the chief complaint will guide your assessment.

This simple and respectful approach can be easily memorized and modified to meet the needs of just about any situation and will go far in helping you establish a positive rapport with your patient.

▶ GERIATRIC FOCUS ◀

Obtaining a thorough and accurate history from an elderly patient can prove to be challenging, especially if the patient suffers from dementia. Rely on family members and caregivers to confirm the information that the patient is telling you or to fill in the gaps left by the patient's own history.

Hearing loss can make gathering a history challenging as well. You may have to speak louder than usual, and it also will help if you speak slowly and clearly.

Now that you have completed your introduction and obtained the chief complaint, what is next? What questions should you ask? How will you remember all that you should ask? Not to worry, there is a tool just for this purpose.

One of the most common tools used for obtaining a patient's medical history at all levels of EMS is called the **SAMPLE history** tool. It is a simple acronym that contains six key reminders. The acronym helps guide the flow of the interview and helps you keep in mind the most important questions to ask your patient. Each letter of the SAMPLE acronym represents a specific element of your interview and should trigger specific questions related to the chief complaint. Below is an explanation with examples for how to use the SAMPLE history tool:

OBJECTIVE

4. Describe the components of the SAMPLE history tool.

SAMPLE history ▶ an acronym used to obtain a patient history during the secondary assessment.

S	—	Signs/symptoms
A	—	Allergies
M	—	Medications
P	—	Past pertinent medical history
L	—	Last oral intake
E	—	Events leading to the illness or injury

The *S* stands for signs and symptoms. It is a reminder to observe the patient for obvious signs of illness or injury and ask or clarify what he may be feeling. One way to address this element would be to ask the patient, "So tell me again: what are you feeling?" or "Tell me again where you hurt the most." If the patient states that he has pain in his right shoulder (symptom), this should trigger you to quickly examine the shoulder, looking for any signs such as deformity or bleeding. So you see, even though you may already know the patient has shoulder pain, it is important to find out more. Are there any obvious signs of injury? Are there signs or symptoms other than those directly related to the chief complaint?

The *A* stands for allergies. Question the patient about any known allergies to things such as medications, food, or bee stings. More important, you want to know about allergies that may be related to the patient's current complaint. It is a good idea to ask if he has recently been exposed to anything to which he is allergic. Most patients have a pretty good idea what they are allergic to, so this is a fairly straightforward question.

The *M* stands for medications. You will want to ask the patient if he is currently taking any medications, prescribed or non-prescribed. If he says yes, then you must ask if he is current with all his medications. In other words, has he been taking them as prescribed up to and including today? Ask to see all of the medications he is taking and gather them together so they are easily accessible for the ambulance crew when they arrive.

The *P* stands for past medical history. To address this component, ask the patient, "Has this happened before?" Also determine the medical history unrelated to the current emergency. You might ask, "Do you have any past history of medical conditions or problems such as heart problems, breathing problems, diabetes, or seizures?" Your job is to discover the history, document it thoroughly, and pass it along to the next level of care.

The *L* stands for last oral intake. For instance, "What have you eaten or had to drink today?" Document what the patient has taken in, when, and an approximate quantity. The primary purpose for this is to alert you to any connection to the current problem (food allergy) as well as alert the next level of care of any stomach contents that may be an issue if the patient needs surgery. Many patients respond to general anesthesia with nausea and vomiting, and the surgical staff will take additional precautions as necessary.

Finally, the *E* stands for events leading to the current problem. In other words, "What were you doing when this began?" The chain of events often can provide important clues to the patient's problem. For example, it is important for the doctor to know if a patient complaining of chest pain was at rest when the pain began or if it started as a result of exertion.

Another very common tool used for obtaining patient histories is called the **OPQRST** tool. Just like the SAMPLE history, each letter of this tool stands for a specific word that is designed to trigger specific questions. The OPQRST tool drives a more detailed assessment related to the chief complaint and can be very helpful in gathering additional information that the SAMPLE tool may miss.

OPQRST is most commonly used for the assessment of pain or discomfort, but it can be used for other problems as well. Those that use the OPQRST tool will slip it in immediately following the *S* in SAMPLE. The letters in OPQRST stand for onset, provocation, quality, region/radiate, severity, and time:

O — *Onset.* The word *onset* is designed to trigger questions pertaining to what the patient was doing when the pain or symptoms began. For example, "What were you doing when the pain began?" or "What were you doing when you first began to feel short of breath?" are questions you might ask related to onset.

P — *Provocation.* The word *provocation* is designed to trigger questions pertaining to what might make the pain or symptoms better or worse. For example, "Does anything you do make the pain better or worse?" or "Does it hurt to take a deep breath or when I push here?" are questions you might ask related to provocation.

Q — *Quality.* The word *quality* is designed to trigger questions pertaining to what the pain or symptom actually feels like. For example, "Can you describe how your pain feels?" or "Is your pain sharp or is it dull?" "Is it steady or does it come and go?" are all questions you might ask related to quality.

KEY POINT

When appropriate, ask someone at the scene for a paper bag and place all of the medications in the bag so that they can be taken to the hospital along with the patient.

OBJECTIVE

5. Describe the components of the OPQRST assessment tool.

OPQRST ▶ a mnemonic used during a secondary assessment to help assess pain; the letters stand for onset, provocation, quality, region/radiate, severity, time.

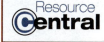

Learn more about interviewing for OPQRST information.

R — *Region/Radiate.* The words *region* and *radiate* are designed to trigger questions pertaining to where the pain is originating and where it may be moving or radiating to. For example, "Can you point with one finger where your pain is the worst?" or "Does your pain move or radiate to any other part of your body?" "Do you feel pain anywhere else besides your chest?" are all questions you might ask related to region and radiate.

S — *Severity.* The word *severity* is designed to trigger questions pertaining to how severe the pain or discomfort is. A standard 1 to 10 scale is typically used and is presented like this: "On a scale of 1 to 10, with 10 being the worst pain you have ever felt, how would you rate your pain right now?" You can take this a step further by asking the patient to describe the severity of the pain when it first began using the same scale. Once you have been with the patient a while and provided care, you will want to ask the severity question again to see if the pain is getting better or worse.

T — *Time.* The word *time* is designed to trigger questions pertaining to how long the patient may have been experiencing pain or discomfort. A simple question such as, "When did you first begin having pain today?" or "How long have you had this pain?" will usually suffice.

It is important to point out that there are many different acronyms and memory tools that can be used to assist the Emergency Medical Responder in performing a more thorough assessment. Only two of the more common tools currently used in EMS have been presented here. Your instructor or EMS system may have different or additional tools. Find the tool or tools that work best for you.

FIRST ON SCENE

continued

"His name is Martin. He says he fell asleep out here and when he woke up, he felt like he was choking on water," Hernandez says, translating the man's short, gurgling words. "He says he didn't have the strength to get up."

"Go ahead and raise the back of that lounge chair, but be careful," Kate says. She holds her watch up, counting the quick but feeble pulse in her patient's wrist. "Respirations are about 36, very shallow with a gurgling sound, and his pulse is 104 and regular, but it's pretty weak."

Kate quickly jots her findings down, noting the time. She attaches the blood pressure cuff and Martin pulls away, saying something quickly and breathy. Kate looks Martin in the eyes and says, "Martin, I'm going to help you as much as I can, okay? Can you help me by answering some questions, please?" Martin listens to the translation Hernandez gives, and he leans back, looking calmer.

"Si. Y gracias."

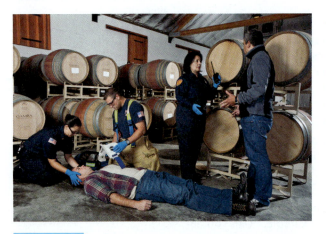

Figure 11.2 • Consider using bystanders or family members when your patient is unresponsive or unable to provide a medical history on his own.

Additional Sources of Information

You may encounter a patient who is unresponsive or unable to answer your questions about his condition or history. If this is the case, you must depend on family members, bystanders, or first responders for information (Figure 11.2). Here are some examples of questions you may want to ask others at the scene if the patient is unable to provide meaningful information:

- *What is the patient's name?* If the patient is a minor, ask if the parents are there or if they have been contacted.
- *Did you* see *what happened?* If the patient fell from a ladder, did he appear to faint or pass out first? Was he hit on the head by something?
- *Did the patient complain of anything before this happened?* You may learn of chest pain, nausea, shortness of breath, a funny odor where the patient was working, and other clues.

Interviewing Family

One technique to consider when interviewing family members is to move them a small distance away from the patient so that they are not distracted by the care being provided. However, do not attempt to isolate them completely from their loved ones.

► GERIATRIC FOCUS ◄

Many elderly patients take prescription medications for various medical conditions. A good trick to help disclose pertinent medical history is to ask to see all the medications the patient is currently taking. Even if you do not know the purpose of each medication, having them handy when the EMTs arrive may help them begin to understand the patient's history sooner.

- *Does the patient have any known illnesses?* Family or friends may know the medical history, such as heart problems, diabetes, allergies, or other problems that may cause a change in his condition.
- *Does the patient take any medications that you know of?*

Medical identification jewelry also can provide important information if the patient is unresponsive and a history cannot be easily obtained by those at the scene. A common example of this type of jewelry is the medallion worn on a necklace, a wrist, or an ankle bracelet. Information on the patient's medical condition or problem is engraved on the reverse side of the medallion, along with a phone number for additional information.

Vital Signs

The term **vital signs** refers to that which is vital to the continuation of life. In EMS, there are five specific vital signs that are commonly observed and measured. They are respiration, pulse, blood pressure, skin signs, and pupils. While it can be argued that not all five are truly "vital" to life, such as pupils and skin signs, the other three are truly necessary for someone to be considered living.

An Overview

Perfusion

In short, perfusion is the adequate supply of well-oxygenated blood to all parts of the body. Each of the five vital signs serves as a window into the patient's perfusion status. For instance, a patient with an abnormally slow pulse or low blood pressure may not be getting enough blood to all parts of the body. A patient with breathing difficulty may not be getting enough air to adequately supply the blood with enough oxygen. Someone with pale skin may be showing signs of shock.

As you learn about the different vital signs, keep in mind that your goal is to paint as complete a picture of your patient as possible. No single vital sign should be used to drive the care that you provide.

Mental Status

Many EMS systems consider **mental status** to be a vital sign. A patient's mental status, also referred to as level of consciousness (LOC), or level of responsiveness, is commonly evaluated using the AVPU scale:

A — Alert
V — Verbal, responsive to verbal stimuli

OBJECTIVES

7. State the characteristics that are obtained and measured when assessing respirations, pulse, blood pressure, skin signs, and pupils.

8. Describe the methods used to assess each of the five vital signs.

vital signs ► the five most common signs used to evaluate a patient's condition (respirations, pulse, blood pressure, skin, and pupils).

mental status ► the general condition of a patient's level of consciousness and awareness.

P — Pain, responsive only to painful stimuli

U — Unresponsive, unconscious, or completely unresponsive

A patient's mental status can provide valuable information about the patient's condition.

Vital signs can alert you to problems that require immediate attention. Taken at regular intervals, they can help you determine if the patient's condition is getting better, worse, or staying the same.

The first set of vital signs taken on a patient is called the **baseline vital signs**. All subsequent vital signs are always compared to the baseline set. This comparison helps determine if the patient is stable or unstable, improving or growing worse, and benefiting or not benefiting from the care that you are providing. For example, comparing baseline vital signs before and after administering oxygen to the patient can give clues as to whether the oxygen is helping the patient.

Trending

One of the values of obtaining and documenting vital signs is that they can be trended. **Trending** is the process of comparing multiple sets of vital signs from the same patient over time. Vitals signs can change for the better or change for the worse, or they can remain generally the same. Each of these represents a trend and can provide valuable information about your patient.

The careful analysis of vital signs can alert you to current or developing problems. For example, the presence of cool, moist skin along with a rapid pulse and increased breathing rate can indicate possible shock in the presence of a significant mechanism of injury. Hot, dry skin with a rapid pulse may indicate a serious heat-related emergency. You can determine which patients are a high priority for immediate transport by taking and closely monitoring their vital signs.

For an adult patient, a continuous pulse rate of less than 60 beats per minute or above 100 beats per minute is considered abnormal. Likewise, a respiratory rate above 28 breaths per minute or below 8 breaths per minute is considered abnormal and may require some intervention. However, vital signs differ for everyone. They also can change. And they are affected by factors other than the patient's medical condition. The temperature of the environment, exercise, and even emotions can all affect a person's vital signs, quickly moving him into what might be considered an abnormal range.

The key with vital signs is to not rush to a conclusion too soon. Usually, it is better to gather as much information as possible before coming to a conclusion about how best to manage your patient. There are exceptions to this rule though. For instance, if you attempt to obtain a pulse and cannot locate one, you would not try to get a blood pressure before starting CPR! You must understand that without a pulse the person will die and time is of the essence. Vital signs will vary significantly by age as well. Familiarize yourself with the normal ranges for different age groups.

▶ GERIATRIC FOCUS ◀

Obtaining accurate vital signs can be challenging with the elderly patient. Small, frail arms can make it painful for them when you try to get a blood pressure. The bones of the chest have become more rigid, making it more difficult to see chest rise and fall. You may have to use other techniques, such as listening for breath sounds or watching the movement of the abdomen, when counting respirations.

Respirations

Respiration is the act or process of breathing in (inhaling) and out (exhaling). You will evaluate several characteristics when assessing a patient's respirations: rate, depth, sound, and ease.

OBJECTIVE

6. Explain the role that monitoring vital signs plays in the overall assessment and care of the patient.

baseline vital signs ▶ the very first set of vital signs obtained on a patient.

trending ▶ the act of comparing multiple sets of signs and symptoms over time to determine patient condition.

respiration ▶ the act of breathing in and out; also, the exchange of oxygen and carbon dioxide within the cells.

TABLE 11.2 | Assessment Signs—Respirations

OBSERVATION	POSSIBLE PROBLEM
Rapid, shallow breaths	Shock, heart problems, heat emergency, diabetic emergency, heart failure, pneumonia
Deep gasping, labored breaths	Airway obstruction, heart failure, heart attack, lung disease, chest injury, diabetic emergency
Slowed breathing	Head injury, stroke, chest injury, certain drugs
Snoring	Stroke, fractured skull, drug or alcohol abuse, partial airway obstruction
Crowing	Airway obstruction, airway injury due to heat
Gurgling	Airway obstruction, lung disease, lung injury due to heat
Wheezing	Asthma, emphysema, airway obstruction, heart failure
Coughing blood	Chest wound, chest infection, fractured rib, punctured lung, internal injuries

A single respiration is one entire cycle of breathing in and out. The respiratory rate is a count of the patient's breaths, one inhalation plus one exhalation, and it is classified as normal, rapid, or slow. The characteristics of breathing are rate, depth, ease, and sounds. While you are counting respirations, note if the depth is normal, shallow, or deep. Breathing depth that is normal is said to be a good tidal volume. Notice if the breathing is easy or whether it appears labored, or difficult. Listen for any abnormal sounds during breathing, such as snoring, gurgling, gasping, or wheezing. If the patient is responsive, ask if he is having any problems or pain while he breathes. Normal breathing is quiet and effortless. A patient who requires effort to breathe is said to have an increased **work of breathing**. Table 11.2 shows some of the problems that are associated with variations in respirations.

work of breathing ▶ the effort that a patient must exert to breathe.

To assess respirations, follow these steps:

1. Grasp the patient's wrist as if you were going to count the pulse rate. Hold his arm firmly against his upper abdomen (Figure 11.3). Do this because many patients will unknowingly alter their respiratory rate when someone is watching them breathe.

2. Observe the patient's abdomen and chest move in and out. Listen for abnormal sounds.

3. Count the number of breaths the patient takes in 15 or 30 seconds. (One breath equals one inspiration plus one expiration.) To obtain the respiratory rate, multiply the number of breaths in 15 seconds by 4, or the number of breaths in 30 seconds by 2.

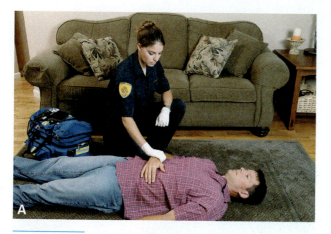 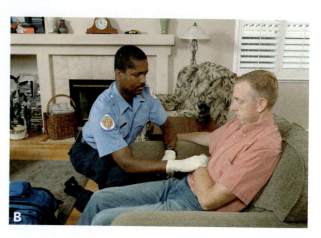

Figure 11.3 • (A) Emergency Medical Responder assessing respirations on a supine patient. (B) EMT assessing respirations on a seated patient.

TABLE 11.3 | Normal Respiration Rates	
NORMAL RESPIRATORY RATES (BREATHS PER MINUTE AT REST)	
Adult	12 to 20. Above 24: serious. Below 10: serious.
Adolescent: 11–14 years	12 to 20
School age: 6–10 years	15 to 30
Preschooler: 3–5 years	20 to 30
Toddler: 1–3 years	20 to 30
Infant: 6–12 months	20 to 30
Infant: 0–5 months	20 to 30
Newborn	30 to 50

4. While counting respirations, note depth and ease of breathing.

5. Record your findings by documenting rate, depth, and ease.

Here are some examples of how you might document respirations:

- 16, good tidal volume (GTV) and unlabored
- 32, shallow and labored
- 8, shallow and unlabored
- 36, deep and labored

OBJECTIVE

10. Differentiate normal and abnormal vital sign values for the infant, child, and adult patient.

The normal range for respirations for an adult who is at rest is from 12 to 20 breaths per minute (Table 11.3). A respiratory rate greater than 28 or less than 8 breaths per minute should be considered serious. Provide care accordingly.

Pulse

pulse ▶ the pulsation of the arteries that is felt with each heart beat.

The presence of a pulse gives us insight into the circulatory status of the patient. A good pulse indicates that blood is moving well throughout the body. The **pulse** is nothing more than a remote heartbeat. It is caused when an artery that lies close to the skin pulsates as the pressure increases and decreases with each heartbeat. There are a number of pulse points that can be used to evaluate heart rate, as well as circulatory status in an extremity such as an arm or a leg. The carotid and femoral pulses are referred to as central pulses because they are in close proximity to the heart (Figure 11.4). The brachial, radial, and pedal pulses are referred to as peripheral pulses because they are further out (peripheral) on the body (Figure 11.5).

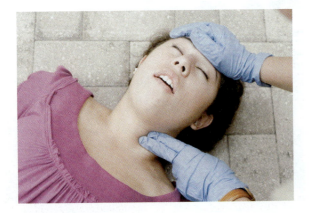

Figure 11.4 • Locating the carotid pulse point in the neck.

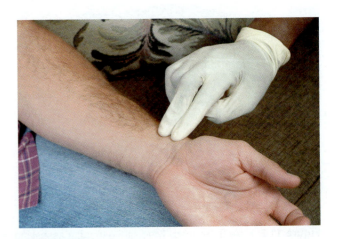

Figure 11.5 • Locating the radial pulse point in the wrist.

When taking a patient's pulse, you must assess for three characteristics: rate, strength, and rhythm. Pulse rate is a count of the number of beats per minute and is used to determine if the patient's pulse is normal, rapid, or slow. Strength is the force of the pulse. It will be either strong or weak. Rhythm is the steadiness of the pulse, which will be either regular or irregular.

When caring for a responsive patient, you can check the radial pulse at the patient's wrist. For an unresponsive patient, the carotid pulse in the neck should be used. The term *radial pulse* refers to the radial artery found in the lateral portion of the forearm, on the thumb side of the wrist. If for any reason you are unable to feel the radial pulse, assess the carotid pulse. The absence of a radial pulse when there is a carotid pulse indicates an abnormally low blood pressure and possible shock. A radial pulse may not be detectable if the patient's blood pressure is too low or if there is an extremity injury that is interrupting blood flow to the distal arm.

To measure a radial pulse rate:

1. Use two or three fingers to locate the pulse. Do not use your thumb, since it has its own pulse, which could be mistaken for the patient's.

2. Place your fingertips on the lateral side of the patient's anterior wrist, just above the crease between hand and wrist. Slide your fingers from this position toward the thumb side of the wrist (lateral side). Keeping the fingertip of the middle finger on the crease between wrist and hand will ensure you are placing the fingertip over the site of the radial pulse.

3. Apply moderate pressure until you feel the pulse. If the pulse is weak, you may have to apply more pressure. Too much pressure can cause the pulse to fade. By having all three fingers in contact with the patient's wrist and hand, you should be able to judge how much pressure you are applying.

4. Once you feel the pulse, count the beats for either 15 or 30 seconds, depending on local practice or protocols.

5. While counting, do your best to note the strength and rhythm of the pulse.

6. Multiply your 30-second count by 2 or your 15-second count by 4 to determine the number of beats per minute.

7. Record your findings by documenting the rate, strength, and rhythm.

Here are some examples of how you might document pulses:

- 72, strong and regular
- 88, strong and irregular
- 104, weak and regular
- 120, weak and irregular

Adults

The normal pulse rate for adults at rest is between 60 and 100 beats per minute (Table 11.4). Any rate above 100 is considered abnormally rapid (tachycardia). Any rate below 60 is considered abnormally slow (bradycardia). One exception to this is a well-conditioned athlete whose normal resting pulse may be about 50 beats per minute or less. In emergency situations, because of anxiety or excitement, it is not unusual for the pulse to be above 100 beats per minute.

Infants

The primary pulse point for obtaining a pulse in infants under the age of one year is the brachial pulse in the upper arm. This is due to the difficulty in isolating the radial pulse and the carotid pulse due to the underdeveloped anatomy of these small children.

To obtain a brachial pulse in an infant, place your index and middle fingers over the brachial artery on the inside of the baby's upper arm, between the elbow and armpit. Press gently with your fingers until you can feel the pulse. You may use the tip of your

KEY POINT ▼

Do not start CPR based only on the absence of a radial pulse. As the blood pressure drops, it becomes very difficult to feel a peripheral pulse such as the radial pulse. Before initiating CPR, *always* confirm the absence of a carotid pulse first.

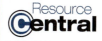

Learn more information about taking a pulse.

OBJECTIVE

9. Differentiate the techniques used to assess a pulse in an infant, child, and adult patient.

TABLE 11.4 | Pulse

NORMAL PULSE RATES (BEATS PER MINUTE AT REST)	
Adult	60 to 100
Adolescent: 11–14 years	60 to 105
School age: 6–10 years	70 to 110
Preschooler: 3–5 years	80 to 120
Toddler: 1–3 years	80 to 130
Infant: 6–12 months	80 to 140
Infant: 0–5 months	90 to 140
Newborn	120 to 160
PULSE QUALITY	**SIGNIFICANCE/POSSIBLE CAUSES**
Rapid	Exertion, anxiety, pain, fever, dehydration, blood loss, shock
Slow	Head injury, drugs, some poisons, some heart problems, lack of oxygen in children
Irregular	Possible abnormal electrical heart activity (arrhythmia)
Absent (no pulse)	Cardiac arrest (clinical death)

Note: In infants and children, a high pulse is not as great a concern as a low pulse. A low pulse may indicate imminent cardiac arrest.

thumb on the opposite side of the arm to apply counter pressure. Be sure to not use the pad of your thumb, because it may be possible to feel your own pulse in your thumb.

Capillary Refill

capillary refill ▶ the time it takes for the capillaries to refill after being blanched; normal capillary refill time is two seconds or less.

Another tool that is used to evaluate circulatory status and perfusion is the capillary refill test. Because the skin is full of very small vessels called capillaries, compressing the skin with a finger or two will temporarily squeeze the blood from the capillaries, causing the normally pink skin to appear blanched or white (Figure 11.6). When the pressure is released, the skin can be observed becoming pink again as blood returns to the capillaries. The time it takes for the blood to return to the capillaries is called the **capillary refill** time and should be two seconds or less.

This test is commonly used on adults to evaluate the circulatory status in an extremity by evaluating capillary refill time in a finger or a toe. In infants and small children, this test can be applied just about anywhere on the body and is used as a test for general perfusion status.

The capillary refill test for older children and adults is best performed using a nail bed or the pad of a finger or toe. Follow these steps to assess capillary refill:

1. Select an appropriate finger or toe (the larger the better).
2. Using your thumb and index finger, squeeze the pad of the patient's finger or toe from both sides. Observe the pad as it blanches.
3. Quickly release the pressure and observe the color return to the pad. Note the time it takes for color to return. Normal color should return in two seconds or less.
4. Document your findings.

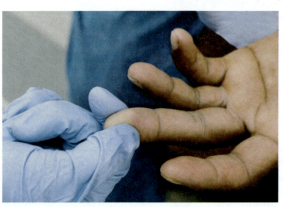

Figure 11.6 • Checking capillary refill time in the fingers.

A delayed capillary refill time may be a sign of impaired circulation due to injury or a sign of poor perfusion due to shock. There are many factors that can affect the reliability of capillary refill time, such as the temperature of the environment, medical conditions, and medications. Capillary refill is just one tool to use in your overall assessment of the patient.

continued

"Now Martin, you said you weren't allergic to anything, but are you taking any medications?" Kate asks, focusing on his skin signs. It seems that sitting him up has improved the ease and tidal volume of his breathing, not to mention his coloring has improved a bit.

"He says yes, he takes medicine for his heart. He doesn't know the names, but he has them up in his room." Hernandez says, standing up. "Should I go grab them?"

"In a minute," Kate says, reaching down to gently lift the pool towel from over Martin's covered legs. "Swollen ankles. This is making more sense of the high blood pressure I recorded a minute ago. Help me ask Martin about his medical history a bit more and then I'll get another set of vitals while you get his medications."

Blood Pressure

Blood pressure is the measurement of the pressure of blood against the walls of the arteries, both when the heart beats and when it is at rest. Blood pressure and perfusion are closely related in that good perfusion requires a good blood pressure. The lower the blood pressure drops below normal, the less effective perfusion is. A single blood pressure reading that is significantly above or below the normal range for a patient can be a valuable tool in determining the current state or condition of the patient. Repeated blood pressure measurements are valuable for trending the patient's condition and also can help to identify changes in the patient's condition over time.

Blood pressure is determined by measuring the pressure changes in the arteries. The pressure generated within the arteries when the heart contracts is called the **systolic** blood pressure. The systolic blood pressure is affected by many factors, such as the force of the heart's pumping action, the resistance and elasticity of the arteries, blood volume (blood loss means lower pressure), blood thickness or viscosity, and the amount of other fluids in the cells.

After the left ventricle of the heart contracts, it relaxes and refills. This relaxation phase is called *diastole*. During diastole, the pressure in the arteries falls. When measured, this pressure is called the **diastolic** blood pressure.

Blood pressure is measured in specific units called *millimeters of mercury (mmHg)*. These are the units on the blood pressure gauge. Since this system of measurement is standard for blood pressure readings, you will not have to say "millimeters of mercury" after each reading. Report the systolic pressure first and then the diastolic, as in "120 over 80" (120/80).

The reading of 120/80 is considered a normal blood pressure reading, which represents the average blood pressure obtained from a large sampling of healthy adults. There is a wide range of "normal" for adults and children. Blood pressures are not usually measured in the field for children under three years of age because it requires specialized equipment.

You will not know the normal blood pressure for a patient unless the person is alert, knows the information, and can tell you what it is. However, there is a general rule for estimating what a patient's blood pressure should be. This rule works for adults up to the age of 40. To estimate the systolic blood pressure of an adult male at rest, add his age to 100. To estimate the systolic blood pressure of an adult female at rest, add her age to 90. To estimate children's systolic blood pressure, use this formula: two times the age in years plus 80 ($2 \times$ age in years $+ 80$). The diastolic estimate will be two-thirds of the systolic measurement.

Since you will not know the normal reading for a particular patient, you will take several readings to identify a trend in the patient's condition.

An initial measurement may show that a patient has a blood pressure within normal limits, but the condition may worsen. For example, a patient going into shock (hypoperfusion)

blood pressure ▶ the measurement of the pressure inside the arteries, both during contractions of the heart and between contractions.

systolic ▶ the pressure within the arteries when the heart beats; the contraction phase of the heart.

diastolic ▶ the pressure that remains in the arteries when the heart is at rest; the resting phase of the heart.

IS IT SAFE?

Many new Emergency Medical Responders feel compelled to obtain a blood pressure reading even when they are unable to actually hear one. This can lead to guessing, which can be bad for patient care. Obtaining blood pressures is a skill that takes lots of practice. Do not feel inadequate if you are unable to obtain a blood pressure on every patient. Simply let others at the scene know that you are unable to clearly hear the blood pressure and ask someone else to make an attempt.

TABLE 11.5 | Normal Blood Pressures

PATIENT	SYSTOLIC	DIASTOLIC
Adult male	100 + age in years to age 40	60 to 90 mmHg
Adult female	90 + age in years to age 40	60 to 90 mmHg
Adolescent	90 mmHg (lower limit of normal)	2/3 of systolic pressure
Child 1–10 years	90 + (2 × age in years) (upper limit of normal); 70 + (2 × age in years)(lower limit of normal)	2/3 of systolic pressure
Infant 1–12 months	70 mmHg (lower limit of normal)	2/3 of systolic pressure

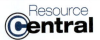
auscultation ▶ the act of listening to internal sounds of the body, typically with a stethoscope.

stethoscope ▶ a device used to auscultate sounds within the body; most commonly used to obtain blood pressure.

palpation ▶ the act of using one's hands to touch or feel the body.

may have a rapid pulse and a normal blood pressure reading when you first arrive at the scene. A few minutes later, the blood pressure may fall dramatically. Taking several readings while you are providing care is a way of identifying changes in the patient's status. Changes in blood pressure are significant and let you know that additional care is needed and transport is a priority.

A systolic blood pressure reading below 90 mmHg is considered lower than normal in most adults (Table 11.5). However, some small adult females and small-build athletes may have a normal systolic blood pressure of 90 mmHg.

A systolic reading above 140 is typically considered high blood pressure, also referred to as *hypertension*. Many patients will show an initial rise in blood pressure at the emergency scene. This is usually due to anxiety, fear, or stress caused by the incident and will return to normal once the situation or condition is under control. You will need more than one reading to confirm high blood pressure. High blood pressure readings are typical in individuals who are obese or who have a history of high cholesterol. There are many other underlying medical conditions that cause high blood pressure that you will be unable to determine at the emergency scene.

Determining Blood Pressure by Auscultation

There are two common techniques used to measure blood pressure in emergency care. The first is by listening, which is called **auscultation** and requires the use of a **stethoscope**. The second is by feeling, which is called **palpation**. The palpation method will only reveal the systolic pressure.

The auscultation method requires the use of a stethoscope to hear the sound of the blood pulsating through the artery. You must begin by adjusting the earpieces so that they fit properly in your ears. Hold the earpieces of the stethoscope between the thumb and index finger of each hand. Adjust the direction of the earpieces by gently turning them so that each piece points slightly forward (away from you) (Figure 11.7). This is to ensure that the opening of the earpieces point directly into your ear canals when placed in the ears and will help ensure that you will hear the pulsations once the blood pressure cuff is inflated.

To determine blood pressure using a blood pressure cuff and a stethoscope, you should:

1. Have the ill or injured person sit or lie down (Figure 11.8). Cut away or remove clothing that is on the arm. Support the arm at the level of the heart. Do not use the arm if there is any possibility of injury.

2. Select the correct-size blood pressure cuff. The average adult cuff can accommodate an arm that is up to 13 inches in circumference. A cuff that is too small will produce falsely high readings, and one that is too large will produce falsely low readings.

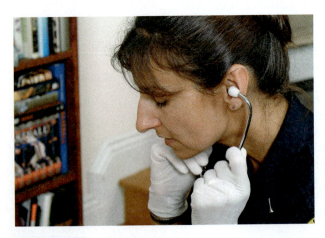

Figure 11.7 • Adjust the earpieces of the stethoscope so they point forward into the ear canal.

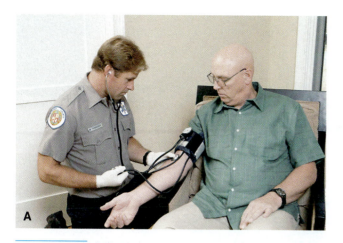
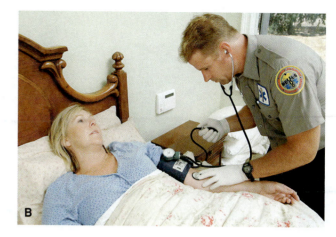

Figure 11.8 • (A) Proper position for taking a blood pressure while seated. (B) Obtaining a blood pressure on a supine patient.

3. Wrap the cuff around the person's upper arm. The lower border of the cuff should be about one inch above the crease in the elbow. The center of the bladder inside the cuff must be placed over the brachial artery in the upper arm (Figure 11.9).

4. Apply the cuff securely but not too tightly. You should be able to place one finger under the bottom edge of the cuff (Figure 11.10).

5. Place the ends of the stethoscope in your ears. Be sure to adjust the earpieces so that they face forward into your ear canals. If you are using a dual-head stethoscope, which has both a bell and a diaphragm, make certain to check that the appropriate side is activated before placing it on the ill or injured person.

6. Use your fingertips to locate the brachial artery at the crease in the elbow.

7. Position the diaphragm of the stethoscope over the brachial artery pulse site. Do not let the head of the stethoscope touch the cuff. If it touches the cuff, the stethoscope will rub against it during inflation and deflation. You will hear the rubbing sounds, which may cause you to record a false reading.

8. Close the valve and inflate the cuff to approximately 180 mmHg for an adult and 120 mmHg for a child.

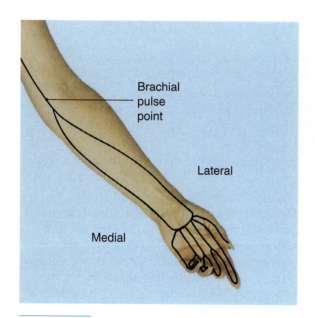

Figure 11.9 • Location of the brachial artery.

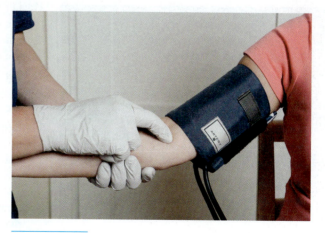

Figure 11.10 • Proper placement of the blood pressure cuff.

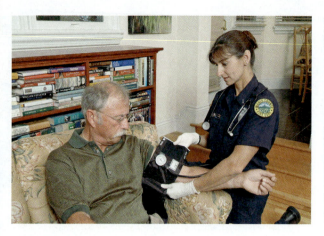

11.1.1 | Place the cuff snugly around the upper arm.

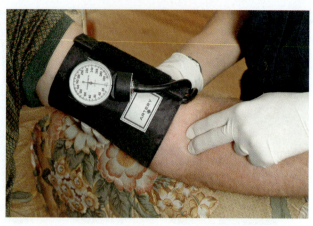

11.1.2 | Palpate the brachial pulse point and place the diaphragm of the stethoscope over the pulse point

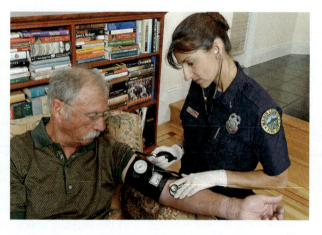

11.1.3 | Quickly inflate the cuff then release the pressure to obtain the blood pressure readings.

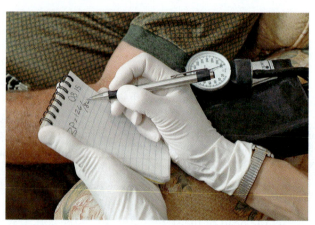

11.1.4 | Document your readings.

9. Once the cuff is inflated, open the valve slowly to release pressure from the cuff. It should fall at a smooth rate of 2 to 3 mmHg per second, or a little faster than the second hand on a watch.

10. Listen carefully as you watch the needle move. Note when you hear the sound of the pulse in the stethoscope. The first significant sound that you hear is the systolic pressure.

11. Let the cuff continue to deflate. Listen for and note when the sound of the pulse (clicking or tapping) fades (not when it stops). When the sound turns dull or soft, this is the diastolic pressure (Figure 11.11).

12. Let the rest of the air out of the cuff quickly. Be sure to squeeze the cuff to release all the air. If practical, leave the cuff in place so you can take additional readings.

13. Record the time, the arm used, the position of the ill or injured person (lying down, sitting), and the pressure readings. Round off the readings to the next highest number. For example, 145 mmHg should be recorded as 146 mmHg. (The markings on the gauge are in even numbers. You may "see" the first sound in between two markings and want to record it as an odd number—145—but all blood pressure readings are recorded in even numbers.)

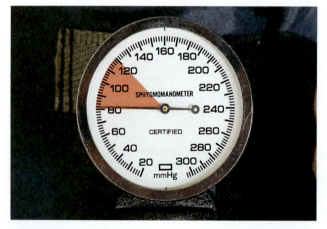

Figure 11.11 • Pulse sounds will be heard between the systolic and diastolic readings.

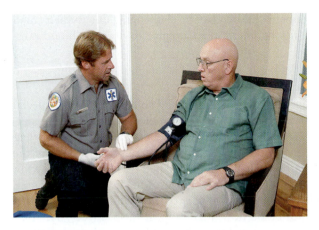

11.2.1 | Place the cuff and locate the radial pulse.

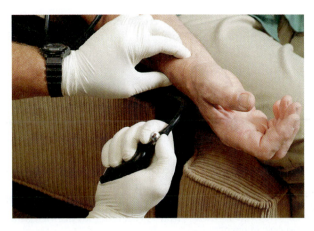

11.2.2 | Inflate the cuff until you feel the radial pulse go away.

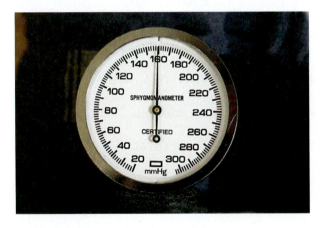

11.2.3 | Continue inflating cuff to approximately 30 mmHg beyond where the pulse went away.

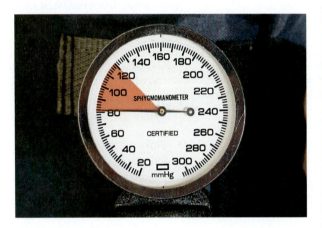

11.2.4 | Release the pressure in the cuff and note the pressure on the gauge when the radial pulse returns.

If you are not certain of a reading, be sure the cuff is totally deflated and wait one or two minutes and try again, or use the person's other arm. Should you try the same arm too soon, you may get a false high reading. (See Scan 11.1.)

Determining Blood Pressure by Palpation

Using the palpation method (feeling the radial pulse) is not a very accurate method. It will provide you with one reading: an approximate systolic pressure. This method is used when there is too much ambient noise, making it difficult to hear with a stethoscope.

To determine blood pressure by palpation, place the cuff in the same position on the arm as you would for auscultation. Then proceed with the following (Scan 11.2.):

1. Find the radial pulse on the arm with the cuff.

2. Close the valve and inflate the cuff until you can no longer feel the pulse.

3. Continue to inflate the cuff to a point 30 mmHg above the point where the pulse disappeared.

4. Slowly deflate the cuff and note the reading when you feel the pulse return. This is the systolic blood pressure. You will not get a diastolic pressure reading by palpation.

5. Record the time, the arm used, the position of the person, and the systolic pressure. Note that the reading was by palpation. If you give this information orally to someone, make sure they know the reading was by palpation, as in, "Blood pressure is 146 by palpation."

Attempting to obtain blood pressure in children can be challenging due to their small size and difficulty sitting still. It may not be practical to attempt to obtain a blood pressure in children under the age of three.

Skin Signs

Skin signs are often the easiest vital signs to assess because they do not require any special skill or equipment. The three characteristics that you will be evaluating are color, temperature, and moisture. All three can be assessed by observing the patient's face and feeling the forehead. When assessing skin color in light-skinned patients, observe the skin of the face, noting if it appears pink (normal) or if it is pale or flushed (reddish) or yellow. In dark-skinned patients, observe the palms, nail beds, and inside of the lips to look for pink appearance. Skin that is not being perfused well will appear pale or **cyanotic** (bluish). Skin that is receiving an abnormal amount of blood flow might appear flushed (red). Skin that is yellow in appearance is said to be jaundiced and may be an indication of an underlying condition related to the liver.

Next, use the back of one hand to assess skin temperature (Figure 11.12). Pull the glove away from the back of your hand and hold it skin-to-skin against the patient's forehead. Note if the skin appears warm (normal), cool, or hot. At the same time you are assessing color and temperature, you can assess for moisture. Note if the skin appears dry (normal) or moist (sweaty). The medical term for sweaty is **diaphoretic**. Moisture can further be classified as mild, moderate, or severe diaphoresis.

Table 11.6 lists some of the problems associated with skin color, relative skin temperature, and moisture.

Here are some examples of how you might document skin signs:

- Pink, warm, dry (PWD)
- Pale, cool, moist
- Flushed, hot, moist
- Flushed, hot, dry

cyanotic ► the bluish coloration of the skin caused by an inadequate supply of oxygen; typically seen at the mucous membranes and nail beds.

diaphoretic ► excessive sweating; commonly caused by exertion or some medical problem, such as heart attack and shock.

TABLE 11.6 | Skin Signs

SKIN COLOR	SIGNIFICANCE/POSSIBLE CAUSES
Pink	Normal in light-skinned patients; normal in inner eyelids, lips, and nail beds of dark-skinned patients
Pale	Constricted blood vessels possibly resulting from blood loss, shock, decreased blood pressure, emotional distress
Blue (cyanotic)	Lack of oxygen in blood cells and tissues resulting from inadequate breathing or heart function
Red (flushed)	Heat exposure, high blood pressure, emotional excitement; cherry red indicates late stages of carbon monoxide poisoning
Yellow (jaundiced)	Liver abnormalities
Blotchiness (mottling)	Occasionally in patients in shock
TEMPERATURE AND CONDITION	**SIGNIFICANCE/POSSIBLE CAUSES**
Cool, moist (clammy)	Shock, heart attack, anxiety
Cold, dry	Exposure to cold, diabetic emergency
Hot, dry	High fever, heat emergency, spine injury
Hot, moist	High fever, heat emergency, diabetic emergency
Goose bumps accompanied by shivering, chattering teeth, blue lips, and pale skin	Chills, communicable disease, exposure to cold, pain, or fear

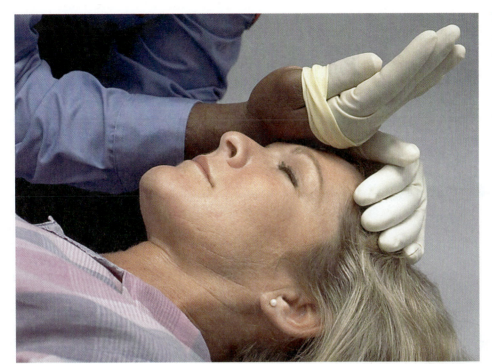

To evaluate skin color in dark-skinned patients, use one or more of these methods:

- *Oral mucosa.* Inspect the inside of the lower lip. This area should be pink and moist.
- *Conjunctiva.* This is the tissue on the inside of the skin that surrounds each eye. By simply pulling down gently on the lower eyelid, you will expose this area. It, too, should be pink and moist.
- *Nail beds.* This is the tissue that lies below each finger and toenail and can typically be seen through the nail. Of course, if the patient is wearing nail polish, this will not be an option.
- *Palms.* The palms of the hands are generally lighter in color regardless of skin pigmentation. They are also full of capillaries, and a simple capillary refill test can provide some indication as to perfusion status in the hand.

Pupils

Whether you realize it or not, you have probably become quite good at assessing a person's condition by looking into their eyes. Emotions such as fear, worry, anxiety, and pain can all be seen in the eyes. As an Emergency Medical Responder, you will be assessing the eyes for the following very specific characteristics: pupil size and shape, equality of pupil size, and reactivity to light (Figure 11.13).

Size and Shape

When you first look at the eyes, note their general condition and identify any obvious injury or deformity. Pay particular attention to the dark circles in the center of each eye known as the pupil. Note the size and shape of each pupil. Many EMS pen lights have a pupil gauge printed on the side to aid in the determination of pupil size. Ensure that both pupils are round.

Equality

Observe both pupils to ensure they are the same size. Keep in mind that dark-colored eyes are much more difficult to assess than light-colored eyes. It is also important to note that

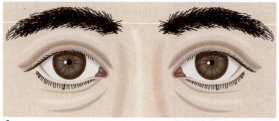

A. Constricted pupils

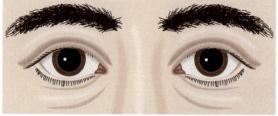

B. Dilated pupils

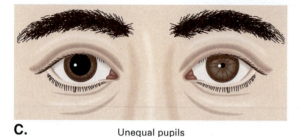

C. Unequal pupils

Figure 11.13 • (A) Constricted pupils. (B) Dilated pupils. (C) Unequal pupils.

unequal pupils are a normal finding in some people. When you encounter a patient with unequal pupils, always ask if this is a normal condition for them.

Reactivity to Light

One of the important signs of good perfusion is pupils that respond briskly to the presence or absence of light. Pupils should respond to the sudden introduction of light by constricting and in contrast should dilate when light to the pupil is blocked. There are at least two methods that can be used to assess pupil reaction, and each depends on the ambient light at the time.

In a well-lit area such as a bright room or on a bright sunny day, it may be of no use attempting to shine a light into someone's eyes. The pupils will likely already be constricted due to the large amount of ambient light. In this situation you will have better results covering each of the patient's eyes, one at a time with your hand for several seconds, and then observing the pupil constrict when you take your hand away. You must learn to be patient when using this method because it may take some time for the pupil to dilate after you cover the eye. It is a good practice to ask at least two or three questions pertaining to the patient's medical history while you cover each eye. This will allow enough time for the pupil to dilate and not appear as an awkward silence.

In situations where there is not a lot of ambient light, an artificial light source such as a penlight or flashlight will be necessary. Ask the patient to stare straight ahead as you hold the light just outside his field of vision. With the light turned on, quickly move the light from the side directly at his pupil. Watch closely for the pupil to constrict as the light hits it. Then move the light away and watch the pupil dilate slightly and return to its original size.

Both pupils should react to the change in light with the same speed. Pupils that respond slowly to the change in light are documented as sluggish. Pupils that do not respond at all are referred to as fixed. When a person goes into cardiac arrest, the pupils gradually become fixed and dilated.

An acronym that is widely used in EMS to help providers remember the characteristics of pupils is PERL. PERL stands for:

P — Pupils
E — Equal
R — Reactive
L — Light

Table 11.7 provides observations you may make when assessing a patient's pupils and lists possible causes.

TABLE 11.7	Pupils	
OBSERVATION	**POSSIBLE PROBLEM**
Dilated, nonreactive pupils	Shock, cardiac arrest, bleeding, certain medications, head injury
Constricted, nonreactive pupils	Central nervous system damage, certain medications
Unequal pupils	Stroke, head injury

"I don't understand," Kate says, looking over the shoulders of the firefighters and ambulance personnel. They are loading Martin onto a stretcher and hooking him up to a heart monitor and oxygen. "Look at his vitals. He was doing better after 10 minutes and then suddenly his skin flashed gray, his pulse was soaring, and he was practically gasping like a fish."

"Ma'am, you did everything just fine," a paramedic says, taking the list of vitals and paper bag of medications from Kate's shaking grip. "Sitting him up, keeping him com-fortable, and keeping track of his vitals as you did probably kept him from getting worse, sooner. We have a better chance of getting him to a doctor because of you."

The loud clatter of the stretcher and the medical chatter of the fire crew drowns out Kate's goodbye to Martin as he is unceremoniously wheeled straight out to the ambulance without a second look back.

Hernandez puts his hand on Kate's shoulder and sighs. "To think I almost called in sick today."

Summary

Gathering information (history) about your patient and his chief complaint and obtaining complete and accurate vital signs are two of the most important aspects of a good patient assessment. Here are some of the key concepts to remember about getting a good medical history and vital signs.

- Properly introduce yourself and get the patient's name right away. Establishing a good rapport from the beginning will make the patient comfortable and more cooperative.

- Whenever possible, direct your questions to the patient.

- Speak clearly and confirm that the patient hears, understands, and answers each question before asking another.

- Utilize the SAMPLE tool to help guide your questions, and always document the patient's answers.

- Obtain a set of vital signs as soon as practical to establish a good baseline for comparison of subsequent vital signs.

- When practical, repeat vital signs and compare them to previous readings to establish trends in the patient's condition.

- Remember that most vital signs have multiple characteristics; document all characteristics for each vital sign for the complete picture of your patient.

Take Action

MAKING HISTORY

You can practice performing a SAMPLE history just about anywhere there are people. Make up a set of flashcards, one for each letter of the SAMPLE acronym. On one side put the letter and the word that it represents. On the opposite side write several questions that pertain to the letter. Now use the flashcards to help you practice performing a SAMPLE history on friends and family members.

PRACTICE MAKES PROFICIENT

Developing proficiency with taking vital signs takes considerable practice. Fortunately, there is rarely a shortage of people to practice on. There are no special tools necessary to practice most vital signs (excluding blood pressure), so there is no reason you cannot practice vital signs every day.

First on Scene Run Review

Recall the events of the "First on Scene" scenario in this chapter and answer the following questions, which are related to the call. Rationales are offered in the Answer Key at the back of the book.

1. What are the signs and symptoms that Kate found, and what might they indicate?

2. What would your treatment be for this patient?

3. Why would sitting Martin up help him?

Quick Quiz

To check your understanding of the chapter, answer the following questions. Then compare your answers to those in the Answer Key at the back of the book.

1. A common tool used in EMS to classify a patient's mental status is the _____ scale.
   a. AVPU
   b. ABC
   c. QRS
   d. TUV

2. In a SAMPLE history, the E represents:
   a. EKG results.
   b. evaluation of the neck and spine.
   c. events leading to illness or injury.
   d. evidence of airway obstruction.

3. When assessing circulation for a responsive adult patient, you should assess:

   a. the carotid pulse.
   b. radial pulses on both sides of the body.
   c. the radial pulse on one side.
   d. the distal pulse.

4. The adequate flow of oxygenated blood to all cells of the body is called:

   a. circulation.
   b. perfusion.
   c. compensation.
   d. systole.

5. When assessing a patient's respirations, you must determine rate, depth, and:

   a. regularity.
   b. count of expirations.
   c. ease.
   d. count of inspirations.

6. The five most important vital signs are pulse, respirations, blood pressure, pupils, and:

   a. oxygen saturation.
   b. skin signs.
   c. mental status.
   d. capillary refill.

7. The first set of vital signs obtained on any patient is referred to as the _____ set.

   a. historical
   b. ongoing
   c. baseline
   d. serial

8. What can be assessed by watching and feeling the chest and abdomen move during breathing?

   a. Pulse rate
   b. Blood pressure
   c. Skin signs
   d. Respiratory rate

9. Characteristics of a pulse include:

   a. rate, depth, and ease.
   b. rate, strength, and rhythm.
   c. rate, depth, and strength.
   d. rate, ease, and quality.

10. The most appropriate location to obtain a pulse for an unresponsive adult is the _____ artery.

    a. brachial
    b. femoral
    c. carotid
    d. radial

11. What are the two pulse points that are referred to as central pulses?

    a. Radial and tibial
    b. Carotid and femoral
    c. Femoral and brachial
    d. Brachial and carotid

12. As blood pressure drops, perfusion is most likely to:

    a. increase.
    b. decrease.
    c. fluctuate.
    d. remain the same.

13. Skin that is bluish in color is called:

    a. pale.
    b. flushed.
    c. cyanotic.
    d. jaundice.

14. The term *diaphoretic* refers to:

    a. pupil reaction.
    b. skin temperature
    c. heart rhythm.
    d. skin moisture.

15. When going from a well-lit room to a dark one, you would expect the normal pupil to:

    a. not react.
    b. dilate.
    c. constrict.
    d. fluctuate.

16. Which one of the following is most accurate when describing a palpated blood pressure?

    a. It provides only the diastolic pressure.
    b. It must be taken on a responsive patient.
    c. It can be obtained without a stethoscope.
    d. It can be obtained without a BP cuff.

17. A respiratory rate that is less than _____ for an adult should be considered inadequate.

    a. 4
    b. 6
    c. 8
    d. 10

18. The pressure inside the arteries each time the heart contracts is referred to as the _____ pressure.

    a. diastolic
    b. pulse
    c. systolic
    d. mean

19. A _____ is something the Emergency Medical Responder can see or measure during the patient assessment.

    a. symptom
    b. history
    c. sign
    d. chief complaint

20. The term *trending* is best defined as the:

    a. ability to spot changes in a patient's condition over time.
    b. name given to the last set of vital signs taken on a patient.
    c. transfer of care from one level of care to another.
    d. the ability to improve a patient's condition over time.

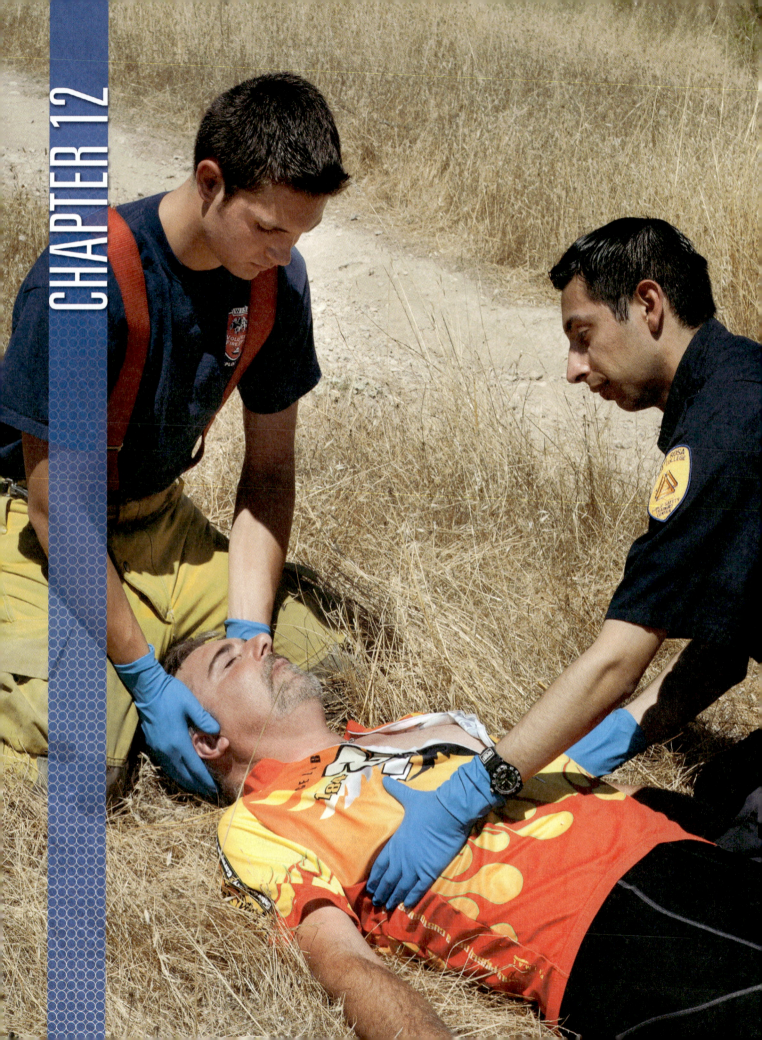

CHAPTER 12

Principles of Patient Assessment

EDUCATION STANDARDS

• Assessment—Scene Size-up, Primary Assessment, Secondary Assessment, Reassessment

COMPETENCIES

• Use scene information and simple patient assessment findings to identify and manage immediate life threats and injuries within the scope of practice of the Emergency Medical Responder.

CHAPTER OVERVIEW

The foundation of all emergency care lies in a good assessment of the patient. One of the most fundamental skills you will learn and develop is that of patient assessment. Patients cannot receive the care they need until their problems are identified. You must assess each patient to detect possible illness or injury and determine the most appropriate emergency care for the patient. This assessment must be done in a structured and orderly fashion to minimize the chance of overlooking an important sign or symptom.

Remember that a good patient assessment almost always leads to good patient care. A poor assessment almost always results in poor patient care. This chapter will assist you in learning a thorough and methodical patient assessment.

Upon successful completion of this chapter, the student should be able to:

COGNITIVE

1. Define the following terms:

   a. ABCs *(p. 251)*

   b. accessory muscle use *(p. 267)*

   c. AVPU scale *(p. 253)*

   d. baseline vital signs *(p. 244)*

   e. brachial pulse *(p. 256)*

   f. BP-DOC *(p. 265)*

   g. capillary refill *(p. 256)*

   h. carotid pulse *(p. 254)*

   i. chief complaint *(p. 244)*

   j. crepitus *(p. 265)*

   k. DCAP-BTLS *(p. 265)*

   l. dorsalis pedis pulse *(p. 268)*

   m. focused secondary assessment *(p. 257)*

   n. general impression *(p. 251)*

   o. guarding *(p. 267)*

   p. immediate life threats *(p. 244)*

   q. interventions *(p. 241)*

   r. jugular vein distention *(p. 267)*

   s. manual stabilization *(p. 251)*

   t. mechanism of injury (MOI) *(p. 248)*

   u. medical patient *(p. 243)*

   v. nature of illness *(p. 248)*

   w. OPQRST *(p. 269)*

   x. paradoxical movement *(p. 267)*

   y. patient assessment *(p. 241)*

   z. primary assessment *(p. 243)*

   aa. radial pulse *(p. 255)*

   bb. rapid secondary assessment *(p. 260)*

   cc. reassessment *(p. 244)*

   dd. SAMPLE history *(p. 262)*

   ee. scene size-up *(p. 241)*

   ff. secondary assessment *(p. 243)*

   gg. signs *(p. 241)*

   hh. symptoms *(p. 241)*

   ii. track marks *(p. 268)*

   jj. trauma patient *(p. 243)*

   kk. tracheal deviation *(p. 267)*

   ll. trending *(p. 271)*

2. Explain the importance that safety plays at the scene of an emergency. *(p. 245)*

3. Describe hazards commonly found at emergency scenes (medical and trauma). *(p. 247)*

OBJECTIVES

4. Explain the role that the Emergency Medical Responder plays in ensuring the safety of all people at the scene of an emergency. *(p. 247)*

5. Describe the components of an appropriate scene size-up and the importance of each component. *(p. 246)*

6. Differentiate between mechanism of injury and nature of illness. *(p. 248)*

7. Differentiate between a significant and non-significant mechanism of injury. *(p. 258)*

8. Explain the purpose of the primary assessment. *(p. 249)*

9. Describe the components of a primary assessment. *(p. 250)*

10. Describe patients who are high and low priority for transport. *(p. 256)*

11. Explain the purpose of the secondary assessment. *(p. 257)*

12. Describe the components of a secondary assessment. *(p. 257)*

13. Describe the components of the SAMPLE history tool. *(p. 262)*

14. Describe the components of the BP-DOC assessment tool. *(p. 265)*

15. Explain the purpose of the reassessment. *(p. 271)*

16. Describe the unique assessment methods used for pediatric and geriatric patients. *(p. 256)*

PSYCHOMOTOR

17. Demonstrate the ability to identify immediate and potential hazards to safety.

18. Demonstrate the ability to properly perform a scene size-up.

19. Demonstrate the ability to properly perform a primary assessment.

20. Demonstrate the ability to properly perform a secondary assessment.

21. Demonstrate the ability to properly perform a reassessment.

22. Demonstrate the ability to properly identify and perform appropriate interventions during a patient assessment.

AFFECTIVE

23. Value the priority that safety plays in the overall assessment and care of the patient.

24. Model a caring and compassionate attitude with classmates and simulated patients.

25. Support the role of the Emergency Medical Responder with respect to patient advocacy.

26. Model an appropriate level of concern for a patient's modesty when exposing the body during an assessment.

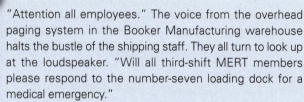

FIRST ON SCENE

"Attention all employees." The voice from the overhead paging system in the Booker Manufacturing warehouse halts the bustle of the shipping staff. They all turn to look up at the loudspeaker. "Will all third-shift MERT members please respond to the number-seven loading dock for a medical emergency."

Two of the warehouse employees remove their leather gloves and face shields and quickly walk to a white locker with "MERT" stenciled on its side in wide red letters. They open the cabinet, remove two nylon bags, and hurry toward the loading docks at the south end of the building.

"I'll be the patient-care person if you'll do scene control," Joanie Sutter says.

"Okay," Renee Murphy replies, fishing a pair of gloves from her bag and putting them on. Renee is actually relieved to be with an experienced Medical Emergency Response Team member. She is new to the company's MERT, and the patient-assessment process is still a little confusing to her.

As the two pass the dock manager's small office and turn left, they are met by a forklift operator whose name, according to his embroidered shirt, is Tariq. "I'm glad you're here," he says quickly. "It's one of the truck drivers. I think he's having a heart attack."

Patient Assessment

Many EMS systems use an assessment-based approach to providing care to patients (Figure 12.1). This is to say that Emergency Medical Responders and other EMS personnel are trained to identify, prioritize, and care for major signs and symptoms. What they will not do is try to diagnose a patient's specific problems. For example, an Emergency Medical Responder will do what he can to make sure a patient with difficulty breathing has an open airway and supplemental oxygen. What he will *not* do is waste critical time attempting to figure out the underlying cause of the patient's difficulty. Once all life threats have been cared for, the Emergency Medical Responder will complete a more

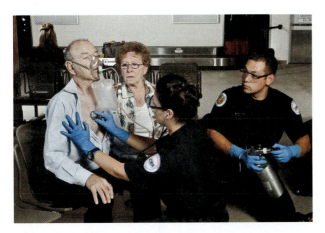

Figure 12.1 • A thorough patient assessment will be the foundation for the care of all patients.

thorough assessment of the patient, identify less obvious **signs** and **symptoms**, and gather a pertinent medical history.

Assessment-Based Care

A typical patient assessment contains four major components (Figure 12.2):

- *Scene size-up*. The **scene size-up** is an overview of the scene to identify any obvious or potential hazards.
- *Primary assessment*. This is a quick assessment of the patient's airway, breathing, circulation, and bleeding undertaken to detect and correct any immediate life-threatening problems.
- *Secondary assessment*. The secondary assessment is a more thorough assessment of the patient and has two subcomponents:
  - *History*. This includes all the information that you can gather regarding the patient's condition as well as any previous medical history.
  - *Physical exam*. This includes using your hands and eyes to inspect the patient for any signs of illness and/or injury.
- *Reassessment*. Monitoring the patient to detect any changes in his condition, this component repeats the primary assessment (usually done en route to the hospital), corrects any additional life-threatening problems, repeats vital signs, and evaluates and adjusts as needed any **interventions** performed, such as repositioning the patient or increasing supplemental oxygen. You will find that the condition of your patient will improve, stay the same, or get worse.

While the responsibilities of the Emergency Medical Responder may differ from one EMS system to another, most use an assessment-based approach to patient care. After ensuring one's own personal safety, an Emergency Medical Responder's first concern is to detect and begin to correct life-threatening problems in his patient. The second concern is to identify and provide care for problems that are less serious or may become serious. The third concern is to constantly monitor the patient's condition to quickly detect any changes that may need attention.

Scene Safety

The components of **patient assessment** and the order in which they are performed may vary from patient to patient based on each patient's problem. But before you study them, you must first address issues related to the safety of the scene.

The conditions at a safe scene allow for rescuers to access and provide care to patients without danger to themselves. An unsafe scene is one that contains hazards that are either immediate or potential. An example may be a motor-vehicle crash site. It is not unusual to find vehicles or objects that can move or shift position (an overturned car and broken

KEY POINT ▼

A patient who appears to be stable can become unstable without warning.

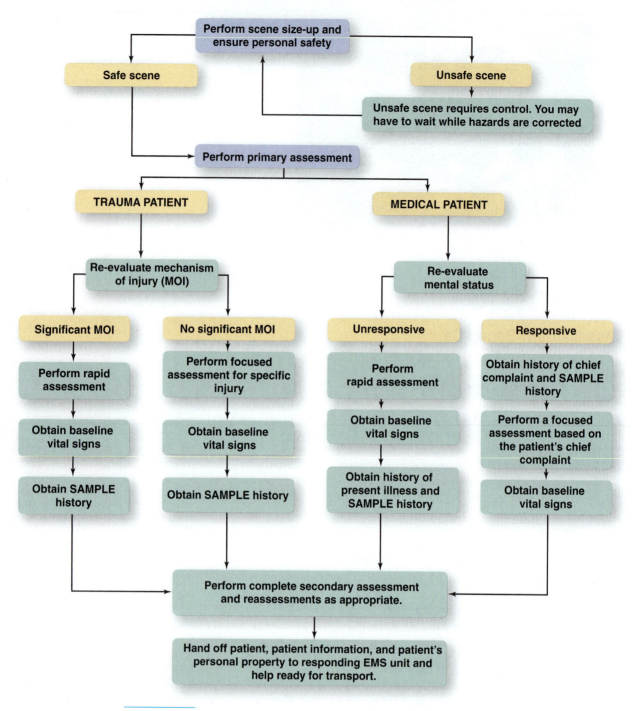

Figure 12.2 • Patient assessment algorithm.

glass are examples of immediate hazards). In addition, fire could break out or fuel and other fluids could leak and increase the danger, causing the scene to become even more unsafe. Those are examples of potential hazards.

Immediate Life Threats

The **primary assessment** is a set of steps meant to detect and correct life-threatening problems. The remaining components of the patient assessment change slightly with each of the four types of patient: (a) responsive **medical patients,** (b) unresponsive medical patients, (c) **trauma patients,** who have a significant mechanism of injury (MOI), and (d) trauma patients who do not have a significant MOI.

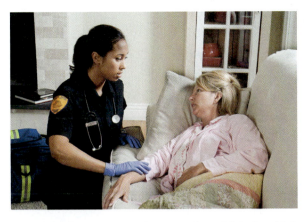

12.1.1 | Perform a scene size-up and establish the chief complaint.

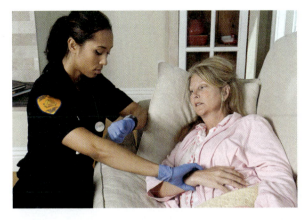

12.1.2 | Perform a primary assessment. Care for immediate life threats first.

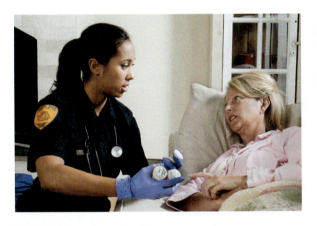

12.1.3 | Obtain a medical history.

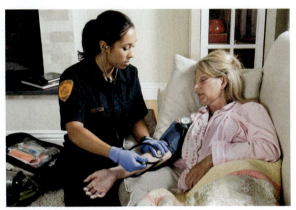

12.1.4 | Perform a secondary assessment including vital signs.

At times, the type of patient you are caring for is not so clearly defined. For example, a patient experiencing a medical problem may fall and injure himself, or a medical problem may have actually caused a car crash. Your patient assessment will need to include elements for both medical and trauma emergencies. What should guide your assessment should be the more serious of the patient's problems.

Medical Patients

For a responsive medical patient, you will (Scan 12.1):

- Perform a scene size-up and a primary assessment.
- Perform a **secondary assessment** based on the patient's **chief complaint**.
- Obtain **baseline vital signs**.
- Perform a **reassessment**, including the patient's vital signs, in order to identify any changes in the patient's condition.

For an unresponsive medical patient, you will (Scan 12.2):

- Perform a scene size-up and a primary assessment. Care for all **immediate life threats** first.
- Perform a rapid secondary assessment to look for signs of illness.
- Obtain baseline vital signs.
- Attempt to interview the patient's family or bystanders to determine the patient's chief complaint and nature of illness (NOI).

primary assessment ▶ a quick assessment of the patient's airway, breathing, circulation, and bleeding to detect and correct any immediate life-threatening problems.

medical patient ▶ one who has or describes symptoms of an illness; a patient with no injuries.

trauma patient ▶ one who has a physical injury caused by an external force.

secondary assessment ▶ a complete head-to-toe physical exam, including medical history.

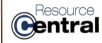

Learn more about safety by viewing a video on domestic violence.

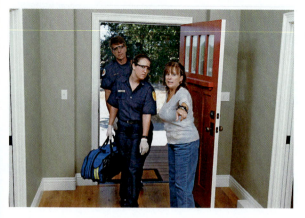

12.2.1 | Perform a scene size-up as you approach the scene.

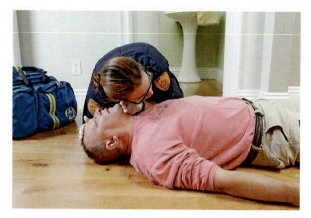

12.2.2 | Perform a primary assessment. Care for immediate life threats first.

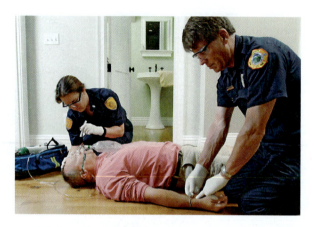

12.2.3 | Perform a rapid secondary assessment to identify signs of illness. Obtain baseline vital signs. Perform reassessments as often as necessary depending on the patient's condition.

chief complaint ▶ the reason EMS was called, in the patient's own words.

baseline vital signs ▶ the first determination of vital signs; used to compare with all further readings of vital signs to identify trends.

reassessment ▶ the last step in patient assessment, used to detect changes in a patient's condition; includes repeating initial assessment, reassessing and recording vital signs, and checking interventions.

immediate life threats ▶ any condition that may pose an immediate threat to the patient's life, such as problems with the airway, breathing, circulation, or safety.

• Perform a reassessment including vital signs to identify any changes in the patient's condition.

Trauma Patients

For a trauma patient with no significant mechanism of injury, you will (Scan 12.3):

• Perform a scene size-up and a primary assessment. Include a size-up of the scene to determine the mechanism of injury (MOI).
• Conduct a secondary assessment based on the patient's chief complaint.
• Obtain baseline vital signs.
• Perform a reassessment, including vital signs, to identify any changes in the patient's condition.

For a trauma patient with a significant mechanism of injury, you will (Scan 12.4):

• Perform a scene size-up. Include a size-up of the scene and make note of the mechanism of injury.
• Perform a primary assessment. Manually stabilize the patient's head and neck. Care for any life threats as you detect them.
• Perform a rapid secondary assessment to look for obvious serious injuries. Simultaneously, begin to question family and bystanders about the incident.

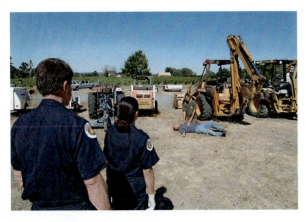

12.3.1 | Perform a scene size-up as you approach the scene.

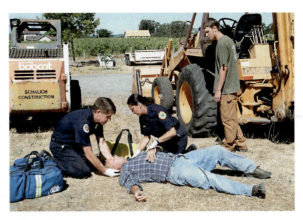

12.3.2 | Perform a primary assessment. Care for immediate life threats first.

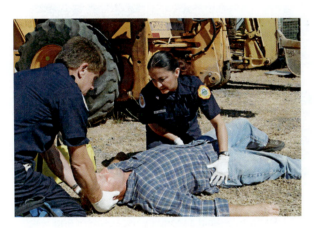

12.3.3 | Perform a focused secondary assessment based on the patient's injuries. Perform reassessments as often as necessary, depending on the patient's condition.

- Obtain baseline vital signs.
- Perform a reassessment, including a reassessment of vital signs, to identify any changes in the patient's condition.

Scene Size-up

Safety is a primary goal of the scene size-up. The scene size-up actually begins with the information you receive from dispatch before you arrive at the emergency scene. While en route, bring to mind the dispatcher's description of the emergency. Think about the types of injuries or hazards you may find at that particular scene.

When you arrive on scene, take appropriate BSI precautions and make sure the scene is safe to enter. When the scene is safe to enter, remain cautious and continue to evaluate scene safety throughout the call. Next, look for the mechanism of injury at calls involving

OBJECTIVE

2. Explain the importance that safety plays at the scene of an emergency.

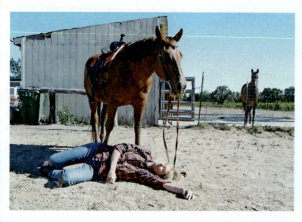

12.4.1 | Perform a scene size-up as you approach the scene.

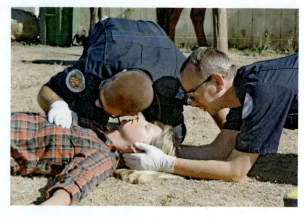

12.4.2 | Perform a primary assessment. Care for immediate life threats first.

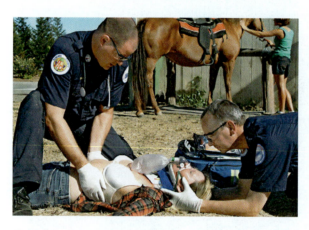

12.4.3 | Perform a rapid secondary assessment and obtain baseline vital signs. Perform reassessments as often as necessary, depending on the patient's condition.

a trauma patient. Identify the nature of illness at medical emergencies (Figure 12.3). Note the number of patients, and anticipate any additional resources that may be needed. For all patients, consider the need for spinal precautions as you approach the scene.

To recap, every patient assessment begins with scene size-up, which includes (Scan 12.5):

- Taking BSI precautions.
- Determining if the scene is safe for you, other responders, the patient, and bystanders.
- Identifying the mechanism of injury or nature of illness.
- Determining the number of patients.
- Identifying any additional resources needed.
- Considering the need for spinal precautions.

BSI Precautions

Always take appropriate BSI precautions when assessing and caring for patients. At the very least, this includes wearing disposable synthetic gloves. Wear eye protection, and use

TRAUMA PATIENT

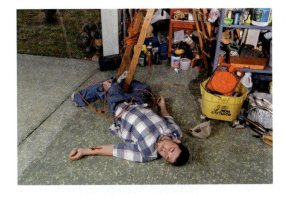

As you approach the trauma patient:

- Take appropriate BSI precautions.
- Determine if the scene is safe for you, the patient, and bystanders.
- Identify and evaluate the mechanism of injury.
- Determine the number of patients.
- Decide if additional resources are needed such as an ambulance, fire department, law enforcement, helicopter, or utility company.
- Consider the need for spinal immobilization.

MEDICAL PATIENT

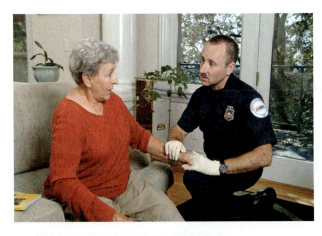

As you approach the medical patient:

- Take appropriate BSI precautions.
- Determine if the scene is safe for you, the patient, and bystanders.
- Identify and evaluate the nature of illness.
- Determine the number of patients.
- Decide if additional resources are needed such as an ambulance, fire department, law enforcement, helicopter, or utility company.

additional personal protective equipment as needed, depending on the patient's problem. Remember, BSI precautions are meant to protect both you and your patient, so take precautions before you make contact.

Scene Safety

A dangerous and sometimes fatal mistake that responders make is entering an unsafe or hazardous scene. Never assume that any scene is safe. Take the time to stop and carefully assess the scene for yourself. If the scene is unsafe, do not enter it. For example, if a scene has the potential for violence, and you are not a law enforcement officer, do not enter it until law enforcement indicates it is safe for you to do so. If there is a potential for a hazardous materials release, remain a safe distance away. In fact, you may never actually enter such scenes. Often, appropriately trained and equipped hazardous-materials team members will bring properly decontaminated patients to you.

Examples of unsafe scenes include those involving vehicle collisions and traffic, the release of toxic substances, violence or crime, any weapon, and unsafe surfaces. Also look for signs of domestic disturbances, electrical hazards, potential for fire or explosions, and guard dogs. Use all your senses to detect unsafe scenes. Remain at a safe distance to keep yourself and others away from harm.

An important rule to remember is this: *Do not become a victim yourself.* Every year many rescuers are injured and some are killed while attempting to care for others at an emergency scene.

OBJECTIVES

3. Describe hazards commonly found at emergency scenes (medical and trauma).

4. Explain the role that the Emergency Medical Responder plays in ensuring the safety of all people at the scene of an emergency.

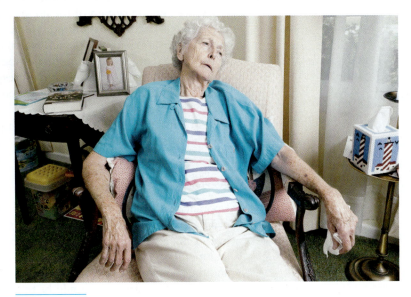

Figure 12.3 • The medical patient's chief complaint may be apparent as you approach.

mechanism of injury (MOI) ▶ the force or forces that may have caused injury.

nature of illness (NOI) ▶ what is medically wrong with the patient; a complaint not related to an injury.

Read about roadside safety issues.

Mechanism of Injury or Nature of Illness

During the scene size-up, you must do your best to identify the mechanism of injury (MOI) for a trauma patient and the nature of illness (NOI) for a medical patient. Information may be obtained from the patient, from family members or bystanders, and by carefully looking at the scene for clues.

The **mechanism of injury (MOI)** is made up of the combined forces that caused the injury. Did the patient fall? Is there a penetrating wound? Was he involved in a motor-vehicle collision? A damaged steering wheel of a vehicle, for example, should lead you to consider the possibility of a chest injury. A cracked windshield could be an indication of a head injury. Consider spine injuries in a patient who experienced a fall.

Identifying the **nature of illness (NOI)** is similar to identifying a mechanism of injury. In most instances the NOI will be directly related to the patient's chief complaint. Common NOIs include chest pain, difficulty breathing, and abdominal pain. Look at the patient and the area in which he is found for clues to his problem. Does the patient look as if he is in distress? Does his position suggest where there might be pain or discomfort? Are there medications or is there home oxygen equipment in view? Do you detect any odors, such as vomit or urine? While diagnosing why the patient is having a particular medical problem is not necessary, the nature of illness will guide you in the appropriate direction for care.

Both the mechanism of injury for trauma patients and the nature of illness for medical patients will allow you to consider what complications may have not yet developed. For example, if the patient is complaining of chest pain, consider the possibility of a heart problem and the potential for cardiac arrest. If the patient experienced a fall, consider the forces involved and the potential for injury.

▶ GERIATRIC FOCUS ◀

It is important to recognize that the elderly may suffer severe injuries from less significant mechanisms of injury than younger patients. Therefore, when caring for the elderly trauma victim, maintain a high index of suspicion regardless of the apparent mechanism.

Number of Patients and Need for Additional Resources

The final part of the scene size-up is to determine the number of patients and whether you have sufficient resources to handle the call.

Once you are certain of the number of patients involved in the emergency, you must determine if additional resources are needed. More than one EMT unit may be required to handle several patients. In fact, you may require additional resources even on calls with only one patient. You may need additional help if a heavy patient must be carried down stairs. You may require a fire services response to help with extrication or to make a collision scene safe. Or the patient may require air transport to a specialty medical facility such as a regional trauma center.

An important part of the scene size-up is recognizing the need for additional resources and calling for them early.

Arrival at the Patient's Side

Upon arrival at the patient's side, begin by identifying yourself, even when initially it appears that the patient may be unresponsive. Simply state your name and then the following: "I am an Emergency Medical Responder." While many people may not know what an Emergency Medical Responder is, the statement should allow you access to the patient and the cooperation of bystanders.

Your next statement should be to the patient: "May I help you?" By answering "yes" to this question, the patient is giving you expressed consent to begin care. The patient may not answer "yes" to your question but instead may simply remain still and allow you to provide care. A patient who is alert and does not refuse your care is said to be providing consent for your care.

Sometimes a patient's fear may be so great that he is confused and will answer "no" or "just leave me alone." Gaining the patient's confidence by talking with him is usually easy. If the patient is unresponsive or unable to give expressed consent, implied consent allows you to care for the patient. This means that if the patient were able to do so, it is assumed that he would consent to care. (Review Chapter 2 for a more detailed discussion of consent.)

Remember, upon arrival and after conducting a scene size-up, you must:

1. State your name and identify yourself as a trained Emergency Medical Responder. Let the patient and bystanders know that you are with the EMS system.
2. Gain consent from the patient to provide care.

If someone is already providing care to the patient when you arrive, identify yourself as an Emergency Medical Responder. If the person's training is equal to or at a higher level than your own, ask if you may assist. You should still identify yourself to the patient and ask if he wishes you to help.

If you have more training than the person who has begun care, respectfully ask to take over care of the patient, and ask him to assist you. Never criticize or argue with anyone who may have initiated care.

continued

FIRST ON SCENE

"Damn it, Tariq!" the driver says loudly. "I told you it's not a heart attack! I think I pulled a muscle in my chest." The older man is sitting on a pallet of low boxes with his hand pressed to the center of his chest.

"Hello, sir," Joanie says as she kneels beside the patient. "I'm Joanie. This is Renee. We're Emergency Medical Responders with the company's MERT team. Do I have permission to make sure that you're okay?"

The driver sighs, rolls his eyes, and says, "Yes, but I'm fine."

"Great," Joanie smiles. "That makes it a good day for both of us, doesn't it? What's your name?" She then touches the driver's wrist with her gloved hand and pauses to feel for a pulse.

"Brad," the driver says between rapid breaths. At first Brad's pulse is weak and somewhat irregular, and Joanie notices that the driver is growing pale and anxious. After a moment, though, his pulse takes on a more regular rhythm and his color returns.

Primary Assessment

The primary assessment is designed to help the Emergency Medical Responder detect and correct all immediate threats to life. Immediate life threats typically involve the patient's airway, breathing, circulation, or bleeding, and each is corrected as it is found. The primary assessment begins as soon as you reach the patient and gain the patient's consent to treat.

OBJECTIVE

8. Explain the purpose of the primary assessment.

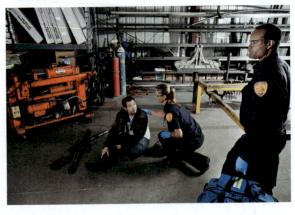

12.6.1 | Size up the scene and form a general impression of the patient.

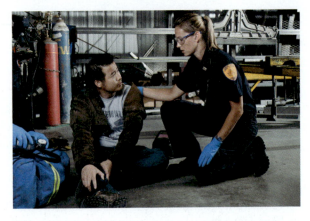

12.6.2 | Evaluate the mental status of the patient.

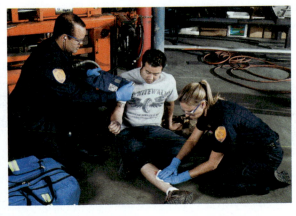

12.6.3 | Address any issues relating to the airway, breathing, and circulation.

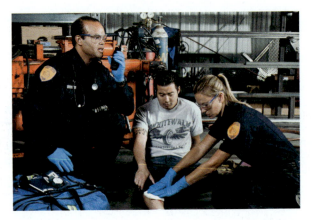

12.6.4 | Determine patient priority for transport.

The primary assessment has seven components (Scans 12.6, 12.7, and 12.8):

- Form a general impression of the patient.
- Assess the patient's mental status. Initially, this may mean determining if the patient is responsive or unresponsive.
- Assess the patient's airway.
- Assess the patient's breathing.
- Assess the patient's circulation.
- Assess for uncontrolled bleeding.
- Make a decision on the priority or urgency of the patient for transport.

While conducting the primary assessment, you will look for life-threatening problems in three major areas:

- *Airway.* Is the patient's airway open?
- *Breathing.* Is the patient breathing adequately?
- *Circulation.* Does the patient have an adequate pulse to circulate blood? Is there serious bleeding? Did the patient lose a large quantity of blood prior to your arrival?

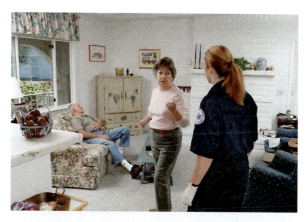

12.7.1 | Size up the scene and form a general impression of the patient.

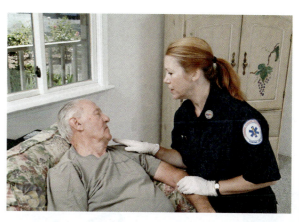

12.7.2 | Assess the patient's mental status.

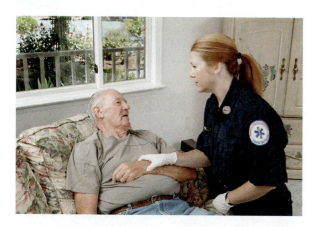

12.7.3 | Assess the patient's airway, breathing, and circulation.

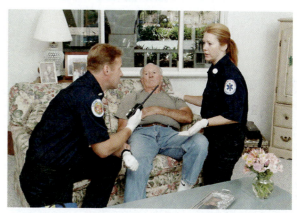

12.7.4 | Determine patient priority for transport.

This assessment and the actions taken are known as the **ABCs** of emergency care, which stand for:

A — Airway
B — Breathing
C — Circulation

During the primary assessment, if a life-threatening problem is detected, it may be necessary to start simultaneous actions focused on the ABCs of emergency care. For example, a trauma patient may require **manual stabilization** of his head and neck at the same time you are opening his airway, providing ventilations, and controlling bleeding. A medical patient may require you to assess his mental status at the same time you are taking a pulse and assessing his breathing. Simultaneous actions can prove to be very challenging. The more you practice your assessment, the better you will become at completing it efficiently.

The General Impression

As you approach your patient you will be forming a general impression of the patient and the patient's environment. Your **general impression** is your first "informal" assessment of the patient's overall condition. The general impression will help you decide the seriousness of the patient's condition based on his level of distress and mental status. You also might be given information by the patient or bystanders at this time, such as the reason

ABCs ▶ the patient's airway, breathing, and circulation as they relate to the primary assessment.

manual stabilization ▶ using your hands to physically hold the body part and keep it from moving.

general impression ▶ the first informal assessment of the patient's overall condition.

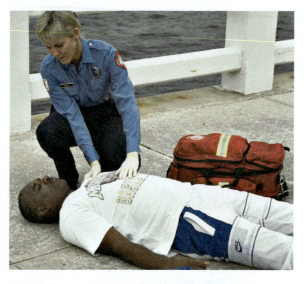

12.8.1 | Determine level of responsiveness.

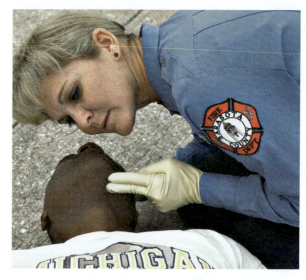

12.8.2 | Ensure an open airway and adequate breathing.

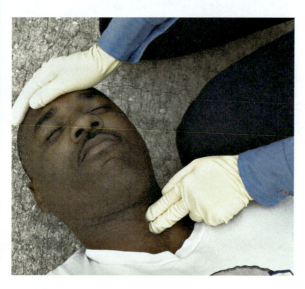

12.8.3 | Check for the presence of a pulse.

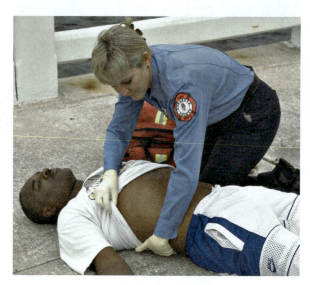

12.8.4 | Look for and control all major bleeding. Determine patient priority for transport.

why EMS was called. In most cases, the reason EMS was called can be determined by identifying the patient's chief complaint.

The general impression contains the following elements: approximate age, sex, and level of distress or responsiveness. Examples of a typical general impression may look something like the following: *I have an approximately 30-year-old male in moderate distress.* Or *I have an approximately 60-year-old female who appears to be unresponsive.*

From the Medical Director

General Impression

Don't be afraid to trust your gut. If the patient's condition makes you worried, uncomfortable, or even nervous, there must be a reason. The patient probably has a serious condition even if you cannot point to any specific finding.

Emergency Medical Responders have always formed a general impression when they first see a patient, even if they are not immediately aware of doing so. With experience, you may form one on intuition alone. You may notice if the patient looks very ill, pale, or cyanotic. You may notice unusual details such as odors, temperature, and living conditions. You may immediately see serious injuries or that the patient looks stable. This impression forms an early opinion of how seriously ill or injured the patient is.

Your decision to request immediate transport or to continue assessing the patient may be based solely on your general impression.

Mental Status

Your actual assessment of a patient begins by determining the patient's level of responsiveness. You must quickly determine if he is responsive or unresponsive. Sometimes this is obvious as you approach. A responsive patient may be obviously awake and interacting with those around him. An unresponsive person may not be so obvious. You must kneel beside the patient, tap his shoulder, and state loudly something like, "Are you okay?" or "Can you hear me?" If he responds, you know he is not totally unresponsive. You will then categorize his level of responsiveness based on the AVPU scale. This will be covered in more detail below.

If it is a trauma patient or you have reason to suspect spine injury, place your hand on his forehead before attempting to illicit a response. This will help stabilize the head and prevent the patient from moving too much in response to your questioning.

Classify the patient's mental status by using the **AVPU scale**, the letters of which stand for *alert, verbal, painful,* and *unresponsive.*

AVPU scale ▶ a memory aid for the classifications of mental status, or levels of responsiveness; the letters stand for *alert, verbal, painful,* and *unresponsive.*

A — *Alert.* The alert patient will be awake, responsive, oriented, and talking with you.

V — *Verbal.* This is a patient who appears to be unresponsive at first but will respond to a loud verbal stimulus from you.

P — *Painful.* If the patient does not respond to verbal stimuli, he may respond to painful stimuli, such as a sternal (breastbone) rub or a gentle pinch to the shoulder. Be careful not to injure the patient when applying painful stimuli. Never forcefully pinch the skin. Never stick the patient with a sharp object.

U — *Unresponsive.* If the patient does not respond to either verbal or painful stimuli, he is said to be unresponsive.

Notice that the term *verbal* does not mean the patient is answering your questions or initiating a conversation. Instead, the patient may speak or grunt, groan, or say "huh." It is possible that the patient may have a medical condition such as a stroke or a problem associated with trauma such as a head injury. Either of those examples may cause the patient to lose the ability to speak. In rare cases, a preexisting condition may have rendered the patient unable to speak prior to the emergency. Often, when such a condition is present, the patient will have a medical identification card or jewelry, such as a bracelet or necklace.

Try to assess mental status without moving the patient. But if the patient is unresponsive, you may need to reposition him to check for breathing, pulse, and serious bleeding or to perform CPR. Follow the procedures shown in Scan 12.9.

▶ GERIATRIC FOCUS ◀

The presence of dementia in the elderly patient can make it very difficult to accurately assess mental status. You must take extra time to ask family members and/or caregivers if the patient's mental status is normal for him or if it is different in some way. With dementia, the patient may appear alert and oriented one minute and completely confused the next. Be aware of the effects of dementia and learn to rely on family and caregivers to help establish a normal mental status baseline for the patient.

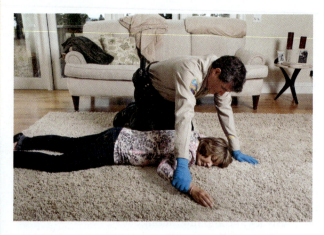

12.9.1 | Move the far arm down to the patient's side.

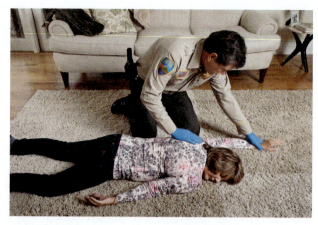

12.9.2 | Move the near arm straight above the patient's head.

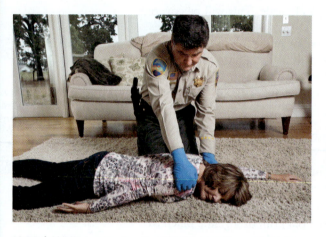

12.9.3 | While supporting the head, move the patient toward you.

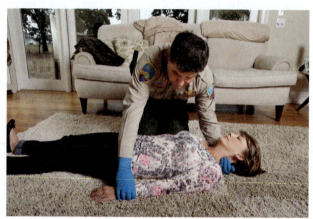

12.9.4 | Now that the patient is supine, perform an appropriate assessment.

Warning: This maneuver is used to initiate basic life support when you must act alone. For all other situations, use a log roll.

Always suspect the presence of neck or spine injuries in the unresponsive trauma patient. Moving this type of patient may cause additional injuries, but it may be necessary to check for life-threatening problems. (Moving a patient safely was covered in Chapter 5.)

Airway and Breathing

If the patient is unresponsive, check for adequate breathing by observing the chest rise and fall. The patient is not breathing if there is no chest movement. Gasping respirations are called *agonal respirations*. They should not be considered normal respirations. If there are no signs of breathing, check for a carotid pulse.

If the patient is breathing, there will be a pulse. At this point, you can check for obvious bleeding.

Circulation

Check for a Pulse

carotid pulse ▶ the pulse that can be felt on either side of the neck.

If the patient is not breathing, check for a **carotid pulse** at the neck to determine if blood is circulating (Figure 12.4). The pulse at the neck is considered more reliable than the

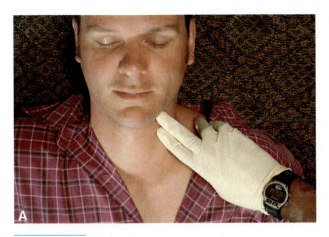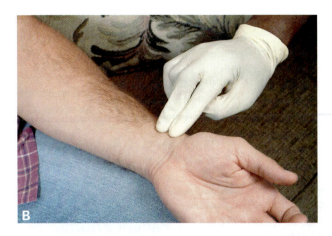

Figure 12.4 • (A) Checking for the presence of a carotid pulse on the neck. (B) Checking for the presence of a radial pulse on the wrist.

pulse at the wrist. A pulse at the wrist—the **radial pulse**—may not be present if the patient is in shock.

radial pulse ▶ the pulse felt on the thumb side of the wrist.

To assess the carotid pulse, first locate the patient's larynx (Adam's apple). Place the tip of your index and middle fingers directly over the midline of this structure. Now, slide your fingertips to the side of the neck closest to you. Do not slide your fingertips to the opposite side of the patient's neck, because this may apply improper pressure and close the airway. Do not attempt to take a carotid pulse on both sides of the neck at the same time. This may interfere with circulation to the brain. You should detect a pulse in the groove between the trachea and the large muscle on the side of the neck. Only moderate pressure is needed to feel it. Check for a carotid pulse for 5 to 10 seconds. Frequent practice will make this skill easy to master.

▶ GERIATRIC FOCUS ◀

The elderly often have an irregular pulse. This is rarely a life-threatening condition. However, the speed of the pulse, both too fast and too slow, can be life threatening and therefore the rate is more important to notice than the regularity.

It is not important during the primary assessment to count the exact rate of the pulse. You only want to confirm the presence of a pulse. If the pulse is very rapid or weak, the patient may be in shock. If there is no pulse, alert dispatch and begin CPR.

If the patient is not breathing but does have a pulse, the patient may have an airway obstruction or he may be in respiratory arrest. You must take immediate action to ventilate the patient before the heart stops. (See Chapter 8.)

KEY POINT ▼

If the patient's pulse is irregular, count the pulse rate for a full minute.

Check for Serious Bleeding

The next step in the primary assessment is checking for serious bleeding. While any uncontrolled bleeding may eventually become life threatening, you will only be concerned with profuse bleeding during the primary assessment. Blood that is bright red and spurting may be coming from an *artery*. Because blood in arteries is under a great deal of pressure, large amounts of blood may be lost in a short period of time. Flowing blood that is darker in color is most likely coming from a *vein*. Even if the bleeding is slow, it may be life threatening if the patient has been bleeding for a long period of time. Look at the amount of blood that has been lost on the ground, in clothing, and in the hair. Your concern is for the total amount of blood that has been lost, not just how fast or slow the bleeding is. (Methods of controlling serious bleeding are covered in Chapter 17.)

Assessing circulation includes checking skin signs—color, temperature, and moisture. An abnormal finding such as pale, cool, moist skin could indicate a serious circulation problem, such as shock.

OBJECTIVE

10. Describe patients who are high and low priority for transport.

OBJECTIVE

16. Describe the unique assessment methods used for pediatric and geriatric patients.

brachial pulse ▶ the pulse that can be felt in the medial side of the upper arm between the elbow and shoulder.

capillary refill ▶ the return (refill) of blood into the capillaries after it has been forced out by fingertip pressure; normal refill time is two seconds or less.

From the Medical Director

Infants and Children

I have found that observing how the infant or child interacts with his or her parents is an excellent gauge of level of responsiveness. Children will maintain eye contact and can usually be soothed when they are not in great distress.

Assessment of circulation may be altered slightly when you immediately see profuse bleeding. In this case, attempt to control the bleeding as soon as it is discovered. Do what you can to control it, but never neglect the patient's airway and breathing status.

Patient Priority

A high-priority patient should be transported immediately, with little time spent on the scene. High-priority conditions include unresponsiveness, breathing difficulties, severe bleeding or shock, complicated childbirth, chest pain, and any severe pain.

Special Considerations for Infants and Children

Your assessment of an infant or child will differ from that of an adult in a few ways. It is important for you to realize that children are not little adults. They react to illness and injury differently.

Infants and children are often shy and distrustful of strangers. A responsive infant or a child who pays no attention to you or what you are doing may be seriously ill. When checking the mental status of an unresponsive infant, talk to him and gently flick the bottoms of his feet.

Opening the airway of an infant involves moving the head into a neutral position, not tilting it back, as with an adult. Opening the airway of a child requires only a slight extension.

Breathing and pulse rates are faster in infants and children than in adults. The pulse to check in an infant or a small child is the **brachial pulse** (Figure 12.5). It is taken at the brachial artery in the upper arm, not at the neck or wrist.

An additional part of checking an infant's or a child's circulation is called **capillary refill**. When the end of a fingernail is gently pressed, it turns white because blood flow is restricted. When the pressure is released, the nail bed turns pink again, usually in less than two seconds. This is a good way to evaluate the circulation of blood in an infant or a child. If it takes longer than two seconds for the nail bed to become pink again or if it does not return to pink at all, there may be a problem with circulation, such as shock or blood loss. If the infant's nail beds are too small, you may perform the same test on the top of his foot or back of his hand. To judge the amount of time it takes for the blood to flow back, count "one-one thousand, two-one thousand," or simply say "capillary refill."

Usually, when adult patients have a serious problem, they become worse gradually. The downward trend often can be spotted in time to take appropriate action. However, an infant's or child's body can compensate so well for a problem such as blood loss that he may appear stable for some time and then suddenly become much worse. Children can actually maintain a near-normal blood pressure up to the time when almost half of their total blood volume is gone. That is why blood pressure is not a reliable assessment of a child's circulation. Checking capillary refill time is more reliable.

A child's condition can change very quickly. It is vital for the Emergency Medical Responder to recognize the seriousness of a child's illness or injury early, before it is too late. You will learn about other considerations in approaching and assessing infants and children in Chapter 23.

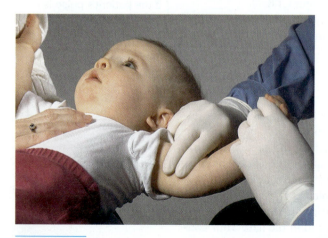

Figure 12.5 • Checking for the presence of a brachial pulse in an infant.

Alerting Dispatch

If you have called for additional resources, such as an ambulance or helicopter, it may be helpful to give them an update of the patient's condition. Your update should include information about the patient such as mental status, age, sex, chief complaint, airway and breathing status, circulation status, and interventions and his results.

Secondary Assessment

A secondary assessment should be performed only after the primary assessment and all immediate life threats have been found and corrected. If you have a patient with a life-threatening problem that you must continually care for (performing CPR on a cardiac-arrest patient, for example), you may not get to complete a secondary assessment.

The main purpose of the secondary assessment is to discover and care for the patient's specific injuries or medical problems. It is a very systematic approach to patient assessment. It also may tell the patient, family, and bystanders that there is concern for the patient and that something is being done for the patient immediately.

The secondary assessment includes a physical examination that focuses in on a specific injury or medical complaint, or it may be a rapid exam of the entire body. It includes obtaining a patient history and taking vital signs. The order in which the steps are accomplished is based on the type of the patient's emergency (Table 12.1).

Some important terms associated with patient assessment are introduced below. There is more about each one later in the chapter. They include:

- *Patient history.* A patient history includes any information relating to the patient's current complaint or condition, as well as information about past medical problems that could be related.
- *Rapid secondary assessment.* This is a quick, less detailed head-to-toe assessment of the most critical patients.
- *Focused secondary assessment.* The **focused secondary assessment** is conducted on stable patients. It focuses on a specific injury or medical complaint.
- *Vital signs.* These include pulse, respirations, skin signs, and pupils. In some areas, Emergency Medical Responders also include assessment of blood pressure. The first set of vital signs taken on any patient is referred to as the *baseline vital signs.* All subsequent vital signs should be compared to the baseline set to identify developing trends.
- *Symptoms.* Reported by the patient, symptoms such as chest pain, dizziness, and nausea are felt by the patient. They are also called *subjective findings.*
- *Signs.* These are what you see, feel, hear, and smell as you examine the patient, such as cool, clammy skin or unequal pupils. They are also called *objective findings.*

OBJECTIVE

11. Explain the purpose of the secondary assessment.

OBJECTIVE

12. Describe the components of a secondary assessment.

focused secondary assessment ▶ an examination conducted on stable patients, focusing on a specific injury or medical complaint.

TABLE 12.1	Secondary Assessment	
TRAUMA PATIENT	**MEDICAL PATIENT**
Significant Mechanism of Injury	**Unresponsive Medical Patient**
• Perform a rapid secondary assessment.	• Perform a rapid secondary assessment.
• Take vital signs.	• Gather a patient history.
• Gather patient history.	• Take vital signs.
No Significant Mechanism of Injury	**Responsive Medical Patient**
• Perform a focused secondary assessment.	• Perform focused secondary assessment.
• Take vital signs.	• Gather a patient history.
• Gather patient history.	• Take vital signs.

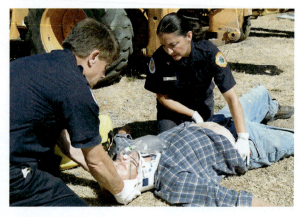

12.10.1 | Examine the area that the patient tells you is injured.

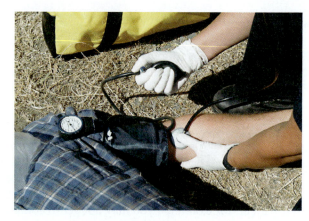

12.10.2 | Obtain baseline vital signs.

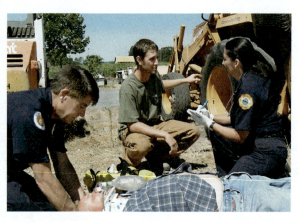

12.10.3 | Gather a patient history.

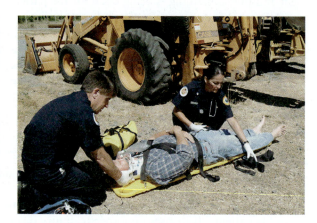

12.10.4 | Provide appropriate care for the injury.

IS IT SAFE?

If you cannot feel a radial pulse, check for the presence of a carotid pulse in the neck. Often when there is no radial pulse, the patient does have a carotid pulse. Never begin CPR without first checking the carotid pulse.

Objective findings can be seen, felt, or in some way measured scientifically. *Subjective findings* are influenced by the person, who in this case is the patient reporting the symptoms. Many of the signs and symptoms you will find during the physical exam are the result of the body's compensating mechanisms. For example, to compensate for blood loss, the body will increase pulse and breathing rates and close down, or constrict, blood vessels in the extremities, all of which results in pale, cool, clammy skin. Those actions are attempts by the body to circulate an adequate amount of oxygenated blood to the vital organs. Adequate flow of oxygenated blood to all cells of the body is called *perfusion*. Inadequate blood flow can lead to shock.

Abnormal findings during your exam indicate a problem that should not be ignored. However, unless the problem is likely to get worse, do not interrupt your assessment. You can stop bleeding from getting worse, but there is little you can do to stop a broken leg from getting worse. It is important to complete your examination.

The Trauma Patient

A trauma patient is one who has received a physical injury of some type. Your assessment of a trauma patient will consist of a physical exam, vital signs, and patient history. The type of physical exam you perform and the order in which you do the various steps will be based on the mechanism of injury.

The trauma patient is classified as either having no significant mechanism of injury (probably not causing a serious injury) or having a significant mechanism of injury (probably causing a serious injury). Your assessment will differ slightly for each type of patient.

OBJECTIVE

7. Differentiate between a significant and non-significant mechanism of injury.

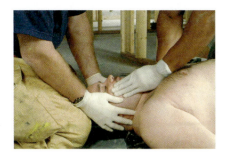

12.11.1 | If appropriate, stabilize the patient's head and neck. Then palpate the head and face.

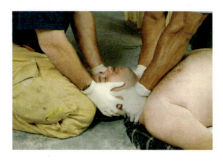

12.11.2 | Palpate the patient's neck. Apply a cervical collar if appropriate.

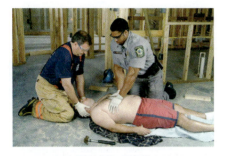

12.11.3 | Palpate the chest.

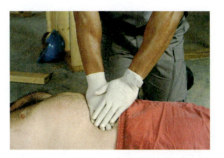

12.11.4 | Palpate each quadrant of the abdomen.

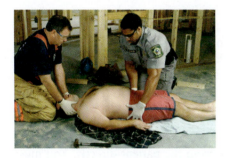

12.11.5 | Palpate the pelvis.

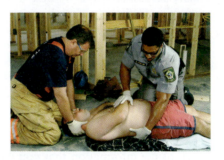

12.11.6 | Palpate the back by sliding your hands under the patient.

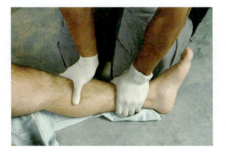

12.11.7 | Palpate the extremities, legs first and then the arms.

To assess a trauma patient with no significant mechanism of injury, begin by performing a focused secondary assessment on the area that the patient tells you is injured (Scan 12.10). Obtain vital signs and gather a patient history. Provide continued care during the reassessment.

To detect and care for serious injuries in a patient with a significant mechanism of injury, perform a rapid secondary assessment looking for obvious injuries (Scan 12.11).

Then obtain vital signs and gather a patient history. If time and the patient's condition allows, perform a complete secondary assessment.

Signs of significant mechanisms of injury for an adult include:

- Ejection from a vehicle
- Death of one or more passengers in a motor-vehicle crash
- Falls greater than 15 feet
- Rollover vehicle collision
- High-speed vehicle collision
- Vehicle-pedestrian collision
- Motorcycle crash
- Unresponsiveness or altered mental status
- Penetrations of the head, neck, chest, or abdomen

Significant mechanisms of injury for a child include:

- Falls of more than 10 feet
- Bicycle collision
- Medium-speed vehicle collision

The Medical Patient

The secondary assessment for a medical patient and a trauma patient are similar, but the order and emphasis are different. For a medical patient, you are more concerned with the medical history of the patient. For the unresponsive medical patient, perform a **rapid secondary assessment** to determine if there are any obvious signs of illness. Obtain baseline vital signs. Gather a patient history, if possible. Provide care as needed.

For the responsive medical patient (Scan 12.12), gather a patient history, observing signs and symptoms while asking about the history of the illness. The patient's chief complaint helps direct the questioning. Perform a focused secondary assessment based on the patient's problem areas. Obtain baseline vital signs. Provide care as needed. Provide continued care during the reassessments.

Patient History

Much of the information that you gather will come from the patient directly. You must become proficient at asking all the appropriate questions depending on the chief complaint.

Interviewing the Patient

An alert patient is your best source of information. Direct your questions to him. Ask questions clearly at a normal rate and in a normal tone of voice. Avoid leading questions. Do not falsely reassure the patient. Do not say things such as "Everything will be fine" or "Take it easy, everything's okay." The patient knows this is not true and will lose confidence in you if you attempt to provide false reassurance. Phrases such as "I'm here to help you" or "I'm doing everything I can to help you" are more appropriate.

When interviewing a patient who is alert, ask the following questions:

- *What is your name?* This is an essential piece of information. It shows your patient that you are concerned for him as a person. Remember his name and use it often. Also, if your patient's mental status decreases, you can call him by name to elicit a response.
- *How old are you?* As an Emergency Medical Responder, you do not need to know more than the general age of your adult patient. But the age of a child is important, because it may determine what type of care is provided. Ask all children their age. It may be appropriate to ask an adolescent his age to be certain that he is a minor. Also ask minors, "How can I contact your parents?" Children may already be upset at being hurt or ill without a parent being there to help them. Always reassure them that someone will contact their parents.

rapid secondary assessment ▶
a quick head-to-toe assessment of the most critical patients.

KEY POINT ▼

The patient history and physical exam can be performed simultaneously. There is no need to wait to take vital signs until the history has been completed. You may obtain the history while performing the physical exam of the patient or while controlling bleeding from a wound. You can do both at the same time.

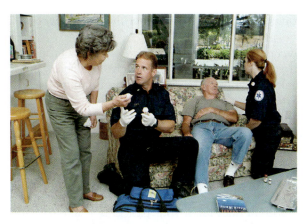

12.12.1 | Gather a patient history.

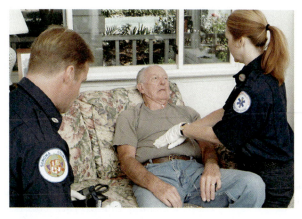

12.12.2 | Perform a focused secondary assessment based on the patient's chief complaint.

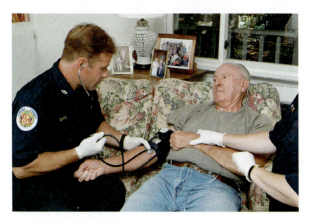

12.12.3 | Obtain baseline vital signs.

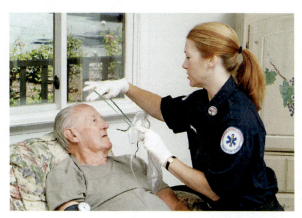

12.12.4 | Provide the appropriate care as indicated.

- *What is going on today?* This usually is the patient's chief complaint. No matter what is wrong, ask if there is any pain. As you learn more about various illnesses and injuries, you also will learn additional questions to ask.
- *How did this happen?* When caring for a trauma patient, knowing how the patient was injured will help direct you to problems that may not be noticeable or obvious to you or the patient. If your patient is lying down, determine if he got into that position himself or was knocked down, fell, or was thrown. Do this for patients with medical problems as well. Remember, the injury to the patient may be the result of a medical problem. This information may indicate the possibility of a spine injury or internal bleeding.
- *How long have you felt this way?* You want to know if the patient's problem occurred suddenly or if it has been developing for the past few days or over a period of time.
- *Has this happened before?* It is especially important to ask this question of medical patients. You want to know if this is the first time or if it is a recurring, or chronic, problem. This question is not usually asked of trauma patients, unless you suspect a recurring problem. If your patient has been hit by a car, it is not necessary to ask him if this has happened before.
- *Are there any current medical problems?* Has the patient been feeling ill lately? Has he seen or is he being treated by a doctor for any problems?
- *Are any medications being taken?* Your patient may not be able to tell you the exact name of a medication he is taking, especially if he is taking several. He may be able to tell you just general medication categories, such as "heart pills" or "water pills." Ask not only about prescription medications but about over-the-counter medications as

well. Routine use of simple medications such as aspirin may alter the treatment the patient receives at the hospital.

Do not use the terms *drugs* or *recreational drugs* in general. They imply misuse or abuse. Some patients may think that you are trying to gather criminal evidence. Instead, ask the patient if he can think of anything else that he might be taking.

- *Do you have any allergies?* Allergic reactions can vary from simple hives or itching to life-threatening airway problems and shock. Knowing that the patient is allergic to a substance will enable you to keep it away from him. Be sure to ask specifically about allergies to medications and latex (as used in gloves), since the patient may come in contact with any of these during care. Also ask the patient what happens when he is exposed to the thing he is allergic to. For instance does he simply develop a rash, get itchy, or does he develop difficulty breathing?
- *When did you last eat?* This is an important question if your patient is a candidate for surgery. It also is important information when dealing with a patient who is having a diabetic emergency.

▶ GERIATRIC FOCUS ◀

Just as it may be difficult to accurately assess mental status in an elderly patient with dementia, obtaining a thorough and accurate history can prove just as challenging. It will become important to rely on family members and caregivers to confirm the information that the patient is telling you or to simply fill in the gaps left by the patient's own history. Hearing loss can make it very challenging when attempting to obtain a history. You may have to speak louder than usual, and it will also help if you speak slowly and clearly.

OBJECTIVE

13. Describe the components of the SAMPLE history tool.

SAMPLE history ▶ a system of information gathering that allows the rescuer to ask questions about past or present medical or injury problems; the letters stand for *signs/ symptoms, allergies, medications, pertinent past medical history, last oral intake,* and *events leading to the illness or injury.*

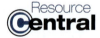

Resource Central

Learn more on obtaining a SAMPLE history.

A common tool used to assist the Emergency Medical Responder in obtaining a patient history is the acronym SAMPLE. The letters serve as a memory aid for the questions that should be asked during a typical medical history. Each letter of the word SAMPLE represents a specific question or series of questions:

S — Signs/symptoms?
A — Allergies?
M — Medications?
P — Pertinent past medical history?
L — Last oral intake?
E — Events leading to the illness or injury?

When taking a history, maintain eye contact with the patient. This will improve personal communication and build the patient's confidence in you. If you look away while asking questions or while listening to answers, it may indicate to your patient that you are not as concerned as you should be or not giving him your full attention. A simple touch also can improve communications. You touch the patient's forehead to note relative skin temperature and moisture and, by touching the patient, you are also showing caring and concern. However, respect a patient's wish not to be touched. Patients are often fearful and anxious. Your calm, caring, and professional attitude often can do as much for the patient as any medical care you provide.

Interview Bystanders

You may encounter a patient who is unresponsive or unable to answer your questions regarding his history. If this is the case, you must depend on family or bystanders for information (Figure 12.6). Ask specific, directed questions to shorten the time required to obtain the information. Questions to bystanders include:

- *What is the patient's name?* If the patient is a minor, ask if the parents are there or if they have been contacted.

- *What happened?* You can receive valuable information when asking this question. If the patient fell from a ladder, did he appear to faint or pass out first? Was he hit on the head by something? Clues from the answers to this question are limitless.
- *Did you see anything else?* For example, was the patient holding his chest before he fell? This gives the bystander a chance to think again and add anything he remembers.
- *Did the patient complain of anything before this happened?* You may learn of chest pain, nausea, shortness of breath, a funny odor where the patient was working, and other clues.
- *Did the patient have any known illness or problems?* Family or friends who know the patient may know his medical history, such as heart problems, diabetes, allergies, or other problems that may cause a change in his condition.
- *Does the patient take any medications?* Again, family or friends who know the patient may be aware of the medications he takes. When talking with the patient, family, friends, or bystanders, remember to use the word *medication* or *medicine* instead of *drugs*. Medicines or medications are considered prescriptions for legitimate medical purposes. The public views drugs as illegal substances. Remember to ask the patient if he is taking over-the-counter medications.

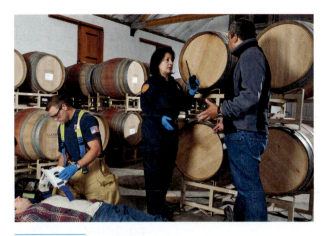

Figure 12.6 • For an unresponsive patient, look to bystanders and family members for additional information.

> **► GERIATRIC FOCUS ◄**

Many elderly patients take prescription medications for various medical conditions. A good trick to help disclose pertinent medical history is to ask to see all the medications the patient is currently taking. Even if you do not know the purpose of each medication, having them handy when the EMTs arrive will help them begin to understand the patient's history sooner.

Most of the questions listed above are questions you would normally ask about someone who is hurt or ill. You would usually introduce yourself and ask for a name, just as you would ask what was wrong and how it happened. Much of your Emergency Medical Responder training is simply formalized common sense.

Locate Medical Identification Jewelry

Medical identification jewelry can provide important information if the patient is unresponsive and a history cannot be obtained from family or bystanders. A common one is the MedicAlert medallion worn on a necklace or a wrist or ankle bracelet. One side of the device has a star-of-life emblem. Information on the patient's medical problem is engraved on the reverse side, along with a phone number for additional information.

Vital Signs

Vital signs can alert you to problems that require immediate attention. Taken at regular intervals, they can help you determine if the patient's condition is getting better, worse, or staying the same (Figure 12.7). For most Emergency Medical Responders, vital signs include pulse, respirations, skin signs, and pupils. In some areas, Emergency Medical Responders also include assessment of blood pressure.

The first set of vital signs is called *baseline vital signs.* Compare all other vital sign readings to the baseline vital signs.

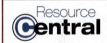

Learn more about evaluating vital signs.

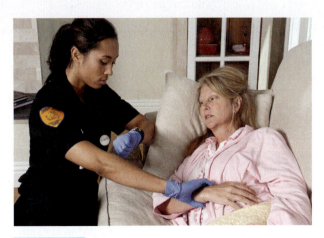

Figure 12.7 • Establishing a baseline set of vital signs is an important aspect of the patient assessment.

This comparison helps determine if the patient is stable or unstable, improving or growing worse, and benefiting or not benefiting from care procedures. For example, comparing baseline vital signs before and after administering oxygen to the patient can tell the EMTs who take over patient care objective information about how that intervention may be affecting the patient.

Certain combinations of vital signs point to possible serious medical or traumatic conditions. For example, cool, clammy skin; a rapid but weak pulse; and increased breathing rate can indicate possible shock in the presence of a significant mechanism of injury. Hot, dry skin with a rapid pulse could indicate a serious heat-related emergency. You can determine which patients are a high priority for immediate transport by taking vital signs.

For an adult, a continuous pulse rate of less than 60 beats per minute or above 100 beats per minute is considered abnormal. Likewise, a respiratory rate above 26 breaths per minute or below 10 breaths per minute is considered serious. You should be concerned about these vital signs because they indicate unstable situations that could become life threatening, and the patient could worsen quickly. Stay alert and monitor the patient closely. Keeping the patient quiet or at rest, caring for shock, and reassuring the responsive patient can make a difference in the outcome.

▶ GERIATRIC FOCUS ◀

Obtaining accurate vital signs can be challenging with the elderly patients. Small, frail arms can make it painful for them when you try to get a blood pressure. The bones of the chest have become more rigid, making it more difficult to see chest rise and fall. You may have to use other techniques, such as listening for breath sounds or watching the movement of the abdomen, when counting respirations.

continued

FIRST ON SCENE

"Are you having trouble breathing, Brad?" Joanie watches the driver's chest and counts his shallow, rapid breaths at 20 per minute.

"A little," the man says. "That's not a big deal though, right? I mean, I was just unloading boxes and all."

"Honestly, Brad, it could be a big deal. I'm not really trained to make that determination." Joanie turns to Renee and says, "Why don't you go ahead and call 911."

"Oh! Hold on a minute," the driver protests as he stands up. "I'm . . . I'm . . . I think . . ." He grows pale again and Joanie helps him sit back on the pallet of boxes.

"Just relax, Brad," Joanie says and places a nonrebreather mask on the driver's face. He can hear Renee talking to the 911 operator through the thin, plywood walls of the dock manager's office.

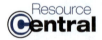

Get more information about performing a detailed physical exam.

The Physical Exam

If your trauma patient has no significant mechanism of injury and appears to have an isolated minor injury (supported by the mechanism of injury and what the patient tells you), perform a focused secondary assessment on the injury site and the area close to it. If the patient has a significant mechanism of injury, a serious injury, or is unresponsive, perform a rapid secondary assessment of the entire body. You must use as many of your five senses as possible when performing your physical exam. Use your eyes, ears, hands, nose, and ears to detect any abnormal findings in your patient.

The physical exam of a medical patient may be brief. If the patient is responsive, perform a focused secondary assessment based on the patient's chief complaint. If the patient is unresponsive, conduct a rapid secondary assessment of the entire body.

When assessing a trauma patient, you may use a memory aid, such as **BP-DOC** or **DCAP-BTLS**, to help you remember what to look for during any physical exam. The letters stand for:

BP-DOC

B	—	Bleeding
P	—	Pain
D	—	Deformities
O	—	Open wounds
C	—	**Crepitus** (a grating noise or sensation)

DCAP-BTLS

D	—	Deformities
C	—	Contusions
A	—	Abrasions
P	—	Punctures and penetrations
B	—	Burns
T	—	Tenderness
L	—	Lacerations
S	—	Swelling

Rapid Secondary Assessment—Trauma Patient with Significant MOI

The rapid secondary assessment is a head-to-toe physical exam of the patient that should take no more than 90 seconds to complete. It is performed on patients who have a significant mechanism of injury (MOI). These patients will most likely have a high priority for transport. Take great care not to move the patient unless absolutely necessary. Neck and spine injuries may be present. To save time, another Emergency Medical Responder may take vital signs while you perform the exam.

It is usually not necessary for the Emergency Medical Responder to remove the patient's clothing during a head-to-toe exam. Of course, you may remove or readjust clothing that interferes with your ability to examine the patient. Cut away, lift, slide, or unbutton clothing covering a suspected injury site, especially the chest, back, and abdomen, so you can fully inspect the area. Also check the patient's clothing for evidence of bleeding. If you have any reason to suspect serious injury or uncontrolled bleeding to the back, you must carefully roll the patient to inspect the back. Use care to keep the head and spine in alignment as you do it.

Suspect internal injuries if your responsive patient indicates pain in the area or pain when you touch the area during your exam. If the patient is unresponsive, you may wish to remove or rearrange clothing covering the chest, abdomen, and back to examine those areas of the body completely. If you must remove or rearrange the clothing of a responsive patient, tell him what you are doing and why. Take great care to respect the modesty of the patient. Also protect him from harsh weather conditions and temperatures.

> ▶ **GERIATRIC FOCUS** ◀
>
> *There are many factors that contribute the high incidence of trauma in the elderly, including arthritis, slower reflexes, poor vision, and hearing loss. Their ability to heal efficiently from injury is also diminished and therefore can lead to much longer recovery times.*

While performing a rapid secondary assessment, avoid contaminating your patient's wounds and aggravating his injuries. Be sure to take the appropriate BSI precautions.

KEY POINT ▼

It is not necessary to learn each and every memory tool for assessment. The important thing is to find one that you understand and are comfortable with and then use it consistently.

OBJECTIVE

14. Describe the components of the BP-DOC assessment tool.

BP-DOC ▶ a memory aid used to recall what to look for in a physical exam; the letters stand for *bleeding, pain, deformities, open wounds,* and *crepitus.*

DCAP-BTLS ▶ a memory aid used to recall what to look for in a physical exam; the letters stand for *deformities, contusions, abrasions, punctures and penetrations, burns, tenderness, lacerations,* and *swelling.*

crepitus ▶ a grating noise or the sensation felt when broken bone ends rub together.

KEY POINT ▼

No matter what other injuries a patient has or does not have, a patient who is unresponsive or who has an altered mental status is a high priority for immediate transport.

IS IT SAFE?

Often there is no way to know for sure if an unresponsive patient has experienced spinal trauma. Therefore, when assessing and caring for an unresponsive patient, maintain a high degree of suspicion for spine injuries. Maintain manual stabilization of the head and spine until you can positively ruled out injury or until you can immobilize the patient on a long spine board.

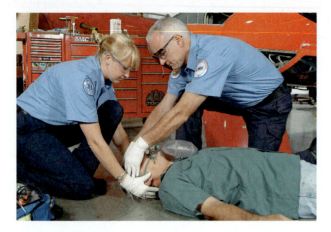

Figure 12.8 • Use both hands to palpate the scalp and inspect the head.

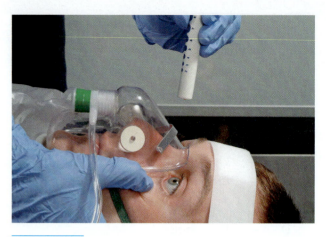

Figure 12.9 • Check the pupils for equality and reaction to light.

KEY POINT ▼

In a rapid secondary assessment for a trauma patient, each area of the body is checked for BP-DOC, plus other problems specific to the area.

To perform a secondary assessment:

1. Check the head for bleeding and deformities (Figure 12.8). Take care not to move the patient's head. Run your fingers through the patient's hair, looking for blood. Check your gloves for blood. Check the face for pain, deformities, or discoloration. Check for symmetry of facial muscles by asking the patient to smile or show his teeth. Look for any fluids that may be leaking from the ears, nose, or mouth.

2. Examine the patient's eyes for signs of injury (Figure 12.9). Check the pupils for size, equality, and reaction to light. A penlight would be helpful for this. If you are outside in bright sunlight, cover the patient's eye with your hand. Remove your hand quickly and watch for reaction of the pupil to the light. Observe the inner surface of the eyelids (conjunctiva). The tissue should be pink and moist. A pale color may indicate poor perfusion.

3. Inspect the ears and nose for drainage, either clear or bloody. Clear or bloody fluids in the ears or nose are strong indications of a skull fracture. Also inspect the nose for singed nostrils, which may indicate the inhalation of toxic smoke. Flaring nostrils may be a sign of respiratory distress.

4. Inspect the mouth for foreign material, bleeding, and tissue damage (Figure 12.10). Look for broken teeth, bridges, dentures, and crowns. Check for chewing gum, food, vomit, and foreign objects.

5. Check the neck front and back for pain and deformity (Figure 12.11). Look for any medical identification jewelry. Also notice if the patient has a stoma, or evidence of

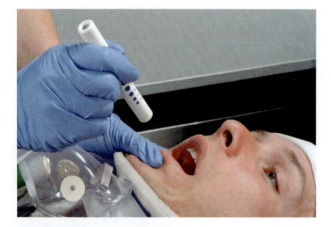

Figure 12.10 • Inspect the mouth for anything that may cause an airway obstruction.

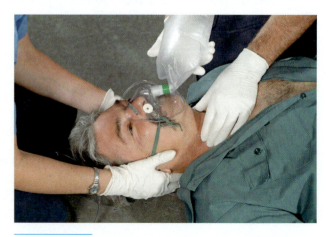

Figure 12.11 • Inspect the neck for pain and deformities.

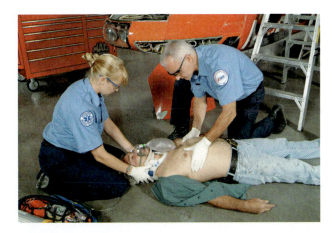

Figure 12.12 • Use both hands to inspect the chest for pain and deformities.

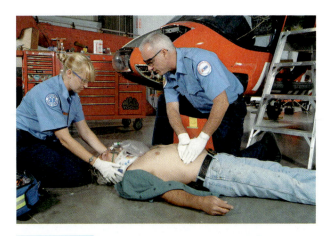

Figure 12.13 • Inspect the abdomen for pain and deformity.

tracheal deviation (any shift of the trachea to one side or the other). Observe for **jugular vein distention (JVD)** and **accessory muscle use**.

6. Use both hands to inspect the chest front and sides for pain and deformities (Figure 12.12). If necessary, bare the chest. Gently apply pressure to all sides of the chest with your hands. Observe for equal expansion of both sides of the chest. Note any portion that appears to be floating or moving in opposite directions to the rest of the chest; this is called **paradoxical movement**. It could indicate an injury called a *flail chest* in which two or more ribs are fractured in two or more places. When baring the chest of female patients, provide them with as much privacy as possible.

7. Inspect the abdomen for an signs or symptoms of trauma such as pain, deformities, distention, rigidity, and **guarding** (Figure 12.13). Gently press on each quadrant of the abdomen with the palm side of the fingers, noting any areas that are rigid, swollen, or painful. As you press on the area, ask the patient if it hurts more when you press down or when you let go.

8. Inspect the pelvis for pain and deformity (Figure 12.14). Note any obvious injury to the genital region. Look for wetness caused by incontinence or bleeding and impaled objects. Do not expose the area unless you suspect there is an injury. In male patients, check for *priapism*, the persistent erection of the penis, which may be a sign of spinal-cord injury.

9. Feel the lower back for pain and deformity (Figure 12.15). Take care not to move the patient. Gently slide your gloved hands into the area of the lower back that is formed by the curve of the spine. Check your gloves for blood. If possible, roll the patient to inspect the entire back for pain and deformity (Figure 12.16).

tracheal deviation ▶ a shifting of the trachea to either side of the midline of the neck caused by the buildup of pressure inside the chest.

jugular vein distention (JVD) ▶ an abnormal bulging of the veins of the neck indicating possible injury to the chest or heart.

accessory muscle use ▶ the use of the muscles of the neck, chest, and abdomen to assist with breathing effort.

paradoxical movement ▶ movement of an area of the chest wall in opposition to the rest of the chest during respiration.

guarding ▶ the protection of an area of injury or pain by the patient; the spasms of muscles to minimize movement that might cause pain.

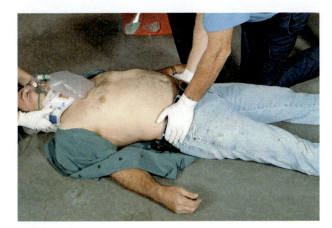

Figure 12.14 • Check the pelvis for pain, deformity, and wetness.

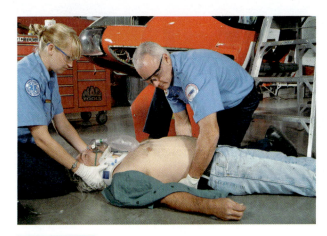

Figure 12.15 • Check the lower back for pain and deformity.

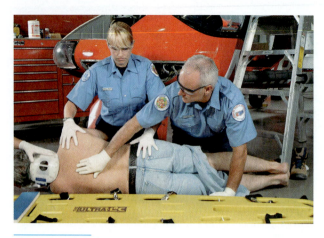

Figure 12.16 • When appropriate, roll the patient to inspect the entire back.

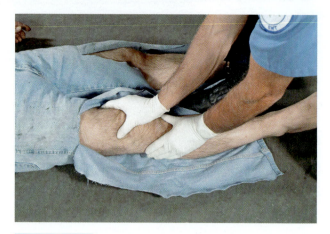

Figure 12.17 • Examine the legs and feet for pain and deformity.

10. Examine each leg and foot individually (Figure 12.17). Compare one limb to the other in terms of length, shape, or deformity.

11. Check for distal circulation, sensation, and motor function (Figure 12.18). Check the **dorsalis pedis pulse**, which is located on top of the foot just lateral to the large tendon of the big toe.

12. Examine the upper extremities from the shoulders to the fingertips (Figure 12.19). Examine each limb separately for pain and deformities.

13. Check for distal circulation, sensation, and motor function in each hand. Note any weakness, numbness, or tingling. Observe for evidence of **track marks** or medical identification jewelry (Figure 12.20).

dorsalis pedis pulse ► the pulse located lateral to the large tendon of the big toe.

track marks ► small dots of infection that form a track along a vein; may be an indication of IV drug abuse.

 Resource **Central**

Learn more about performing an abdominal assessment.

Secondary Assessment—Trauma Patient with No Significant MOI

When your trauma patient has no significant mechanism of injury, the steps of the secondary assessment are appropriately simplified. Instead of examining the patient from head to toe, focus your assessment on just the areas that the patient tells you are painful or that you suspect may be injured because of the mechanism of injury. The assessment includes a physical exam, vital signs, and a patient history.

Your decision on which areas of the patient's body to assess will depend partly on what you see and partly on the patient's chief complaint. Be sure to consider potential injuries based on the mechanism of injury. For example, if the patient's chief complaint is pain in his leg after falling down several stairs, consider possible back or neck injuries and care for the patient accordingly. Use the memory aid BP-DOC to help you properly perform your assessment.

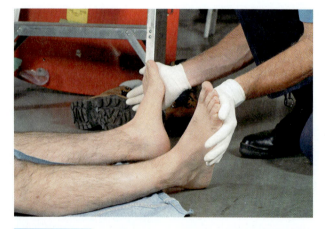

Figure 12.18 • Assess distal circulation, sensation, and motor function in each leg.

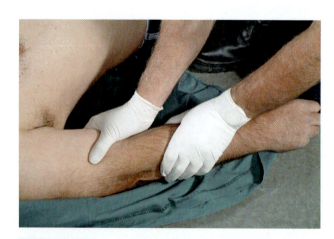

Figure 12.19 • Check the arms and hands for pain and deformities.

Rapid Secondary Assessment—Unresponsive Medical Patient

The rapid secondary assessment of an unresponsive medical patient is almost the same as the rapid assessment of a trauma patient with a significant mechanism of injury (MOI). You will rapidly assess the patient's head, neck, chest, abdomen, pelvis, extremities, and posterior. As you assess each area of the body, look for signs of illness:

- *Neck.* Look for neck vein distention and medical identification jewelry.
- *Chest.* Check presence and equality of breath sounds.
- *Abdomen.* Assess for distention, firmness, or rigidity.
- *Pelvis.* Check for incontinence of urine or feces.
- *Extremities.* Check circulation, sensation, motor function, and for a medical identification jewelry.

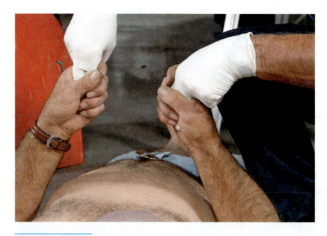

Figure 12.20 • Assess distal circulation, sensation, and motor function in each arm.

Secondary Assessment—Responsive Medical Patient

The secondary assessment of a responsive medical patient is usually brief. The most important assessment information is obtained through the patient history and the taking of vital signs. Focus the exam on the body part that the patient has a complained about. For example, if the patient complains of abdominal pain, focus your exam on that area of the body. Another memory aid used to help assess the responsive medical patient is known as the **OPQRST** assessment. Just as with the acronym SAMPLE, each of the letters represents a word, and each of the words is designed to trigger specific questions that the Emergency Medical Responder should ask. OPQRST is especially helpful when the chief complaint is related to pain or shortness of breath:

OPQRST ▶ a memory device used for assessing the responsive medical patient; the letters stand for *onset, provocation, quality, region/radiate, severity,* and *time.*

O — *Onset.* This letter is designed to trigger questions pertaining to what the patient was doing at the onset of pain (when the pain or symptoms began). For example, "What were you doing when the pain began?" or "What were you doing when you first began to feel short of breath?"

P — *Provocation.* Ask questions pertaining to what provokes or affects the pain. For example, "Does anything you do make the pain better or worse?" or "Does it hurt to take a deep breath or when I push here?"

Q — *Quality.* Ask about the quality of the pain; that is, find out what does the pain or symptom actually feels like. For example, ask, "Can you describe how your pain feels?" or "Is the pain sharp or is it dull?" or "Is it steady or does it come and go?"

R — *Region and radiate.* Ask where the pain is originating and to where it may be moving or radiating. For example, "Can you point with one finger to where your pain is the worst?" "Does your pain move or radiate to any other part of your body?" "Do you feel pain anywhere else besides your chest?"

S — *Severity.* Ask how severe the pain or discomfort is. A standard scale is typically presented like this: "On a scale of 1 to 10, with 10 being the worst pain you have ever felt, how would you rate your pain right now?" Using the same scale, also ask the patient to describe the severity of his pain when it first began. Once you have been with the patient a while and provided care, you will want to ask the severity question again to see if his pain is getting better or worse.

T — *Time.* Ask the patient how long he may have been experiencing the pain or discomfort. A simple question such as, "When did you first begin having pain today?" or "How long have you had this pain?" will usually suffice.

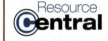

Learn more about assessing a patient's pain.

▶ GERIATRIC FOCUS ◀

Many elderly patients have a much higher tolerance for pain and may not always feel the result of a significant injury or illness. A thorough and methodical assessment may reveal areas of involvement that were not initially seen or part of the chief complaint.

Avoid leading questions, which tend to "put words into the patient's mouth." Instead, provide the patient with choices and then allow him to choose. It also is important to use the patient's own words when documenting the call or transferring care of the patient to more highly trained personnel. For example, if the patient tells you he feels as though an anvil is sitting on his chest, quote his words to describe the pain. Do not paraphrase or attempt to translate what he said into medical terminology.

"Okay, Brad," Joanie says and kneels in front of the driver. "While we wait for the ambulance, let's talk about your chest pain." The driver, now frightened by his symptoms, nods with wide eyes. "I already know that you were unloading the truck when the pain started, right?"

"Yes," Brad says, his voice somewhat muffled by the oxygen mask.

"Does anything make it better or worse? You know, like if you move a certain way or push on it?"

The driver moves his upper body back and forth and presses harder on his chest. "No," he answers.

The sound of sirens quickly approaches the parking lot next door to the loading dock. "Okay." Joanie is now writing in a small notebook. "What does the pain feel like?"

The driver thinks for a moment and pulls the mask up to speak. "Like a pressure. Like a heavy weight or something right on my chest."

Completing the Exam

Upon completing the physical exam of the patient, you must consider all the signs and symptoms found that could indicate an illness or injury. Certain combinations of signs and symptoms can point to one specific problem. A finding as simple as pain in a certain region of the body may be significant. The lack of certain findings also may lead you to a conclusion. For example, if a patient has an obvious injury but feels no pain at the site, you must consider problems such as spine injury, brain damage, shock, or drug abuse.

During your assessment of the patient and throughout the time you are caring for him, remember the first rule of emergency care: *Do no further harm*. Be sure to do only what you have been trained to do. Avoid adding injury and aggravating existing injuries and problems. (See a summary of Rules for Patient Examination in Table 12.2.) Later in your training, you will learn what you can do to help the patient based on the findings in your physical exam.

TABLE 12.2	Rules for Patient Assessment
1	Do no further harm.
2	If anything about the patient's awareness or behavior does not seem "right," consider that something is seriously wrong.
3	Patients who appear stable may worsen rapidly. You must be alert to all changes in a patient's condition.
4	Monitor the patient's skin for color changes.
5	Look over the entire patient and note anything that appears to be wrong.
6	Unless you are certain that the patient is free of spine injury, assume every trauma patient has a spine injury.
7	Tell the patient that you are going to examine him, what you will be doing, and why you are doing it. Stress the importance of the exam.
8	Monitor vital signs.
9	Conduct a head-to-toe exam. If anything looks, sounds, feels, smells, or "seems" wrong to you or the patient, assume that there is something seriously wrong with the patient.
10	Failure of the patient to respond properly on any test for sensation or motor function in the leg or arm must be considered a sign of spine injury.

TABLE 12.3 | Elements of the Reassessment

- Ensure that ABCs are intact.
- Reassess vital signs and compare with baseline.
- Check and adjust interventions as appropriate handoff to EMTs.

Reassessment

When performing the reassessment either at the scene or en route to the hospital, repeat the primary assessment, reassess vital signs, and check any interventions to ensure they are still effective. Reassess the patient, watching closely for any changes in his condition (Table 12.3). Repeating assessments and noting any changes in patient condition are ways of **trending** a patient's condition. Remember that patients will get better, get worse, or stay the same. Seriously ill or injured patients should be reassessed every five minutes. A good rule to follow is that by the time you finish a reassessment from start to finish, it is time to start over with the beginning of the next reassessment. Patients who are not seriously ill or injured should be reassessed every 15 minutes.

When additional EMS providers arrive at the scene, it is important to communicate with them well. Give the responding EMTs a verbal report, including:

- Name and age of patient
- Chief complaint
- Mental status
- Airway, breathing, and circulatory status
- Physical findings
- Patient history
- Interventions applied and the patient's response to them

Some EMS systems also require the Emergency Medical Responder to provide a written report to the EMT crew. It usually includes the same information as the verbal report. The written report and the information in it will become part of the EMT crew's patient care report. Accuracy is vital in any verbal or written report because care given by the responding EMTs and the hospital emergency department staff may be based, in part, on your evaluation of the patient.

OBJECTIVE

15. Explain the purpose of the reassessment.

trending ▶ monitoring the patient's signs and symptoms and documenting any changes, both good and bad.

WRAP-UP

FIRST ON SCENE

Before Joanie can ask the next question, Renee, her partner in this incident, leads a group of firefighters to the loading dock. They are carrying several bags and a bright green AED. "Okay," the firefighter in the lead says, pulling on a pair of purple exam gloves. "Who do we have here?"

Joanie introduces Brad and explains the situation. Just as she finishes, an ambulance crew arrives, noisily rolling a wheeled stretcher across the metal grating of the loading dock floor. In one fluid motion, the ambulance crew has obtained a set of vitals, loaded the patient onto the wheeled stretcher, switched the nonrebreather mask onto their own oxygen tank, and rolled him out to the waiting ambulance. Joanie and Renee stand and watch the firefighters and ambulance crew load up into their vehicles and disappear from the parking lot.

"Boy," Renee says as the women turns and returns to the building. "That went just like clockwork."

"Yes it did." Joanie holds the door open for Renee and pats her on the shoulder as they walk back into the darkness of the loading dock. "And next time, you get to do patient care."

Summary

- Patient assessment is one of the most important skills you will learn as an Emergency Medical Responder. Even though it may seem time-consuming, it is necessary to properly and completely examine the patient if you are to determine what care the patient requires.

- You must detect life-threatening problems and correct them as quickly as possible. Then you must detect problems that may become life threatening if left without care.

- Always perform a scene size-up. Always make sure the scene is safe to enter before you enter it. Then gain information quickly from the scene, the patient, and bystanders. If possible, determine the patient's nature of illness or mechanism of injury.

- During the primary assessment, determine if the patient is responsive. If you suspect a spine injury, maintain manual stabilization of the head and neck. Make certain that the patient has an open airway, adequate breathing, and a pulse. Control all serious bleeding.

- During the secondary assessment, look over the patient. Check for medical identification jewelry. Begin gathering information by asking questions and listening. The more organized your interview and physical exam are, the better your chances of gaining the needed information. Utilize the SAMPLE, BP-DOC, and OPQRST assessment tools as appropriate.

- Take the patient's vital signs. Remember that baseline vital signs—plus repeated vital signs over time—are valuable to the personnel who take over patient care.

- The physical exam of a patient varies somewhat depending on whether the patient is a medical or trauma patient. A head-to-toe exam consists of the following:
  - *Head*. Check the scalp for cuts, bruises, and swellings and the skull and facial bones for deformities, depressions, and other signs of injury. Inspect the eyelids and the eyes for injury and check pupil size, equality, and reactions to light. Note the color of the inner surface of the eyelids. Look for blood, clear fluids, or bloody fluids in the nose and ears. Examine the mouth for airway obstructions, blood, and any odd odors.
  - *Neck*. Examine the cervical spine for tenderness and deformity. Recheck to see if the patient has a stoma. Note obvious injuries and look for medical alert jewelry.
  - *Chest*. Examine the chest for cuts, bruises, penetrations, and impaled objects. Check for possible bone fractures. Look for equal expansion and note chest movements.
  - *Abdomen*. Examine the abdomen for cuts, bruises, penetrations, and impaled objects. Check for local and general pain as you examine the abdomen for tenderness.
  - *Lower back*. Feel for point tenderness, deformity, and other signs of injury. Check the rest of the back last and only if it is safe to roll the patient (no suspected spine injuries).
  - *Pelvis*. Press in and down to check for possible fractures and note any signs of injuries.
  - *Genital region*. Note any obvious injuries. Look for wetness. Note the presence of priapism when examining male patients.
  - *Extremities*. Examine for deformities, swelling, bleeding, discoloration, bone protrusions, and obvious fractures. Check for point tenderness on all suspected closed fracture sites. Check for distal pulse. In pediatric patients, check for capillary refill. Determine motor function and sensation as appropriate. Remember to look for medical identification jewelry.

- While EMTs usually complete a more detailed secondary assessment en route to the hospital, in some systems Emergency Medical Responders may assist by repeating the primary assessment and vital signs. If you also assist with the reassessment, note any changes in patient condition or the need for additional interventions.

Take Action

HIDE AND SEEK

Developing a thorough and efficient patient assessment can take years and hundreds of patients. For that reason, it is important to practice this skill often, especially if you are not in a job where you are responding to and assessing patients regularly.

For this exercise, gather several small to medium-size items such as an oral airway (OPA), a nasal airway (NPA), bite stick, pencil or pen, eraser, and so on. Use some tape and secure several items in random places on your body beneath your clothing. You might hide them at the lower back, behind the knee, under the arm, and inside the ankle. Once you have several items secured beneath your clothing, find a fellow classmate who is willing and ready to practice patient assessment. Do not let them know that you have items hidden on your body.

Now lie down and think of a simple scenario that you can use to set the stage for your practice session. Let your partner perform a complete assessment and see how many of the objects he can find. If he finds an item, just tell him that it represents a deformity and to continue on with the exam. When he is finished with the exam, reveal all the items for him. Was he able to locate all of them? Why do you suppose he may have missed some? This is a great way to reinforce the importance of a thorough physical exam.

First on Scene Run Review

Recall the events of the "First on Scene" scenario in this chapter and answer the following questions, which are related to the call. Rationales are offered in the Answer Key at the back of the book.

1. Why should you ask permission to help a person?

2. For this call why would scene control be important?

3. As an Emergency Medical Responder, how could you help this patient with these signs and symptoms?

4. Why might this patient not want the ambulance called?

Quick Quiz

To check your understanding of the chapter, answer the following questions. Then compare your answers to those in the Answer Key at the back of the book.

1. For most patients, an Emergency Medical Responder's assessment begins with performing a scene size-up followed by:

  a. a secondary assessment.
  b. a primary assessment.
  c. obtaining vital signs.
  d. determining the nature of illness.

2. After arriving on scene, but before making patient contact, you should:

  a. perform a primary assessment.
  b. contact medical direction.
  c. perform a secondary assessment.
  d. take BSI precautions.

3. There are six components to the primary assessment, beginning with:

  a. assessing the patient's mental status.
  b. assessing the patient's airway.
  c. forming a general impression.
  d. evaluating patient's circulation.

4. The assessment of a patient's mental status or responsiveness includes using the _____ scale.

  a. AVPU
  b. ABC
  c. SAMPLE
  d. BP-DOC

5. In a SAMPLE history, the *E* represents:

  a. EKG results.
  b. evaluation of the neck and spine.
  c. events leading to illness or injury.
  d. evidence of airway obstruction.

6. When assessing circulation for a responsive adult patient, you should assess the:

  a. carotid pulse.
  b. radial pulses on both sides of the body.
  c. the radial pulse on one side.
  d. distal pulse.

7. When assessing a trauma patient with NO significant mechanism of injury, perform a focused secondary assessment, followed by:

  a. rapid physical exam.
  b. SAMPLE history.
  c. rapid trauma assessment.
  d. vital signs.

8. There are 10 rules for a patient examination, the first of which is always:

  a. if patient behavior does not seem "right," consider that something is seriously wrong.
  b. do no further harm.
  c. take vital signs.
  d. watch for skin color changes.

9. Below is a list of steps carried out during a rapid secondary assessment. They are not listed in the correct order. On a separate sheet of paper, write in a column the numerals 1 to 22. Then copy the steps below in the correct order.

  a. Inspect chest for penetrations, cuts, bruises and impaled objects.
  b. Feel pelvis for possible fractures.
  c. Inspect scalp for cuts and bruises.
  d. Check each upper extremity for injury and paralysis.
  e. Inspect the back surfaces.
  f. Examine the eyes (including the pupils).
  g. Inspect the mouth for possible airway obstructions.
  h. Inspect genital region (groin) for obvious injury.
  i. Examine chest for possible rib fracture.
  j. Feel lower back for point tenderness and look for deformity.
  k. Inspect ears and nose for blood, clear fluids, or bloody fluid.
  l. Check the lower extremities for sensation and motor function.
  m. Observe and feel for equal expansion of both sides of the chest.
  n. Inspect abdomen for cuts, bruises, penetrations.
  o. Check for distal pulses in the feet.
  p. Look at inner surface of eyelids (conjunctiva).
  q. Feel abdomen for tenderness.
  r. Check the cervical spine for point tenderness and deformity.
  s. Examine the legs and feet.
  t. Check the front of neck for injury and deformity.
  u. Check the face and skull for deformity and depressions.
  v. Examine the chest for possible collarbone or breastbone fractures.

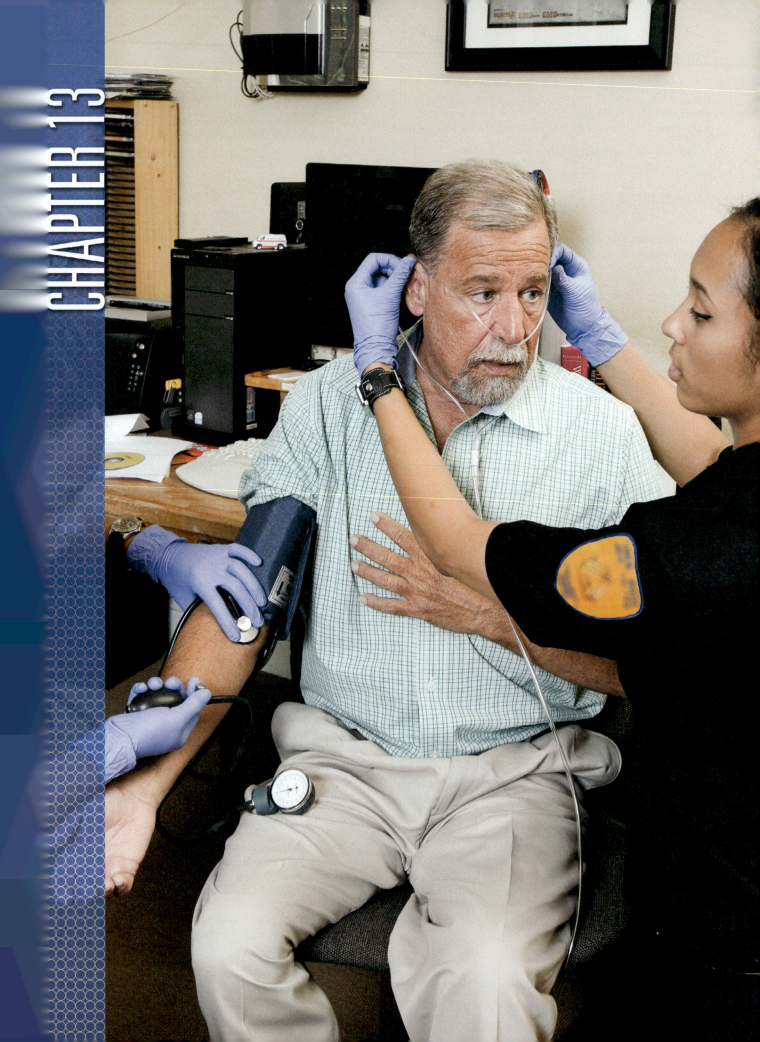

CHAPTER 13

Caring for Cardiac Emergencies

EDUCATION STANDARDS
- Medicine—Cardiovascular

COMPETENCIES
- Recognizes and manages life threats based on assessment findings of a patient with a medical emergency while awaiting additional emergency response.

CHAPTER OVERVIEW
According to the most recent statistics from the Centers for Disease Control and Prevention (CDC), heart disease is the number one killer among adults in the United States. As discussed earlier in this textbook, the heart is at the center of the cardiovascular system, which also includes the blood vessels and blood. The cells of the body require a constant supply of well-oxygenated blood to function properly. This is known as perfusion. Good perfusion depends on the heart's ability to circulate blood throughout the body at a constant and steady pressure, also called blood pressure. When the heart's function is affected by illness or injury, it is unable to maintain a pressure necessary to support adequate perfusion. This chapter discusses some of the more common conditions that affect the heart's ability to pump adequately, the consequences that will often result, and the care that you as an Emergency Medical Responder will need to provide to support these patients.

OBJECTIVES

Upon successful completion of this chapter, the student should be able to:

COGNITIVE

1. Review cardiovascular anatomy and physiology in Chapter 4.
2. Define the following terms:
   a. angina *(p. 278)*
   b. cardiac compromise *(p. 277)*
   c. conduction pathway *(p. 277)*
   d. heart failure *(p. 279)*
   e. myocardial infarction *(p. 279)*
3. Describe the normal flow of blood through the heart. *(p. 276)*
4. Explain common causes of cardiac compromise. *(p. 277)*
5. Describe the signs and symptoms of a patient experiencing cardiac compromise. *(p. 277)*
6. Differentiate and explain the pathophysiology of angina, myocardial infarction, and heart failure. *(p. 278)*
7. Explain the appropriate assessment and care for a patient experiencing cardiac compromise. *(p. 281)*

PSYCHOMOTOR

8. Demonstrate the ability to appropriately assess and care for a patient experiencing cardiac compromise.

AFFECTIVE

9. Value the importance of caring for all patients with chest pain as though it were cardiac compromise.

Police officer Taylor Revell forgot his lunch on the kitchen table before leaving for work this morning. It was a move he regretted the moment one of the dispatchers advised him, while stifling a giggle, that his wife had dropped it off at the front desk. The giant smiley face scrawled on the brown paper bag and his wife's childish block letters spelling out his name made his face flush hot and sent quiet laughter through the department's administrative staff. This was Alexandra's way of ensuring that he never forgot his lunch again.

He is just walking out the lobby doors toward his patrol car, lunch bag in hand, when the squeal of tires catches his attention. A small, blue subcompact car skitters across the lanes in front of the police station and slides to a halt about 10 feet from where Taylor is standing. A panicked woman stumbles from the driver's side yelling for help.

"My dad!" she shouts, pointing back at the car. "He's turning blue. I think it's his heart!"

Taylor drops his lunch onto the pavement and rushes to the car's passenger door. An elderly man is slumped against the window, eyes partially open but clearly not seeing.

Normal Heart Function

When functioning properly, the heart is an amazingly efficient pump that beats an average of 100,000 times per day. It also circulates approximately 6,000 to 7,500 liters of blood each day. Blood flows through the heart beginning with the right atrium (Figure 13.1). It then flows down into the right ventricle. From there it flows into the lungs, where it drops

Figure 13.1 • Cross-section of the heart.

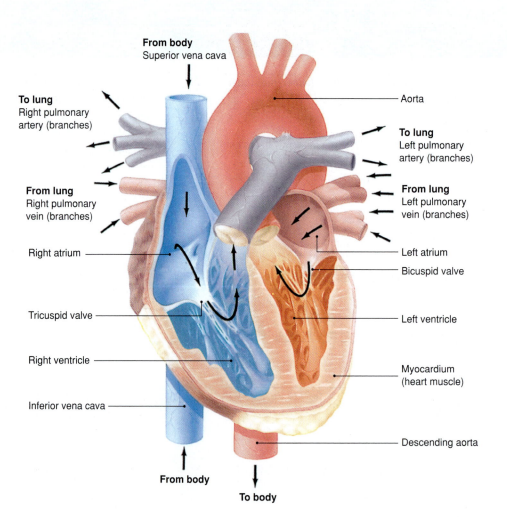

off carbon dioxide and picks up oxygen. It returns from the lungs and enters the left atrium and then flows down into the left ventricle. The left ventricle is the largest and strongest chamber of the heart and must force blood out to the entire body. The heart muscle itself receives its blood supply from tiny vessels called *coronary arteries*. Many of the problems related to the heart are the result of the coronary arteries becoming narrowed or blocked, causing a decrease in the normal blood flow to the heart muscle.

The heart contains a sophisticated electrical system that keeps it beating every minute of every day (Figure 13.2). At the core of this electrical system is the **conduction pathway**. This is an electrical pathway that begins at the top of the heart in the atria and continues down the center of the heart, eventually branching out to the right and left ventricles. Each normal beat of the heart begins with an electrical impulse that flows downward along the conduction pathway, causing a coordinated contraction of the heart. Damage to the conduction pathway can lead to an abnormal heart rhythm and is a common cause of poor circulation and perfusion.

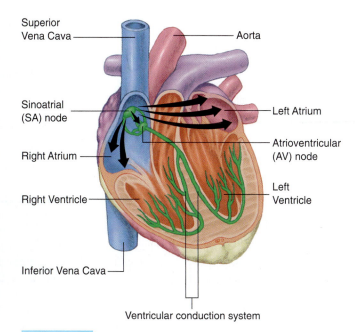

Figure 13.2 • The cardiac conduction pathway, highlighted in green.

Cardiac Compromise

The term **cardiac compromise** is used to describe specific signs and symptoms that indicate some type of emergency relating to the heart. Medical conditions such as myocardial infarction (MI)(also known as a heart attack), angina pectoris, and heart failure are some of the most common causes of cardiac compromise. The following is a list of common signs and symptoms of cardiac compromise:

- Chest discomfort, which is typically described as pain or a dull pressure, tightness, or a squeezing sensation in the chest. The discomfort also may radiate to the arms, shoulders, back, neck, or jaw.
- Diaphoresis (sudden onset of sweating)
- Dyspnea (shortness of breath)
- Nausea/vomiting
- Anxiety, irritability
- Feeling of impending doom
- Abnormal pulse (may be rapid, slow, and/or irregular)
- Abnormal blood pressure (may be high or low)

Cardiac compromise has many causes and can present with any one or all of the above signs and symptoms. As an Emergency Medical Responder, you must use your assessment skills to quickly gather a patient history and perform a physical exam to identify the potential for cardiac involvement. When in doubt, provide care for the worst possible scenario and call for an advanced life support (ALS) ambulance.

conduction pathway ▶ the electrical pathway within the heart.

cardiac compromise ▶ a general term used to describe specific signs and symptoms that indicate some type of emergency relating to the heart.

OBJECTIVES

4. Explain common causes of cardiac compromise.

5. Describe the signs and symptoms of a patient experiencing cardiac compromise.

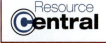

Learn about congenital heart defects, as well as coronary artery disease.

From the Medical Director

Signs and Symptoms
Always assume that chest pain is cardiac in origin. Although there are several non-cardiac causes of chest pain, you must assume the worst until the patient undergoes a more extensive evaluation.

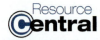

angina ▶ pain in the chest caused by a lack of sufficient blood and oxygen to the heart muscle.

KEY POINT ▼

Care for all patients who display the signs and symptoms of cardiac compromise as unstable and request immediate transport to an appropriate hospital. If available, request an ALS unit.

KEY POINT ▼

Many times, cardiac chest pain is associated with other signs and symptoms suggestive of a heart attack. They include shortness of breath, nausea, sweating, and weakness.

OBJECTIVE

6. Differentiate and explain the pathophysiology of angina, myocardial infarction, and heart failure.

Cardiac arrest is the ultimate form of cardiac compromise and results in stoppage of the heart. Cardiac arrest can occur for many reasons, such as trauma, allergic reaction, overdose, etc. Sudden cardiac arrest is most common in adults and is most commonly caused by a heart attack. Cardiac arrest and care for patients in cardiac arrest are covered in detail in Chapter 10.

Angina Pectoris

A common cause of cardiac compromise is known as angina pectoris, or as it is more commonly called, **angina**. Literally translated, *angina pectoris* means pain in the chest. Angina occurs when one or more of the coronary arteries are unable to provide an adequate supply of oxygenated blood to the heart muscle (myocardium). Although this may sound like what happens in a heart attack, the similarity ends there. With angina, there is no actual damage to the heart muscle. The supply of oxygenated blood is never cut off entirely, and the pain is caused by the muscles starving for more blood and oxygen. Angina can be caused by a partial blockage or spasm of a coronary artery.

Chest pain caused by a heart attack and angina is often triggered by exertion. Exertion such as physical activity creates a demand on the heart muscle that the coronary arteries are unable to meet. The pain increases until the patient stops the activity and rests. In the case of angina, when the demand on the heart returns to normal, the pain begins to subside, and eventually it goes away. Some patients are prone to angina attacks and must take medication such as nitroglycerin to help increase circulation to the heart. (Nitroglycerin is discussed in more detail later in this chapter.)

The signs and symptoms of angina are nearly identical to those of a heart attack. For that reason, it is important to care for all suspected cardiac-related pain as though the patient is having a heart attack and to seek immediate advanced medical care.

Myocardial Infarction

The medical term for what is commonly known as a heart attack is **myocardial infarction (MI)**. *Myo-* meaning muscle, *cardial-* meaning heart, and *infarction* meaning a deadening of tissue due to a loss of adequate blood supply. The heart muscle (myocardium) must have an adequate supply of well-oxygenated blood to continue to function properly. The heart receives its blood supply through vessels known as *coronary arteries* (Figure 13.3). When these arteries become excessively narrow or blocked from disease (atherosclerosis) or a clot and can no longer supply the myocardium with enough oxygenated blood, the tissue of the heart begins to die.

It is important to understand that a heart attack, or MI, and cardiac arrest are not the same thing. Patients suffering a cardiac arrest are unresponsive, not breathing (apneic), and have no pulse. Those patients should receive immediate CPR and the application of an automated external defibrillator (AED). Although it is true that most cardiac arrests are the result of an MI, most MIs do not result in a cardiac arrest.

There are many factors that will ultimately determine whether a heart attack will result in a cardiac arrest. The most common are the location of the damage on the heart and how much heart muscle actually dies. Damage that occurs over an important electrical pathway or to the left ventricle is more likely to cause a cardiac arrest.

The following are common signs and symptoms of a heart attack (Figure 13.4):

- Chest or upper abdominal sensations of pain, pressure, tightness, or heaviness. Some patients describe a burning sensation that can easily be mistaken for indigestion.
- The pain or discomfort may be described as behind the sternum (substernal) and radiate to either one of the arms or shoulders. In some cases, the pain may extend to the back, neck, jaw, or upper abdomen.

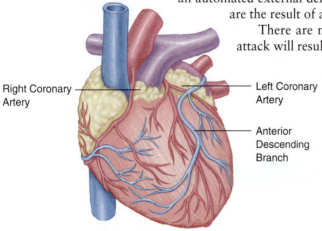

Right Coronary Artery

Left Coronary Artery

Anterior Descending Branch

Figure 13.3 • The coronary arteries supply blood to the heart muscle.

DISTINGUISHING ANGINA PECTORIS FROM MYOCARDIAL INFARCTION

	Angina Pectoris	Myocardial Infarction
Location of Discomfort	Substernal or across chest	Same
Radiation of Discomfort	Neck, jaw, arms, back, shoulders	Same
Nature of Discomfort	Dull or heavy discomfort with a pressure or squeezing sensation	Same, but maybe more intense
Duration	Usually 2 to 15 minutes, subsides after activity stops	Lasts longer than 10 minutes
Other symptoms	Usually none	Perspiration, pale gray color, nausea, weakness, dizziness, lightheadedness
Precipitating Factors	Extremes in weather, exertion, stress, meals	Often none
Factors Giving Relief	Stopping physical activity, reducing stress, nitroglycerin	Nitroglycerin may give incomplete or no relief

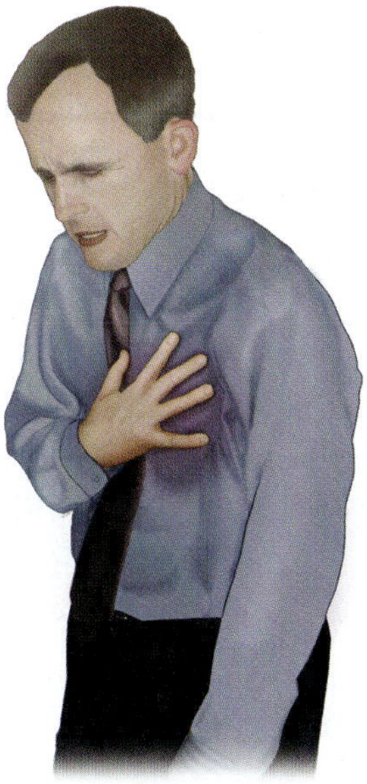

Figure 13.4 • Both myocardial infarction and angina can present with symptoms of chest pain. Treat all cases of chest pain as true cardiac emergencies.

Those are the "classic" signs and symptoms of a cardiac-related event. However, there are other ways that a cardiac event can present. Patients most likely to display signs and symptoms other than those noted above are women, diabetics, and the elderly. Although they often do present with common signs and symptoms, it is important to remain suspicious even if the more classic signs and symptoms are absent. During a cardiac event, those populations may experience what appear as "flulike" signs and symptoms, such as nausea and vomiting, indigestion, or a feeling of general weakness. The patient may simply tell you, "I don't feel right," or "Something is wrong with me, but I don't know what it is."

As an Emergency Medical Responder, you must be very aware of all possible presentations of cardiac compromise and not just the typical "Hollywood" presentation of the man who suddenly grasps his chest and falls to the ground. You must be very suspicious of the elderly, female, or diabetic patient who may be insisting that they just have the flu. Provide care as if they are suffering cardiac compromise.

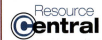

View a video about angina.

myocardial infarction (MI) ▶ a condition that results when the blood supply to a portion of the heart is interrupted. Also known as a *heart attack*.

continued

After requesting an ambulance on his shoulder microphone, Taylor carefully opens the car door and lowers the unresponsive man to the ground.

"He wasn't feeling well, and I was taking him to the doctor." The woman stands above Taylor, hands intertwined in her hair and tears streaming down her cheeks.

Taylor checks carefully for any signs of breathing or a pulse. There are none. "Go into the lobby and tell them that you need the AED," Taylor says to the woman, firmly accentuating each letter.

As she turns and runs toward the glass doors, he places his hands on the man's chest and begins compressions.

FIRST ON SCENE

heart failure ▶ a condition that develops when the heart is unable to pump blood efficiently, causing a backup of blood and other fluids within the circulatory system. Also may be referred to as *congestive heart failure*.

Heart Failure

Sometimes called congestive heart failure (CHF), **heart failure** is a term used to describe a condition that develops when the heart is unable to pump blood efficiently. Heart failure can occur slowly over time as part of the normal aging process. It also can occur suddenly following a heart attack. Because the heart muscle is weakened, it is unable to manage the normal amount of blood volume. When this happens, fluid backs up within the circulatory system. This backup of fluids, if left untreated, can cause fluid to be pushed into the alveoli within the lungs, resulting in difficulty breathing. The backup also can result in swelling in the lower extremities (pedal edema). Although some patients with heart failure have a chief complaint of chest pain, many more have a chief complaint of difficulty breathing.

Heart failure can be both chronic and acute. Some of the causes of chronic heart failure include diseased heart valves, high blood pressure (hypertension), and various lung diseases. A patient also can experience a sudden (acute) episode of heart failure following a heart attack.

Much like angina and heart attack, the acute heart failure patient may complain of chest pain, difficulty breathing, or both. These patients typically have a history of cardiac problems and for that reason will likely have a long list of prescribed medications. Many patients with this condition have difficulty breathing while lying down. The patient will tell you that he cannot lie down and needs to sit upright, or he will tell you that he has to sleep in a recliner in order to breathe.

> ### ▶ GERIATRIC FOCUS ◀

Just as with chest pain, the elderly patient suffering from congestive heart failure may have vague complaints, with fatigue being one of the most common.

If the patient is in a seated position, you are likely to see obvious swelling of the feet and ankles (pedal edema) because gravity pulls the excess fluids to those areas. If the patient is confined to a bed, you may see edema in the sacral area (sacral edema), because this is typically the lowest part of the body, and once again, gravity pulls the excess fluid downward. Depending on the amount of fluid in the lungs, the patient may experience increased shortness of breath while lying down. Be alert for this and be prepared to place the patient in a position of comfort. You also may see some jugular vein distention (JVD) as a result of the increased pressure inside the circulatory system.

The signs and symptoms of heart failure include (Figure 13.5) the following:

- Shortness of breath
- Chest pain/discomfort
- Rapid pulse rate
- Pedal edema (swollen ankles)
- Jugular vein distention (JVD)
- Pale, moist skin
- Altered mental status due to a decrease in perfusion to the brain

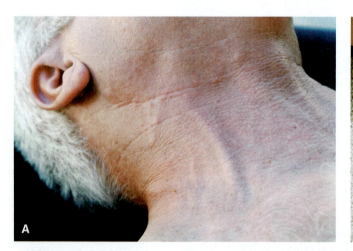 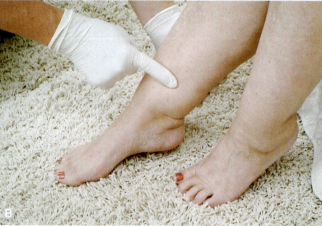

Figure 13.5 • Signs of congestive heart failure include (A) bulging neck veins and (B) swollen ankles.

Police officer Taylor Revell was never happier to hear ambulance sirens fast approaching as he rhythmically drives the heel of his hand into the man's chest, sweat dripping down his face and falling onto the dark fabric of his uniform as he counts out loud. 17...18...19...20...21....

"Here. Here. Here!" The man's daughter shouts as she approaches, carrying the AED. She is being trailed by several records clerks with worried looks on their faces.

Taylor quickly pulls the man's shirt open, exposing a pale, sunken chest, and touches the power button on the cardiac device. The verbal directions from the machine are almost drowned out by the arrival of thundering diesel engines followed by numerous slamming doors.

Emergency Care for Cardiac Compromise

Assessment

When your patient's chief complaint is chest pain, gather a patient history first, focusing your questions on the chief complaint. The mnemonic OPQRST is a common tool used to assess chest pain. Be sure to look the patient in the eyes as you ask questions to be certain he understands and is not distracted by what is happening to him. Remember that the patient is likely to be frightened. Be very clear with each question, and allow plenty of time for him to respond. Following is a review of OPQRST and some sample questions for each component:

O — *Onset.* What were you doing when the pain/discomfort began? With this question you are trying to determine if the patient was at rest or may have been involved in some physical activity when the pain began. Although it may not change how you treat the patient, this information will be valuable to the physician who will be treating the patient at the hospital.

P — *Provocation.* Does anything you do make the pain/discomfort better or worse? This question helps determine if anything the patient does in terms of movement or positioning makes the pain get better or worse. Cardiac-related chest pain is typically a constant pain that will not change with palpation or position. Although the patient may feel as though he can breathe easier in one position or another, the pain/discomfort will not usually change.

Q — *Quality.* Can you describe how your pain/discomfort feels? Try to get the patient to describe his pain/discomfort in his own words. Be careful, because it is easy to accidentally lead the patient. That is, if the patient is having difficulty finding words to describe what he is experiencing, he may agree with the first suggestion you offer him. Instead, a better way to explore what he is feeling is to offer contrasting choices and allow him to select the most appropriate word. For example, you might ask, "Is your pain/discomfort sharp or dull?" or "Is your pain/discomfort steady, or does it come and go?" You must remember that he may be distracted by what is happening to him, so be patient and allow the patient enough time to process the question and provide an appropriate response.

R — *Region and radiate.* Can you point with one finger to where the pain/discomfort is the most intense? Does your pain/discomfort move or radiate anywhere else? The focus of those questions is to determine where the pain/discomfort is located. Watch the patient carefully after you ask. See if he is able to pinpoint the pain, or if he motions with an open hand over his chest or other area, suggesting that the pain is spread out and perhaps radiating.

OBJECTIVE

7. Explain the appropriate assessment and care for a patient experiencing cardiac compromise.

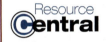

Resource **Central**

Watch a video on cardiac compromise.

S — *Severity.* On a scale of 1 to 10, with 10 being the worst pain you have ever felt, how would you rate your pain/discomfort? This question will help you determine just how much pain/discomfort the patient is experiencing from the event. It will be important to ask it three different times. The first time you ask, you are trying to determine the level of discomfort at that moment. You must then ask, "What level was the pain when it first began?" This will provide insight into whether the pain has gotten better, worse, or stayed the same. You will then want to ask the question again after you have provided some care and comfort to the patient.

T — *Time.* When did you first begin feeling this pain/discomfort? In many cases of cardiac compromise, time plays an important factor. Although it will not and should not affect the way you care for your patient, it will be an important part of the history you obtain. Ask when the pain/discomfort first began. Also find out if the patient felt bad or had any other symptoms prior to its onset. Many patients may begin experiencing nausea, lightheadedness, shortness of breath, and fatigue long before the pain or discomfort begin.

The emergency care for a patient with signs and symptoms of cardiac compromise is similar to other medical complaints: Maintain an open airway. Make certain that someone activates the EMS system and requests ALS services, if available. Position the patient to provide the greatest ease when breathing, which is usually an upright position. If the patient is alert, he should be assisted into a sitting position. Administer oxygen if allowed to do so. Reassure the patient and calm him if possible (Figure 13.6).

If the patient is in cardiac arrest (no pulse and not breathing), have someone activate EMS and begin CPR. Otherwise, complete the assessment as required, carefully noting the patient's signs and symptoms (Figure 13.7). If the patient is unresponsive when you arrive, gain what information you can from bystanders.

Emergency Care

When caring for a patient with signs and symptoms indicating cardiac compromise, you should:

1. Take appropriate BSI precautions.
2. Perform a primary assessment and support the ABCs (airway, breathing, and circulation) as necessary.
3. Obtain a medical history.
4. If allowed, provide oxygen per local protocols.
5. Keep the patient at rest. Provide emotional support and reassure the patient.

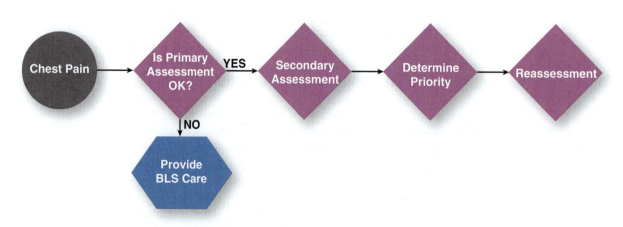

Figure 13.6 • Algorithm for the emergency care of medical patients.

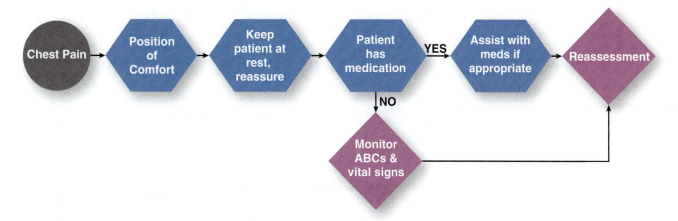

Figure 13.7 • Algorithm for assessment of patients with chest pain.

6. Allow the patient to maintain a position of comfort. That usually is sitting up.

7. Obtain vital signs.

8. Assist the patient with the prescribed dose of nitroglycerin, if your protocols permit. Consult medical direction.

9. Continue to monitor vital signs.

Remember to conduct yourself in a calm, professional manner when caring for your patient. That is of particular importance in caring for patients with chest pain. These patients can be anxious, restless, or in denial. Their chances for survival may be increased if they can be calm and kept at rest.

A patient may ask if he is having a heart attack. It is best to respond by saying, "Your pain could be a lot of things, but let's not take chances." Do all you can to keep the patient calm and still. Remain calm yourself and talk to your patient. Let the patient know that resting is an important part of his care.

Continue to comfort the patient as long as he is in your care. Assure the patient that more highly trained help is on the way. Tell him that you are a trained Emergency Medical Responder and that you will stay with him until further help arrives.

Medications

Some patients with a history of heart problems have been prescribed medications by their physicians to take when having chest pain. Always ask if a physician has given the patient any medications for the current problem. If medications have been prescribed, then assist the patient in taking them only if your local protocols allow.

▶ GERIATRIC FOCUS ◀

Many elderly patients have been prescribed multiple medications for a wide variety of medical problems. Whenever possible, gather all the medications together and place them in a paper bag for transport to the hospital with the patient.

From the Medical Director

Oxygen
Recent studies indicate that high-concentration oxygen may be harmful to the heart even in the case of myocardial infarction. Some organizations recommend oxygen only if the patient is in respiratory distress. Follow your Medical Director's recommendations.

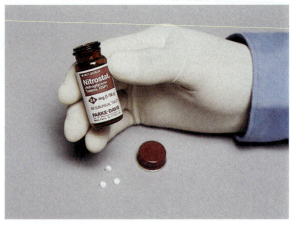

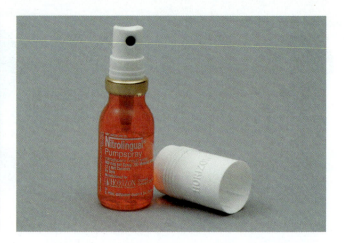

Medication Name

1. Generic: nitroglycerin
2. Trade: Nitrostat, NitroTab, Nitrolingual

Indications

All of the following conditions must be met:

1. Patient complains of chest pain.
2. Patient has a history of cardiac problems.
3. Patient's physician has prescribed nitroglycerin.
4. Systolic blood pressure is greater than 100 systolic. (Local protocols may vary.)
5. Medical direction authorizes administration of the medication.

Contraindications

1. Patient has a systolic blood pressure below 100 mmHg. (Local protocols may vary.)
2. Patient has a head injury.
3. Patient has already taken the maximum prescribed dose.

Medication Form

Tablet or sublingual spray

Dosage

One dose is equal to 0.4 mg. Repeat it in three to five minutes. If no relief, systolic blood pressure remains above 100 (local protocols may vary), and if authorized by medical direction, up to a maximum of three doses. Spray is typically prescribed for one metered spray followed by a second in 15 minutes.

Steps for Assisting the Patient

1. Perform a focused assessment for the cardiac patient.
2. Take blood pressure. (Systolic pressure must be above 100. Local protocols may vary.)
3. Contact medical direction, if there are no standing orders.
4. Ensure right medication, right patient, right dose, right route, and right time. Check the expiration date.
5. Ensure that the patient is alert.
6. Question the patient on the last dose taken and any effects.
7. Ask the patient to lift his tongue and place a tablet or spray dose on or under tongue. If you are assisting, be sure you are wearing gloves.
8. Have the patient keep his mouth closed with the tablet under his tongue (without swallowing) until dissolved and absorbed.
9. Recheck blood pressure within two minutes.
10. Record administration, route, and time.
11. Perform a reassessment.

Actions

- Dilates blood vessels.
- Decreases workload of heart.

Side Effects

- Hypotension (lowers blood pressure)
- Headache
- Pulse rate changes
- Dizziness, lightheadedness

Reassessment Strategies

- Monitor blood pressure.
- Ask patient about affect on pain relief.
- Seek medical direction before re-administering.
- Document changes in the patient's condition.
- Provide oxygen as appropriate.

KEY POINT ▼

Continue to monitor the cardiac patient and provide care, even if the pain stops. Do not cancel your request for an EMT or more advanced EMS response just because the patient states he is feeling better.

Patients who suffer from angina pectoris usually have nitroglycerin tablets or spray to take when having chest pain (Scan 13.1). Their chest pain could indicate that the heart muscle needs more oxygen. Placing a nitroglycerin tablet or giving one spray under the patient's tongue will allow the drug to rapidly enter the bloodstream. Nitroglycerin dilates (enlarges) blood vessels, allowing an increase in blood flow to the heart muscle. It also reduces the workload of the heart. In doing so, the patient's blood pressure may be lowered. This can cause the patient to become dizzy or lightheaded. Patients receiving nitroglycerin should be sitting or lying down to avoid fainting.

In the form of *transdermal patches*, nitroglycerin can pass through the skin and be picked up by the circulatory system. However, the patches are too slow to be of use in a cardiac emergency. The manufacturers state specifically that the patches are prescribed for use to help "prevent angina, not for the treatment of an acute angina attack."

In recent years, the use of aspirin for the treatment of suspected heart attack has become commonplace in hospitals and EMS systems. In fact, several pharmaceutical companies have created television and radio commercials encouraging the use of aspirin for this purpose. As an Emergency Medical Responder, you may encounter patients who have recently taken aspirin or who may want to take some while in your care. Follow your local protocols when assisting any patient with the administration of medication.

WRAP-UP

FIRST ON SCENE

The AED fires once, shaking the elderly man briefly, and then the paramedic from the ambulance touches Taylor's shoulder. "You've done perfectly, officer," she says. "I can take it from here."

Taylor stands and watches as the EMS personnel apply electrodes and provide oxygen to the man who is now breathing weakly on his own, eyelids fluttering.

"Oh thank you, thank you," the woman shouts, wrapping her arms around Taylor's midsection. She then kisses his cheek and rushes over to where her moaning father is being loaded into the ambulance.

Taylor sighs, wipes the sweat from his face, and picks up his hurriedly discarded lunch, smiling now at the big cartoon face scrawled on the side. Regardless of what is in the bag, he knows that it will be the best lunch ever.

Summary

- A properly functioning heart is at the core of a healthy cardiovascular system.

- Blood flows through the heart beginning at the right atrium, then to the right ventricle, and then to the lungs. It returns to the left atrium and down to the left ventricle. From there it is pumped to the body.

- Each heartbeat is generated by an electrical impulse that flows along the conduction pathway.

- When normal heart function is disrupted, the patient will display signs and symptoms of cardiac compromise.

- Signs and symptoms of cardiac compromise include chest pain or discomfort that begins in the chest and may radiate to the shoulders, arms, neck, or jaw; shortness of breath; pale, moist skin; nausea; and weakness.

- Angina is caused by a lack of sufficient supply of oxygenated blood to the myocardium.

- A myocardial infarction results when a portion of the myocardium dies due to inadequate blood supply.

- Heart failure, also known as congestive heart failure (CHF), occurs when the heart is weakened by illness such as a heart attack and can no longer pump blood efficiently. Blood and other fluids then back up in the system, causing pedal edema and fluid in the lungs.

- Care for cardiac compromise involves support of the ABCs, supplemental oxygen, obtaining a thorough medical history, and monitoring of vital signs.

- Patients with signs and symptoms of cardiac compromise should be considered unstable and in need of immediate transport. Initiate ALS transport if available.

Take Action

There are many causes of cardiac compromise. Most of them share at least one common symptom: pain. While you will likely care for anyone with chest pain as though he is having a heart attack, there are subtle and not so subtle differences in the three most common causes of cardiac compromise: angina, myocardial infarction, and heart failure.

This activity will help you learn the specific signs and symptoms for each of the three conditions. Using either 3 × 5 or 4 × 6 index cards, write the name of each condition on one side of a card—one card per condition for a total of three cards. Now, using your textbook and the Internet, research the specific signs and symptoms of each one. Write as many signs and symptoms as you can find on the reverse of each respective card.

You will now have a very effective study tool for learning the different presentations for the three conditions. It is important to remember that as an Emergency Medical Responder, you will always provide care for the worst possible cause of chest pain and not waste time trying to figure out the exact cause.

First on Scene Run Review

Recall the events of the "First on Scene" scenario in this chapter and answer the following questions, which are related to the call. Rationales are offered in the Answer Key at the back of the book.

1. Should Taylor have checked the scene for safety first? Why or why not?

2. Why should you look at the chest when you give rescue breaths?

3. What information would you give the paramedics when they arrive?

Quick Quiz

To check your understanding of the chapter, answer the following questions. Then compare your answers to those in the Answer Key at the back of the book.

1. Blood that is returning to the heart from the lungs enters the heart at the:
   a. right atrium.
   b. left atrium.
   c. right ventricle.
   d. left ventricle.

2. You are caring for a 44-year-old male patient who began experiencing chest pain and shortness of breath while jogging. His pain went away completely about 20 minutes after stopping to rest. The most likely cause of his chest pain is:
   a. myocardial infarction.
   b. heart failure.
   c. angina.
   d. muscle strain.

3. Your patient is a 65-year-old female who has a long history of cardiac problems. She is complaining of chest pain and difficulty breathing. You should:

   a. lay her in a supine position.
   b. administer oxygen.
   c. obtain a past medical history.
   d. take her vital signs.

4. The myocardium receives its blood supply from:

   a. coronary arteries.
   b. myocardial arteries.
   c. the conduction pathway.
   d. the aorta.

5. You have responded to a 53-year-old male who suddenly collapsed while mowing his lawn. Your assessment reveals that he is pulseless and apneic. His condition is best described as:

   a. angina pectoris
   b. myocardial infarction.
   c. cardiac arrest.
   d. heart failure.

6. Which one of the following statements best describes the relationship between a heart attack and sudden cardiac arrest?

   a. A heart attack and sudden cardiac arrest are the same thing.
   b. Sudden cardiac arrest is a leading cause of heart attack.
   c. Heart attack results in tissue damage; sudden cardiac arrest does not.
   d. Heart attack is a leading cause of sudden cardiac arrest.

7. You have arrived on the scene of an unresponsive female who is pulseless and apneic. You should:

   a. begin CPR.
   b. administer oxygen.
   c. obtain a set of vital signs.
   d. place her in the recovery position.

8. You are caring for a 52-year-old female with a chief complaint of nausea and general fatigue. She is pale and sweaty and has a history of diabetes. You should:

   a. administer oxygen.
   b. administer oral glucose.
   c. obtain vital signs.
   d. perform a secondary assessment.

9. Your patient is experiencing chest pain and shortness of breath and has a history of angina. He took one nitroglycerin tablet 15 minutes ago. Vital signs are respirations 20, pulse 104, and blood pressure 144/88. You should:

   a. have the patient rest until the pain subsides.
   b. assist the patient in taking another dose of nitro.
   c. do nothing until ALS arrives.
   d. apply the AED.

10. You are caring for a 72-year-old female with a chief complaint of shortness of breath. You observe pedal edema and distended neck veins. She states that it is more difficult to breathe while lying down. Her signs and symptoms are most likely caused by:

    a. a myocardial infarction.
    b. angina pectoris.
    c. heart failure.
    d. congestive infarction.

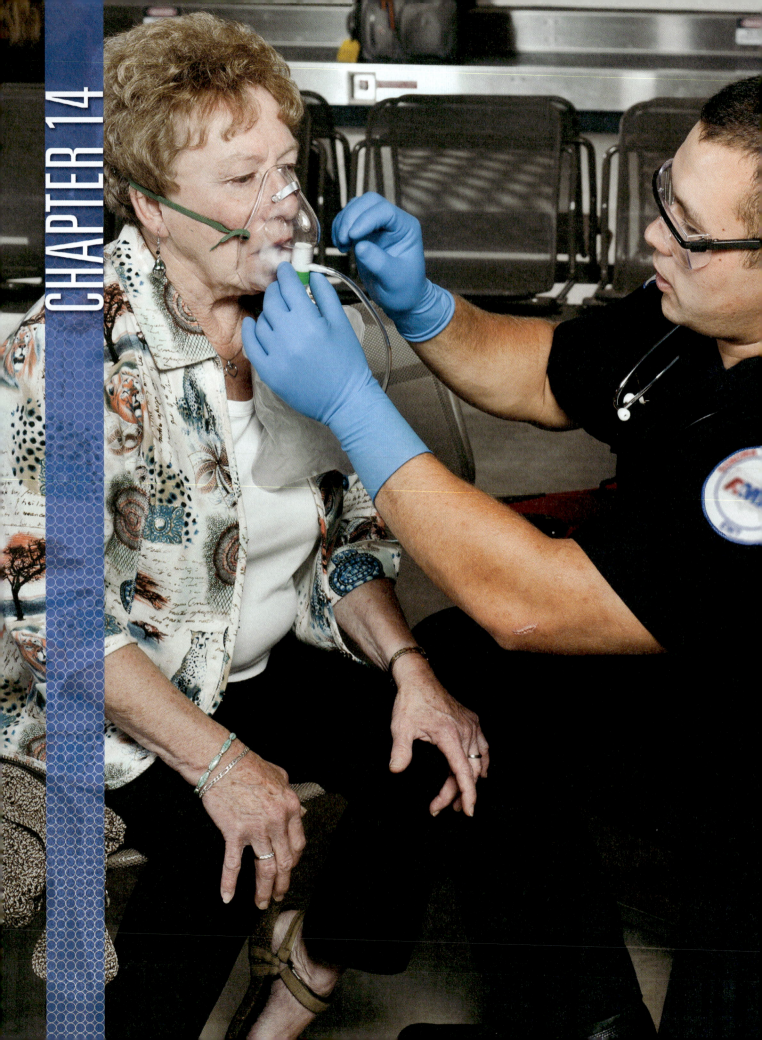

Caring for Respiratory Emergencies

OBJECTIVES

Upon successful completion of this chapter, the student should be able to:

COGNITIVE

1. Review respiratory anatomy and physiology in Chapter 4.

2. Define the following terms:
   a. accessory muscles *(p. 293)*
   b. asthma *(p. 295)*
   c. bronchitis *(p. 296)*
   d. chronic obstructive pulmonary disease (COPD) *(p. 294)*
   e. cyanosis *(p. 298)*
   f. dyspnea *(p. 291)*
   g. emphysema *(p. 298)*
   h. hypercarbia *(p. 291)*
   i. hyperventilation *(p. 298)*
   j. hypoxia *(p. 291)*
   k. respiratory compromise *(p. 291)*
   l. respiratory distress *(p. 291)*
   m. respiratory failure *(p. 291)*
   n. tripod position *(p. 293)*
   o. wheezing *(p. 295)*

3. Explain common causes of respiratory compromise. *(p. 291)*

4. Describe the signs and symptoms of a patient experiencing respiratory compromise. *(p. 294)*

5. Explain the pathophysiology of respiratory compromise. *(p. 294)*

6. Describe the appropriate assessment and care for a patient experiencing respiratory compromise. *(p. 299)*

PSYCHOMOTOR

7. Demonstrate the ability to appropriately assess and care for a patient experiencing respiratory compromise.

AFFECTIVE

8. Recognize the fear that a respiratory emergency can cause.

9. Value the importance of reassurance when caring for a patient with a respiratory emergency.

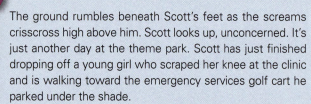
The ground rumbles beneath Scott's feet as the screams crisscross high above him. Scott looks up, unconcerned. It's just another day at the theme park. Scott has just finished dropping off a young girl who scraped her knee at the clinic and is walking toward the emergency services golf cart he parked under the shade.

Scott looks longingly at the ice cream cart that sits beside the carousel. "Wow, no lines," he thinks. "A slight 45-degree turn is all it would take to walk over and get a double scoop of my favorite ice cream." Suddenly his radio sounds off. "Dispatch to Medical One. What is your location?"

"Medical One at the carousel," Scott responds, just a little disappointed that he would not soon be enjoying a large scoop of mint chocolate chip ice cream.

"Medical One, Park Services is requesting a response at the Crusher roller coaster. Sounds like a young female with difficulty breathing. You will be meeting Cal from security."

Scott leaps into the front seat of the golf cart, puts it in drive, and speeds off in the direction of the Crusher.

Overview of Respiratory Anatomy

The respiratory system includes the pathways where air enters the body (nose and mouth) and the areas at the back of the throat, which are called the *nasopharynx* and *oropharynx*. (See Figure 14.1.) The oropharynx leads down the throat into the structure at the top of the *trachea* called the *larynx*. It is in the larynx where the vocal chords are positioned. All spaces and structures above the vocal chords make up the upper airway, and all structures and spaces below the vocal chords make up the lower airway.

Once air passes through the larynx it enters the trachea and travels down to the carina. The *carina* is the point at which the trachea splits into the right and left *main stem bronchi*. These large air passages get smaller as the air passes down into the lungs. The smaller airways are called *bronchioles* and eventually terminate into the *alveoli*. You will remember from Chapter 4 that it is within the *alveoli* that the exchange of oxygen and carbon dioxide takes place. The alveoli are surrounded by tiny blood vessels that drop off the carbon dioxide while picking up fresh oxygen.

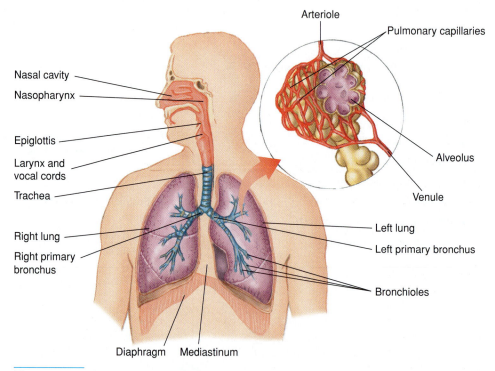

Figure 14.1 • Overview of the respiratory system.

The control center for the respiratory drive is located deep within the brain. It carefully monitors the level of carbon dioxide in the blood and adjusts both rate and volume as necessary.

Respiratory Compromise

Any time a person experiences a condition that affects his ability to breathe adequately, it is referred to as **respiratory compromise**. Respiratory compromise can be the result of any number of conditions that can come on suddenly or develop slowly over time (Scan 14.1). When breathing becomes compromised, the patient is unable to receive an adequate supply of oxygen. If left untreated, this could lead to a condition known as **hypoxia**. Hypoxia occurs when the body's cells do not receive an adequate supply of oxygen. Signs of hypoxia include altered mental status, pale skin, and cyanosis of the nail beds and mucous membranes. As hypoxia occurs, another condition called hypercarbia develops. **Hypercarbia** is the condition of having too much carbon dioxide in the blood.

Respiratory Distress

Respiratory distress, also known as **dyspnea**, is the body's normal response to not getting an adequate supply of oxygen and an increase in the levels of carbon dioxide in the blood. It is characterized by an increased work of breathing, increased respiratory rate, and the use of accessory muscles to promote breathing. In most cases it is easy to spot a patient in respiratory distress because you can see that he has an increased work of breathing.

If the cause of the respiratory compromise is not corrected, respiratory distress can lead to respiratory failure. **Respiratory failure** occurs when the body's normal compensatory mechanisms fail and breathing rate begins to slow and tidal volume begins to get shallower. The patient in respiratory failure will almost always have an altered mental status. If not corrected, respiratory failure will quickly lead to respiratory arrest and death.

While there are many reasons a patient may experience dyspnea, a few of the more common causes that you are likely to encounter as an Emergency Medical Responder include:

- Hyperventilation
- Asthma
- Chronic bronchitis
- Emphysema

In addition to the medical conditions listed above, difficulty in breathing may stem from being exposed to a poison or something to which the patient is allergic. Management of those medical complaints will be discussed in detail in Chapter 15.

The first step in the management of a patient with respiratory compromise is to be able to differentiate adequate breathing from inadequate breathing.

Normal Breathing

Normal breathing is breathing that is sufficient to support life. It is easy and effortless and sometimes referred to as adequate breathing. Patients should not have to work hard to breathe. Patients should be able to speak full sentences without having to catch their

---

From the Medical Director

Adequate Breathing

The level of carbon dioxide in the bloodstream is the primary factor that controls respiratory rate and depth. As the level of CO_2 rises, the brain increases the rate and depth of breathing to enhance the elimination of carbon dioxide. Technology allows providers to measure the amount of carbon dioxide exhaled using a device called a capnograph. *In the absence of this technology, the provider must rely on his understanding of the body's response to carbon dioxide levels to appreciate whether the patient is breathing adequately.*

KEY POINT ▼

One of the first things the body does when it recognizes an increase in carbon dioxide in the blood is to increase the breathing rate. This will serve to blow off excess carbon dioxide and stabilize the balance between oxygen and carbon dioxide.

respiratory compromise ▶ a general term referring to the inability of a person to breathe adequately.

hypoxia ▶ an inadequate supply of oxygen.

hypercarbia ▶ an abnormally high level of carbon dioxide in the blood.

OBJECTIVE

3. Explain common causes of respiratory compromise.

KEY POINT ▼

When caring for a patient with respiratory distress, you must monitor his breathing status continually. You must assess breathing rate, depth, and work of breathing and be ready to change your care if the patient doesn't improve quickly.

respiratory distress ▶ the body's normal response to not getting an adequate supply of oxygen. Also called *dyspnea*.

dyspnea ▶ shortness of breath.

respiratory failure ▶ a respiratory condition characterized by altered mental status, slow respiratory rate, and shallow tidal volume; occurs when the body's normal ability to compensate for inadequate oxygen fails.

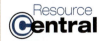

Learn more about breath sounds and assessment tips.

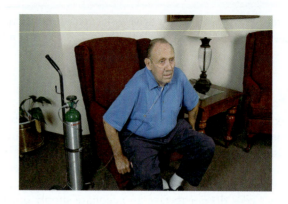

Signs and Symptoms

Difficulty breathing

Shortness of breath

Rapid deep breathing

Noisy breathing

Altered mental status

Restlessness, anxiety, or confusion

Use of accessory muscles: neck, chest, abdomen

Pursed lips or mouth open wide to aid breathing

Pale or blue (cyanotic) skin color

Sharp chest pains

Numbness or tingling in the hands or feet

Spasm of the fingers and toes (possible hyperventilation)

Emergency Care

1. Perform a primary assessment and support the ABCs as necessary.
2. Ensure an open airway. Check for an airway obstruction.
3. Administer oxygen per local protocols.
4. Obtain a patient history.
5. Check to see if the patient is allergic to anything at the scene.
6. Keep patient at rest and try to calm him.
7. Monitor the ABCs and vital signs.
8. Assist with inhaler per local protocols and medical direction.

Chronic Obstructive Pulmonary Disease (COPD)

Signs and Symptoms

History of respiratory problems

Cough

Shortness of breath

Tightness in chest

Swelling in lower extremities

Rapid pulse

Barrel chest

Dizziness

Pale or blue (cyanotic) skin

Desire to sit upright at all times

Emergency Care

Provide the same care as you would for respiratory distress. Do what you can to reduce stress.

NOTE

If you are allowed to provide oxygen, follow local guidelines for the COPD patient.

breath. Adequate breathing is characterized by a normal respiratory rate, depth, and very little effort or work of breathing. The diaphragm is the primary muscle of respiration. It gently and smoothly moves down when we breathe in and upward when we breathe out.

To get a better understanding of what normal breathing looks like, take a moment now to notice the character of your own breathing. In all likelihood you are sitting somewhere quiet as you are studying this textbook. Close your eyes for a few moments and notice the natural movement of air as it enters your nose and mouth. Notice the movement of your chest and abdomen as the air fills your lungs. Pay attention to the air as it rises up through the airways and exits your nose and mouth. Notice how quiet and calm this process is. Now, if you are seated near other people, try to observe their breathing. Are they breathing through their nose or mouth, or perhaps both? Can you see the movement of their chest and abdomen? Which area seems to be moving more, their chest or their abdomen? This may differ from person to person, depending on what positions they are in. As you will see, normal breathing for a person who is not ill seems very subtle. To the untrained eye, normal breathing could easily be described as shallow.

Characteristics of normal breathing include:

- *Normal rate* (number of breaths per minute), which is 12 to 24 for an adult, 16 to 32 for a child, and 24 to 48 for an infant.
- *Normal depth* (the size of each breath), which is also described as *tidal volume*. Normal breaths are not too shallow and not too deep. Your best indicator is good rise and fall of the chest with each breath.
- *Work of breathing*. Work of breathing has to do with how much effort it takes for the patient to move each breath in and out. Normal respirations are effortless and unlabored as the diaphragm muscle moves up and down with each breath.

Along with assessing rate, depth, and work of breathing, you must assess the rhythm of a patient's breathing. Respiratory rhythm should be regular. Breaths should occur at regular intervals and last the same amount of time. Exhaling (breathing out) should take about twice as long as inhaling (breathing in).

Abnormal Breathing

Abnormal breathing, also known as inadequate breathing, is breathing that is not sufficient to support life. Left untreated, such a condition will eventually result in death. For most patients, the most obvious sign of inadequate breathing is an increase in the work of breathing. In other words, breathing will appear labored and difficult. Common signs of inadequate breathing include:

- Increased work of breathing
- Increased respiratory rate (early sign)
- Decreased respiratory rate (late sign)
- Respirations that are too deep or too shallow
- Irregular breathing rhythm
- Audible breath sounds, such as gurgling, snoring or wheezing

When breathing becomes difficult, the patient may have to work extra hard to move air in and out of his lungs. Labored breathing is usually obvious because the patient will be sitting upright, mouth open, and struggling to breathe. People experiencing dyspnea often will maintain what is known as a **tripod position**. This is a position where they are seated or standing with their hands on their knees, shoulders arched upward, and their head forward. This position allows for unrestricted movement of the muscles used for respiration. Other muscles such as the ones between the ribs (intercostal) and those in the neck and abdomen begin to assist the diaphragm. These are called **accessory muscles** because they assist only when the diaphragm alone is not able to move enough air.

tripod position ▶ a body position characterized by the person sitting forward with hands on knees.

accessory muscles ▶ muscles of the neck, chest, and abdomen that can assist during respiratory difficulty.

▶ GERIATRIC FOCUS ◀

The elderly patient does not have the same ability to compensate for inadequate breathing as a younger adult does. Be sure to intervene quickly if breathing becomes inadequate.

Respiratory difficulty may be caused by a variety of conditions, ranging from ongoing medical problems such as asthma to sudden illnesses such as a blood clot in the lung. Always listen to what a patient tells you about how he perceives the problem before attempting to make a determination of a patient's condition.

The patient may have special medications that need to be inhaled. He will want to take the medication but may be too upset or frightened to use the inhaler properly. Some

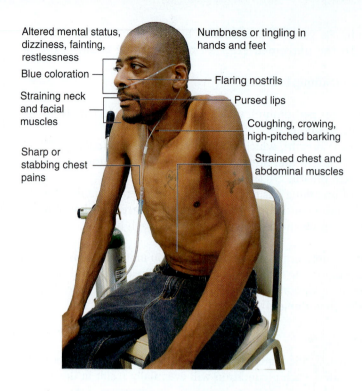

Figure 14.2 • Signs and symptoms of respiratory distress.

Altered mental status, dizziness, fainting, restlessness

Blue coloration

Straining neck and facial muscles

Sharp or stabbing chest pains

Numbness or tingling in hands and feet

Flaring nostrils

Pursed lips

Coughing, crowing, high-pitched barking

Strained chest and abdominal muscles

From the Medical Director

Rapid Breathing

If the breathing is rapid, it is most likely a result of a combination of hypoxia and an elevated carbon dioxide level (hypercarbia). You should not attempt to slow the patient's breathing down because the rate and depth together is a symptom of an underlying condition, not the cause.

---

jurisdictions allow Emergency Medical Responders to help such patients use an inhaler. Check local protocols, and always call for medical direction before assisting a patient with medications.

Signs and Symptoms of Respiratory Compromise

For most cases of respiratory compromise, any or all of the following signs and symptoms may be noticed (Figure 14.2):

- Labored or difficulty breathing; a feeling of suffocation
- Audible breathing sounds
- Rapid or slow rate of breathing
- Abnormal pulse rate (too fast or too slow)
- Changes in skin color, particularly of the lips and nail beds
- Tripod position
- Altered mental status

Chronic Obstructive Pulmonary Disease

A variety of respiratory conditions can be classified as **chronic obstructive pulmonary disease (COPD)**. Such conditions include asthma, chronic bronchitis, and emphysema.

The signs and symptoms of COPD may include:

- History of heavy cigarette smoking
- Persistent cough

OBJECTIVES

4. Describe the signs and symptoms of a patient experiencing respiratory compromise.

5. Explain the pathophysiology of respiratory compromise.

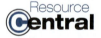

View a video on chronic obstructive pulmonary disease (COPD).

chronic obstructive pulmonary disease (COPD) ▶ a general term used to describe a group of lung diseases that commonly cause respiratory distress and shortness of breath.

- Chronic shortness of breath
- Pursed-lip breathing
- Maintaining a tripod position
- Fatigue
- Tightness in the chest
- Wheezing

In advanced cases, there may be altered mental status, barrel-chest appearance, a strong desire to remain sitting even when asleep, and pale or blue discoloration of the skin, lips, and nail beds.

COPD can be difficult to distinguish from heart failure. However, you do not have to make that distinction. For Emergency Medical Responders, emergency care is the same.

continued

▶ GERIATRIC FOCUS ◀

The elderly patient may become short of breath with even the slightest amount of exertion. It will be important for you to make sure the cause of the increased work of breathing is not due simply to exertion. The OPQRST assessment tool may be helpful with making this determination.

FIRST ON SCENE

Scott pulls up to the roller coaster and finds a large group of park guests surrounding a teenage girl sitting in the grass. He grabs his response bag and runs up to the young woman, who is gasping loudly with each breath. Two other girls are on either side, holding her forward.

"Can anyone tell me what happened here?" Scott says as he opens his jump bag.

"Her name is Karyn," one of the girls says. "I told her not to go on this stupid ride, but of course, since Cor was going on it..."

"She's hyperventilating," the other girl shouts, "I've seen this before. I'm a babysitter, and am first aid certified!"

"Okay, okay, thank you," Scott says, trying to concentrate on Karyn, who is steadily turning white as a sheet, letting her eyes close slowly. "Karyn, I am going to help you, but before I can, can you tell me what you were doing when you started having trouble breathing?"

"I was just, standing in line, for the ride." Karyn says in short bursts of words between breaths.

"Do you have any breathing problems, such as asthma?" Scott asks as he prepares an oxygen cylinder.

Karyn shakes her head no.

"Has this ever happened before?"

Once again Karyn shakes her head no.

"Are you allergic to anything? Maybe a bee sting, or food?" Scott continues.

Once again, Karyn shakes her head no.

Asthma

Asthma is probably the most common form of chronic obstructive pulmonary disease, affecting millions of people in the United States. Asthma is a disease of the lower airway caused by an increased sensitivity to a variety of irritants such as pollen, pollutants, and even exercise. When irritated, the bronchioles begin to spasm and constrict. Once irritated they also begin to swell and produce excess mucus. Those factors all contribute to making the air passages smaller, resulting in an acute onset of respiratory distress (Figure 14.3). The narrowing of the air passages will often cause the presence of wheezing.

Wheezing is a high-pitched whistling sound that is created when the air passes through the narrowed airways. It is most often heard when the lungs are auscultated with a stethoscope. In extreme cases, wheezing can be heard without a stethoscope.

The good news is that most asthma sufferers have little or no symptoms between attacks. Most known asthma patients carry medication in the form of a *metered-dose inhaler* that they breathe into their lungs when they feel an asthma attack coming on. The

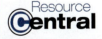
Resource Central

Watch a video about asthma.

asthma ▶ a condition affecting the lungs, characterized by narrowing of the air passages and wheezing.

wheezing ▶ a course whistling sound often heard in the lungs when a patient with respiratory compromise exhales. May also be heard on inspiration.

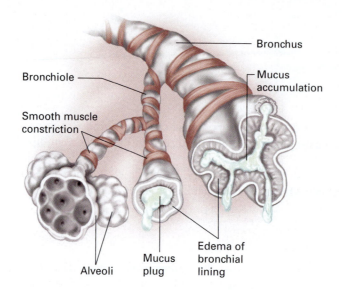

Figure 14.3 • Asthma causes the bronchioles to become narrow and filled with mucus.

Bronchus

Bronchiole

Mucus accumulation

Smooth muscle constriction

Alveoli

Mucus plug

Edema of bronchial lining

Read more about asthma triggers.

medications are called *bronchodilators* because they help dilate the bronchiole passages to help make breathing easier. However, if left untreated, an asthma attack can be severe enough to cause respiratory arrest and even death (Scan 14.2).

The signs and symptoms of asthma include the following:

- Moderate to severe shortness of breath
- Wheezing
- Anxiety
- Nonproductive cough

Bronchitis

bronchitis ▶ a condition of the lungs characterized by inflammation of the bronchial airways and mucus formation; a form of chronic obstructive pulmonary disease (COPD).

Bronchitis is a disease process that causes swelling and thickening of the walls of the bronchi and bronchioles. In addition to swelling of the tissues, bronchitis causes an overproduction of mucus in the air passages. Both of these conditions cause the airways to become restricted, resulting in difficulty breathing for the patient. Some people suffer from a condition called *chronic bronchitis*. Chronic bronchitis is defined as a productive cough that continues for three consecutive months and occurs for at least two consecutive years (Figure 14.4).

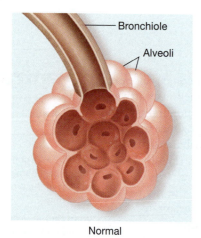
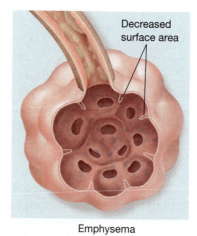
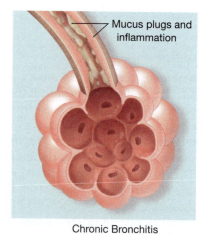

Bronchiole

Alveoli

Normal

Decreased surface area

Emphysema

Mucus plugs and inflammation

Chronic Bronchitis

Figure 14.4 • Emphysema affects the alveoli, and bronchitis affects the bronchioles.

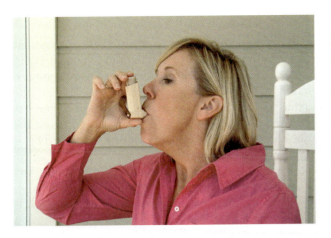
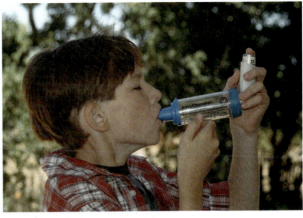

Metered-Dose Inhaler
Medication Name

1. Generic: albuterol, ipratropium, metaproterenol
2. Trade: Proventil, Ventolin, Atrovent, Alupent, Metaprel

Indications

Meets all of the following criteria:

1. Patient exhibits signs and symptoms of respiratory difficulty.
2. Patient has physician-prescribed inhaler.
3. Medical direction gives Emergency Medical Responder specific authorization to use.

Contraindications

1. Altered mental status (such that the patient is unable to use the device properly).
2. No permission has been given by medical direction.
3. Patient has already taken maximum prescribed dose prior to rescuer's arrival.

Medication Form

Handheld metered-dose inhaler

Dosage

Number of inhalations based on medical direction's order or physician's order

Steps for Administration

1. Obtain order from medical direction.
2. Confirm patient is alert enough to use inhaler.
3. Ensure it is the patient's own prescription.
4. Check expiration date of inhaler.
5. Check if patient has already taken any doses.
6. Shake inhaler vigorously several times.
7. Have patient exhale deeply.
8. Have patient put lips around the opening of the inhaler.
9. Have patient depress the handheld inhaler when beginning to inhale deeply.
10. Instruct patient to hold breath for as long as is comfortable so that medication can be absorbed.
11. Allow patient to breathe a few times and repeat second dose if so ordered by medical direction.
12. If patient has a spacer device for use with the inhaler (device for attachment between inhaler and patient to allow for more effective use of medication), it should be used.
13. Provide oxygen as appropriate.

Actions

Dilates bronchioles, reducing airway resistance

Side Effects

1. Increased pulse rate
2. Anxiety
3. Nervousness

Reassessment Strategies

1. Monitor vital signs.
2. Adjust oxygen as appropriate.
3. Reassess level of respiratory distress.
4. Observe for deterioration of patient. If breathing becomes inadequate, provide artificial ventilations.

The typical patient with a history of chronic bronchitis is overweight and has a pale or bluish complexion due to inadequate oxygen. Classic signs and symptoms of chronic bronchitis include:

- Overweight
- Mild to moderate shortness of breath
- Pale complexion
- Productive cough
- Wheezes

Emphysema

Most often associated with cigarette smoking, **emphysema** is a disease of the lungs that causes permanent damage to the alveoli. Emphysema is also common in individuals who have been exposed to environmental toxins over a long period of time, such as coal miners.

Emphysema causes the destruction of the alveoli, making them useless for the exchange of oxygen and carbon dioxide. In addition, it causes the lungs to become less elastic, causing carbon dioxide to become trapped. The loss of lung elasticity and the resulting accumulation of air cause the chest wall to become extended over time. This is often described as a "barrel chest" appearance.

Another classic sign of the advanced emphysema patient is what is called "pursed-lip" breathing. The patient will hold his lips tight while forcing his exhaled air out. This increases the exhalation phase and causes a back pressure deep within the lungs, which is believed to assist with gas exchange.

The majority of emphysema patients are middle aged and older and spend most of their energy just trying to breathe. Common signs and symptoms of emphysema include:

- Moderate to severe shortness of breath
- Very thin in appearance
- Large chest (barrel chest)
- Nonproductive cough
- Extended exhalations
- Pursed-lip breathing

Hyperventilation Syndrome

Breathing can often be affected by an emotional response or a sudden onset of anxiety. When this happens, breathing often becomes rapid, deep, and difficult to control. The body needs a proper balance of both oxygen and carbon dioxide. **Hyperventilation** occurs when the person breathes out and eliminates an excess amount of carbon dioxide. Most cases of hyperventilation are caused by anxiety and do not represent a true medical emergency.

In some instances, hyperventilation can be a sign of something more serious, such as an impending heart attack or other serious medical condition. Activate the EMS system and provide care for respiratory distress. Be alert for **cyanosis** (blue discoloration of the skin, lips, and nail beds) or other signs and symptoms of inadequate breathing. Monitor the patient for changes in vital signs, which may indicate serious medical problems. Suspect the worst, and be prepared to respond appropriately.

Regardless of the underlying cause, your priority in the care of these patients is to reduce anxiety by reassuring and comforting them. Though hyperventilation is rarely life threatening, it can be very frightening for patients. They have a feeling of not being able to breathe, and this often makes the situation worse. Signs and symptoms of common anxiety-driven hyperventilation include:

- Moderate to severe shortness of breath
- Anxiety
- Numbness or tingling of the fingers, lips, and/or toes
- Dizziness
- Spasm of the fingers and/or toes
- Chest discomfort

From the Medical Director

Hyperventilation

Your patient may be hyperventilating because he is anxious, but you should assume that his breathing is a reflexive response to either hypoxia or too much carbon dioxide, and rather than trying to slow his breathing, provide emotional support and attempt to calm him.

The care of the patient with hyperventilation should focus on calming the patient. You may need to remove him from an environment that may be contributing to his anxiety and assist him with slowing his breathing. It is not recommended that you have him breathe into a paper bag or similar device, because this could make the situation worse if there is an underlying medical problem. If your local protocols allow, you may use low-flow oxygen while helping to calm down the patient and slow his breathing.

▶ GERIATRIC FOCUS ◀

Be very cautious of the elderly patient who you think may be hyperventilating. There is a high likelihood he may have an underlying medical condition that could be causing the hyperventilation. Do not withhold oxygen from any elderly patient with breathing difficulty. Always follow local protocols.

continued

FIRST ON SCENE

"Okay," Patrick says, unraveling his oxygen tubing. "I just want to rule out an allergic reaction. I'm going to get this oxygen ready, so can you work on slowing your breathing for me?"

Karyn opens her eyes and nods, though her breathing is almost uncontrollable.

"Karyn, you're doing great," Scott says, holding the oxygen mask close to her mouth and nose. She forcefully pushed the mask away when he tried to attach it, so he holds it as close to her face as she will allow. Her face is dripping with sweat and her hands are shaking as she grips the grass down by her knees.

"She needs a paper bag!" one of her friends shouts. "I told you she's hyperventilating."

"Thanks again," Scott says automatically as he counts Karyn's breaths again. Her respiratory rate is 32, and she is crying weakly. "Karyn, I know this coaster was scary, but it's okay. You're safe now. Can you breathe with me?"

She nods and watches Scott carefully. He breathes in slowly and breathes out even slower. Karyn tries copying his breathing but keeps cutting each breath with a sharp intake. "You're doing fine," Scott encourages. "Just keep breathing with me."

Emergency Care for Respiratory Compromise

Your assessment of the patient with respiratory compromise will begin as you enter the scene and first lay eyes on the patient. You must begin by observing his body language. Is he sitting, standing, or lying down? Does he appear conscious or unresponsive? Your assessment of an unresponsive patient will need to be much more aggressive than that for a responsive patient. You must kneel beside the patient and place your ear next to his nose and mouth to confirm he has a patent airway. You also must determine the characteristics of his breathing (rate, depth, and work of breathing). You must provide positive pressure ventilations if you determine breathing is inadequate.

When assessing a responsive patient, pay attention to the level of distress and facial expression. Does he appear anxious and frightened? If so, his situation is likely getting worse. Introduce yourself and immediately begin to reassure the patient. Tell him that you are going to help him breathe easier. As you begin to gather a history about the present situation, pay attention to his ability to speak clearly and in full sentences. One of the classic signs of moderate to severe distress is the inability to speak in full sentences. A patient in moderate to severe distress will only be able to speak a few words before having to stop for a breath.

Listen for sounds as he breathes. Noisy breathing is always a sign of some form of airway obstruction. It can sound like gurgling, which usually indicates the presence of fluid in the airway. If the sound is more like snoring, either swelling of the upper airway or partial blockage caused by the tongue may be the cause. The problem usually can be corrected with proper positioning of the head. Another common sound heard with breathing is that of wheezing. Wheezing usually is heard with a stethoscope, but severe cases of wheezing can be heard without one.

OBJECTIVE

6. Describe the appropriate assessment and care for a patient experiencing respiratory compromise.

KEY POINT ▼

A patient who can only speak a few words at a time is in serious distress. These patients are in need of more advanced care and rapid transport.

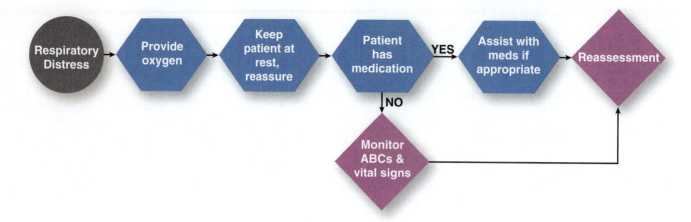

Figure 14.5 • Algorithm for emergency care of patients with respiratory distress.

The general care for anyone with respiratory compromise is the same regardless of the cause. When caring for cases of respiratory compromise, perform the following steps (Figure 14.5):

1. Take appropriate BSI precautions.
2. Perform a primary assessment and support the ABCs as necessary.
3. Ensure a patent airway. Administer oxygen per local protocols.
4. Allow the patient to maintain a position of comfort.
5. Arrange for ALS response if available.
6. Assist with prescribed medication per local protocols and medical direction. (See Appendix 2.)
7. Obtain vital signs.
8. Continue to monitor the patient and provide reassurance.

Positive Pressure Ventilations

When the normal breathing rate for a patient becomes too slow or too shallow, it may be necessary to provide positive pressure ventilations. Simply applying supplemental oxygen by a mask or cannula will not be enough (Figure 14.6). Use an appropriate bag-mask device to provide rescue breaths when breathing is determined to be inadequate. Place the mask firmly over the patient's face and provide rescue breaths at a rate appropriate for the patient's age.

Figure 14.6 • When breathing is inadequate, provide positive pressure ventilations with a bag-mask device.

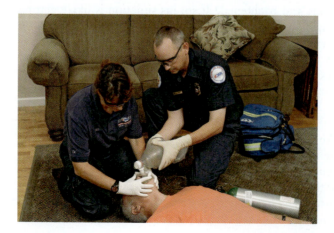

Metered-Dose Inhalers

Patients with a history of respiratory problems usually have been prescribed medication in the form of a metered-dose inhaler (MDI). An MDI is a small device that stores and delivers medication that the patient inhales into the lungs. The patient places his lips around the opening of the device and squeezes the device to deliver one carefully measured "puff," or dose, of medication. Whenever possible, encourage the patient to take his medication exactly as prescribed by his doctor. Like all medications, MDIs have an expiration date. Prior to allowing the patient to self-administer her medication, check the expiration date to ensure that it has not expired. It is not recommended that you allow the patient to self-administer any medication that has expired. More information regarding metered-dose inhalers can be found in Appendix 2.

IS IT SAFE?

It is not advisable to allow a patient to administer any medication that has expired. If you encounter a medication that has expired, ask the patient if he has another MDI available. In many cases, patients have more than one MDI available to them.

WRAP-UP

FIRST ON SCENE

"She won't need transport," the EMS crew says after assessing Karyn. She sits on the grass, holding the mask close to her face, her breathing quickly returning to normal. "Her breathing rate is about 18 now, and her pulse rate and blood pressure have returned to normal. She's been advised not to go on any more coasters today."

"That's good. I wasn't sure if I could get her to catch her breath before she passed out altogether."

"You did fine, Scott," the medic assures, "and anyway, her friends said they watched the medical drama Grey's Anatomy last night on television and were ready to save Karyn if you couldn't."

Scott laughs, "That's reassuring. Now I can breathe easier myself."

CHAPTER REVIEW

Summary

- Respiratory compromise (difficulty breathing) is one of the most common calls you will encounter as an Emergency Medical Responder.

- There are many causes of respiratory compromise including asthma, bronchitis, emphysema, and hyperventilation.

- Respiratory distress is the body's normal response to an inadequate supply of oxygen and is characterized by increased work of breathing, increased breathing rate, and the use of accessory muscles.

- If left untreated, respiratory distress can lead to respiratory failure and eventually respiratory arrest and death.

- Common causes of respiratory compromise include asthma, bronchitis, emphysema, and hyperventilation.

- Asthma is a disease of the lower airways characterized by spasm and swelling of the bronchioles, resulting in the narrowing of the airways. Asthma can be triggered by many things, such as allergies, dust, stress, and exercise.

- Bronchitis is an inflammation of the bronchi and bronchioles and results in an overproduction of mucus over the inside lining of the airways. In some cases it is chronic and may last for months at a time. Bronchitis is also characterized by a productive cough.

- Emphysema causes a loss of elasticity of the lung tissue as well as destruction of the alveoli. The result is poor gas exchange and a trapping of excess carbon dioxide within the lungs. Emphysema is a slow, progressive disease that results in severe respiratory distress.

- Hyperventilation syndrome is most often associated with situations of high stress or anxiety. It begins when the stress of a situation causes the patient to begin breathing fast. If not controlled, it will result in a loss of too much carbon dioxide, and other signs and symptoms will appear. It usually can be treated by helping the patient calm down and control breathing.

- Care for respiratory compromise is the same regardless of the cause. It includes support of the ABCs, providing supplemental oxygen, and calming and reassuring the patient.

- Allow the patient to maintain a position of comfort and do not force the patient to lie down unless he becomes unresponsive.

- Respiratory compromise is often a true emergency, and rapid transport by an ALS ambulance is often the most appropriate care.

- If available, encourage the patient to self-administer his prescribed meter-dose inhaler exactly as the doctor has prescribed.

Take Action

SNEEK A PEEK

Being able to observe a patient from a distance and quickly make an assessment of his breathing status is an important skill that all experienced Emergency Medical Responders should have. It can be a bit challenging, so for this activity, practice assessing the respiratory status of people around you, without their ever knowing.

You can begin right at home. While you and others are sitting around quietly watching television, pick someone and try to count his or her respirations. Remember, one inspiration plus one expiration equals one respiration. Continue to count the respirations for everyone in the room, getting their minute rate each time.

You also can do this for people who are asleep. You will soon notice that the tidal volume for your subjects may appear shallow. This is quite normal for most people, so you will have to adjust your definition of *shallow* to something less than what you observe in normal people.

First on Scene Run Review

Recall the events of the "First on Scene" scenario in this chapter and answer the following questions, which are related to the call. Rationales are offered in the Answer Key at the back of the book.

1. Did Scott ask all the proper questions to find out the problem? Why or why not?

2. How would you treat this patient if she were hyperventilating?

3. Should Scott have called an ambulance? Why or why not?

Quick Quiz

To check your understanding of the chapter, answer the following questions. Then compare your answers to those in the Answer Key at the back of the book.

1. You are caring for a patient with difficulty breathing. She states that she has a history of asthma. You understand asthma to be a disease of the:

   a. upper airway.
   b. lower airway.
   c. alveoli.
   d. trachea.

2. The respiratory control center located deep within the brain primarily monitors the level of _____ to maintain proper respiratory rate and volume.

   a. carbon dioxide
   b. carbon monoxide
   c. oxygen
   d. glucose

3. Your patient has been in respiratory distress for approximately 30 minutes. Your assessment reveals pale skin and cyanosis of the nail beds. These are signs of:

   a. respiratory failure.
   b. asthma.
   c. hypoxia.
   d. respiratory arrest.

4. You are caring for a patient complaining of shortness of breath. Her respiratory rate is 24 with good tidal volume. Following the primary assessment, you should:

   a. provide supplemental oxygen.
   b. take a set of vital signs.
   c. perform a rapid secondary assessment.
   d. place her in the recovery position.

5. You are caring for a 17-year-old female who began experiencing difficulty breathing during a soccer practice. You find her on her knees in the tripod position with a respiratory rate of 24 and shallow. She has taken two puffs from her inhaler with no relief. Her condition is most likely caused by:

   a. bronchitis.
   b. asthma.
   c. emphysema.
   d. hyperventilation.

6. You are caring for a patient with a history of chronic bronchitis. He is sitting upright in a chair and in obvious distress. His respirations are 26 and shallow, and he is still able to speak in full sentences. The ABCs are intact. You should:

   a. place him in the recovery position.
   b. suction his airway.
   c. perform a secondary assessment.
   d. provide supplemental oxygen.

7. Which medical condition listed below causes inflammation of the bronchioles and excess mucus production within the airways? It is also characterized by a productive cough.

   a. Asthma
   b. Bronchitis
   c. Emphysema
   d. Hyperventilation

8. You have been dispatched to a call for respiratory distress and find a 67-year-old male in severe distress. He has a history of emphysema and is on home oxygen at 2 Lpm by cannula. His respirations are 32, and he is unable to speak more than two or three words at a time. His airway is clear. You should:

   a. increase the home oxygen to 6 Lpm.
   b. place him on a nonrebreather mask at 15 Lpm.
   c. provide positive pressure ventilations.
   d. remove the home oxygen.

9. You are caring for a 22-year-old female with difficulty breathing. She has no prior medical history and states that she began having trouble breathing following an argument with her boyfriend. She states that her fingers are numb and tingly. You should:

   a. provide low-flow oxygen and attempt to calm her down.
   b. provide high-flow oxygen and transport.
   c. not provide oxygen and transport.
   d. massage her hands and fingers while calming her down.

10. Which one of the medical conditions listed below results in the loss of elasticity of the lungs and the retention of carbon dioxide?

    a. Asthma
    b. Bronchitis
    c. Emphysema
    d. Hyperventilation

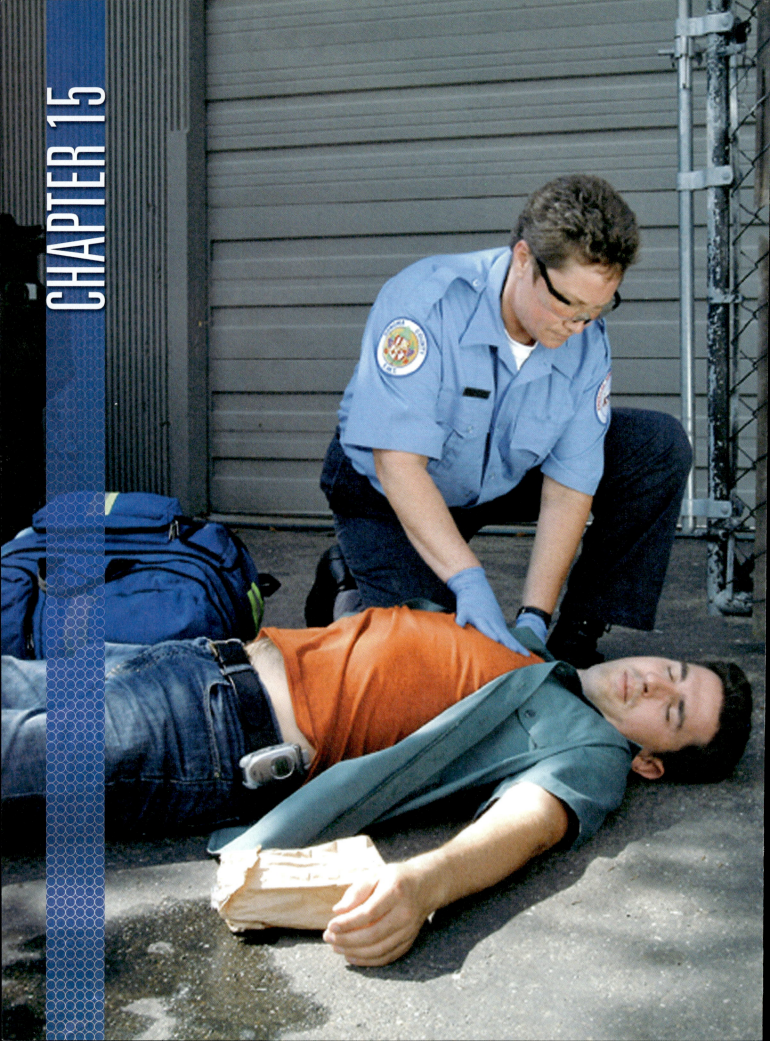

CHAPTER 15

Caring for Common Medical Emergencies

EDUCATION STANDARDS

- Medicine—Neurology, Immunology, Endocrine Disorders, Psychiatric, Toxicology, Genitourinary/Renal

COMPETENCIES

- Recognizes and manages life threats based on assessment findings of a patient with a medical emergency while awaiting additional emergency response.

CHAPTER OVERVIEW

All patient emergencies can be categorized one of two ways: medical or trauma. Emergencies that result in injury, such as from a fall or a vehicle crash, are categorized as trauma. However, this chapter focuses on the illnesses and conditions that can affect the body. Those illnesses and conditions are known as medical emergencies. You must be prepared to provide appropriate emergency care to the various medical patients you encounter. While some situations require you to intervene with specific skills, others will be referred to as common medical complaints.

This chapter provides an overview of several common medical emergencies, such as altered mental status, stroke, seizures, diabetes, poisoning, and overdose. It also addresses the appropriate emergency care for those emergencies.

Upon successful completion of this chapter, the student should be able to:

COGNITIVE

1. Define the following terms:
   a. altered mental status (p. 307)
   b. behavioral emergency (p. 326)
   c. convulsions (p. 310)
   d. diabetes (p. 314)
   e. epilepsy (p. 310)
   f. febrile (p. 311)
   g. generalized seizure (p. 310)
   h. hemodialysis (p. 325)
   i. hyperglycemia (p. 314)
   j. hypoglycemia (p. 316)
   k. overdose (p. 316)
   l. partial seizure (p. 310)
   m. postictal (p. 311)
   n. sepsis (p. 324)
   o. stroke (brain attack) (p. 311)
2. Explain the common causes of altered mental status. (p. 307)
3. Describe the signs and symptoms of a patient with an altered mental status. (p. 309)

4. Explain the appropriate assessment and care for a patient with an altered mental status. (p. 309)
5. Describe the signs and symptoms of a patient experiencing a generalized seizure. (p. 310)
6. Explain the appropriate assessment and care for a patient experiencing a generalized seizure. (p. 311)
7. Describe the signs and symptoms of a patient experiencing a stroke (brain attack). (p. 311)
8. Explain the appropriate assessment and care for a patient experiencing a stroke (brain attack). (p. 313)
9. Describe the signs and symptoms of a patient experiencing a diabetic emergency. (p. 314)
10. Differentiate between the signs and symptoms of hyperglycemia and hypoglycemia. (p. 314)
11. Explain the appropriate assessment and care for a patient experiencing a diabetic emergency. (p. 315)
12. Describe the signs and symptoms of a patient experiencing an overdose or poisoning. (p. 317)
13. Describe the signs and symptoms of a patient experiencing carbon monoxide poisoning. (p. 320)
14. Explain the appropriate assessment and care for a patient experiencing an overdose or poisoning. (p. 317)
15. State when it is most appropriate to contact the poison control center. (p. 317)
16. Describe the signs and symptoms of a patient experiencing an emergency related to renal failure. (p. 325)

OBJECTIVES

17. Explain the special considerations when caring for a hemodialysis patient. *(p. 326)*

18. Describe the signs and symptoms of a patient experiencing a generalized infection (sepsis). *(p. 324)*

19. Explain the appropriate assessment and care for a patient experiencing a generalized infection (sepsis). *(p. 324)*

20. Describe the signs and symptoms of an allergic reaction. *(p. 325)*

21. Explain the appropriate assessment and care for a patient experiencing a severe allergic reaction. *(p. 325)*

22. Describe the signs and symptoms of a patient experiencing a suspected behavioral emergency. *(p. 326)*

23. Explain the appropriate assessment and care for a patient experiencing a suspected behavioral emergency. *(p. 326)*

PSYCHOMOTOR

24. Demonstrate the ability to appropriately assess and care for a patient experiencing an altered mental status.

AFFECTIVE

25. Value the significance of an altered mental status as a sign of an unstable patient.

FIRST ON SCENE

"Jordan! Jordan, will you wake up!" Jordan Garibaldi shoots up in his bed and quickly looks around the dorm room. Nothing seems out of place. His vacationing roommate's movie posters still hang at odd angles from multicolored pushpins. Clothing and books are still scattered around in piles. The filter on the little octagon-shaped goldfish tank is still humming away, even though the fish are long gone. Just as he was starting to lie back down, someone pounds on the door, rattling it with each booming impact.

"Jordan! Are you in there?" Jordan slides out of bed and stomps across the room to the door.

"What?" he shouts as he pulls the door open. The look on that new freshman Kaden Kline's face tells him immediately that something really is wrong.

"There's this girl down in our room." Kaden is wide-eyed and whispering hoarsely. "And she's like, like having some sort of, I think she's dying or something!" Jordan, the dorm "doctor" ever since completing an Emergency Medical Responder course, quickly grabs a robe and throws it on as he runs down the hall.

Medical Emergencies

Patients may request EMS for a variety of medical complaints. *Medical emergencies* may be caused by infections, poisons, or the failure of one or more of the body's organ systems. You must assess each patient and determine the chief complaint as well as any signs and symptoms that might be present. The patient or a bystander may be able to tell you of an existing disease or condition. However, in most cases, what you observe and what the patient describes will be your main clues to the patient's problems.

A patient's medical emergency may be hidden because of an injury. For example, a diabetic patient may collapse because of very low blood sugar or may be involved in a vehicle crash and become injured. As an Emergency Medical Responder, your primary job will be to provide care for the patient's most obvious problem, in this case his injuries. The medical problem, however, should not go unnoticed. During your assessment of a trauma patient, keep in mind that there also may be an underlying medical problem.

Signs and Symptoms of a General Medical Complaint

To detect a medical emergency, you have to be aware of common signs and symptoms, such as:

- Altered mental status
- Abnormal pulse rate and rhythm

- Abnormal breathing rate and character
- Abnormal skin signs
- Abnormal pupil size or response
- Unusual breath odors
- Tenderness or rigidity in the abdomen
- Abnormal muscular activity such as spasms or paralysis
- Bleeding or discharges from the body

A patient may complain of some of the following symptoms:

- Pain
- Shortness of breath
- Fever or chills
- Upset stomach and/or vomiting
- Dizziness or feeling faint
- Chest or abdominal pain
- Unusual bowel or bladder activity
- Thirst, hunger, or odd tastes in the mouth

Assessment

Emergency care for medical emergencies is based on the patient's signs and symptoms. That is why it is so important to complete an appropriate patient assessment. For general medical complaints, you should:

1. Take appropriate BSI precautions and complete a scene size-up before you begin emergency medical care.
2. Perform a primary assessment.
3. Perform a secondary assessment, including patient history and physical exam.
4. Complete appropriate reassessments.
5. Comfort and reassure the patient while awaiting additional EMS resources.

When assessing the patient, keep in mind the following: If the patient appears or feels unusual in any way, suspect that there is a medical emergency. If the patient has abnormal vital signs, conclude that there is a medical emergency.

Altered Mental Status

As an Emergency Medical Responder, altered mental status is one of the most common complaints that you will respond to. For this reason it is important that you are familiar with the basic causes of, as well as the assessment and care for, a patient with an altered mental status. Although there are many potential causes for altered mental status, remember that regardless of the cause, your assessment and emergency care will follow the same basic steps.

Evaluating Mental Status

A normal mental status is characterized by a complete and accurate awareness of one's surroundings. For instance, at any point in time, a person with a normal mental status would be aware of who they are, (person) where they are (place), the day and time (time), and the events going on around them (events). When alert and oriented to all four elements, a person is said to be alert and oriented times four, or simply "A & O × 4." A person who can tell you who he is and where he is but is unsure of the time, day, or events is described as "A & O × 2."

An **altered mental status (AMS)** is characterized by a decrease in the patient's alertness and responsiveness to his surroundings. Several conditions can cause a patient to

altered mental status ▶ a state characterized by a decrease in the patient's alertness and responsiveness to his surroundings.

OBJECTIVE

2. Explain the common causes of altered mental status.

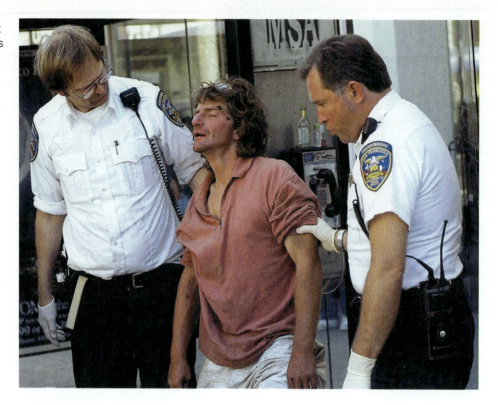

Figure 15.1 • Often a patient with an altered mental status is not aware of his surroundings.

experience an altered mental status, including trauma to the head (Figure 15.1). Other common causes of an altered mental status are (Figure 15.2):

- Seizures
- Stroke (brain attack)
- Diabetic emergencies
- Poisonings and overdose
- Hypoxia
- Shock
- Infection

Figure 15.2 • Common causes of an altered mental status.

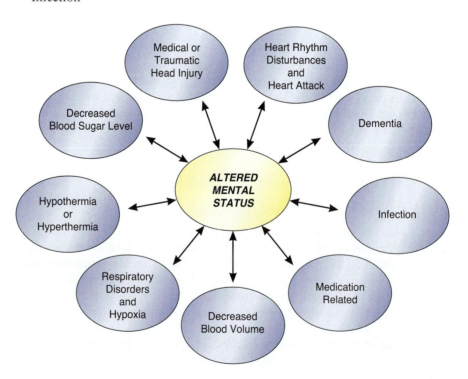

- Trauma
- Psychiatric condition
- Liver failure

Before you can begin to evaluate a person's mental status and determine if it is altered, you need to understand his normal mental status, also referred to as his baseline mental status. Many people with chronic illnesses may have an altered mental status normally. You must rely on family, friends, and caregivers to provide you with a description of the person's normal mental status. They will usually be able to tell you if the person appears altered or if his status is normal for him.

> ▶ **GERIATRIC FOCUS** ◀

An elderly patient with dementia may not fully comprehend the seriousness of his situation and may not want you to provide care. In other words, the elderly patient with dementia may not be competent to make decisions about his own medical care. When presented with an elderly patient who is showing signs of disorientation, a short attention span, confusion, or hallucinations, obtain a detailed history from family members or caregivers. It will be important to determine if his mental status is normal for him or if it has gotten worse. Do not allow a patient who is showing signs of dementia to refuse care without further investigation into his normal state of mind.

Signs and Symptoms of Altered Mental Status

Some of the most common signs and symptoms of altered mental status include:

- Confusion
- Seizures
- Inappropriate behavior (verbal, physical)
- Lack of awareness of surroundings
- Combativeness
- Syncope (collapse or fainting)
- Unresponsiveness (Figure 15.3)

OBJECTIVE

3. Describe the signs and symptoms of a patient with an altered mental status.

Assessing the Patient with an Altered Mental Status

The assessment of patients with an altered mental status should be focused on observation and obtaining as complete a medical history as possible. This is where having a basic understanding of the common causes of altered mental status becomes important. As you examine the patient's surroundings and communicate with both the patient and any family members, friends, or caregivers, you usually will be able to determine whether the patient's condition is being caused by a medical issue (diabetes, stroke, poisoning, etc.) or a trauma-related issue such as a head injury. One tool that is used to categorize the mental status of patients is called the AVPU scale. It provides for four general categories for a patient's mental status: alert, verbal, painful, and unresponsive (Table 15.1).

OBJECTIVE

4. Explain the appropriate assessment and care for a patient with an altered mental status.

The more altered a patient appears, the more aggressive your care may need to be. For instance, if a patient is unresponsive, he will not be able to manage his own airway very well. In this case you will need to monitor and manage his airway and be alert for vomiting. If the patient is behaving violently, you must ensure your safety and call for additional resources such as law enforcement.

General guidelines for the emergency care of the patient with an altered mental are as follows:

1. Take BSI precautions and perform a primary assessment.

2. Monitor the patient's airway and breathing.

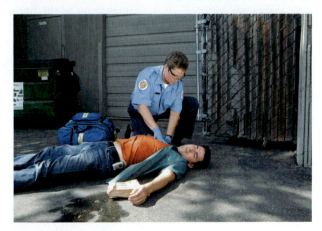

Figure 15.3 • Some cases of altered mental status can be caused by traumatic injury.

TABLE 15.1 | The AVPU Scale

Patient is awake and aware of his surroundings. Often, it is stated that a patient is alert and oriented times four (A & O × 4), which means the patient is:

A—Alert	A & O × 1 to person—He can tell you his name.
	A & O × 2 to place—He also can tell you where he is.
	A & O × 3 to time—He also can tell you exactly or approximately what time it is.
	A & O × 4 to event—He also can tell you about the event.
V—Verbal	Patient responds only to verbal stimuli (yelling or raised voice).
P—Painful	Patient responds only to painful stimuli.
U—Unresponsive	Patient does not respond to any stimuli.

3. Administer oxygen as per local protocols.

4. Monitor vital signs

5. Provide emotional support.

6. Position the patient properly for comfort and protection.

7. Do not administer anything by mouth.

8. Continue to monitor the patient while awaiting EMS arrival.

OBJECTIVE

5. Describe the signs and symptoms of a patient experiencing a generalized seizure.

convulsions ▶ uncontrolled muscular contractions.

generalized seizure ▶ a type of seizure characterized by a loss of consciousness and full-body muscle contractions.

partial seizure ▶ a seizure characterized by a temporary loss of awareness with no dramatic body movements.

epilepsy ▶ a disorder of the brain that causes seizures.

Seizures

Irregular electrical activity in the brain that can cause a sudden change in mental status and behavior is called a *seizure*. Seizures can cause both a change in mental status and uncontrolled muscular movements known as **convulsions** (Figure 15.4). When a seizure causes the entire body to convulse, it is referred to as a **generalized seizure**. Other seizures characterized by a temporary loss of awareness with no dramatic body movements are known as **partial seizures**. Older terms, still in use, are *grand mal* for the generalized seizure and *petit mal* for the partial seizure.

Seizures can be frightening for a patient's family, friends, and others to witness. Even though most seizures last less than a minute, it can seem much longer to a bystander. Talk to witnesses to determine what the patient was doing prior to the seizure and whether this has happened in the past. Although some people have seizures on a regular basis, anyone experiencing a seizure should be evaluated by someone with advanced medical training. Approximately 250,000 people in the United States have some form of epilepsy. **Epilepsy** is a disorder of the brain that causes seizures.

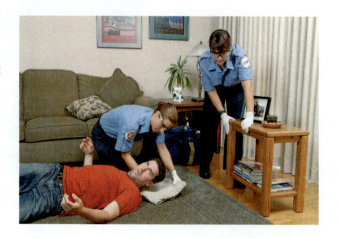

Figure 15.4 • Protect the patient from injury by removing objects that he may strike and by placing something soft beneath his head.

A seizure is not a disease but a sign of an underlying condition. The following are some of the common causes of seizures:

- Epilepsy
- Ingestion of drugs, alcohol, or poisons
- Alcohol withdrawal
- Brain tumors
- Infections, high fever (called **febrile** seizures)
- Diabetic problems
- Stroke
- Heat stroke
- Head injury

In cases of generalized seizure, any or all of the following may be present:

- Sudden loss of responsiveness
- Patient may report bright light, bright colors, or the sensation of a strong odor prior to losing responsiveness
- Convulsions
- Loss of bladder and/or bowel control
- Labored breathing, and there may be frothing at the mouth
- Patient may complain of a headache prior to or following a seizure
- Following the seizure, the patient's body completely relaxes

Basic care for a generalized seizure includes:

1. Take BSI precautions and perform a primary assessment.
2. Protect the patient from further injury. Move objects away from the patient and place something soft under his head if necessary.
3. Do not attempt to restrain the patient or force anything into his mouth.
4. Loosen restrictive clothing.
5. After convulsions have stopped, place the patient in the recovery position.
6. Administer oxygen as per local protocols.

Protect the patient from embarrassment by asking onlookers to step away and give the patient some privacy. Patients with a history of seizures will often refuse care once they regain consciousness. If they refuse care, suggest that they contact a friend or family member so they can be observed following the seizure. After a seizure, the patient will generally feel tired and weak and may not be fully alert. This is called the **postictal** stage of a seizure. Talk to the patient and provide reassurance as he gradually becomes more responsive. Provide emotional support to the patient and family members until additional medical help arrives.

Stroke

One potentially serious cause of altered mental status is a **stroke**, or cerebrovascular accident (CVA), also known as "brain attack." A stroke occurs when blood flow to the brain is disrupted. Common causes of stroke include an obstruction of a blood vessel or ruptured blood vessel. During a stroke, a portion of the brain does not receive an adequate supply of oxygenated blood and brain cells begin to die. In some cases, this damage is so great that it may lead to death (Scan 15.1).

Some of the common signs and symptoms of stroke include:

- Headache
- Syncope (fainting)
- Altered mental status
- Numbness or paralysis, usually to the extremities or to the face
- Difficulty with speech or vision
- Confusion, dizziness

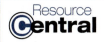

CAUSES OF CEREBROVASCULAR ACCIDENTS: STROKE

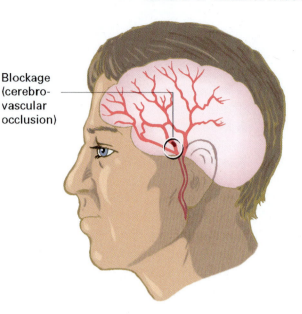

Blockage (cerebro-vascular occlusion)

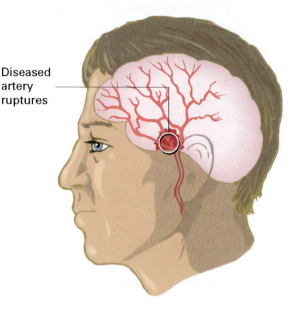

Diseased artery ruptures

Cerebral Thrombosis (Clot)

Blockage in arteries supplying oxygenated blood will result in damage to affected parts of the brain.

Cerebral Hemorrhage (Rupture)

An aneurysm or other weakened area of an artery ruptures. This has two effects:
* An area of the brain is deprived of oxygenated blood.
* Pooling blood puts increased pressure on the brain, displacing tissue and interfering with function. Cerebral hemorrhage is often associated with arteriosclerosis and hypertension.

Signs and Symptoms of Stroke

* Headache
* Confusion and/or dizziness
* Loss of function or paralysis of extremities (usually on one side of the body)
* Numbness (usually limited to one side of the body)
* Collapse
* Facial paralysis and loss of expression (often to one side of the face)
* Impaired speech
* Unequal pupil size
* Impaired vision

* Rapid or slow pulse
* Abnormal respirations
* Nausea, vomiting
* Convulsions
* Loss of bladder and bowel control
* High blood pressure (may have history of hypertension)

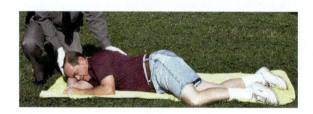

Emergency Care of Stroke Patients

* Ensure an open airway.
* Administer oxygen per local protocols.
* Keep the patient calm.
* Monitor vital signs.
* Give nothing by mouth.
* Provide care for shock.
* Place the patient into the recovery position on affected side to protect extremities.

* Seizures
* Altered breathing patterns
* Unequal pupils
* Altered vision
* Weakness typically to one side of the body
* Loss of bowel and bladder control
* High blood pressure

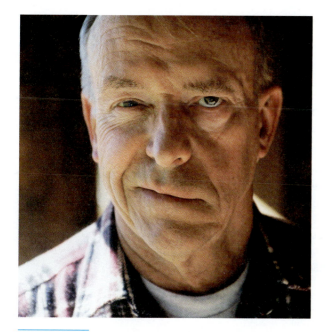

Figure 15.5 • A patient suffering a stroke may have facial droop on one side or the other.

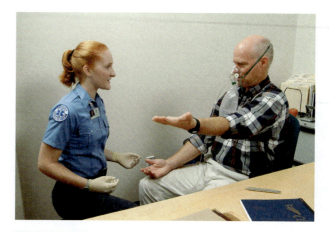

Figure 15.6 • An inability to hold both arms up may be a sign of possible stroke.

There are several assessment tools that can be helpful when responding to a responsive patient suspected of having a stroke. One of the most common of those tools is the Cincinnati Prehospital Stroke Scale (CPSS). The CPSS uses three assessment characteristics to evaluate for the likelihood of a stroke:

- *Facial droop.* Have the patient look directly at you and smile or show his teeth. Observe if the facial muscles do not move symmetrically or if there is facial droop on one side or the other (Figure 15.5).
- *Arm drift.* Have the patient hold both arms straight out in front of him and close his eyes. Observe for arm drift, one arm that drops down while the other remains up. It is also significant if the patient cannot bring both arms up together (Figure 15.6).
- *Abnormal speech.* Observe for slurred speech, inappropriate words, or an inability to respond verbally.

Presence of an abnormality in any one of the three areas of the CPSS indicates a strong likelihood of a stroke.

When providing emergency care for a possible stroke patient, you should:

1. Take BSI precautions and perform a primary assessment.
2. Maintain an open airway. Be prepared to provide ventilations or CPR if needed.
3. Administer oxygen as per local protocols.
4. Keep the patient at rest, and protect all paralyzed parts.
5. Provide emotional support.
6. Place the patient in the recovery position.
7. Do not administer anything by mouth.
8. Continue to monitor the airway and vital signs until EMS arrives.

Prompt recognition is important when dealing with patients exhibiting the signs and symptoms of stroke. There are specific medications that can be given to stroke patients. If they are given soon enough, they can greatly decrease the long-term effects of the stroke. Those medications are called thrombolytics and are most commonly given in the hospital setting. Because of the importance of prompt delivery of the medications, some EMS systems are allowing them to be delivered by paramedics in the field setting.

OBJECTIVE

8. Explain the appropriate assessment and care for a patient experiencing a stroke (brain attack).

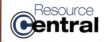

Learn more about how to assess stokes and stroke prevention.

The girl, a teen too young to be a student at the college, is convulsing on the dorm room's dirty carpet. Her arms and legs are pulling and pushing slowly in all directions, her back arched severely, and her head snapping rhythmically from side to side, sending foamy splatters of saliva back and forth on the carpet.

"What did you guys give her?" Jordan demands of the small group of terrified young men.

"Nothing!" Kaden shouts, holding his palms out in an unconscious effort to show that he didn't possess anything that would have had this effect on the girl. "We were just drinking some beer and playing video games! We didn't do anything!"

Jordan looks down at the girl and sees that her lips are now bluish and her breathing is coming in hitches and gasps as she convulses. "How long has she been like this?" he asks.

"Since just before I knocked on your door." Kaden keeps looking from the girl to his friends and then back to Jordan. "Just a couple of minutes."

Jordan suddenly feels useless. The freshmen had the sense to pull furniture away so the girl wouldn't crash into anything, and one of them put a sweatshirt under her head, but as long as she is seizing, there is nothing he can do.

"Kaden," Jordan says, pointing to the cowering young man. "Bring me a phone right now. She needs an ambulance, and I have to let campus security know what's going on."

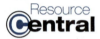

Learn more about diabetes.

diabetes ▶ usually refers to diabetes mellitus, a disease that prevents individuals from producing enough insulin or from using insulin appropriately.

hyperglycemia ▶ an abnormally high blood-sugar level.

OBJECTIVES

9. Describe the signs and symptoms of a patient experiencing a diabetic emergency.

10. Differentiate between the signs and symptoms of hyperglycemia and hypoglycemia.

Diabetic Emergencies

Glucose, a form of simple sugar, is the main source of energy for the body's cells. It is carried to the cells by way of the bloodstream. However, to enter the cells, *insulin*, a hormone secreted by the pancreas, must be present. Insulin allows glucose to enter the cells so the glucose can be used effectively.

Diabetes is a disease that prevents individuals from producing enough insulin or from using insulin effectively. Although some patients can manage their condition with a balanced diet, others require the administration of oral medications, or in severe cases, the patient must inject himself with insulin (Scan 15.2).

Hyperglycemia

High blood sugar, or **hyperglycemia**, is usually a gradual event, taking many hours to several days to develop. It can occur when the patient eats normally but fails to take a normal dose of insulin or eats too much for the amount of insulin being taken.

The onset of signs and symptoms will be gradual. If left untreated, hyperglycemia can lead to unresponsiveness and a condition known as diabetic coma.

The signs and symptoms of hyperglycemia include:

- Extreme thirst
- Abdominal pain
- Dry, warm skin, although sometimes the skin may become reddened
- Rapid, weak pulse
- Sweet or fruity odor on the patient's breath, which is called *ketone breath*; ketones smell like acetone, the same compound found in fingernail-polish remover
- Dry mouth
- Restlessness
- Altered mental status, including coma

▶ GERIATRIC FOCUS ◀

The elderly patient with diabetes is usually taking pills to control his blood sugar and also may be taking insulin. While you may administer glucose, his blood sugar might drop again, sometimes many hours later because the pills he takes are long lasting. For this reason it is generally advised that all elderly diabetic events result in transport to the hospital.

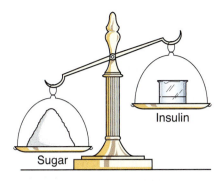

Hyperglycemia

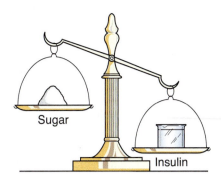

Hypoglycemia

Hyperglycemia
Causes

- Diabetic condition has not been diagnosed or treated.
- Diabetic has not taken his insulin.
- Diabetic has overeaten, taking in more food than the supply of insulin can manage.
- Diabetic suffers an infection or other stress that disrupts his glucose/insulin balance.

Signs and Symptoms

- Gradual onset of signs and symptoms over hours or days.
- Patient complains of dry mouth and intense thirst.
- Abdominal pain and vomiting.
- Gradually increasing restlessness and confusion.
- Unresponsiveness with these signs: deep, sighing respirations; weak, rapid pulse; dry, red, warm skin; eyes that appear sunken; breath smells of acetone—sickly sweet, similar to nail polish remover.

Emergency Care

- Monitor ABCs.
- Provide oxygen per local protocols.

Hypoglycemia (Insulin Shock)
Causes

- Diabetic has taken too much insulin.
- Diabetic has not eaten enough to provide her normal sugar intake.
- Diabetic has overexercised or overexerted herself, reducing her blood glucose level.
- Diabetic has vomited following a meal.

Signs and Symptoms

- Rapid onset of signs and symptoms
- Dizziness and headache
- Altered mental status
- Aggressive behavior
- Fainting, convulsions, and occasionally coma
- Rapid weak pulse
- Hunger, drooling
- Pale, cold, clammy skin with profuse perspiration

Emergency Care

- For a responsive patient with a gag reflex, administer oral glucose or a substitute such as honey, candy, soft drink, or orange juice.
- For an unresponsive patient, place in the recovery position, administer oxygen per local protocols, and consider oral glucose per local protocols and medical direction

When faced with a patient who may be suffering from either hyperglycemia or hypoglycemia:

- Determine if the patient is diabetic. Look for a medical identification device or information cards. Interview patient and family members.
- If the patient is a known or suspected diabetic, and hypoglycemia (insulin shock) cannot be ruled out, conclude that it is possible hypoglycemia and administer glucose.

Often, a patient suffering from those conditions may appear drunk. Always check for underlying conditions—such as diabetic complications—when caring for someone who appears to be intoxicated.

Emergency care for hyperglycemia consists of the following:

1. Take BSI precautions and perform a primary assessment.
2. Maintain an open airway and ensure adequate breathing.
3. Administer oxygen per local protocols.
4. Keep the patient at rest. If the patient is alert, try to gain additional information through a secondary assessment. Ask if the patient is diabetic. Find out if the patient has taken insulin and has eaten recently.

OBJECTIVE

11. Explain the appropriate assessment and care for a patient experiencing a diabetic emergency.

5. If the patient is alert and you are not certain if the problem is too much sugar (hyperglycemia) or too little sugar (hypoglycemia), give the patient sugar, candy, orange juice, or a soft drink. Make certain that the patient can swallow without difficulty before giving anything by mouth. Ensure that the substance you give contains real sugar, not an artificial sweetener. Some jurisdictions may allow Emergency Medical Responders to give oral glucose. Check local protocols and always call for medical direction before assisting a patient with medications.

Hypoglycemia

The diabetic who has taken too much insulin, eaten too little sugar, overexerted himself, or experienced excessive emotional stress or any combination of these may develop **hypoglycemia** (low blood sugar). Hypoglycemia usually comes on quickly over a period of several minutes or more slowly over a few hours.

Signs and symptoms of hypoglycemia include:

hypoglycemia ▶ an abnormally low blood-sugar level.

- Altered mental status
- Pale, cool skin; often it is moist as well
- Rapid, strong pulse
- Dizziness
- Headache
- Normal or shallow breathing
- Very hungry
- Some patients will develop seizures if they do not receive early care.

Emergency care for hypoglycemia consists of the following:

1. Take BSI precautions and perform a primary assessment.

2. Maintain an open airway and provide ventilations as necessary.

3. If the patient is alert, provide oral glucose or a suitable substitute.

4. Keep the patient comfortable and administer oxygen per local protocols.

FIRST ON SCENE

continued

As Jordan hangs up the cell phone and tosses it onto the dorm's old brown couch, he turns to Kaden. "Go down to the grass common in front of the building and wait for the ambulance."

As the young man runs from the room, obviously happy to get out, the girl's seizure tapers off and then stops altogether. She is still unconscious but is now snoring loudly. Jordan squats next to her, not wanting to kneel in the pools of saliva, and gently opens her airway by placing one hand on her cool, moist forehead and the other under her jaw. The girl's snoring immediately stops and her lips fade from blue to the same paleness as the rest of her face.

With the help of two of the remaining freshmen, Jordan is able to roll the girl into the recovery position. It is then that he notices something glimmering inside the collar of her denim jacket. He reaches into it and pulls out a MedicAlert necklace indicating that the girl is an insulin-dependent diabetic.

Overdose and Poisoning

Any substance that can be harmful to the body is known as a *poison*. There are more than 2 million incidents of poisoning reported annually in the United States. An **overdose** occurs when a person takes in more of a medication than is normal. This can happen either intentionally or by accident.

overdose ▶ an incident that occurs when a person takes in more of a medication than is normal.

Routes of Exposure

We usually think of a poison as a liquid or solid chemical that has been ingested (swallowed), but there are actually four routes of exposure, or ways that a substance can enter the body. They are *ingestion*, *inhalation*, *absorption*, and *injection*. The following is a description of each:

- *Ingestion.* Substances taken into the body by way of the mouth are said to be ingested. Ingested poisons include various household and industrial chemicals, improperly prepared foods, plant materials, petroleum products, medications (particularly if taken in improper doses), and poisons made specifically to control rodents, insects, and crop diseases.
- *Inhalation.* Substances taken in by breathing are said to be inhaled. Inhaled poisons take the form of gases, vapors, and sprays, including carbon monoxide (from car exhaust, kerosene heaters, and wood-burning stoves), ammonia, chlorine, volatile liquid chemicals (including many industrial solvents), and insect sprays.
- *Absorption.* Substances taken into the body through the skin and body tissues are said to be absorbed. Many such poisons damage the skin and then are slowly absorbed into the bloodstream. Some insecticides, agricultural chemicals, and corrosive chemicals may damage the skin and then are absorbed by the body. A wide variety of plant materials and certain forms of marine life can cause allergic reactions and/or damage to the skin, with the poison (toxin) being absorbed into the underlying tissues.
- *Injection.* Substances delivered directly into the bloodstream are said to be injected. Insects, spiders, snakes, and certain marine life are able to inject poisons into the body. Injection also may be self-induced by a hypodermic needle. Unusual industrial accidents producing cuts or puncture wounds also can be a source of injected poisons.

Table 15.2 lists some of the types of poisons that could require emergency care.

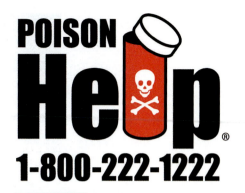

Figure 15.7 • The American Association of Poison Control Centers maintains an easy to remember 800 number.

Poison Control Centers

There are over 60 regional poison control centers in the United States, most of which are staffed 24 hours a day. The staff at each center is trained to advise you on what should be done for most cases of poisoning. There are several ways the Emergency Medical Responder can access a poison control center. The first is by calling the national poison control center number at 1-800-222-1222 (Figure 15.7). Another way is by contacting the EMS dispatcher who, in most cases, can put you in direct contact with the poison control center. In this case the dispatcher will typically stay on the line and dispatch the appropriate resources if necessary.

To aid the poison control center or medical direction, note and report any containers at the scene of the emergency. Let them know if the patient has vomited and describe the vomit. (Check the vomit for pill fragments.) When possible, and if it can be done quickly, gather information from the patient or from bystanders before you call the center.

Ingested Poisons

In cases of possible ingested poisoning, you must gather information quickly. If at all possible, do so while you are conducting the primary assessment. Note any containers that

OBJECTIVE

15. State when it is most appropriate to contact the poison control center.

KEY POINT ▼

In your jurisdiction, Emergency Medical Responder care for ingested poisons may include giving the patient activated charcoal. Check local protocols and always call for medical direction before administering activated charcoal.

OBJECTIVES

12. Describe the signs and symptoms of a patient experiencing an overdose or poisoning.

14. Explain the appropriate assessment and care for a patient experiencing an overdose or poisoning.

From the Medical Director

Poison Control

Poison control centers can be a wealth of knowledge and can help you determine the significance of the poisoning, which you can relay to arriving EMS providers. However, do not delay emergent care of the patient to contact poison control. Follow your Medical Director's protocols regarding any poison control center recommendations.

TABLE 15.2 Commonly Abused Substances

UPPERS

Amphetamine (Benzedrine, bennies, pep pills, ups, uppers, cartwheels)	Methamphetamine (speed, meth, crystal, diet pills, Methedrine)
Biphetamine (bam)	Methylphenidate (Ritalin)
Cocaine (coke, snow, crack)	Preludin
Desoxyn (black beauties)	
Dextroamphetamine (dexies, Dexedrine)	

DOWNERS

Amobarbital (blue devils, downers, barbs, Amytal)	Nonbarbiturate sedatives (various tranquilizers and sleeping pills; Valium or diazepam, Miltown, Equanil, meprobamate, Thorazine, Compazine, Librium or chlordiazepoxide, reserpine, Tranxene or clorazepate, and other benzodiazepines)
Barbiturates (downers, dolls, barbs, rainbows)	
Chloral hydrate (knockout drops, Noctec)	
Ethchlorvynol (Placidyl)	
Glutethimide (Doriden, goofers)	
Methaqualone (Quaalude, ludes, Sopor, sopors)	

NARCOTICS

Codeine (often in cough syrup)	Heroin (H, horse, junk, smack, stuff)
Meperidine	Paregoric (contains opium)
Demerol	Methadone (dolly)
Morphine	Fentanyl
Dilaudid	Oxycodone (perc), OxyContin
Opium (op, poppy)	

HALLUCINOGENS AND MIND-ALTERING DRUGS

Hallucinogenics	Nonhallucinogenics
Psilocybin (magic mushrooms)	Mescaline (peyote, mesc)
DMT	Marijuana (grass, pot, weed, dope)
STP (serenity, tranquility, peace)	Morning glory seeds
LSD (acid, sunshine)	Hash
	PCP (angel dust, hog, peace pills)
	THC

VOLATILE CHEMICALS

Amyl nitrate (snappers, poppers)	Nail polish remover
Glue	Furniture polish
Butyl nitrate (locker room, rush)	Paint thinner
Hair spray	Gasoline
Cleaning fluid (carbon tetrachloride)	

may hold poisonous substances (Figure 15.8). See if there is any vomit. Check for any substances on the patient's clothes or if the patient is wearing clothing that indicates the nature of work (farmer, miner, and so on). Can the scene be associated with certain types of poisonings? Question the patient and any bystanders.

The signs and symptoms of ingested poisons can be gathered during the scene size-up and primary assessment. They may include any one or all of the following:

- Burns or stains around the patient's mouth
- Unusual breath odors, body odors, or odors on the patient's clothing or at the scene
- Abnormal breathing
- Abnormal pulse rate and rhythm
- Sweating
- Dilated or constricted pupils
- Excessive saliva formation or foaming at the mouth
- Burning in the mouth or throat or painful swallowing
- Abdominal pain
- Upset stomach or nausea, vomiting, diarrhea
- Convulsions
- Altered mental status, including unresponsiveness

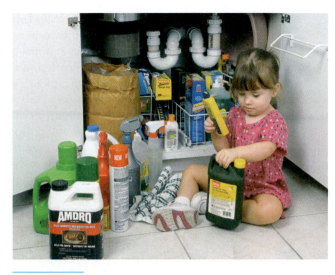

Figure 15.8 • Poisons come in colorful containers that are appealing to children.

Contact your local poison control center to obtain advice on appropriate care for specific poisons. But do not provide any care, other than for the ABCs to ensure control of life-threatening situations, until you have contacted medical direction.

Emergency care directions from a poison control center may consist of diluting the poison or using activated charcoal to absorb the poison. Never attempt to dilute the poison or give activated charcoal if the patient is not fully alert. The patient who is unresponsive may not have an intact gag reflex. Follow your local guidelines and the instructions given by the poison control center.

For responsive patients, emergency care typically includes the following:

1. Take BSI precautions and perform a primary assessment.
2. Ensure an open airway and adequate breathing.
3. Call the poison control center or medical direction for instructions.
4. You may be directed to dilute the poison by having the patient drink one or two glasses of water or milk, or you may be directed to give activated charcoal. Check local protocols, and always call for medical direction before assisting a patient with medications. The poison control center or medical direction may tell you to have the patient consume the fluids in sips to prevent vomiting. Do not give anything by mouth if the patient is having convulsions or is gagging, unless otherwise directed by a physician or the poison control center.
5. Administer oxygen as per local protocols. Assist ventilations as necessary.
6. If supplies are available and you are directed to do so, give activated charcoal. For an adult, give 25 to 50 grams. For a child, give 12.5 to 25 grams.
7. In case of vomiting, position the patient so that no vomit will be aspirated (inhaled). Put him on one side or in a semi-sitting position with the head turned to the side.
8. If possible, save vomit for later analysis by hospital staff.

Inhaled Poisons

Poisons that are inhaled can reach the circulatory system directly through the lungs. Gases, fumes, vapors, and dust are all forms of inhaled poisons. Gather information from the patient and bystanders as quickly as possible. Look for indications of inhaled poisons.

KEY POINT ▼

Providing liquids by mouth to ingested-poisoning patients may be dangerous for some victims. This is especially true if the patient has been convulsing or if the source of the poison is a strong acid, alkali, or petroleum product such as gasoline or diesel fuel. Included in those groups of substances are oven cleaners, drain cleaners, toilet bowl cleaners, lye, ammonia, bleach, and kerosene. Always check for burns around the patient's mouth and for the presence of unusual odors on the patient's breath. Follow the poison control center's instructions.

KEY POINT ▼

In addition to the usual risks, if the patient has ingested a highly concentrated dose of certain poisons, such as arsenic or cyanide, and if deposits remain on the patient's lips, there is a chance the rescuer may be harmed. The current recommendation is to use a pocket face mask with HEPA filter or a bag-mask device on all poisoning patients who need rescue breathing.

Possible sources include automobile exhaust systems, stoves, charcoal grills, industrial solvents, and spray cans.

Signs and symptoms of inhaled poisons vary depending on the source of the poison. Shortness of breath and coughing are common indicators. Pulse rate is usually fast or slow. Often, the patient's eyes will appear irritated.

Emergency care consists of safely removing the patient from the source of the inhaled poison, maintaining an open airway, administering oxygen, providing life-support measures, contacting the poison control center or medical direction, and making certain that the EMS system has been activated. Remember to gather information from the patient and bystanders such as substance inhaled, length of time exposed, early care measures, and patient's initial reactions and appearance.

Fire presents problems other than thermal burns. One such problem is smoke inhalation. The smoke from any fire source contains poisonous substances. Modern building materials and furnishings often contain plastics and other synthetics that release toxic fumes when they burn or overheat. It is possible for the substances found in smoke to burn the skin, irritate the eyes, injure the airway, cause respiratory arrest, and in some cases cause cardiac arrest. Do not attempt a rescue a victim unless you have been trained to do so and have all the required personnel and equipment.

As an Emergency Medical Responder, you will probably see irritation to the eyes and airway associated with smoke. Irritations to the skin and eyes may be cared for by flushing with water. But your first priority will be the patient's airway. In cases of smoke inhalation, you should:

1. Move the patient to a safe, smoke-free area.
2. Perform a primary assessment and assist with breathing as necessary.
3. Administer oxygen, if allowed to do so.
4. If the patient is responsive and without signs of neck or spine injury, place him in a sitting or semi-sitting position. The patient may find it easier to breathe in a different position, so let him assume a position of comfort. Always provide support for the back, and be prepared if the patient becomes unresponsive.

OBJECTIVE

13. Describe the signs and symptoms of a patient experiencing carbon monoxide poisoning.

Carbon monoxide poisoning is often present at fire scenes. This gas enters the patient's bloodstream, where it is picked up by red blood cells that should be carrying oxygen. The patient will complain of headache and dizziness and may experience confusion, seizures, and coma. Proper care requires moving the patient away from the source and following the same basic procedures as would be provided for any smoke inhalation or inhaled-poison victim. EMT-level care and transport are required in all cases of carbon monoxide poisoning. Look for soot around the nose and/or mouth. This may be a sign of smoke inhalation along with inhalation of the superheated gases from the combustion process of fire.

Absorbed Poisons

As mentioned earlier in this chapter, absorbed poisons usually irritate or damage the skin or eyes. However, there are cases in which a poison can be absorbed with little or no damage to the skin. The patient, bystanders, and other clues at the scene will help you determine if you are dealing with such cases.

Signs and symptoms of absorbed poisoning include any or all of the following:

- Skin reactions, ranging from mild irritations to severe burns
- Hives
- Itching
- Eye irritation
- Headache
- Increased skin temperature

Emergency care for absorbed poisons includes moving the patient from the source of the poison (when it is safe to do so) and immediately flooding with water all the areas of the patient's body (including the eyes) that have been exposed to the poison. After flushing with water, remove all contaminated clothing (including shoes and jewelry), and wash the affected areas of the patient's skin with soap and water. If no soap is available, continue to flush the exposed areas of the patient's skin. Be certain to have someone contact the poison control center or medical direction and activate the EMS system.

If the poison is in the form of a powder, you may have to brush it from the patient's clothing, skin, and hair. It is best done with you wearing gloves and eye protection. If available, protect the patient's eyes as well. Take precautions so that no one—you, the patient, or onlookers—inhales the powder.

Injected Poisons

Insect stings, spider bites, stings from marine life, and snakebites can all be sources of injected poisons. Some of these poisons cause very serious emergencies in all patients. Others are only problems for those patients sensitive to the poison. In all cases of injected poisons, be alert for anaphylactic (allergy) shock.

Poisons also can be injected into the body by a hypodermic needle. Drug overdose and drug contamination can produce serious medical emergencies. Gather information from the patient, bystanders, and the scene. Signs and symptoms of injected poisoning may include:

- Noticeable stings or bites to the skin (puncture marks)
- Pain at or around the wound site
- Itching
- Weakness, dizziness, or collapse
- Difficulty breathing and abnormal pulse rate
- Headache
- Nausea
- Anaphylactic (allergy) shock

Since a patient may go into anaphylactic (allergy) shock, alert the poison control center and the EMS system or medical direction as soon as possible for all cases of injected poisoning.

Emergency care for injected poisons includes:

1. Take BSI precautions and perform a primary assessment.
2. Administer oxygen as per local protocols.
3. Scrape away bee and wasp stingers and venom sacs. Do not pull out stingers. Always scrape them from the patient's skin. A plastic credit card works well as a scraper.
4. Place an ice bag or cold pack over the bitten or stung area.

Some patients sensitive to stings or bites carry medication to help prevent anaphylactic shock. Help all such patients to take their medications. Your Emergency Medical Responder course may include training in how to administer medications by injection when the patient cannot inject himself. Do only what you have been trained to do.

Alcohol Abuse

Alcohol is a drug, socially acceptable in moderation, but still a drug. Abuse of alcohol, as with any other drug, can lead to illness, poisoning of the body, abnormal behavior, and even death. A patient under the influence of alcohol is at risk for causing harm to himself or others.

As an Emergency Medical Responder, try to provide care to the patient suffering from alcohol intoxication as you would any other patient. It is often difficult to determine that the problem has been caused by alcohol and if alcohol abuse is the only problem. Even trained mental health professionals can miss making a dual diagnosis. If the patient allows you to do so, conduct a secondary assessment that includes a thorough history. In some cases, you will have to depend on bystanders for meaningful information. Also, remember that diabetes, epilepsy, head injuries, high fevers, and other medical problems can make a patient appear drunk.

For all situations involving patients with alcohol or other drug emergencies, perform a thorough scene size-up and remain alert for changes in mental status. Once you can approach the patient, let him know who you are and what you are going to do before you start a patient assessment. You may have to modify your approach and communication techniques as you try to determine whether the situation also involves a medical or a trauma problem. It may be difficult to perform a physical exam or any care procedures until you can calm the patient and gain his confidence.

Signs of alcohol intoxication may include:

- Odor of alcohol on the patient's breath or clothing. This is not enough by itself unless you are sure that this is not "acetone breath," a sign of the diabetic patient.
- Swaying and unsteady, uncoordinated movements
- Slurred speech and the inability to carry on a conversation. Do not be fooled into thinking that the situation may not be serious because the patient jokes or clowns around.
- Flushed appearance, often with sweating and complaining of being warm
- Nausea and vomiting or feeling the need to vomit

A patient suffering from alcohol intoxication may be going through withdrawal from having been without alcohol. *Delirium tremens (DTs)* may result from sudden withdrawal. In such cases, look for:

- High blood pressure, rapid heart rate
- Confusion and restlessness
- Abnormal behavior
- Hallucinations
- Tremors (obvious shaking) of the hands
- Convulsions

As you see, some of the signs displayed in alcohol intoxication are similar to those found in other medical emergencies. Be certain that the only problem is alcohol intoxication. Remember, persons who abuse alcohol also may be injured or ill. The effects of the alcohol might mask the typical signs and symptoms observed during assessment. Also, be on the alert for other signs, such as abnormal vital signs.

The basic care for the alcohol abuse patient consists of the following:

- Take appropriate BSI precautions and perform a primary assessment.
- Ensure a clear airway and adequate breathing.
- Perform a thorough secondary assessment to detect any signs of illness or injuries. Remember that alcohol may mask pain. Look carefully for mechanisms of injury and the signs of illness.
- Monitor vital signs, staying alert for respiratory problems.
- Help the patient when he is vomiting, so the vomit will not be aspirated (inhaled).
- Protect the patient from further injury.

Drug Abuse

Drugs may be classified as uppers, downers, narcotics, hallucinogens, and volatile chemicals. *Uppers* are stimulants affecting the nervous system to excite the user. *Downers* are depressants meant to affect the central nervous system to relax the user. *Narcotics* affect the nervous system and change many of the normal activities of the body. Often they produce an intense state of relaxation and feelings of well-being. *Hallucinogens*, or mind-altering drugs, act on the nervous system to produce an intense state of excitement or distortion of the user's surroundings. *Volatile chemicals* give an initial rush but then depress the central nervous system.

Drug Abuse

Do your best to be nonjudgmental of the patient with a drug or alcohol addiction. Your view of the patient may cloud your ability to treat him appropriately. Regardless of the underlying cause of the addiction, the patient is suffering an acute emergency that requires immediate and often life-saving intervention.

Some courses that train rescuers and EMS personnel have spent considerable time in the past teaching specific drug names and reactions. As an Emergency Medical Responder, you will not need such knowledge. For you, it is important to be able to detect possible drug abuse at the overdose level and to relate certain signs to certain types of drugs.

Your care for the drug abuse patient will be basically the same as for any drug that may have been used. Your care will not change unless you are ordered to change it by medical direction or a poison control center. lists some of the names of common drugs that are abused. You do not need to memorize them.

The signs and symptoms of drug abuse and drug overdose can vary from patient to patient, even for the same drug. The scene, bystanders, and the patient may be your only sources of finding out if you are dealing with drug abuse and what the substance is. When questioning the patient and bystanders, you will get better results if you ask if the patient has been taking any medications, rather than using the word *drugs*. If you have any doubts, then ask if the patient has taken drugs or is "using anything." Patients may not give information about their drug use.

Some significant signs and symptoms related to specific drugs include:

- *Uppers.* Uppers can cause excitement, increased pulse and breathing rates, rapid speech, dry mouth, dilated pupils, sweating, and the complaint of having gone without sleep for long periods.
- *Downers.* The use of downers can cause the patient to be sluggish or sleepy, lack normal coordination of body movements, and have slurred speech. Pulse and breathing rates are low, often to the point of a true emergency.
- *Hallucinogens.* These can cause a fast pulse rate, dilated pupils, and a flushed face. The patient often sees things and hears voices or sounds that do not exist, has little concept of real time, and may not be aware of the true environment. Often, the patient makes no sense when speaking. Many show signs of anxiety and fearfulness. They have been described as paranoid. Some patients become very aggressive. Others tend to withdraw.
- *Narcotics.* Reduced pulse and breathing rates and a lowered skin temperature often are seen in the patient who is abusing narcotics. The pupils are constricted, muscles are relaxed, and sweating is heavy. The patient is very sleepy and does not wish to do anything. In overdoses, coma is a common event. Respiratory arrest may occur.
- *Volatile chemicals.* The user may seem dazed or show temporary loss of contact with reality. This patient may go into a coma. The inside of the nose and mouth may show swollen membranes. The patient may complain of numbness or tingling inside the head or a headache. The face may be flushed and the pulse rate accelerated. There may be a chemical odor to the patient's breath, skin, or clothing.

These signs and symptoms have a lot in common with many medical emergencies. Never just assume drug abuse by itself.

Withdrawal from drugs varies from patient to patient and from drug to drug. In most cases of withdrawal, you will see shaking, anxiety, nausea, confusion, irritability, sweating, and increased pulse and breathing rates.

When providing care for drug abuse patients, you should:

1. Take BSI precautions and perform a primary assessment.
2. Maintain an open airway and ensure adequate breathing.

KEY POINT ▼

The most commonly abused substance in the United States is alcohol (ethanol). In addition to its direct effects, alcohol is often mixed with other abused substances, worsening effects on the body.

KEY POINT ▼

Always consider PCP users dangerous, even when they appear to be calm. PCP usage leads to aggressive behavior. The drug can build up in the body and cause a violent reaction without warning. If PCP is the cause of the problem, wait for the police to arrive, unless the patient is unresponsive or in need of immediate life support measures.

IS IT SAFE?

Always consider PCP users dangerous, even when they appear to be calm. PCP usage leads to aggressive behavior. The drug can build up in the body and cause a violent reaction without warning. If PCP is the cause of the problem, wait for police to arrive, unless the patient is unresponsive or in need of immediate life support measures.

3. Administer oxygen as per local protocols.

4. Monitor vital signs and be alert for respiratory arrest.

5. Talk to the patient to gain his confidence and to maintain his level of responsiveness.

6. Protect the patient from further harm.

7. Continue to reassure the patient throughout all phases of care.

For all cases of possible drug overdose, it is good practice to contact medical direction and your local poison control center.

Generalized Infections (Sepsis)

We all get infections from time to time. Most commonly they are from a cut or scrap on the skin. Infections can also form deep within the body. If an open wound is not cleaned properly it can lead to redness, swelling, and pain commonly referred to as an infection. If an infection does not receive proper care, it can spread throughout the body. This is called a generalized infection, or **sepsis**.

The signs and symptoms of sepsis include:

- Fever
- Chills
- Rapid breathing
- Rapid heart rate
- Low blood pressure
- Altered mental status

Although sepsis can have numerous causes, the following types of patients are more susceptible to a generalized infection:

- Transplant patients
- Infants and elderly patients
- Radiation or chemotherapy patients
- Burn patients
- Diabetes patients
- AIDS patients

The general care for a patient with signs and symptoms of sepsis include:

1. Take appropriate BSI precautions and perform a primary assessment.

2. Ensure a clear airway and adequate breathing.

3. Administer oxygen as per local protocols.

4. Monitor vital signs.

5. Continue to reassure the patient throughout all phases of care.

Allergic Reactions

Allergic reactions occur when people come into contact with a substance to which they are allergic. The body considers the substance an invader and reacts to counteract it. In minor reactions there may only be mild swelling of the skin and itching. Extreme cases can cause a life-threatening emergency known as anaphylactic shock. There is no way of knowing if patients will stabilize, grow worse slowly or rapidly, or overcome the reaction on their own. Many patients become worse rapidly. For some, death is a certain outcome unless special care is provided quickly. Anaphylaxis causes the air passages to constrict, making it difficult for the patient to breath. It also causes the blood vessels to dilate, which results in a dangerously low blood pressure.

There are many different causes of anaphylactic shock, such as insect bites and stings; foods (nuts, spices, shellfish); inhaled substances, including dust and pollens; chemicals, inhaled or when in contact with the skin; and medications, injected or taken by mouth, including penicillin.

Signs and symptoms of am anaphylactic reaction are as follows:

- Burning, itching, or breaking out of the skin (such as hives or some type of rash)
- Breathing that is difficult and rapid
- Altered mental status, such as fainting or unresponsiveness
- Pulse that is rapid and weak
- Cyanosis of the lips and nail beds
- Swelling of the tongue and throat
- Restlessness

OBJECTIVE

20. Describe the signs and symptoms of an allergic reaction.

When you interview a patient who you suspect may be having an allergic reaction, ask if he is allergic to anything and if he has been in contact with that substance. If unresponsive, look for medical identification jewelry, which might indicate that there is a history of allergies.

Some people who have known allergies carry prescribed medications to take in case of an emergency. Those medications (usually an epinephrine autoinjector) may be administered by the patient. (See Appendix 2.) Your jurisdiction may allow Emergency Medical Responders to assist. Epinephrine is a form of adrenaline that helps to open the air passages and constrict the blood vessels.

State laws and protocols will govern if you can assist the patient in administering the medication. Your instructor will inform you of local policies for the care of these patients.

Emergency care for anaphylactic shock:

OBJECTIVE

21. Explain the appropriate assessment and care for a patient experiencing a severe allergic reaction.

1. Take appropriate BSI precautions and perform a primary assessment.
2. Ensure a clear airway and adequate breathing.
3. Administer oxygen as per local protocols.
4. Assist the patient with his prescribed epinephrine autoinjector. (Follow local protocols.)
5. Monitor vital signs and ABCs until EMS units arrive.

Kidney (Renal) Failure

Kidney failure, also known as renal failure, occurs when a person's kidneys fail to function normally. The kidneys serve as complex filters for the blood and are essential for the removal of excess water and waste products from the blood. The kidneys can fail for a wide variety of reasons, such as injury, blood loss, disease, and reactions to medications.

Patients most at risk for renal failure include those over the age of 60 and those with a history of diabetes, high blood pressure, a family member with kidney failure, and heart disease.

Common signs and symptoms of renal failure include:

- Weakness
- Altered mental status
- Generalized swelling
- Increased heart rate
- Increased blood pressure
- Decrease in urination

OBJECTIVE

16. Describe the signs and symptoms of a patient experiencing an emergency related to renal failure.

Dialysis is the process of artificially removing excess water and waste products from the blood. The most common type of dialysis is called **hemodialysis**. A patient with renal failure must receive dialysis at frequent intervals to keep the blood clean and functioning properly.

Hemodialysis requires that the patient be connected to a specialized machine that filters the blood. The patient is connected to the machine through a surgically implanted access point beneath the skin of the arm. This access point is called a shunt or fistula (Figure 15.9). The patient's blood is run through the dialysis machine where it is filtered and then returned to the body.

hemodialysis ▶ the process of mechanically filtering the blood to remove wastes and excess fluid.

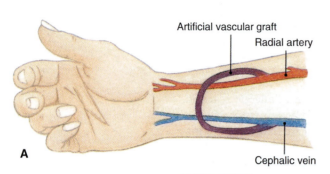

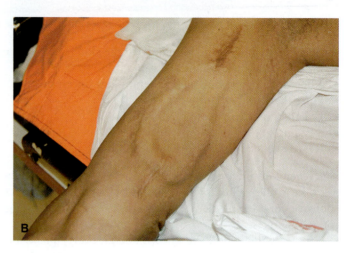

Artificial vascular graft
Radial artery

Cephalic vein

A

B

Figure 15.9 • During hemodialysis the dialysis machine is connected to an access site such as a shunt beneath the skin.

Emergency care of the patient with renal failure includes:

1. Take appropriate BSI precautions and perform a primary assessment.
2. Ensure a clear airway and adequate breathing.
3. Control any bleeding from the access point with direct pressure and elevation.
4. Administer oxygen as per local protocols.
5. Monitor vital signs until EMS units arrive.

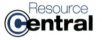

Learn more about caring for patients with behavioral disorders.

Behavioral Emergencies

Behavior is the manner in which a person acts or performs. This includes any or all of a person's activities, including physical and mental activity. The behavior of most people is considered typical or normal because it is accepted by their families and society. It does not interfere with the daily activities of life. Behavior that is unacceptable or intolerable to others is known as abnormal (atypical) behavior. Although caring for this type of patient might be challenging, it is crucial that you remain professional and provide appropriate care.

A **behavioral emergency** exists in situations where the patient exhibits abnormal behavior that is unacceptable or intolerable to the patient, family, or community. Such behavior may occur because of extremes of emotion or a psychological or medical condition. Other causes of behavioral changes include situational stress (patient reacting to events at the scene), mind-altering substances, psychiatric problems, and psychological crises, including panic or paranoia.

Assessment and Emergency Care

Follow these guidelines when performing an assessment on behavioral emergency patients:

- Approach with caution and observe for signs of agitation or violence. Do not approach the patient if it is not safe!
- Identify yourself and let the patient know you are there to help.
- Inform the patient of what you are doing at all times.
- Ask questions in a calm, reassuring voice.
- Without being judgmental, allow the patient to tell what happened.
- Show that you are listening by rephrasing or repeating part of what is said.
- Be aware of your posture and body language and the message it may be sending to the patient.

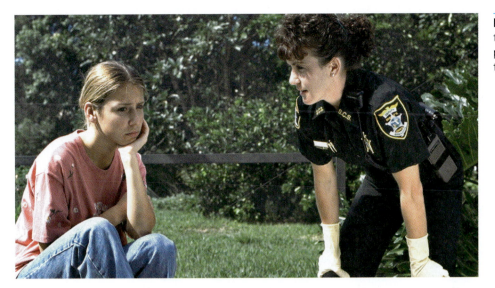

Figure 15.10 • Encourage the emotionally distraught patient to tell you what is troubling her.

- Assess the patient's mental status: appearance, activity, speech, and orientation to person, place, time, and event.
- Always consider the need for law enforcement.

Emergency care of a patient with a behavioral emergency includes the following:

- Perform a scene size-up and consider the need for law enforcement.
- Perform a primary assessment by observing the patient from a safe distance.
- Acknowledge that the patient seems upset and restate that you are there to help.
- Inform the patient of what you are doing.
- Ask questions in a calm, reassuring voice.
- Encourage the patient to state what is troubling him (Figure 15.10).
- Do not make quick moves.
- Answer questions honestly.
- Do not threaten, challenge, or argue with disturbed patients.
- Do not "play along" with hallucinations or auditory disturbances.
- Involve trusted family members or friends, if appropriate.
- Be prepared for an extended scene time.
- Avoid unnecessary physical contact.
- Leave yourself a way out. Never let the potentially violent patient come between you and your exit.

Assessing the Potential for Violence

Sometimes patients experience conditions that cause them to become violent and uncooperative. As an Emergency Medical Responder, your priority is to prevent the patient from harming himself or others, while also protecting yourself. Consider contacting law enforcement (Figure 15.11) and note the following:

- *Scene size-up.* Use caution when approaching a scene. Observe the patient and the surroundings for any indication that he might be a danger to himself or others. Ensure that he has no weapons or anything that may be used as a weapon.
- *History.* Often, patients who have exhibited violent behavior in the past will repeat it. Take such past history into consideration during your assessment.
- *Posture.* How is the patient standing? Is he in an offensive stance? What does his body language tell you? Are you positioned at a safe distance?
- *Verbal activity.* Often, verbal abuse is a precursor to violence. If a patient continues to use foul language or raise his voice, consider such action as a possible warning sign of violent behavior.

IS IT SAFE?

Responding to a behavioral emergency can present many risks for responders. Although most patients want your care, behavioral emergency patients may not want any part of it. Consider the need for law enforcement early in the call, and do not get yourself cornered in a room with the patient.

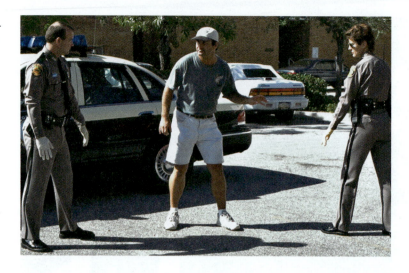

- *Physical activity.* Patients may begin to pace or wave their arms in the air with increased activity. Such movements may escalate into more violent behavior.

Restraining Patients

In some cases, behavioral emergency patients might become violent to the point that it is necessary to physically restrain them. Although this task should be avoided, it is often necessary to protect the patient, yourself, and others. In those situations, follow your local guidelines for contacting police and consulting medical direction. Remember the emotional disturbance may be caused by an underlying medical condition that the patient is not aware of, does not understand, or cannot control. Because of this, emotionally disturbed patients may threaten those who are trying to help and will often resist emergency care.

You cannot provide emergency care to a patient without proper consent, so you must have a reasonable belief that the patient will harm himself or others and would want help if he were able to understand and consent to it. Contact medical direction for guidance before attempting to provide care for a patient without consent. Local protocols may require you to contact law enforcement for assistance.

Do not approach a violent patient alone. While waiting for assistance, try the following:

- Talk and listen to the patient to divert his focus and keep him from harming himself and others.
- Sit or stand passively but remain alert to the patient's actions and responses.
- Avoid any action that may alarm the patient and cause him to react violently.
- Wait for law enforcement assistance to arrive if restraining the patient is necessary, and let police officers take the lead in restraining the patient.
- Use reasonable force only to defend yourself against attack.

From the Medical Director

Restraining Patients

Physically restraining a patient should be the last resort taken only when it is clear that without doing so the patient may harm himself. Your personal safety is paramount. If you are injured, then the number of patients on the scene is doubled. Use the least amount of restraint necessary to protect the patient from harm, and do not be afraid to stop and evaluate whether your actions are making things better or worse. There is nothing wrong with a tactical retreat and reassessment of the situation. It may be better to wait until additional help arrives.

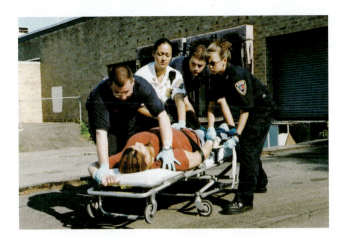

Figure 15.12 • Use restraint only as a last resort.

Do not attempt to restrain a patient except only as a last resort. Make certain you have enough resources and have a coordinated plan of action (Figure 15.12). Review the section on patient restraint in Chapter 5.

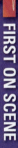

The small room is bustling with firefighters, ambulance personnel, campus security, and two police officers from the city. Jordan described the patient's seizure and pointed out the medical identification necklace to the firefighters who were the first on scene.

"Who took care of this patient before we got here?" the paramedic from the ambulance asks as he starts an IV on the unconscious girl. A firefighter points at Jordan.

"You did a great job!" The paramedic is now administering a clear fluid into the IV line with a huge syringe. "You kept her airway open and got her into the lateral recumbent position. I couldn't have asked you to do better than that."

Jordan smiles and feels his face get hot at the compliment. Before he walks from the room, he is happy to see the girl blink her eyes several times and begin to ask questions of the Paramedic.

Summary

- Several conditions can cause a patient to experience an altered mental status, including seizures, strokes, diabetic emergencies, poisonings, breathing problems, and cardiac events.

- Altered mental status can present with a wide range of signs and symptoms, from confusion and dizziness to seizures and even syncope (fainting).

- The assessment and care of a patient with an altered mental status is dependent on the Emergency Medical Responder observing the patient's environment and asking questions.

- Seizures can present with sudden unresponsiveness, convulsions, headaches, and unusual breathing patterns. Clearing the area around a seizing patient is the primary way that an Emergency Medical Responder can help while waiting for the seizure to subside.

- A patient suffering a stroke will commonly have some of the following signs and symptoms: syncope, confusion, partial or full paralysis, headache, difficulty speaking or swallowing, and altered mental status.

- Stroke patients should be closely monitored since they may experience airway compromise, breathing difficulty, or even cardiac arrest.

- Diabetic emergencies can present with difficult or unusual breathing, abdominal pain, seizures, dry mouth, extreme thirst, fruity breath odor, altered mental status, and even unresponsiveness.

- Hyperglycemia (high blood sugar) can cause a patient to complain of abdominal pain, extreme thirst and dry mouth, whereas hypoglycemia (low blood sugar) can result in extreme hunger, strong, rapid pulse, shallow breathing, seizures, and pale, cool, and moist skin.

- When the Emergency Medical Responder cannot determine if the diabetic emergency is caused by hypo- or hyperglycemia, the care for both should be the same. Administer real sugar (if appropriate), provide oxygen, and activate the EMS system. While waiting for advanced medical personnel, monitor the patient's ABCs and make him as comfortable as possible (in the recovery position if unresponsive).

- Common signs and symptoms of a patient who has been poisoned are altered mental status, vomiting, abdominal pain, sweating, abnormal pulse and/or breathing, unresponsiveness, pain when breathing or swallowing, dilated or constricted pupils, and weakness or dizziness.

- Carbon monoxide poisoning may present with headaches, dizziness, confusion, seizures, and even coma. The primary indicator of this type of poisoning is the patient's surroundings. If a patient presents with the signs and symptoms and he has been near any sort of combustion (fire, automobile, heater, etc.), you should suspect carbon monoxide poisoning.

- Caring for the poisoning or overdose patient is primarily about protecting the patient's airway, administering oxygen (if allowed), activating the EMS system, and monitoring the ABCs.

- A local, regional, or national poison control center should be contacted (per local protocols) once you have established that the patient has been exposed to poison and you have determined the type of poison encountered.

- A patient who is already suffering from either a serious infection or a suppressed immune system can develop sepsis. Sepsis is a condition whereby a once isolated infection spreads through the patient's bloodstream to become a system-wide problem. Fever, chills, confusion, unresponsiveness, rapid breathing, rapid heart rate, and low blood pressure are all common indicators of sepsis.

- Septic patients must be treated at a hospital as soon as possible. The Emergency Medical Responder should ensure activation of the EMS system, provide oxygen (if allowed), and monitor the patient's ABCs closely while awaiting advanced care.

- Anaphylaxis is a life-threatening allergic reaction characterized by altered mental status, difficulty breathing, and swelling of the throat. Support the ABCs and assist with the prescribed autoinjector if available.

- Renal failure occurs when the kidneys no longer function normally. Dialysis is the process of artificially filtering the blood and removing excess water and waste products.

- Any time a patient is behaving in a manner that is intolerable to himself, his family, or the community, he is said to be having a behavioral emergency. Emergency Medical Responders should first and foremost ensure their own safety and the safety of others near the patient. Following that, they should clearly and calmly identify themselves to the patient, ensure that the EMS system is activated, and engage the patient with clear, effective communication until assistance arrives.

Take Action

20 QUESTIONS

Assessing the general medical patient, especially the one with an altered mental status, can be very challenging, especially if the patient is unable to provide any clues to what may be going on. Getting some practice with asking questions when you do not know what is wrong will be very helpful when you encounter your first real live patient.

Pair up with another student in your class. One of you will serve as the patient and use this chapter as a reference while the other one asks the questions. Use this chapter to select a specific medical problem such as stroke, hyperglycemia, and so on. As the person playing the role of the patient, take a few minutes to refer to the specific signs and symptoms of the complaint. When you are ready, instruct the person acting as the Emergency Medical Responder to begin asking questions. The goal is to identify the specific medical condition in as few questions as possible.

First on Scene Run Review

Recall the events of the "First on Scene" scenario in this chapter and answer the following questions, which are related to the call. Rationales are offered in the Answer Key at the back of the book.

1. When a person has had a seizure, what information should you get from the patient and/or bystanders?

2. What should your treatment be after a person has had a seizure?

3. If a person is an insulin-dependent diabetic, why might he have a seizure?

Quick Quiz

To check your understanding of the chapter, answer the following questions. Then compare your answers to those in the Answer Key at the back of the book.

1. Altered mental status is best defined as a patient who:
   a. is unresponsive.
   b. cannot speak properly.
   c. cannot tell you what day it is.
   d. is not alert or responsive to surroundings.

2. A patient who is unresponsive and having full body muscle contractions is likely experiencing:
   a. stroke.
   b. seizure.
   c. heart attack.
   d. respiratory distress.

3. Which one of the following is the best example of appropriate care for a seizure patient?
   a. Keep him from injuring himself and place him in the recovery position following the seizure.
   b. Place him in a semi-sitting position and apply oxygen following the seizure.
   c. Place him in a prone position and provide oxygen by nasal cannula.
   d. Restrain him and assist ventilations with a bag-mask device.

4. A patient who presents with abnormal behavior that is unacceptable to family members and others is said to be experiencing a(n):
   a. psychosis.
   b. mental breakdown.
   c. altered behavioral state.
   d. behavioral emergency.

5. One of the best techniques for dealing with a patient experiencing a behavioral emergency is to:
   a. not let the patient know what you are doing.
   b. not believe a thing the patient says.
   c. speak in a calm and reassuring voice.
   d. acknowledge the "voices" he is hearing.

6. Which one of the following is NOT evaluated as part of the Cincinnati Prehospital Stroke Scale?
   a. Abnormal speech
   b. Equal circulation
   c. Facial droop
   d. Arm drift

7. Your patient is presenting with an altered mental status and a history of diabetes. He states that he took his normal dose of insulin this morning but has not had anything to eat. His most likely problem is:
   a. hyperglycemia.
   b. anaphylaxis.
   c. hypoglycemia.
   d. a stroke.

8. Activated charcoal is only recommended for what type of poisoning?
   a. Ingested
   b. Inhaled
   c. Topical
   d. Absorbed

9. When called to assist with a responsive person who has taken PCP, you should first:
   a. assess her vital signs.
   b. determine if she is experiencing any hallucinations.
   c. gently restrain her.
   d. ensure the scene is safe.

10. What is the most commonly abused chemical in the United States?
    a. Arsenic
    b. Amyl nitrate
    c. Butane
    d. Alcohol

11. A diabetic who forgets to take her insulin and continues to eat a meal will most likely become:
    a. hypoglycemic.
    b. responsive.
    c. hyperglycemic.
    d. short of breath.

12. What is caused by either a clot or a rupture?

   a. Diabetic coma

   b. Narcotic overdose

   c. Stroke

   d. Hallucination

13. Once a seizure has ended, the patient is said to be in the _____ state.

   a. REM

   b. postictal

   c. syncopal

   d. recovery

14. The process of sending a patient's blood through an artificial filter is referred to as:

   a. photodialysis.

   b. syncope.

   c. hemodialysis.

   d. autodialysis.

15. All of the following are common causes of renal failure EXCEPT:

   a. angina.

   b. injury.

   c. diabetes.

   d. blood loss.

16. You are caring for a 10-year-old boy who was stung by a bee. He is crying in pain and able to move air without difficulty. You observe a small red dot where the sting occurred and he states that it itches. This is most likely a:

   a. severe reaction requiring immediate transport.

   b. mild reaction requiring immediate transport.

   c. mild reaction that may not require transport.

   d. severe reaction that does not require transport.

17. A severe allergic reaction causes the air passages:

   a. and blood vessels to dilate.

   b. and blood vessels to constrict.

   c. to dilate and the blood vessels to constrict.

   d. to constrict and the blood vessels to dilate.

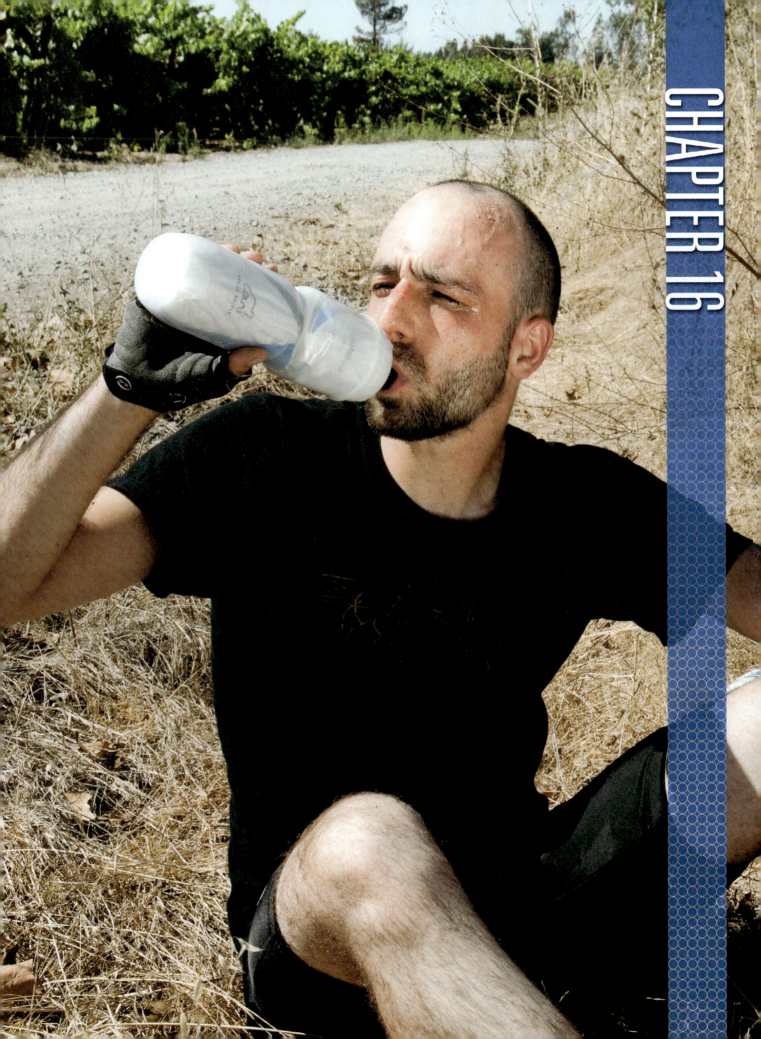

CHAPTER 16

Caring for Environmental Emergencies

EDUCATION STANDARDS
- Trauma—Environmental Emergencies
- Medicine—Toxicology

COMPETENCIES
- Uses simple knowledge to recognize and manage life threats based on assessment findings for an acutely injured patient while awaiting additional emergency medical response.
- Recognizes and manages life threats based on assessment findings of a patient with a medical emergency while awaiting additional emergency response.

CHAPTER OVERVIEW
This chapter provides an overview of some of the more common environmental emergencies that you are likely to encounter as an Emergency Medical Responder. They include a wide variety of conditions such as exposure to extremes of heat and cold as well as bites, stings, and water- and ice-related emergencies.

OBJECTIVES

Upon successful completion of this chapter, the student should be able to:

COGNITIVE

1. Define the following terms:
   a. anaphylaxis (p. 344)
   b. conduction (p. 336)
   c. convection (p. 336)
   d. core temperature (p. 336)
   e. drowning (p. 346)
   f. evaporation (p. 336)
   g. frostbite (p. 341)
   h. heat cramps (p. 337)
   i. heat exhaustion (p. 337)
   j. heat stroke (p. 339)
   k. hyperthermia (p. 336)
   l. hypothermia (p. 339)
   m. radiation (p. 335)

2. Explain the four ways the body loses excess heat. (p. 335)

3. Describe the signs and symptoms of a patient experiencing a heat-related emergency. (p. 336)

4. Explain the appropriate assessment and care for a patient experiencing a heat-related emergency. (p. 336)

5. Differentiate the signs and symptoms of heat stroke and heat exhaustion. (p. 337)

6. Describe the signs and symptoms of a cold-related emergency. (p. 339)

7. Explain the appropriate assessment and care for a patient experiencing a cold-related emergency. (p. 339)

8. Describe the signs and symptoms of emergencies related to bites and stings. (p. 343)

9. Explain the appropriate assessment and care for a patient experiencing an emergency related to a bite or sting. (p. 343)

10. Describe common factors leading to submersion injuries. (p. 349)

11. Describe common methods used for water-related rescue. (p. 346)

12. Explain the hazards related to water rescue. (p. 346)

13. Describe the signs and symptoms of a submersion injury. (p. 349)

14. Explain the appropriate care for a victim of a submersion injury. (p. 350)

PSYCHOMOTOR

15. Demonstrate the ability to appropriately assess and care for a patient experiencing a heat-related emergency.

16. Demonstrate the ability to appropriately assess and care for a patient experiencing a cold-related emergency.

17. Demonstrate the ability to appropriately assess and care for a patient experiencing a bite or sting emergency.

AFFECTIVE

18. Value the importance of proper training when attempting to conduct a water rescue.

"It's got to be coming from over here," AJ thinks as he makes his way toward the sound of sobbing that is coming from somewhere on the hiking path. The day is unseasonably hot, and AJ squints in the bright sunlight that beats against the dirt and rock, creating thick, watery-looking waves against the ground.

"Help, somebody!" a raspy voice calls out at AJ's immediate left. In the shade are two women, one of them lying semiconscious on the ground.

"What's wrong?" AJ asks, although he is pretty sure he knows what is happening. He unzips his backpack and pulls out the three water bottles he stored in preparation.

"We were hiking out here and Melody said she was getting too hot. She just started breathing funny and saying funny things. She was sweating so much. We both are."

AJ looks down and feels Melody's skin at her forehead, which is burning hot. He checks her neck and core area but she doesn't seem to be sweating anymore. "I think she might be having a heat stroke." As soon as the words leave his mouth, Melody's body starts to convulse.

"What's going on?" shrieks her friend.

Temperature and the Body

The human body operates within a very narrow temperature range. It is capable of closely and carefully regulating its own temperature in a wide range of environmental conditions. The process of maintaining proper body temperature is called *temperature regulation* and is performed by the brain through various processes.

Hypothermia (abnormally low body temperature) and hyperthermia (abnormally high body temperature) may result when the body is not able to regulate temperature effectively. Hypothermia can occur when the body loses heat faster than it can produce heat. Hyperthermia can occur when heat gain occurs faster than the body can shed heat.

Heat is lost through a number of means (Figure 16.1):

- *Radiation*. With **radiation**, body heat is emitted into the environment. This is the heat that is lost to the surrounding air as it radiates off our bodies.

OBJECTIVE

2. Explain the four ways the body loses excess heat.

radiation ▶ loss of body heat to the atmosphere or nearby objects without physical contact.

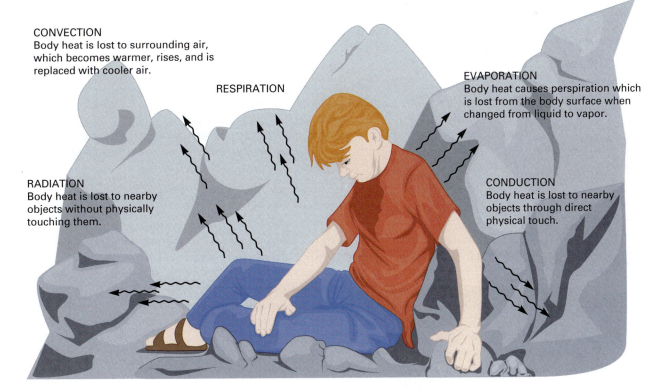

CONVECTION
Body heat is lost to surrounding air, which becomes warmer, rises, and is replaced with cooler air.

RESPIRATION

EVAPORATION
Body heat causes perspiration which is lost from the body surface when changed from liquid to vapor.

RADIATION
Body heat is lost to nearby objects without physically touching them.

CONDUCTION
Body heat is lost to nearby objects through direct physical touch.

Figure 16.1 • Mechanisms of heat loss for the body.

conduction ▶ the loss of body heat through direct contact with another object or the ground.

convection ▶ the loss of body heat when air that is close to the skin moves away, taking body heat with it.

evaporation ▶ the loss of body heat through the evaporation of moisture in the form of sweat on the skin.

- *Conduction.* Body heat is transferred to an object with which the body is in contact. **Conduction** occurs when our bodies are in contact with a cool or cold surface such as the ground or when immersed in water.
- *Convection.* With **convection**, body heat is lost to surrounding air that becomes warmer, rises, and is replaced with cooler air. This occurs when cool air is warmed by our bodies and then moves away. That air is replaced by cooler air and the cycle continues. Wind can greatly increase the affects of convection.
- *Evaporation.* Body heat is lost when perspiration is changed from liquid to vapor. Sweating is a normal body function. As the sweat on our skin evaporates, it carries heat with it. Wind can also greatly increase the effectiveness of **evaporation**.
- *Respiration.* Heat leaves the body with each breath. Our breath contains a considerable amount of moisture. As we breathe out, we expel warm moist air from within our bodies.

You must consider each of these methods of heat loss when you are caring for patients with emergencies related to heat or cold.

Heat Emergencies

The human body is a finely tuned machine. It is capable of maintaining an ideal internal temperature in a wide variety of environments. Overexposure to hot and humid environments can cause the body to generate too much heat, which can create an abnormally high body **core temperature** known as **hyperthermia**. Such a condition could result from a patient being outside on a hot, humid afternoon for a prolonged period of time, or from exposure to excessive heat while indoors, such as a boiler room. Left unchecked, hyperthermia can lead to a serious emergency and even death.

The body generates heat in many ways. Some of the body's normal processes, such as digestion, metabolism, and movement, generate heat. Heat is also lost through breathing and sweating. The entire process is controlled by a structure deep in the brain called the hypothalamus. The hypothalamus serves as the body's thermostat, carefully regulating all processes to maintain a normal core body temperature of approximately 98.6°F (37°C).

core temperature ▶ the temperature in the core of the body. Typically 98.6 degrees Fahrenheit or 37 degrees Celsius.

hyperthermia ▶ an increase in body core temperature above its normal temperature.

OBJECTIVE

3. Describe the signs and symptoms of a patient experiencing a heat-related emergency.

IS IT SAFE?

Extreme environments can be dangerous for emergency personnel as well as patients. Use caution when entering these environments, and always wear the appropriate clothing for the environment.

OBJECTIVE

4. Explain the appropriate assessment and care for a patient experiencing a heat-related emergency.

▶ **GERIATRIC FOCUS** ◀

The elderly are particularly prone to both extremes of temperature. Sweating may be reduced due to aging of their skin as well as the effects of their medications. The normal response to a loss of fluids is to increase the heart rate to maintain blood pressure. This reflex is often weaker in the elderly and can easily lead them to passing out before reaching a cooler place.

Sweating is one of the body's ways of ridding itself of excess heat. On a really hot day, you can lose up to one liter (about two pints) of sweat per hour. The sweat, in turn, evaporates from the skin, taking with it excess heat. The effects of heat loss through evaporation are greatly reduced when the humidity is high.

Dry heat (low humidity) can often fool individuals, causing them to continue to work in or be exposed to heat far beyond the point that can be accepted by their bodies. For this reason, the problems caused by dry heat exposure are often far worse than those seen in moist heat exposure.

When dealing with problems created by exposure to excessive heat, you must perform a thorough history and physical exam (Figure 16.2). A previous history of medical problems may quicken the effects of heat exposure. The very young, the very old, and

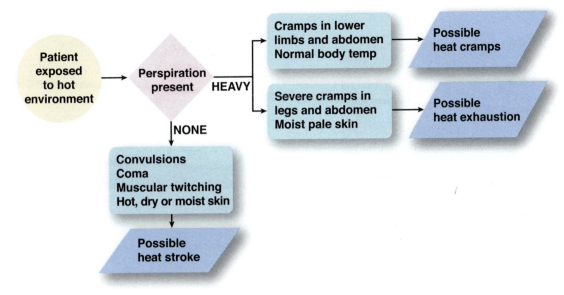

Figure 16.2 • Algorithm for the assessment of patients with a heat emergency.

those with chronic illnesses are especially susceptible to the effects of heat and cold (Scan 16.1).

Heat Cramps

Heat cramps are painful muscle spasms following strenuous activity in a hot environment. Heat cramps are usually caused by an electrolyte imbalance. Sometimes the cramps are accompanied by signs and symptoms of heat exhaustion. In most cases, however, the patient will be fully alert and sweaty with a normal to warm skin temperature. The care for these patients is to move them to a cool environment and replenish fluids by having them drink water.

Heat Exhaustion

Heat exhaustion is a condition that can occur when an otherwise healthy individual is exposed to excessive heat for a prolonged period of time. The body's normal cooling mechanisms become overworked and begin to fail due to excessive fluid loss. Heat exhaustion occurs when the body is barely able to shed as much heat as it is generating. The typical patient experiencing heat exhaustion will present with skin that is moist, pale, and normal to cool to the touch.

Signs and symptoms of heat exhaustion include:

- Mild to moderate perspiration
- Warm or cool skin temperature
- Skin color may be normal to pale
- Weakness, exhaustion, or dizziness
- Nausea and vomiting
- Muscle cramps (usually in legs)
- Rapid, weak pulse
- Rapid, shallow breathing
- Altered mental status (extreme cases)

Emergency care for heat exhaustion includes (Figure 16.3):

1. Take appropriate BSI precautions.
2. Perform a primary assessment and ensure that breathing is adequate.
3. Move the patient to a cool area.
4. Loosen or remove excess clothing.
5. Cool the patient by fanning. Be careful not to overcool the patient.

heat cramps ▶ common term for muscle cramps in the lower limbs and abdomen associated with the loss of fluids and salts while active in a hot environment.

heat exhaustion ▶ prolonged exposure to heat, which creates moist, pale skin that may feel normal or cool to the touch.

OBJECTIVE

5. Differentiate the signs and symptoms of heat stroke and heat exhaustion.

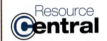

Learn more about heat-related conditions.

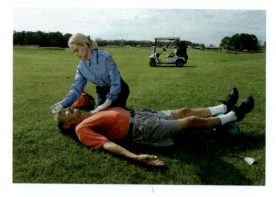

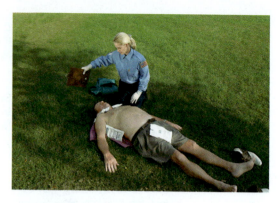

Heat Cramps/Exhaustion

Heat cramps and heat exhaustion are typically early signs of a heat emergency.

Signs and Symptoms

- Mild to severe muscle cramps in legs and abdomen
- Exhaustion, possible altered mental status (dizziness, faintness, and unresponsiveness)
- Weak pulse and rapid, shallow breathing
- Heavy perspiration
- Normal to pale skin color

Emergency Care

- Move patient to nearby cool place. Loosen or remove clothing. Do not chill. Watch for shivering.
- Provide oxygen at 15 liters per minute by nonrebreather mask if allowed.
- Give water to the responsive patient.
- Position the responsive patient on his back with legs elevated; unresponsive patient on the left side, monitoring airway and breathing.
- Help ease cramps by applying moist towels over cramped muscles or, if the patient has no history of circulatory problems, apply gentle but firm pressure on the cramped muscle.

Heat Stroke

Heat stroke is a true life-threatening emergency.

Signs and Symptoms

- Altered mental status
- Skin that is hot to the touch
- Rapid, shallow breathing
- Strong and rapid pulse
- Weakness, unresponsiveness
- Little to no perspiration
- Dilated pupils
- Seizures or muscular twitching

Emergency Care

- Rapidly cool the patient in any manner. Move to a cool place. Remove clothing. Keep skin wet by applying wet towels. Fan the patient.
- Wrap cold packs or ice bags, if available, and place them at the neck, armpits, wrists, and groin (latest protocols often request only positions that touch trunk). Fan the patient to increase heat loss.
- If transport is delayed, find tub or container and immerse patient in cool water. Monitor to prevent drowning.
- Continue to monitor the patient's vital signs.
- Provide oxygen at 15 liters per minute via nonrebreather mask if allowed.

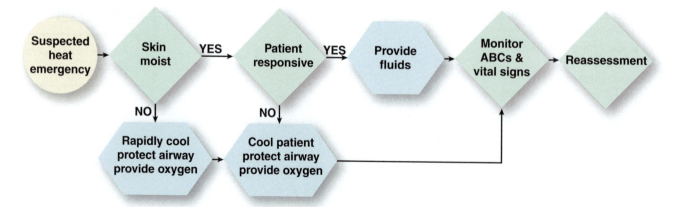

Figure 16.3 • Algorithm for the emergency care of patients with a heat emergency.

6. Place the patient in the recovery position.

7. Provide oxygen as per local protocol.

Heat Stroke

Sometimes the body's temperature-regulating mechanism fails and is unable to rid the body of excess heat. The body's core temperature is allowed to rise uncontrolled, causing the body to overheat. This condition is known as **heat stroke** and is a life-threatening emergency. A patient's body temperature may increase to 105°F (40.5°C) or higher. The skin will typically be hot and dry. The patient with heat stroke will almost always present with an altered mental status. If you are caring for a patient with a heat emergency and he has an altered mental status, assume that it is heat stroke and provide care accordingly.

Patients suffering from heat stroke may have the following signs and symptoms:

- Altered mental status
- Skin hot to the touch
- Skin slightly moist to dry
- Rapid, shallow breathing
- Rapid pulse
- Weakness, exhaustion, or dizziness
- Nausea and vomiting
- Convulsions

Emergency care for heat stroke includes the following:

1. Take appropriate BSI precautions.

2. Perform a primary assessment and ensure that breathing is adequate.

3. Move the patient to a cool area and remove excess clothing.

4. Aggressively cool the patient by dowsing or immersing the patient in cool water. Be sure not to overcool the patient.

5. Wrap cold packs or ice bags, if available, and place under the armpits, on the groin, and on each side of the neck. Follow your local protocol.

6. Place the patient in the recovery position.

7. Provide oxygen as per local protocol.

8. Monitor vital signs.

Cold Emergencies

Hypothermia

When the body loses heat faster than it can be generated, a condition known as generalized **hypothermia** may result. To prevent this condition from occurring, the body will attempt to compensate by increasing muscle activity (shivering) to increase metabolism and maintain body heat. But as the core temperature continues to drop, shivering stops and the body can no longer warm itself (Figure 16.4).

As with heat exposure, young children and the elderly are more susceptible to cold emergencies. Those with previous medical conditions are also at greater risk for hypothermia. The risk for hypothermia is sometimes obvious, such as a victim who is working or playing outside in a cold environment during the winter months. Sometimes, however, the risk for hypothermia can be much less obvious. For example, elderly patients who do not maintain the home thermostat at a proper level during the winter are often affected by cold exposure. Refrigeration accidents and incidents in mild climates also occur.

The patient experiencing a generalized cold emergency will present with cool or cold abdominal skin temperature. Place the back of your ungloved hand against the patient's abdomen to assess general temperature. In healthy adults, the abdomen should be warm.

Signs and symptoms of a generalized hypothermia may include the following:

- Cool or cold skin temperature
- Shivering

heat stroke ► prolonged exposure to heat, which creates dry or moist skin that may feel warm or hot to the touch.

IS IT SAFE?

Do not give the patient with an altered mental status anything by mouth. He may not be able to manage his own airway and may vomit.

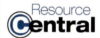

Get more information on hypothermia.

OBJECTIVE

6. Describe the signs and symptoms of a cold-related emergency.

hypothermia ► a general cooling of the body. Also called *generalized cold emergency*.

OBJECTIVE

7. Explain the appropriate assessment and care for a patient experiencing a cold-related emergency.

KEY POINT ▼

The environmental temperature does not have to be below freezing for hypothermia to occur.

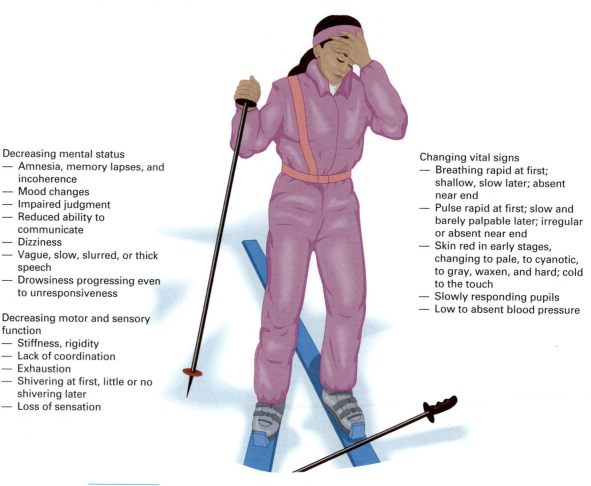

Decreasing mental status
— Amnesia, memory lapses, and incoherence
— Mood changes
— Impaired judgment
— Reduced ability to communicate
— Dizziness
— Vague, slow, slurred, or thick speech
— Drowsiness progressing even to unresponsiveness

Decreasing motor and sensory function
— Stiffness, rigidity
— Lack of coordination
— Exhaustion
— Shivering at first, little or no shivering later
— Loss of sensation

Changing vital signs
— Breathing rapid at first; shallow, slow later; absent near end
— Pulse rapid at first; slow and barely palpable later; irregular or absent near end
— Skin red in early stages, changing to pale, to cyanotic, to gray, waxen, and hard; cold to the touch
— Slowly responding pupils
— Low to absent blood pressure

Figure 16.4 • Signs and symptoms of hypothermia.

- Altered mental status
- Abnormal pulse (initially rapid, then slow)
- Lack of coordination
- Muscle rigidity
- Impaired judgment
- Complaints of joint/muscle stiffness

Emergency care for generalized hypothermia includes:

1. Take appropriate BSI precautions.

2. Perform a primary assessment and ensure adequate breathing.

3. Remove the patient from the cold environment, but do not allow the patient to walk or exert himself in any way.

4. Protect the patient from further heat loss.

5. Remove any wet clothing and place a blanket over and under the patient. Remember to handle the patient gently.

6. Administer oxygen as per local protocols.

7. Monitor vital signs.

8. Do not give the patient anything to eat or drink (including hot coffee or tea or alcohol).

Some cases of generalized hypothermia are extreme. The patient might be unresponsive with skin that is cold to the touch and show no vital signs. You cannot assume that this patient is dead. Assess the pulse for at least 30-45 seconds. If there is no pulse, begin

KEY POINT ▼

Do not allow the patient to smoke or drink alcohol or caffeine. These substances may affect blood vessels and worsen the patient's condition.

CPR immediately and arrange for immediate transport. In most instances a patient will not be pronounced dead until the hospital team can bring the patient's core temperature to within a normal range.

Localized Cold Injury

Another common cold-related injury is characterized by the freezing or near freezing of a body part. This is referred to as a localized cold injury or **frostbite** (Figure 16.5). It is caused by a significant exposure to cold temperature (below 32°F or 0°C). It mainly occurs in the extremities and most commonly affects the fingers, toes, ears, face, and nose.

A typical scenario where a localized cold emergency can occur is someone who is outdoors during the winter and unprotected by scarves, gloves, or boots for a prolonged period of time. The core of the body remains warm, but the exposed extremities are susceptible to the impact of cold and wind. Most patients will describe a localized cold injury as starting with a cold sensation to the extremities that leads to pain, followed by numbness. This is the classic progression of symptoms (Scan 16.2).

Signs and symptoms of a localized cold injury may include the following:

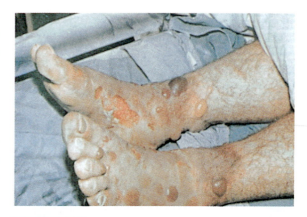

Figure 16.5 • Severe frostbite.

frostbite ▶ localized cold injury in which the skin is frozen.

Early Signs

- Numbness and tingling to the exposed area
- Slow or absent capillary refill
- Skin remains soft
- If thawed, tingling and pain are present

Late Signs

- White, waxy skin (in light-skinned patients)
- Firm to frozen feeling upon palpation
- Swelling may be present
- Blisters may be present
- If thawed, may appear flushed with areas of purple and blanching

Emergency care for a localized cold injury is as follows:

1. Take appropriate BSI precautions.

2. Perform a primary assessment and ensure adequate breathing.

3. Remove the patient from the cold environment and protect from further cold exposure.

4. Remove any wet or constrictive clothing.

5. If it is an early injury:

- Manually stabilize the extremity or affected part.
- Cover the affected part.
- Do not rub or massage it.
- Do not re-expose the injured part to cold.

From the Medical Director

Localized Cold Injury

If you are providing care to a frostbite victim in a remote area where there is a long delay in receiving care, you should avoid warming if there is any chance the injury might refreeze.

CONDITION	SKIN SURFACE	TISSUE UNDER SKIN	SKIN COLOR
Early, superficial	Soft	Soft	White
Late, deep	Hard	Initially soft, progressing to hard	White and waxy, progressing to blotchy white, then to yellow-gray to blue-gray

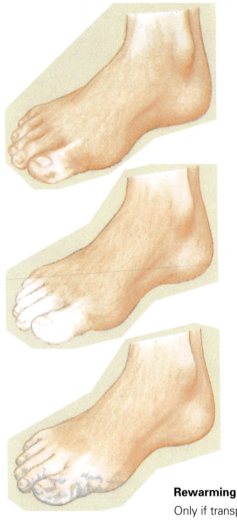

Early, Superficial

Slow onset with numbing of affected part. Have the patient rewarm the part with his own body heat. Tingling and burning sensations are common during rewarming.

Late, Deep

Tissues below the surface initially will have their normal bounce. Protect the entire limb. Handle gently. Keep the patient at rest and provide external warmth to injury site. Untreated, this will progress to where the tissue below the surface will feel hard. Provide the same care you would for early superficial cooling. Immediate EMS transport is recommended.

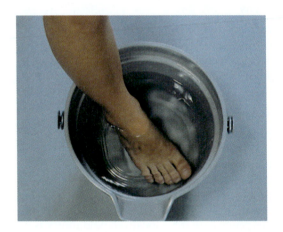

Rewarming

Only if transport is delayed in case of late or deep local cooling and if medical direction allows, rewarm the affected part by immersing it in warm water (100°F to 105°F [37.7°C to 40.5°C]). Do not allow the body part to touch the container bottom or side. After rewarming, gently dry the part and pad between fingers or toes. Dress the affected area, cover and elevate the limb, and keep the patient warm. *Do not rewarm* if there is any chance that the tissue may refreeze, usually due to extended exposure.

6. If it is a late injury:

- Remove jewelry from the injured part.
- Cover the injured part with dry, sterile dressings. Place dressing between fingers and toes prior to covering.
- Do not break blisters.
- Do not rub or massage the injured part.
- Do not apply heat.
- Do not rewarm. (Some jurisdictions allow rewarming. Check with medical direction.)
- If legs are affected, do not allow the patient to walk.

"My name is Aubree," AJ hears the woman say behind him as he lifts Melody's arm and gently rolls her into the recovery position. "My friend, she, she just had some kind of seizure, and we think she is having a heat stroke. We're in the middle of the main hiking trail at Armstrong Woods."

As Aubree continues to describe their location to dispatch, AJ checks Melody's breathing and her pulse, both of which are rapid. Melody has already removed most of her clothing, which are piled nearby. AJ opens two of the water bottles and soaks her remaining clothes and skin.

"I think I'm going to throw up," Aubree says as she sits down by Melody. Her coloring is becoming pinker as she begins fanning herself.

"Here," AJ says, passing her the last water bottle. "Slowly drink some of this and stay right there in the shade. Help will be here soon, and you can help me keep Melody cool."

Bites and Stings

Our environment contains many insects and animals that can pose a threat when people come in contact with them. Insect stings, spider bites, stings from marine life, and snakebites can all be sources of injected poisons. Some of those poisons cause very serious emergencies, while others cause only a minor local reaction such as redness and swelling.

Assessment of a patient who has suffered a bite or sting involves an inspection of the injury site. Look for redness and swelling directly at the site (Figure 16.6). The patient will usually report pain, itching, or discomfort at the site. Localized redness and swelling is quite normal. If you observe the area of redness expanding, involving hives or increased swelling—especially involving the face, neck, and chest—the patient may be developing anaphylaxis. Be alert for other indications of anaphylaxis, such as difficulty breathing, hoarseness, difficulty swallowing, wheezing, and altered mental status.

It will be important to determine if the patient has a history of past reactions to similar bites or stings. In the event the patient has a history of severe allergic reactions, remain alert for anaphylaxis.

OBJECTIVES

8. Describe the signs and symptoms of emergencies related to bites and stings.

9. Explain the appropriate assessment and care for a patient experiencing an emergency related to a bite or sting.

Assessment and Emergency Care

Gather information from the patient, bystanders, and the scene. Signs and symptoms of a reaction to a bite or sting may include:

- Noticeable puncture marks on the skin
- Pain at or around the injury site
- Redness and itching at the injury site
- Weakness, dizziness
- Difficulty breathing
- Headache
- Nausea
- Altered mental status

Emergency care for a localized reaction includes:

1. Take appropriate BSI precautions.
2. Perform a scene size-up and ensure that the scene is safe for both you and the patient.
3. Perform a primary assessment and ensure adequate breathing.

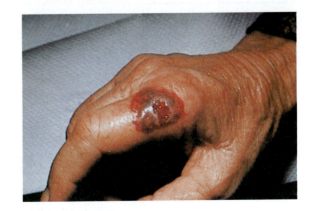

Figure 16.6 • The local reaction caused by a brown recluse spider several days after the initial bite.

Figure 16.7 • If the insect stinger is still present, remove it by scraping it away with the edge of a credit card or similar object.

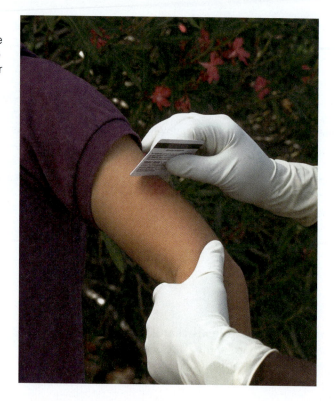

4. Scrape away noticeable bee and wasp stingers and venom sacs. Do not attempt to pinch or pull out stingers because it may force more venom into the wound. A plastic credit card works well as a scraper (Figure 16.7).

5. Place a cold pack over the injury site.

6. Administer oxygen as per local protocols.

Anaphylactic Shock

anaphylactic shock ▶ a severe allergic reaction in which a person goes into shock. Also called *anaphylaxis* or *allergy shock*.

Anaphylactic shock, or allergy shock, occurs when people come into contact with a substance to which they are severely allergic. The body considers the substance an invader and reacts to counteract it. This is a life-threatening emergency. There is no way of knowing if patients will remain stable, grow worse slowly or rapidly, or overcome the reaction on their own. For some, death is a certain outcome unless special care is provided quickly.

There are many different causes of anaphylactic shock, such as insect bites and stings, including bee stings; foods (nuts, spices, shellfish); inhaled substances, including dust and pollens; certain chemicals; and medications.

Signs and symptoms of anaphylactic shock include:

- Burning, itching, or breaking out of the skin (such as hives or some type of rash)
- Breathing that is difficult and rapid, with possible chest pains and wheezing
- Pulse that is rapid, very weak, or not detected
- Lips that turn blue (cyanosis)

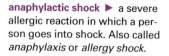

Learn more about allergic reactions to stings.

From the Medical Director

Anaphylactic Shock

Anaphylaxis is not a simple allergic reaction but a life-threatening condition. It must be treated quickly and aggressively if the patient is to survive.

- Swelling of the face and tongue
- Restlessness
- Changes in mental status, such as fainting or unresponsiveness

As you perform your primary assessment, ask if the patient is allergic to anything and if so, has he been in contact with that substance. Remember to always look for medical identification jewelry, which may indicate that there is an allergy problem.

To provide emergency care to patients with anaphylaxis, follow the same procedures used for shock. (See Chapter 18.) In some jurisdictions, EMTs and Emergency Medical Responders are authorized to carry and administer the epinephrine autoinjector for cases of anaphylaxis. Check local protocols, and always call for medical direction before assisting a patient with medications.

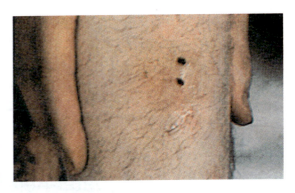

Figure 16.8 • A typical rattlesnake bite.

Snakebites

Between 7,000 and 8,000 people in the United States are bitten by poisonous snakes each year, with fewer than 20 deaths being reported annually (Figure 16.8). (In the United States, more people die each year from bee and wasp stings than from snakebites.) Signs and symptoms of poisoning may take several hours to develop. Death from a snakebite is usually not a rapidly occurring event unless anaphylactic shock also occurs. Keeping the patient calm will be an important part of your care. There is usually time to activate the EMS system and to provide care for the patient.

Consider all snakebites to be from poisonous snakes. The patient or bystanders may indicate that the snake was not poisonous. They could be mistaken. If you see the live snake, do not approach it to determine its species. Only if safe to do so from a distance, note its size and coloration.

Signs and symptoms of snakebite may include:

- Noticeable bite to the skin. This may appear as nothing more than a discoloration.
- Pain and swelling in the area of the bite. This may be slow to develop, taking 30 minutes to several hours.
- Rapid pulse and labored breathing
- Weakness
- Vision problems
- Nausea and vomiting

Emergency care for snakebite includes:

1. Take appropriate BSI precautions.
2. Perform a scene size-up and ensure the scene is safe for you and the patient
3. Perform a primary assessment and ensure that breathing is adequate.
4. Locate the fang marks and clean this site with soap and water.
5. Remove from the bitten extremity any rings, bracelets, and other constricting items.
6. Keep the extremity immobilized. Try to keep the bitten area at or below the level of the heart.
7. Provide supplemental oxygen if available.
8. Provide care for shock, and monitor vital signs.

If you know that the patient will not reach a medical facility within 30 minutes after having been bitten, or if the signs and symptoms of the patient begin to worsen, some experts suggest the application of a constricting band proximal to the fang marks. The band should be about two inches wide, placed about two inches from the wound, or above the swelling. (Never place a band directly on a joint.)

The constricting band should be placed so that you can slide your finger underneath it. Do not place it so tight that it cuts off arterial flow. Monitor for a distal pulse at the wrist or ankle, depending on the extremity involved. Many EMS systems recommend constricting bands for all cases of snakebite. Check with your instructor regarding your local protocol.

Do not place an ice bag or cold pack on the bite unless you are directed to do so by a physician or the poison control center.

Recent research suggests the application of a pressure bandage around the entire length of the affected extremity. When properly applied, it can be a safe and effective means of slowing the spread of the venom. The bandage should be applied comfortably tight and snug. It is tight enough if a finger can be easily slipped between the bandage and the skin.

Water-Related Incidents

Most people, when they think of water-related incidents, tend to think only of **drowning**. Injuries occur on, in, and near the water. Boating, waterskiing, and diving incidents produce airway obstructions, fractures, bleeding, and soft-tissue injuries. Other types of incidents, such as falls from bridges and watercraft collisions, also involve the water. In these cases, the victims suffer injuries normally associated with the underlying mechanism of injury plus the effects of the water hazard (drowning, hypothermia, delayed care because of complicated rescue, and so on).

Sometimes, the mishap or drowning may have been caused by a medical emergency that took place while the patient was in the water or on a boat. Knowing how the incident occurred may give you clues to detecting the medical emergency. As with all aspects of Emergency Medical Responder care, consider the mechanism of injury or nature of illness and perform a thorough patient assessment. They may be critical in deciding the procedures to be followed when caring for a patient.

Learn to associate the problems of drowning with scenes other than swimming pools and beaches. Remember, bathtub drownings do occur. Only a few inches of water are needed for a person to drown. As an Emergency Medical Responder, take particular care to look for the following when your patient is the victim of a water-related mishap:

- Airway obstruction may be from water, foreign matter in the airway, or a swollen airway (often seen if the neck is injured in a dive). Spasms along the airway are common in cases of submersion in water.
- Cardiac arrest is usually related to respiratory arrest.
- Injuries to the head and neck are to be expected in boating, waterskiing, and diving incidents, but they also occur in cases of drowning.
- While performing a patient assessment, be alert for suspected fractures, soft-tissue injuries, and internal bleeding. Constantly monitor patients for the signs and symptoms of shock.
- The water does not have to be very cold and the length of stay in the water does not have to be very long for hypothermia to occur.

Reaching the Victim

The U.S. Coast Guard, the American Red Cross, and the YMCA offer water safety and rescue courses. Unless you are trained in water rescue, do not go into the water to save someone.

If the patient is close to shore or poolside, attempt to reach and pull the patient from the water. If unable to reach the victim with your hand, attempt to use a branch, a fishing pole, an oar, a stick, or other such object. A towel, a shirt, or an article of your own clothing may work as well. In cases where there is no object near at hand or conditions are such that you may only have one opportunity to grab the person (e.g., strong currents), lie down flat on your stomach and extend your arm or leg (not recommended for the nonswimmer). In all cases, make sure that your position is secure and that you will not be pulled into the water. This is critical if you are extending an arm or leg to the person. If the person is alert but too far away to be pulled from the water, then you must carefully throw an object that will float. A personal flotation device (PFD), life jacket, or ring buoy (life preserver) is ideal, but those objects may not be at the scene. If that is the case, then the best course of action is to throw anything that will float. Objects you might use include inflated automobile tubes, foam cushions, plastic jugs, logs, boards, plastic picnic containers, surfboards, pieces of wood, large balls, and plastic toys. Two empty, capped plastic milk jugs can keep an adult afloat for hours. It is best to tie rope to the objects so that they can be retrieved if they do not land near the patient. You may have to add some water to lightweight plastic jugs so that you can throw them the required distance.

Once you are sure that the person has a flotation device or floating object to hold on to, try to find a way to tow the patient to shore. Throw the patient a line or another flotation device attached to a line. Make sure that your own position is a safe one. If you must reduce the distance for throwing the line, and if conditions are safe and you are a strong swimmer, wade no deeper than your waist.

Again, in water-rescue situations (Figure 16.9), begin by trying to pull the patient from the water. If this cannot be done, throw objects that will float and try to tow the patient from the water. Unless you are a good swimmer and trained in water rescue and lifesaving, do not swim to the patient. Even so, have on a personal flotation device.

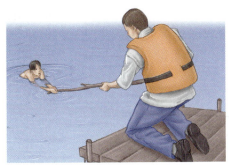
Reach

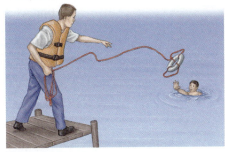
Throw

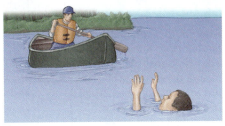
Then go

Figure 16.9 • Reach for the victim. Throw an object to him. If necessary, go to the victim if you are trained to do so.

Care for the Patient

Patient with No Neck or Spine Injuries

Once the patient is safely removed from the water, you should:

1. Perform a primary assessment.
2. If needed, provide mouth-to-mask resuscitation as quickly as possible. Check for airway obstruction.
3. Provide CPR, if needed. As in all such cases, make certain that someone has activated the EMS system.
4. If the patient is breathing and has a pulse, check for bleeding and attempt to control any serious bleeding that you find.
5. If there is breathing and a pulse, perform a patient assessment. But first cover the patient to conserve body heat. Also be sure to put something under the patient to prevent heat loss. Uncover only those areas of the patient's body involved in assessment. Care for any problems you may find. If hypothermia is suspected, remove excess wet clothing to minimize heat loss.
6. If the patient can be moved, take him to a warm place. Do not allow the patient to walk. Handle the patient gently at all times.
7. Provide care for shock.

You may encounter water in the airway of a patient who was pulled from the water. Turn the patient on his side and allow excess water to exit the mouth. Watch the patient's chest rise and fall with each breath.

Many times, a patient with water in the airway will also have water in the stomach. Current American Heart Association and American Red Cross guidelines indicate that you should not attempt to relieve water or air from the patient's stomach (unless immediate suctioning is available) due to the risk of forcing material from the stomach into the patient's airway, even to the point of entering the lungs. When gastric distention occurs, reposition the airway and continue with resuscitation, making sure the breaths are slow and full.

Human beings have a reaction in cold water that is similar to other mammals. This reaction is called the *mammalian diving reflex*. When the face of a person or other mammal is submerged in cold water, the mammalian diving reflex slows down the body's metabolism, which results in a decrease in oxygen consumption. At the same time, the reflex causes a redistribution of blood to more vital organs—the brain, heart, and lungs. The diving reflex is more pronounced in infants and children, and they may fare better in cold-water drowning

KEY POINT ▼

Drowning victims who are resuscitated are very likely to vomit. Rescuers should have suction ready and be prepared to clear the airway when this occurs.

than adults. Start CPR on all drowning victims as soon as they are pulled from the water. Cases have been reported in which cold-water drowning victims, especially children, were revived and fully recovered after being in the water for longer than 30 minutes.

Patient with Neck or Spine Injuries

Injuries to the neck (cervical spine) and the rest of the spinal column can occur during many water-related incidents. For Emergency Medical Responder care, you will not be expected to know how to use long spine boards and other floating, rigid devices for rescue situations.

When a patient with possible neck and spine injuries is responsive and you are in shallow warm water, stabilize the patient until the EMS system responds with personnel trained to remove the patient from the water. Keep the patient floating in a face-up position while you support the back and stabilize the head and neck.

If a patient is unresponsive, neck and spine injuries may not be easily detected. In such a situation, assume that the patient has them and provide care accordingly. Also assume neck and spine injuries whenever you find a patient with head injuries.

If you arrive at the scene and find the unresponsive patient has already been removed from the water, have someone activate the EMS system and begin your primary assessment. Provide life support care as needed, using the jaw-thrust maneuver rather than the head-tilt/chin-lift maneuver. After breathing and circulation are ensured, and bleeding is cared for, perform a secondary assessment, providing care as needed. Keep the patient warm and provide care for shock.

If the patient is still in the water, do not attempt a rescue unless you are a good swimmer, are trained to do so, and have others at hand who can help you. Providing care for a possible spine-injury patient still in the water requires you to do the following (Scan 16.3):

KEY POINT ▼

Attempt to remove the patient from the water yourself *only* if trained rescue personnel will not arrive soon and the patient has problems with the ABCs. You must make every effort to maintain in-line stabilization of the patient's body.

1. Turn the patient face up in the water. This should be done while you are in the water and wearing a personal flotation device. To turn the patient, you should:
   a. Position yourself at patient's side. Grasp the patient's arms midway between the elbow and shoulder and gently float them above the patient's head.
   b. Clasp the patient's arms firmly against his head to brace the neck and keep the head in line. Move forward in the water to bring the patient's body to the surface and in line.
   c. Rotate the patient by pushing down on the near arm and pulling the far arm toward you, making sure you brace the patient's head firmly with his arms. Do not lift the patient.
   d. Once the patient is face up, maintain pressure on the patient's arms to brace the head.
   e. In shallow water, you can hold the patient's arms with one hand and support the hips with the other.
   f. In deeper water, continue to move toward shallow water where you can stand or can be supported by someone else.

2. If necessary, begin your primary assessment while the patient is still in the water.

3. If needed, provide rescue breathing as soon as possible. Use the jaw-thrust maneuver to protect the patient's neck and spine. CPR will not be effective while the patient is in the water.

4. If someone is there to help you, have him support the patient along the midline of the back while you provide support to the patient's head and neck. Float the patient to shore and continue to provide back and neck support. Wait for trained rescue personnel equipped with a backboard and cervical collar to remove the patient from the water.

5. Once the patient is out of the water, attempts at resuscitation can begin. In some cases, depending on the boat's stability and water conditions, you may be able to provide effective CPR in the boat until other rescuers arrive.

6. If the patient is breathing, check for and control all serious bleeding. Cover the patient to conserve body heat and perform a patient assessment, caring for any injuries you may find.

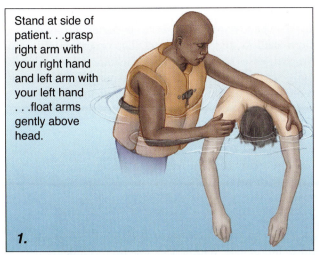

1. Stand at side of patient. . .grasp right arm with your right hand and left arm with your left hand . . .float arms gently above head.

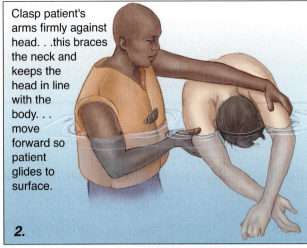

2. Clasp patient's arms firmly against head. . .this braces the neck and keeps the head in line with the body. . . move forward so patient glides to surface.

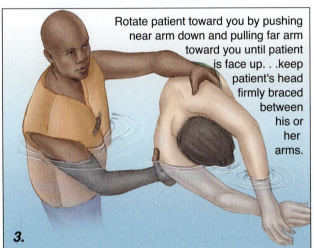

3. Rotate patient toward you by pushing near arm down and pulling far arm toward you until patient is face up. . .keep patient's head firmly braced between his or her arms.

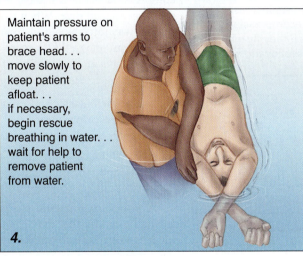

4. Maintain pressure on patient's arms to brace head. . . move slowly to keep patient afloat. . . if necessary, begin rescue breathing in water. . . wait for help to remove patient from water.

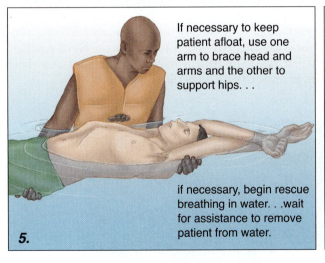

5. If necessary to keep patient afloat, use one arm to brace head and arms and the other to support hips. . .

if necessary, begin rescue breathing in water. . .wait for assistance to remove patient from water.

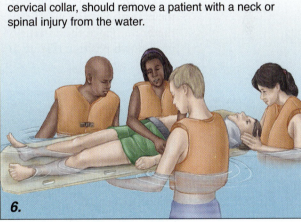

6. Only specially trained personnel, using a backboard and cervical collar, should remove a patient with a neck or spinal injury from the water.

Submersion Injuries

Other injuries related to submersion in water are commonly associated with the sport of scuba diving. Incidents involving scuba diving can produce a variety of injuries resulting in a temporary loss of consciousness or even death. Two common problems seen in submersion incidents related to scuba diving are gas bubbles in the diver's blood and the "bends."

Small bubbles of gas can form in the bloodstream when a diver ascends too quickly. These bubbles can form an *air embolism* that will obstruct blood flow wherever they form and cause severe pain and even death. This happens for many reasons, though it is most

OBJECTIVES

10. Describe common factors leading to submersion injuries.

13. Describe the signs and symptoms of a submersion injury.

often associated with divers who hold their breath because of inadequate training, equipment failure, underwater emergency, or when trying to conserve air during a long dive.

Air embolism can develop in both shallow and deep waters. The onset is rapid, with signs of personality changes and distorted senses sometimes giving the impression of drunkenness. The patient may have convulsions and rapidly become unresponsive. You should suspect possible air embolism when the patient has any of the following signs or symptoms:

- Personality changes
- Distorted senses; blurred vision is most common
- Chest pain
- Numbness and tingling sensations in the arms and/or legs
- General weakness, or weakness of one or more limbs
- Frothy blood in the mouth or nose
- Convulsions

KEY POINT ▼

Scuba divers increase the risk of decompression sickness if they fly within 12 hours following a dive.

The *bends* are really part of what is called *decompression sickness*. Patients with decompression sickness usually are those individuals who have come up too quickly from a deep, prolonged dive. When they do this, nitrogen gas is trapped in their tissues and may find its way into the bloodstream. The onset of the bends is usually slow for scuba divers, taking from one to 48 hours to appear.

The signs and symptoms of decompression sickness include:

- Fatigue
- Pain to the muscles and joints (the bends)
- Numbness or paralysis
- Choking, coughing, and/or labored breathing
- Chest pains
- Collapse and unresponsiveness
- Blotches on the skin (mottling); sometimes these rashes keep changing appearance

OBJECTIVE

14. Explain the appropriate care for a victim of a submersion injury.

If you think a patient has gas bubbles in the blood or decompression sickness due to a dive, be certain that the dispatcher is aware of the problem. Dispatch may wish to direct the EMTs to take the patient to a special facility (hyperbaric trauma center) where a patient is exposed to oxygen under greatly increased pressure conditions. This procedure is done in a sealed hyperbaric chamber.

While waiting for the EMTs to arrive, provide care for shock and constantly monitor the patient. Positioning of the patient is critical to avoid gas bubbles in the blood reaching the brain. Place the patient on his left side. The patient may also be placed in a slight head-down position (Figure 16.10). Provide oxygen as per local protocols.

Figure 16.10 • For scuba accidents, position the patient head down.

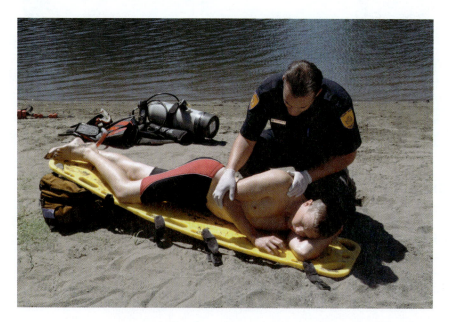

Ice-Related Incidents

Ice rescues require special training. Unless you are trained specifically to work on ice, do not attempt a rescue. You may walk on an undetected thin spot, fall through the ice, and quickly drown. All rescuers who are on or at the edge of the ice must wear personal flotation devices.

The major problem faced in ice rescue is reaching the victim. Never walk out to the person or attempt to enter the water through a hole in the ice to find the victim. Never attempt an ice rescue by yourself unless you have some basic equipment, such as a personal flotation device and a ladder, and you are specifically trained in one-rescuer techniques. Never go onto ice that is rapidly breaking up. Your best course of action will be to work with others from a safe ice surface or the shore (Figure 16.11).

As the first choice of action, throw a line to the victim or reach out with a stick or a pole. If the victim is not holding onto the ice but trying to keep afloat in open water, throw anything that will float. Do not try to go onto the ice to rescue the victim. Call for help immediately. Ice rescues require special training, protective clothing, and rescue equipment.

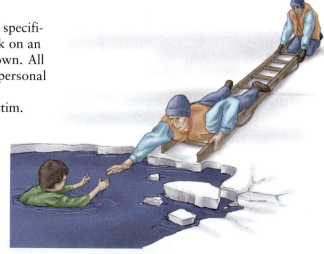

Figure 16.11 • A safe ice rescue requires teamwork from specially trained responders.

If you have had specialized training and the necessary equipment and personnel and you have to go onto the ice to get the patient, it is strongly recommended that you work with other trained help. Pushing a long ladder out onto the ice and then crawling along the ladder is a very effective method of safe rescue, providing someone is holding the ladder from a safe position. If enough people are on hand, a human chain can be formed to reach the patient; however, these rescuers should be trained and wearing PFDs.

Expect to find injuries with any patient who has fallen through the ice. Broken leg bones are common. Hypothermia is often a problem and should always be considered. Do not attempt to actively rewarm a severely hypothermic patient. Simply get him to a warm environment, remove wet clothing, and cover him with blankets to minimize further heat loss.

Activate the EMS system for all patients who have had incidents on ice or have been in cold water. There may be injuries that are difficult to detect and problems because of the cold that may be delayed.

CHAPTER REVIEW

Summary

- The body losses heat through the following five ways: radiation, conduction, convection, evaporation, and respiration.

- A hot and humid environment may cause the body to generate too much heat, which can create an abnormally high body temperature, known as hyperthermia.

- Early signs and symptoms of hyperthermia include cramps, excessive sweating, rapid weak pulse, weakness.

- Heat cramps are sudden and sometimes severe muscle cramps, most often occurring in the legs.

- Heat exhaustion results from prolonged exposure to heat, which creates moist, pale skin that may feel normal or cool to the touch.

- Heat stroke results from prolonged exposure to heat and causes hot, dry or moist skin; altered mental status; and rapid breathing. This is a life-threatening emergency.

- Emergency care for heat emergencies includes removing patients from the hot environment, cooling them with water, and fanning them.

- In cold environments, body heat may be lost quicker than it can be generated. Rapid heat loss creates a state of low body temperature known as hypothermia, or a generalized cold emergency.

- Patients suffering from hypothermia will have cool skin temperature, shivering, decreased mental status, stiff or rigid posture, and poor judgment. The environmental temperature does not have to be below freezing for hypothermia to occur.

- Frostbite is characterized by the freezing or near freezing of a body part. Frostbite patients will experience a feeling of cold followed by pain and finally numbness or tingling.

- Emergency care for frostbite includes removing the patient from the cold environment, removing any wet clothes, keeping the patient calm and warm, and stabilizing any cold extremity.

- When providing care for injected poisons other than snakebite, care for shock, scrape away stingers and venom sacs, and place an ice bag or cold pack over the area.

- For snakebite, keep the patient calm and lying down, clean the site, keep bitten extremities immobilized, alert the dispatcher, and provide care for shock.

- Anaphylactic shock, or allergy shock, is a life-threatening emergency. It is brought about when people come into contact with a substance to which they are allergic (bee stings, insect bites, chemicals, foods, dusts, pollens, drugs).

- Signs of anaphylactic shock may include burning or itching skin, hives, difficulty breathing, rapid, weak pulse, swelling of the face and tongue, cyanosis, and altered mental status.

- Care for anaphylactic shock is the same as for other cases of shock. Transport the patient to a hospital as soon as possible and care for the patient according to local protocol. Ask the patient about allergies during the interview. Be certain to look for a medical identification device.

- Many submersion injuries are related to the sport of scuba diving and result when a person ascends too quickly.

- The "bends" result when tiny gas bubbles form in the tissues, causing pain.

- In severe cases, these bubbles can form an air embolism that can obstruct blood flow, resulting in death.

Take Action

TWO STINGS DON'T MAKE A BITE

Environments vary widely depending on where you live. In addition to differences in climate and weather, there are differences in the types of creatures that inhabit the areas where we live. In this activity, identify at least two creatures that are common to your environment or region. They can be things that sting or bite and are venomous to some degree, but they must be common to your area.

1. Identify two creatures. They can be animals, reptiles, or insects that are venomous to humans.

2. Utilizing the Internet, research the common signs and symptoms that result when someone is bitten or stung.

3. Research the most appropriate care that the Emergency Medical Responder can provide for a bite/sting. How does the care differ once the patient gets more advanced care?

4. Share your results with your fellow classmates to learn about other creatures that you did not research. Did your results match what your fellow classmates found?

First on Scene Run Review

Recall the events of the "First on Scene" scenario in this chapter and answer the following questions, which are related to the call. Rationales are offered in the Answer Key at the back of the book.

1. Recall the events of the "First on Scene" scenario in this chapter. How would Melody's friend know that she was suffering from heat stroke?

2. Does AJ need to ask permission before helping Melody? Why or why not?

3. What information does AJ need to give the EMS responders?

Quick Quiz

To check your understanding of the chapter, answer the following questions. Then compare your answers to those in the Answer Key at the back of the book.

1. In which one of the following situations is the patient losing body heat primarily by conduction?
   a. A 66-year-old male is found lying on the frozen ground without a coat.
   b. A 14-year-old male is wearing wet clothing after falling out of his boat while fishing.
   c. A 23-year-old female is outside in cool, windy weather.
   d. An elderly female patient is breathing into the cool night air.

2. More serious heat-related injuries should be suspected when the patient presents with:
   a. feeling lightheaded.
   b. muscle cramps.
   c. hot, dry skin.
   d. weakness.

3. Your patient is a 34-year-old male who has been working outside in a hot, humid climate. He is alert and oriented, complaining of feeling weak and dizzy. His skin is cool and moist, and he has a heart rate of 104, a blood pressure of 110/70, and respirations of 16. You should:
   a. place cold packs at the groin, armpits, and neck.
   b. move the patient to a cool area in the shade.
   c. offer the patient some salt tablets.
   d. wet the skin, turn the air conditioning on high, and vigorously fan the patient.

4. A patient who is experiencing an abnormally low body core temperature is said to be:
   a. hyperthermic.
   b. cyanotic.
   c. hypothermic.
   d. hyperglycemic.

5. An injury characterized by the freezing or near freezing of a body part is known as:
   a. frostbite.
   b. frostnip.
   c. hypothermia.
   d. cold bite.

6. All of the following are appropriate steps in the management of a patient with a generalized cold emergency, EXCEPT:
   a. removing the patient from the cold environment.
   b. protecting him from further heat loss.
   c. providing warm liquids to drink.
   d. monitoring his vital signs.

7. A patient who presents with warm, moist skin; weakness; and nausea is likely experiencing.
   a. heat exhaustion.
   b. heat stroke.
   c. heat cramps.
   d. mild heat stroke.

8. Your patient was hiking and was bitten on the ankle by a rattlesnake. When caring for this patient, you should:
   a. keep the foot lower than the level of the patient's heart.
   b. elevate the foot on pillows.
   c. apply a tourniquet above the bite.
   d. apply ice to the area of the bite.

9. It is late winter and you respond to an alley to find a homeless man lying on the ground. Your patient presents with confusion, shivering, and muscle stiffness. Based on his presentation, this man's likely problem is:
   a. a localized cold injury.
   b. frostnip.
   c. generalized frostbite.
   d. generalized hypothermia.

10. You are caring for a person who fell from a rope swing, landed in the water, and is now unresponsive. She has a large laceration on the top of her head. You should:
   a. suspect spine injury.
   b. begin CPR in the water.
   c. drag her by one arm to shore.
   d. wait for EMS before beginning care.

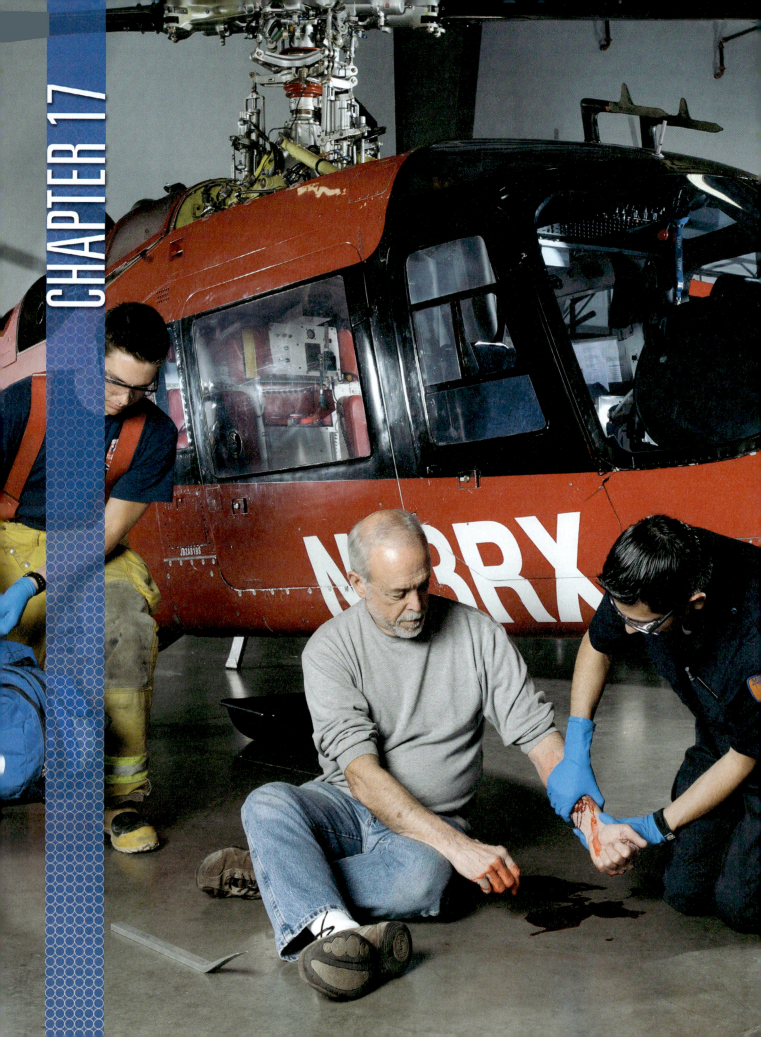

CHAPTER 17

Caring for Soft-Tissue Injuries and Bleeding

EDUCATION STANDARDS

• Trauma—Bleeding, Soft-Tissue Trauma

COMPETENCIES

• Uses simple knowledge to recognize and manage life threats based on assessment findings for an acutely injured patient while awaiting additional emergency medical response.

CHAPTER OVERVIEW

The leading cause of death in the United States for people under the age of 40 is trauma. As an Emergency Medical Responder, you will be called on to provide emergency care to trauma patients with injuries that range from minor to life threatening. Early assessment and intervention is crucial to the proper care of these patients. As an Emergency Medical Responder, you must be familiar with the care of soft-tissue injuries and how to help keep bleeding under control. This chapter introduces you to many of the most common types of soft-tissue injuries, including burns, as well as how to manage the bleeding that is so often associated with these injuries.

OBJECTIVES

Upon successful completion of this chapter, the student should be able to:

COGNITIVE

1. Define the following terms:
   a. amputation *(p. 374)*
   b. artery *(p. 357)*
   c. avulsion *(p. 373)*
   d. bandage *(p. 360)*
   e. blunt trauma *(p. 369)*
   f. capillary *(p. 358)*
   g. dressing *(p. 361)*
   h. hemostatic dressing *(p. 365)*
   i. multisystem trauma *(p. 370)*
   j. penetrating trauma *(p. 369)*
   k. shock *(p. 358)*
   l. tourniquet *(p. 363)*
   m. vein *(p. 357)*

2. Explain the importance of utilizing appropriate body substance isolation (BSI) precautions when caring for a patient with external bleeding. *(p. 358)*

3. Identify the characteristics of multisystem trauma. *(p. 370)*

4. Differentiate the characteristics of arterial, venous, and capillary bleeding. *(p. 358)*

5. Explain the proper care for a patient with active external bleeding. *(p. 360)*

6. Describe the signs and symptoms of internal bleeding. *(p. 367)*

7. Explain the proper care of a patient with suspected internal bleeding. *(p. 370)*

8. Describe common types if external soft-tissue injuries. *(p. 372)*

9. Explain the proper care for a patient with an impaled object. *(p. 375)*

10. Explain the proper care for an amputation injury. *(p. 376)*

11. Explain the proper care for nosebleed. *(p. 381)*

12. Explain the proper care for an injury to the eye. *(p. 378)*

13. Differentiate superficial, partial-thickness, and full-thickness burns. *(p. 384)*

14. Explain the process for determining percentage of body surface area (BSA) affected by a burn. *(p. 385)*

15. Explain the proper care for a patient with a superficial, partial-thickness, and full-thickness burn. *(p. 386)*

16. Differentiate the care for electrical, chemical, and thermal burns. *(p. 386)*

17. Explain the purpose of a dressing. *(p. 366)*

18. Explain the purpose of a bandage. *(p. 366)*

PSYCHOMOTOR

19. Demonstrate the proper care for a patient with suspected internal bleeding.

20. Demonstrate the proper techniques for controlling external bleeding.

21. Demonstrate the proper care of a patient with an impaled object.

22. Demonstrate the proper care of a patient with an amputation injury.

AFFECTIVE

23. Value the importance of proper body substance isolation (BSI) precautions when caring for patients with soft-tissue injuries.

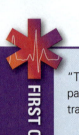

FIRST ON SCENE

"This darn fifth wheel lock is sticking," Casey shouts to his partner, Taine, as he crouches with his left arm under the trailer. "Rock the tractor a little."

Sitting in the driver's seat of the big rig watching his partner in the side mirror, Taine slips the transmission into reverse and eases off the clutch. The semi lurches backward, thundering into the empty trailer as Casey pulls on the handle to unlock it. Taine then pulls the stick down into a low forward gear and eases the clutch again.

The truck bounces forward this time, and the fifth wheel lock snaps free. Taine pulls the tractor forward about 10 feet, puts it in neutral, and sets the noisy parking brake. As he climbs down out of the cab, he notices Casey rolling around on the ground, holding his left hand close to his

body. It takes Taine a second before he sees the blood. And there is a lot of it.

"Ah, man. What happened, Casey?" He jogs over to his friend, careful not to step in the bright blood.

Casey, his face contorted in pain, just keeps cursing under his breath and rolling from side to side in the parking lot.

"Let's see your hand." Taine bends over and touches the other man's arm. Casey holds his left hand up for a moment, long enough for Taine to see that all of the skin and most of the flesh is gone from the ring finger. From the tip to where it meets the hand is now nothing more than a spindly red bone. Casey then buries his hand back close to his body and curses through clenched teeth.

Heart, Blood, and Blood Vessels

The Heart

The heart is the center of the circulatory system. It is responsible for pumping blood through the many miles of vessels and to all the body's tissues, organs, and systems. When an injury occurs and the soft tissues are damaged, blood will be forced out of the circulatory system with each beat of the heart (Figure 17.1).

Blood

Blood performs many functions necessary to sustain life. Blood carries oxygen to the body's cells and carries away carbon dioxide (Figure 17.2). It transports nutrients to the cells and carries away certain waste products. The blood contains cells that destroy bacteria and produce substances that help resist infection. There are elements in the blood that act with calcium and chemical factors to combine blood cells, forming sticky clots around cuts to help control bleeding. Without an adequate supply of blood circulating through your body, vital organs begin to starve for oxygen and nutrients and will eventually shut down. When organ systems begin to fail, death will soon follow.

The functions of blood are:

- To carry oxygen and carbon dioxide
- To carry food to the tissues (nutrition)
- To carry wastes from the tissues to the organs of excretion—kidneys, lungs, and liver
- To carry hormones, water, salts, and other compounds needed to keep the body's functions in balance (body regulation)
- To protect against disease-causing organisms (defense)

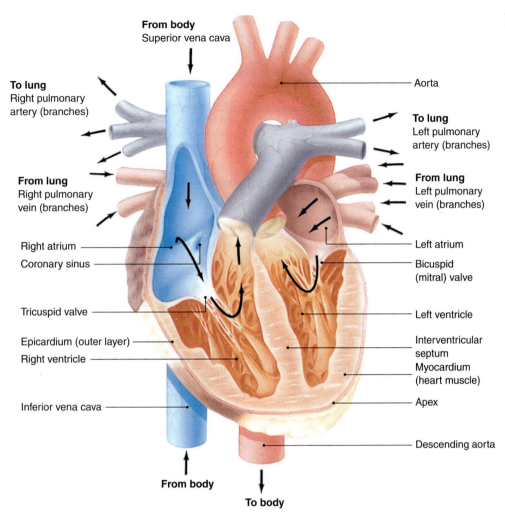

Figure 17.1 • The heart.

From body
Superior vena cava

To lung
Right pulmonary
artery (branches)

Aorta

To lung
Left pulmonary
artery (branches)

From lung
Right pulmonary
vein (branches)

From lung
Left pulmonary
vein (branches)

Right atrium

Coronary sinus

Left atrium

Bicuspid
(mitral) valve

Tricuspid valve

Left ventricle

Epicardium (outer layer)

Interventricular
septum

Right ventricle

Myocardium
(heart muscle)

Inferior vena cava

Apex

Descending aorta

From body

To body

Blood contains red blood cells, white blood cells, and elements involved in forming blood clots. These are carried by a watery, salty fluid called *plasma*. The volume of blood in the typical adult's body is approximately six liters (about 12 pints). When bleeding occurs, the body not only loses blood cells and clotting elements, but it also loses plasma and total fluid volume. This loss can be significant because the volume of blood must be maintained at a certain level to ensure good perfusion and nutrient exchange for the body's cells and vital organs. The body has more blood than is needed to produce minimum circulation. During bleeding, once this reserve is gone, the patient experiences circulatory system failure, followed very quickly by death. See Table 17.1 for blood volumes and lethal blood loss volumes for adults, children, and infants.

artery ▶ a vessel that carries blood away from the heart, typically carrying oxygenated blood.

vein ▶ a vessel that returns blood to the heart, typically carrying deoxygenated blood.

Blood Vessels

Arteries carry blood away from the heart and to the tissues, organs, and systems of the body. The largest artery is the *aorta*. The smallest artery is called an *arteriole*. At certain points in the body, where arteries are close to the skin surface, you can feel the blood pumping through the artery. These points are called *pulse points*, places where you can feel the pressure caused by the pumping heart and assess the heart rate.

Veins carry blood from the tissues, organs, and systems of the body back to the heart. The largest veins are the superior and inferior *vena cava*. The smallest vein is called a *venule*. The sizes in between are just referred to as *veins*. On some parts of the body you can see the blue of veins showing through skin where they are close to the surface.

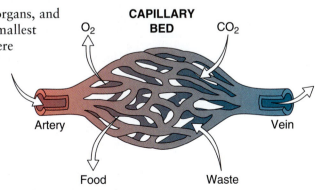

CAPILLARY BED

O_2

CO_2

Artery

Vein

Food

Waste

Figure 17.2 • Gas exchange.

TABLE 17.1	Blood Volumes and Serious Blood Loss		
PATIENT	**TOTAL BLOOD VOLUME**	**LETHAL BLOOD LOSS (RAPID)**
Adult male (154 pounds)	6.6 liters	2.2 liters
Adolescent (105 pounds)	3.3 liters	1.3 liters
Child (early to late childhood: depends on size)	1.5 to 2.0 liters	0.5 to 0.7 liters
Infant (newborn, normal weight range)	300+ milliliters	30 to 50 milliliters

capillary ▶ the smallest of the body's blood vessels.

The oxygen and nutrients carried by arteries are passed off to the body's cells when the blood reaches a small system of vessels called **capillaries**. Capillaries act as an exchange point for nutrients and wastes. Some of our organs act as disposal and maintenance organs, such as the kidneys and liver, but the heart is the organ that works with the lungs to replenish oxygen. Once the blood has dropped off its supply of oxygen for the body's cells to use, it travels from the capillary system into the veins and back to the heart, through the lungs to pick up oxygen, and back to the heart again to be pumped through vessels to the body. By the time blood reaches the capillaries, pressure and speed are greatly reduced and the beating action of the heart no longer causes pulsations. The adequate supply of well-oxygenated blood to the vital organs and tissues is called *perfusion*. Good perfusion is essential to life.

Bleeding

Understanding the circulatory system and how it functions will assist you in assessing and caring for patients with soft-tissue injuries. Keep the following general considerations in mind while you learn how to provide emergency care for patients with soft-tissue injuries:

- *Body substance isolation (BSI) precautions.* The risk of infectious disease should always be assessed and minimized when caring for bleeding patients. BSI precautions must be taken routinely to avoid direct contact with blood and other potentially infectious body fluids. Gloves should be worn during every patient encounter. Additional equipment (goggles, gown, mask) also should be used when there is an increased risk of contact with blood or other body fluids, such as in cases of childbirth or when a patient is spitting or vomiting blood.

- *Severity of blood loss.* The severity of blood loss should be based on the patient's signs and symptoms and an estimation of visible blood loss. If signs and symptoms of **shock** are present, bleeding should be considered serious. Shock will be discussed in more detail in Chapter 18.
- *Body's normal response to bleeding.* The body's automatic response to bleeding is blood vessel constriction and clotting. In cases of major bleeding, however, clotting may not occur because the flow of blood from the wound is too great to allow for the formation of a clot.

Uncontrolled bleeding always should be taken seriously. If not stopped, it will lead to shock and eventually death.

External Bleeding

Bleeding can be classified as external or internal. The assessment and care of both kinds of bleeding are presented in this chapter. External bleeding may be classified as (Figure 17.3):

- *Arterial bleeding.* Arterial bleeding occurs when the arteries carrying blood away from the heart are damaged. The bleeding is often characterized by a spurting action with each beat of the heart. The color of arterial blood is bright red because it

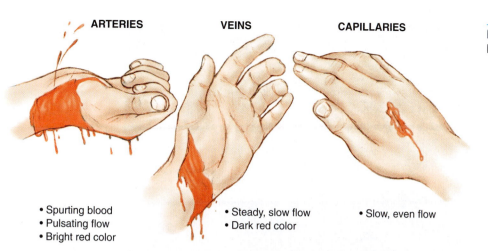

ARTERIES   VEINS   CAPILLARIES

- Spurting blood
- Pulsating flow
- Bright red color

- Steady, slow flow
- Dark red color

- Slow, even flow

Figure 17.3 • Three types of bleeding.

contains oxygen. Depending on the size of the artery that has been damaged, a great deal of blood can be lost in a short amount of time.

- *Venous bleeding.* Venous bleeding occurs when vessels that return blood to the heart have been damaged. Veins often lie close to the surface of the skin. Venous bleeding is characterized by a steady flow of dark red blood. Depending on the size of the vein affected, venous bleeding can also be serious.
- *Capillary bleeding.* Capillaries are tiny blood vessels that are contained within the skin. Capillary bleeding is characterized by a slow oozing of bright red blood from tissues. Capillary bleeding is common with minor scrapes and abrasions to the skin.

Evaluating External Bleeding

Of the three types of external bleeding, arterial bleeding is usually the most serious. This is because the blood within the arteries is under much higher pressure than that contained within the veins. The pressure created with each beat of the heart can prevent blood clot formation. Arterial bleeding can take several minutes or more to clot. Because arteries are typically located deep within body structures, capillary and venous bleeding is seen more often than arterial bleeding.

Venous bleeding can range from very minor to very severe. Some veins are located near the surface of the body, and many are large enough to be seen through the skin. Other veins are deep in the body and can be as large as arteries. Bleeding from a deep vein can produce rapid blood loss. Surface bleeding from a vein can be profuse, but blood loss is not as rapid as that seen from arteries and deep veins because of their smaller diameters and lower pressure. Veins have a tendency to collapse as soon as they are cut. This often reduces the severity of venous bleeding.

Most individuals experience little difficulty with capillary bleeding. The blood oozes slowly, and clotting is very likely to occur within a few minutes. However, the larger the area of the wound, the more likely is the chance of infection. Capillary bleeding requires care to stop blood flow and reduce contamination.

In emergency care, arterial and large vein bleeding are given priority over small vein and capillary bleeding. If bleeding is severe and considered an immediate threat to life, bleeding control has to begin during the primary assessment. Even though it may prove awkward, an Emergency Medical Responder may be faced with the task of stopping severe bleeding while also evaluating airway and breathing.

Estimating external blood loss requires some experience (Figure 17.4). It is important in cases where slow bleeding has been occurring for a long time or in cases where both internal and external bleeding are present. To get a good idea of how to estimate blood volume loss, pour a pint of water on the floor next to a fellow student or a mannequin. Also, try soaking an article of clothing with a pint of water and then note how much of the article is wet and how wet it feels.

KEY POINT ▼

Large veins may produce serious bleeding, but there is no pulsation as is typically seen with arterial bleeding. Rate of flow and pulsation are more significant factors than color in determining if the bleeding is arterial or venous.

IS IT SAFE?

Do not be fooled by capillary bleeding. Even though it is rarely life threatening, patients can fall prey to severe infection if the wound is not cared for properly. Always be sure to use proper BSI precautions when caring for a patient with open wounds.

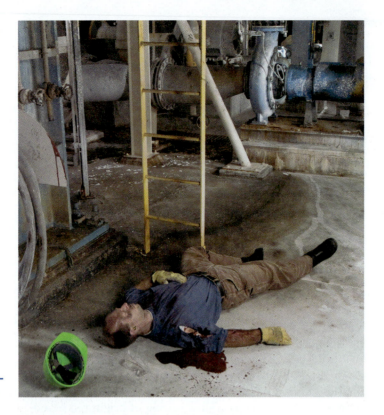

OBJECTIVE

5. Explain the proper care for a patient with active external bleeding.

bandage ▶ a device used to secure a dressing in place on the body, typically made of cloth or similar material.

Controlling External Bleeding

There are three steps to controlling external bleeding (Figure 17.5 and Scan 17.1): direct pressure, including the use of a pressure **bandage**; elevation combined with direct pressure; and the tourniquet, which may be used when all other bleeding control steps have failed.

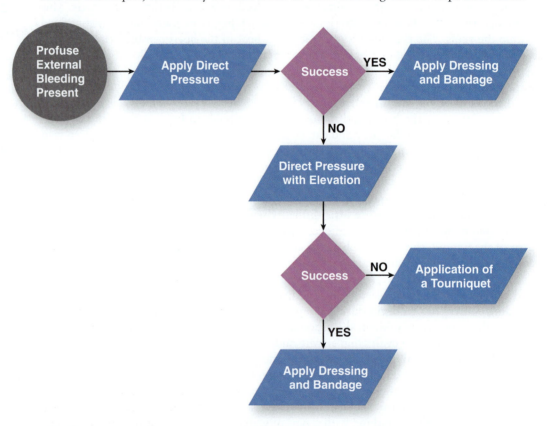

Figure 17.5 • Algorithm for control of external bleeding.

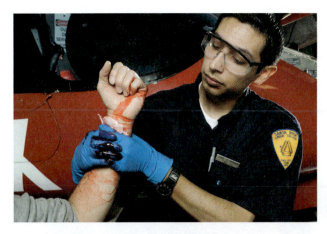

17.1.1 | Use BSI precautions.

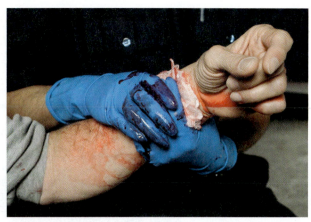

17.1.2 | Apply direct pressure.

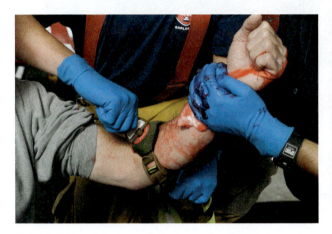

17.1.3 | If bleeding does not stop, apply tourniquet.

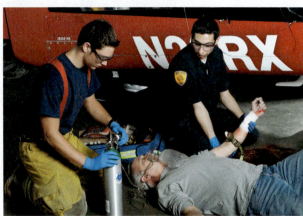

17.1.4 | Administer oxygen and monitor patient. Assess for shock.

Direct Pressure

Most cases of external bleeding can be controlled by applying *direct pressure* to the site of the wound. Ideally, a clean **dressing** should be used. If profuse bleeding is found during the primary assessment and you do not have dressings immediately available (Figure 17.6):

dressing ▶ a device used to cover an open wound, typically made of absorbent gauze that may be sterile or nonsterile.

1. Place your gloved hand(s) directly over the wound and apply pressure.
2. Keep applying steady, firm pressure.

If dressings are immediately available, then do the following (Figure 17.7):

1. Apply firm pressure using clean dressings or a clean cloth.
2. Apply pressure until bleeding is controlled. In some cases, this may take several minutes. Resist the temptation to remove pressure repeatedly to determine if the bleeding has stopped. Assume it has stopped only when you do not see bleeding through or around the dressing and bandage.
3. Secure the dressing in place with a bandage to create a pressure bandage.

Never remove or attempt to replace any dressing that is applied directly to the wound. To do so may interrupt clot formation and restart bleeding. If an outer dressing becomes soaked with blood, replace it with another dressing. Make sure you do not disturb the dressing that is immediately against the wound.

Figure 17.6 • In cases of profuse bleeding, use your gloved hand. Do not waste time hunting for a dressing.

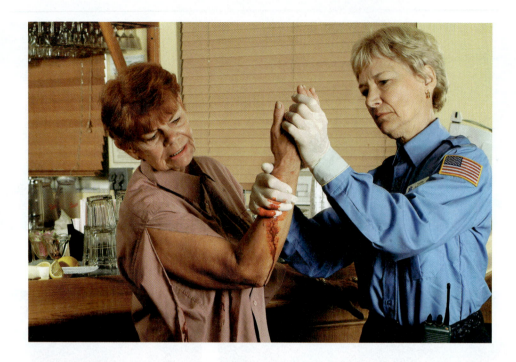

> ► **GERIATRIC FOCUS** ◄

Often, the elderly are taking medications that contain "blood thinners" such as Coumadin. This prevents their blood from clotting. As a result, minor cuts may bleed profusely. Be prepared to aggressively treat any bleeding in the elderly with direct pressure and pressure bandages.

The application of a pressure bandage can be helpful during the early stages of attempting to control bleeding. To apply a pressure bandage, follow these steps:

1. Place several layers of clean dressings directly on the wound. Maintain pressure with your gloved hands.
2. Use a *roller bandage* or *cravat* (folded triangular bandages) to secure the dressings in place. It should be wrapped firmly over the dressing and above and below the wound.
3. Wrap the bandage to produce enough pressure to control the bleeding.
4. Check for a distal pulse to be certain that the pressure has not restricted circulation beyond the wound.

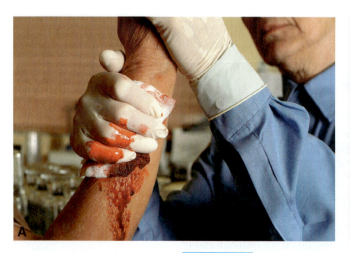
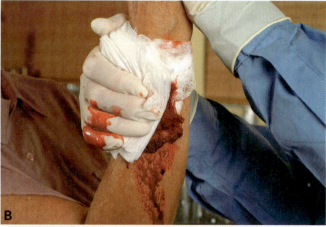

Figure 17.7 • (A) To control bleeding, place several (a small stack) 4 × 4s on the wound and apply direct pressure. (B) If the wound bleeds through the dressings, apply several more 4 × 4s.

A pressure bandage should not be removed once it is in place. If bleeding continues, add more pressure by using the palm of your gloved hand or applying more dressing pads, and continue the process of bandaging. (Do not remove the bandage to add more pads.) You also may apply more bandages to increase the direct pressure.

If you use your gloved hand or a dressing to apply direct pressure, you can apply a pressure bandage once the bleeding is controlled. If you are dealing with bleeding from the chest, abdomen, or neck, attempting to apply a pressure bandage may not be of any real use. Your best approach to such situations is to maintain direct pressure on the wound using a dressing held in place by your gloved hand.

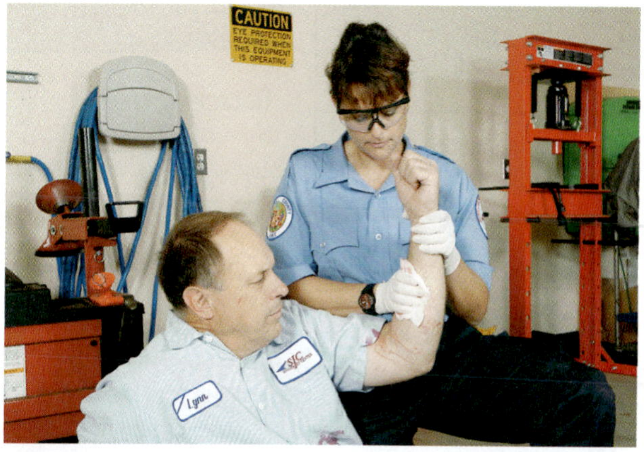

Figure 17.8 • Combine elevation and direct pressure for an arm or leg.

Elevation

Elevation may be used in combination with direct pressure when dealing with bleeding from an arm or leg (Figure 17.8). The effects of gravity may help reduce blood pressure at the wound and slow the bleeding. Do not elevate if you suspect fractures to the extremities or possible spine injury.

To use elevation, follow these steps:

1. While maintaining direct pressure over the wound, elevate the injured extremity. When practical, raise it so that the wound is above the level of the heart.

2. Continue to apply direct pressure to the site of bleeding.

For bleeding from the forearm:

1. Make sure someone activates the EMS system.
2. Take appropriate BSI precautions.
3. Perform a primary assessment, supporting the ABCs as necessary.
4. Apply direct pressure to the wound.
5. Elevate the limb as appropriate.
6. Provide care for shock. Calm and reassure the patient, maintain normal body temperature, and administer oxygen as soon as possible as per local protocols.

For bleeding from the leg:

1. Make sure someone activates the EMS system.
2. Take appropriate BSI precautions.
3. Perform a primary assessment, supporting the ABCs as necessary.
4. Apply direct pressure to the wound.
5. Elevate the limb as appropriate.
6. Provide care for shock. Calm and reassure the patient, maintain normal body temperature, and administer oxygen as soon as possible as per local protocols.

Tourniquet

Sometimes bleeding is so severe that no amount of direct pressure will control it. When this occurs, do not wait too long to move to the next step. If you are unable to control bleeding using direct pressure within two to three minutes, or if bleeding is very severe from the beginning, your best course of action is to place a **tourniquet** just above the injury site. A partial amputation of the arm or leg may leave you with no other choice but to use a tourniquet. In cases in which there is profuse bleeding from an arm or leg wound, a tourniquet should be applied to stop life-threatening bleeding after direct pressure and elevation have failed.

KEY POINT ▼

If there are no indications of spine injury or possible fractures of the extremity, direct pressure and elevation can be combined to control bleeding. Any patient who has suffered moderate to severe blood loss will benefit from receiving oxygen. Follow local protocols.

KEY POINT ▼

A tourniquet should be used only when other methods of controlling life-threatening bleeding such as direct pressure and elevation have failed.

tourniquet ▶ a device used to cut off all blood supply past the point of application.

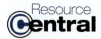

Resource Central

Get more information about tourniquets.

Tourniquet

Once banned from EMS use, tourniquets have gained favor again after military studies showed success in saving lives of those with extremity injuries secondary to explosions.

FIRST ON SCENE

continued

Taine runs across the busy parking lot and crashes through the doors of the truck stop. He is breathing too heavily to say anything, and, as the store's tinny overhead speakers play an upbeat tune, all eyes turn silently toward him. He catches his breath and shouts, "Somebody call an ambulance! A guy just tore his finger off out back."

He then turns, heads back out the door, and stumbles across the parking lot. A woman standing in line at the register sets a soft drink down on a candy display and runs out the door after him. They both reach the semi at the same time.

The woman kneels down and puts her hand on Casey's shoulder. "Sir," she says. "My name is Gina, and I'm an Emergency Medical Responder. I'm trained to provide emergency care for injuries. May I help you?"

"Oh God." Casey is still squeezing his left hand, trying to make the overwhelming pain go away. "Only if you can knock me out!"

KEY POINT ▼

For years the use of tourniquets fell out of favor for many EMS systems. Recent research by the military suggests that a tourniquet can be an effective tool for controlling severe bleeding and ultimately saving lives. The use of a tourniquet does not mean the person will lose the injured limb. In the vast majority of cases the patient will get to the hospital in time to save the limb.

If all other methods have failed and you must apply a tourniquet, carefully follow these steps (Figure 17.9):

1. Place the tourniquet just above (proximal) to the wound, but as close to the wound as possible without interfering with it.

2. Place a four-inch roller gauze or similar material on the site you have selected over the artery. This pad also can be a folded handkerchief or similar material.

3. If you are using a manufactured tourniquet, carefully place it around the limb just above the wound. Pull the free end of the band through the friction catch or buckle and draw it tightly over the pad. Tighten the tourniquet to the point where bleeding is stopped. Do not tighten it beyond this point.

If you do not have a commercially manufactured tourniquet or would have to leave the patient to retrieve one, use a necktie, stocking, or long bandage material. Flat materials are best. The band should be at least one inch wide. Do not use any material that could cut into the patient's skin. Carefully slip the tourniquet around the patient's limb and tie a half knot on the top side of the limb. A device such as a long stick, wooden dowel, or metal rod should then be placed over the half knot. Next, tie a full knot over the stick or rod. Then turn the device until bleeding has been stopped. Do not tighten the tourniquet beyond this point.

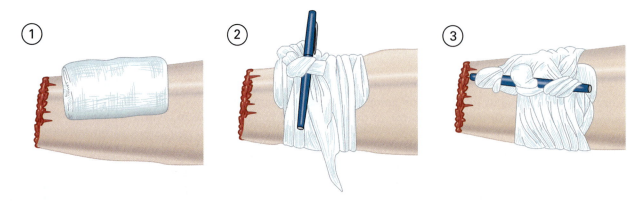

Figure 17.9 • Application of a tourniquet.

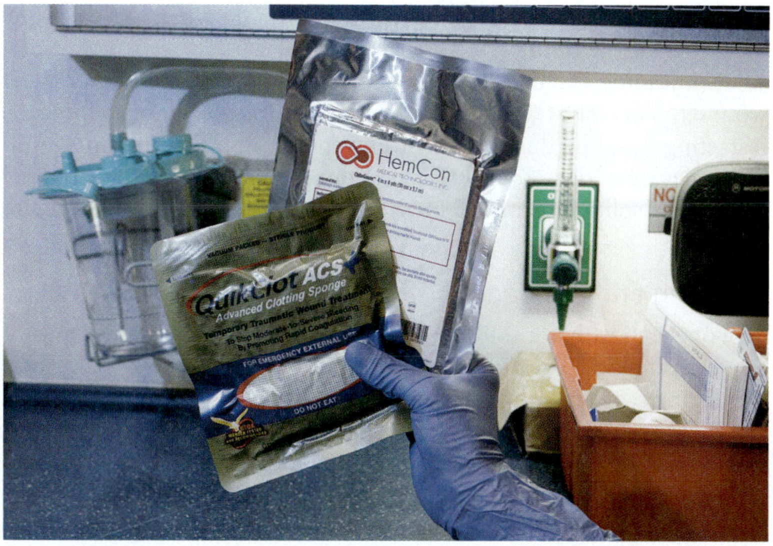

Figure 17.10 • Examples of hemostatic dressings.

4. Once the tourniquet is in place, do not loosen it. Tie it or tape it in place.

5. Attach a tag to the patient. Write on it that a tourniquet has been applied and the time at which it was applied (for example: T/K—5:11 p.m.). If you do not have a tag, write the information in ink on the patient's forehead. If you do not have a pen, write in lipstick, blood, or whatever is available at the scene. This information must be written so that the tourniquet does not go unnoticed and so that the hospital staff will know how long it has been in place.

6. Provide care for shock, but do not cover the tourniquet. This is an additional safeguard to prevent it from being missed by others who provide care for the patient.

Hemostatic Dressings and Agents

EMS has begun to see the introduction of specialized dressings called **hemostatic dressings** for the management of bleeding wounds (Figure 17.10). These are typically traditional gauze dressings that have been treated with specialized chemicals called hemostatic agents, which help promote the formation of clots directly at the wound site.

In addition to hemostatic dressings, there are hemostatic agents in the form of a powder-like substance that can be poured directly into an open wound to help promote clotting. Both of these approaches to bleeding control have been used successfully for years by the military and are just now starting to become commonplace in EMS.

hemostatic dressing ▶ a dressing that has been treated with a specialized chemical that when placed onto a wound promotes clotting.

Splinting

Splinting is not usually considered an Emergency Medical Responder-level method for controlling bleeding. However, some Emergency Medical Responders are trained to use air-inflatable splints. For long wounds on an arm or leg, the application of an air splint can help control bleeding. This is actually a form of direct pressure. Using an air splint requires special training in its application and knowledge of its limitations.

From the Medical Director

Hemostatic Dressings

Military experience in the Middle East has expanded our understanding of the potential role of tourniquets. They were traditionally the measure of last resort. Improved surgical techniques now allow us to consider their use. It is important to realize that this tool still carries the risk of significant complications and should be used according to your Medical Director's recommendation.

(See Chapter 19.) The air splint can be used even when there is no suspected fracture to the bones of the limb.

Combining the use of an air splint and elevation can work well on long, bleeding wounds. The splint also serves to immobilize the limb, helping reduce the chance of restarting bleeding due to patient movement. Because obtaining and applying air splints consumes time, this procedure is best done in cases of minor bleeding. The skilled rescuer can use air splints to control more serious bleeding if the splint is immediately at hand.

Dressing and Bandaging

OBJECTIVES

17. Explain the purpose of a dressing.

18. Explain the purpose of a bandage.

One of the most basic skills an Emergency Medical Responder must learn is that of properly dressing and bandaging wounds. If you follow the basic principles of dressing and bandaging, you will provide effective emergency care for the patient.

A dressing is any material (preferably sterile) placed over a wound to help control bleeding and prevent additional contamination. A bandage is any material used to hold a dressing in place.

Dressings, whenever possible, should be sterile. This means that they have been processed so that all germs and spores are killed. Commercially prepared dressings are usually sterile. They come in a variety of sizes. The most common size is four inches square. Dressings are referred to according to size, such as 2 × 2s, 4 × 4s, 5 × 9s, and 10 × 30s.

Throughout this text, you will find reference to *bulky dressings*, or multi-trauma dressings. They are thick dressings, often large enough to allow for the complete covering of large wounds. They are used to help control very serious bleeding and to stabilize impaled objects. Sanitary pads can be used in their place. They are available individually wrapped and are very clean. Bulky dressings also can be formed by applying many layers of smaller dressings.

There are a variety of specialized dressings available for use in EMS. One such dressing is the *occlusive dressing*. Occlusive dressings are typically made of sterile gauze that has been saturated with petroleum jelly. These dressings are used to create an airtight seal over a wound that penetrates a body cavity. Commercially prepared occlusive dressings are available. If they are not on hand, you can use folded plastic wrap or a plastic bag to help seal off an open wound to the chest or abdomen.

As an Emergency Medical Responder, you may not have any dressing materials at the scene of an emergency. In such cases, you might have to use clean handkerchiefs, towels, sheets, or a piece of clothing or other similar materials. When you improvise a dressing, it will not be sterile, but it can be used to help provide proper emergency care for the patient. Because the patient's wound has already been contaminated, your task is to avoid further contamination by using the cleanest material available. In the field, you must be concerned with controlling bleeding and minimizing contamination.

To be most effective, dressings must be secured in place over the wound. In most instances the dressing should be secured to the wound using a bandage. Common bandages include roller gauze, cravats, a handkerchief, strips of cloth, or any other material that will not cut into the patient's skin. Avoid the use of elastic bandages, as they can restrict circulation to the tissues if applied improperly.

The use of the self-adherent, form-fitting roller bandage makes the task of bandaging much easier (Figure 17.11). It clings to itself, making the task of wrapping around a dressing easier, quicker, and more efficient.

The following rules apply to dressing wounds:

- A dressing and bandage are of little value if they do not help control bleeding. Continue to apply dressing material and pressure as needed to control bleeding.
- Use sterile or clean materials. Avoid touching dressings in the area that will come into contact with the wound.
- Cover the entire surface of the wound and, if possible, the immediate area surrounding the wound.
- Once a dressing is applied to a wound, it must remain in place. Add new dressings on top of blood-soaked dressings. When a dressing is removed from a wound, bleeding may restart or increase in rate.

CSM Assessment

It is vital that you evaluate circulation, sensation, and motor function (CSM) before and after bandaging. Swelling may increase and cause the bandage to become too tight. If this occurs, loosen the bandage without completely removing it and recheck distal CSM.

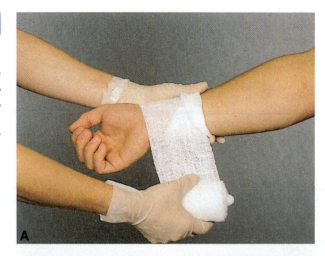

The following rules apply to bandaging:

- Do not bandage too tightly. It should hold the dressing snugly in place but not restrict blood supply to the distal extremity.
- Do not bandage too loosely. The dressing must not be allowed to slip from the wound or move while on the wound.
- Do not leave loose ends. Loose ends of tape, dressing, or cloth might get caught on objects when the patient is being moved.
- Do not cover fingers and toes unless they are injured. These areas must be left exposed for you to watch for color changes that indicate a change in circulation. Blue skin, pale skin, and complaints of numbness, pain, and tingling sensations all indicate that the bandage may be too tight.
- Wrap the bandage around the limb starting at its far (distal) end and working toward its origin or near (proximal) end. Taking such action will help reduce the chances of restricting circulation.
- Always check distal circulation, sensation, and motor function before and after bandaging.

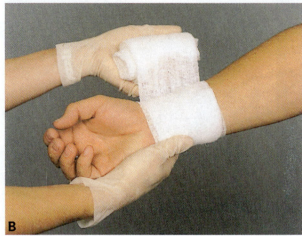

See Scan 17.2 for examples of general dressing and bandaging techniques.

Internal Bleeding

Internal bleeding can range from a minor bruise to a major life-threatening problem. Most small, simple bruises are examples of minor internal bleeding. Such minor blood loss is not of great significance. Of primary concern to Emergency Medical Responders is internal bleeding that brings about shock, heart and lung failure, and eventual death. Some cases of internal bleeding are so severe that the patient dies in a matter of seconds. Other severe cases of internal bleeding take minutes to hours before death. Emergency Medical Responder-level care may keep these patients alive until the EMTs arrive.

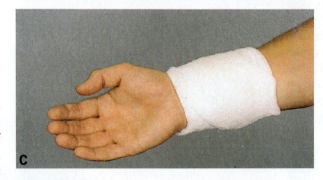

Figure 11.11 • (A) Begin by securing the end of the bandage with several overlapping wraps, (B) Continue to wrap so that the entire dressing is covered. (C) Secure the end of the bandage with tape.

The care you provide for internal bleeding, even when the bleeding is not severe, may save the patient's life. Because you have no way to know the severity of internal bleeding, always assume it is severe and care for the patient aggressively.

OBJECTIVE

6. Describe the signs and symptoms of internal bleeding.

▶ GERIATRIC FOCUS ◀

The signs and symptoms of internal bleeding in the elderly are often different from those in a younger patient. The survival reflexes that the younger body uses, such as increased heart rate, may be blunted due to cardiac disease or medication the elderly patient is taking. The elderly patient's level of consciousness is the most reliable sign to monitor for shock.

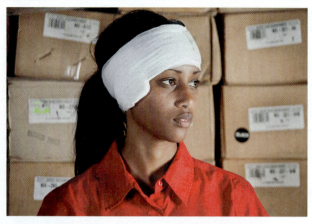

17.2.1 | Head

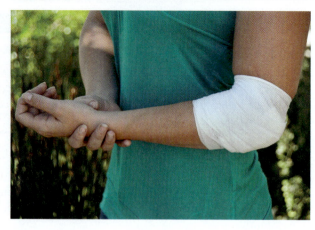

17.2.2 | Elbow

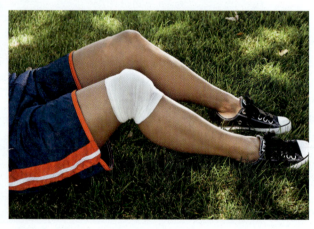

17.2.3 | Knee

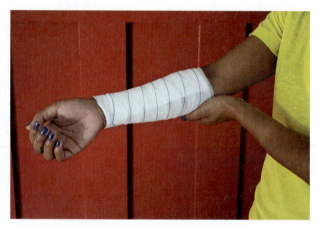

17.2.4 | Forearm

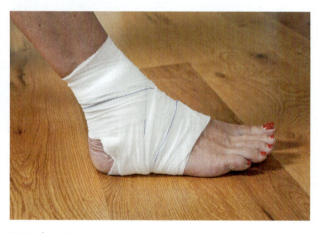

17.2.5 | Ankle

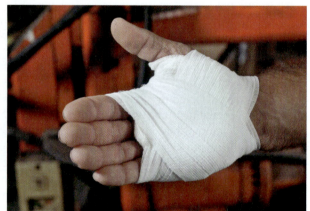

17.2.6 | Hand

Detecting Internal Bleeding

Internal bleeding can occur in many ways. It can be caused by wounds that are deep enough to sever major blood vessels or the vessels within an organ, such as a deep wound to the chest or abdomen. Open wounds that have cut through major vessels to produce profuse internal bleeding may show only minor external bleeding. Many cases of internal bleeding occur even when there are no cuts in the skin. Internal organs and blood vessels may have been ruptured or crushed by a severe blow to the body that did not produce any external wounds. This is an example of **blunt trauma**, an injury caused by an object that was not sharp enough to penetrate the skin. Blunt objects can be fairly large, such as the steering wheel of an automobile. Even though they do not tend to cause penetrating wounds, blunt objects can deliver a great deal of force to the body, causing life-threatening internal bleeding.

Pay special attention to bruises on the neck, chest, and abdomen. Severe injury with internal bleeding may show no more than a bruise at first, to be followed by the rapid decline of the patient's condition. Bruise detection can be particularly important in assessing possible internal bleeding when the patient is unresponsive and thus unable to complain of pain that would clearly indicate the problem.

Conclude that there is internal bleeding whenever you detect any of the signs listed below:

- Wounds that have penetrated the skull
- Blood or clear fluids draining from the ears and/or nose
- Vomiting or coughing up blood (coffee-grounds or frothy red appearance)
- Bruises on the neck
- Bruises on the chest, possible fractured ribs, and wounds that have penetrated the chest
- Bruises or penetrating wounds to the abdomen
- Pain, rigidity, or distention of the abdomen
- Bleeding from the rectum or vagina
- Possible fractures (with special emphasis on the pelvis, the long bones of the upper arm and thigh, and the ribs)

Always suspect internal bleeding if the patient has been injured and the signs and symptoms of shock are present (Figure 17.12). The symptoms of shock associated with internal

blunt trauma ► injury to the body caused by the impact with large objects or surfaces; non-penetrating trauma.

penetrating trauma ► injury to the body caused by any object that punctures the skin.

KEY POINT ▼

Internal bleeding may be difficult to detect. It can occur in cases where external bleeding is absent or minor and away from the site of noticeable injury. In fact, it can occur where there is no obvious external injury. Considering the mechanism of injury (falls, steering wheel injuries, and the like) and conducting a proper patient assessment are of major importance in detecting internal bleeding.

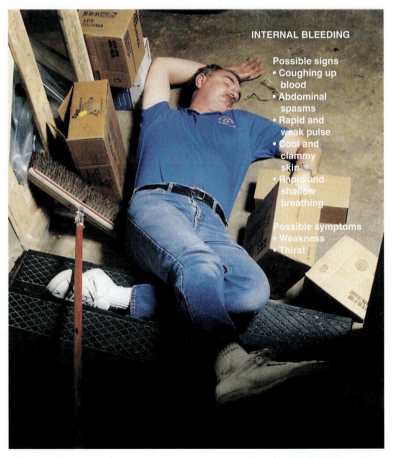

INTERNAL BLEEDING

Possible signs
- Coughing up blood
- Abdominal spasms
- Rapid and weak pulse
- Cool and clammy skin
- Rapid and shallow breathing

Possible symptoms
- Weakness
- Thirst

Figure 17.12 • Signs and symptoms of shock associated with internal bleeding.

bleeding are restlessness or anxiety, increased pulse rate, thirst, feeling cold, and rapid breathing. However, during the early stages of internal bleeding, there may not yet be signs or symptoms. Do not wait for signs and symptoms to develop. Treat the patient based on the mechanism of injury and/or history.

The signs of shock associated with internal bleeding include:

- Decreasing level of responsiveness
- Restlessness or combativeness
- Shaking and trembling
- Shallow and rapid breathing
- Rapid and weak pulse
- Pale, cool, moist skin
- Dilated (enlarged) pupils, which may respond sluggishly

Remember, none of these signs or symptoms may be present in the early stages of internal bleeding. If the mechanism of injury is severe enough to make you think that there may be internal bleeding, assume that there is such bleeding and provide the necessary care.

Management of Internal Bleeding

OBJECTIVE

7. Explain the proper care of a patient with suspected internal bleeding.

In general, the steps in the emergency care of patients with suspected internal bleeding include:

1. Take appropriate BSI precautions
2. Perform a primary assessment. Support the ABCs as necessary.
3. Provide high-flow oxygen if allowed. Follow local protocols.
4. Keep the patient lying flat and still, loosen restrictive clothing, and provide care for shock.
5. Do not give the patient anything by mouth. Be alert in case the patient starts to vomit.
6. Reassure the patient and keep him calm.
7. Facilitate rapid transport to an appropriate trauma center.

If you are an Emergency Medical Responder who is allowed to administer oxygen, remember that any patient with possible internal bleeding will benefit from receiving it. Provide oxygen per local protocols.

Internal bleeding is very serious, often leading to death, even in cases in which the bleeding begins once the patient is at the hospital. You may provide excellent Emergency Medical Responder care for a patient with internal bleeding, only to have him die later. To be a good Emergency Medical Responder, accept the fact that there are limits to emergency care at all levels.

Multisystem Trauma

OBJECTIVE

3. Identify the characteristics of multisystem trauma.

multisystem trauma ▶ trauma to the body that affects multiple organ systems.

At this point it is important to understand how multiple injuries to different body systems (musculoskeletal, respiratory, nervous, etc.) can impact patients and their care. When your patient has suffered a significant mechanism of injury (MOI), such as an automobile collision on the highway, a fall from great height, or a gunshot wound to the torso, you should suspect that numerous body systems have been impacted.

Multisystem trauma creates a much more critical situation for the patient and the Emergency Medical Responder because a combination of injuries to multiple body systems can quickly overwhelm the patient's ability to compensate, leading to shock and death.

The best way to anticipate multisystem trauma is to evaluate the mechanism of injury and actively assume that the patient has suffered all possible injuries. Proper treatment involves activation of the EMS system, supporting the ABCs, and treating each life threat as you identify it. It is necessary to understand the importance of rapid transport to an appropriate trauma center for victims of multisystem trauma. Be sure to request transport as soon as possible and consider the need for air medical transport if available.

Gina looks at Casey's bloody hand and notices that it isn't actively bleeding. She turns to Taine, who is still trying to catch his breath from the run to and from the convenience store, and asks if there is a first aid kit in the truck. Taine thinks for a moment and brightens, "Oh yeah! We have one next to the emergency triangles in the side box!"

He then turns and hurries to the truck. As he digs the first aid kit from among the spare bulbs, rags, and jumper cables, he sees the skin of Casey's finger hanging limply from the fifth wheel lock handle. It is dangling from some-thing that flickered like gold, so he steps closer. It is Casey's wedding ring. It got caught on the lock handle, and when it finally popped open, the action of the lock handle must have pulled the finger right off the bone.

Taine turns, feeling queasy, and hurries back over with the dirty first aid kit. Casey is extremely pale now, and Taine can see that he has thrown up on the pavement.

"Quick," Gina says, grabbing the kit from Taine's shaking hands. "I need you to cover him with your jacket and keep him from getting cold."

Soft-Tissue Injuries

The *soft tissues* of the body include the skin, muscles, nerves, blood vessels, fatty tissues, and cells (Figure 17.13). As children growing up, people learn about soft-tissue injuries such as bruises, scratches, and cuts the hard way. The idea of amputations and crush injuries are at least known, if not witnessed. Your own experiences and those of the people around you have led to a general understanding of injuries.

This prior knowledge will be useful to you. To be an Emergency Medical Responder, you will have to refine that knowledge, learning how to recognize and provide emergency care for various injuries. Most of your patients will, at best, have the same level of understanding that you had when you started this course. Remembering this will help you with patient interviews and in providing explanations and reassurance. Also, recalling what you knew about injuries as you went through childhood will help when dealing with children who have suffered injuries.

Except for cases of spine injury and certain types of internal injury, most adults can look at someone and often tell if there is an injury. Your training will build on this ability so that you will not miss detectable injuries. This is why there has been so much emphasis on patient assessment. As you progress through this course, you will be trained to determine the extent of an injury and the emergency procedures needed to care for it.

▶ GERIATRIC FOCUS ◀

Because the elderly have thin skin that is easily damaged, one of the more common soft-tissue injuries is called a "skin tear." This occurs when a twisting or shearing action is applied to the skin. You will often find a large flap of thin skin similar to a burn hanging from the wound. Treatment for this includes gently laying the flap of skin back into its original position and applying pressure bandages over it to prevent bleeding from the numerous small blood vessels that may be damaged.

Types of Injuries

Soft-tissue injuries can be categorized as either closed wounds or open wounds.

Closed Wounds

A *closed wound* is an injury in which the skin is not broken. Such injuries are usually caused by the impact of a blunt

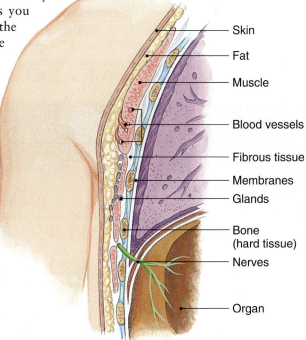

Skin
Fat
Muscle
Blood vessels
Fibrous tissue
Membranes
Glands
Bone (hard tissue)
Nerves
Organ

Figure 17.13 • Soft tissues and associated underlying structures

Figure 17.14 • Bruises are the most common form of closed wounds

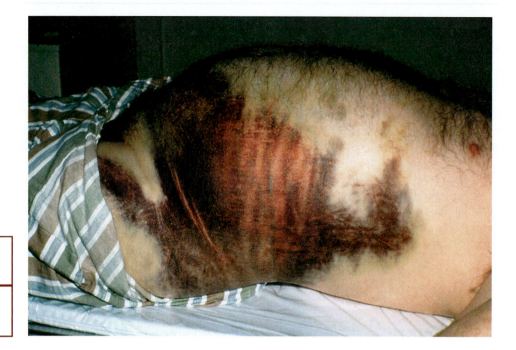

OBJECTIVE

8. Describe common types if external soft-tissue injuries.

object. Bleeding can range from minor to major, while the extent of injury can range from a simple *bruise* to the rupturing of internal organs.

One of the most obvious signs of a closed wound is the presence of swelling and/or bruises (contusions) (Figure 17.14). There is always some internal bleeding associated with a bruise. Because the outer skin is not broken, the blood leaks between tissues, causing discoloration over time ranging from black and blue to a brownish-yellow. Keep in mind that large bruises can mean serious blood loss and that there may be fractures or extensive tissue damage under the site of the bruise.

Open Wounds

In the case of an *open wound*, the skin has been damaged and there will be obvious bleeding. The extent of injury can range from a mild scrape (abrasion) to a tearing or cutting open of the skin (laceration). A simple scraping of the skin may produce no bleeding, while more severe open wounds may be associated with minor to life-threatening bleeding.

Open wounds may be classified as:

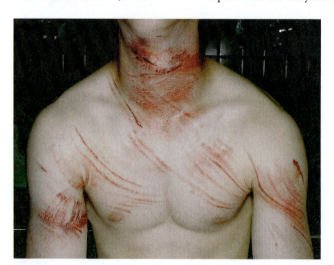

Figure 17.15 • Abrasions are the least serious form of all open wounds.

- *Abrasions.* Wounds such as skinned elbows and knees, "road rash," and "rug burns," are minor open wounds known as abrasions (Figure 17.15). Although such scrapes may be painful, tissue injury is usually not serious because the skin is not fully penetrated and the force causing the injury does not crush or rupture underlying structures. Wound infection tends to be the most serious problem faced when caring for abrasions to the skin.
- *Lacerations.* With lacerations, the skin is fully penetrated, with injury also occurring to tissues lying under the skin. Lacerations may be classified as:
  - Smooth cuts, or *incisions* (Figure 17.16). These types of lacerations are produced by very sharp objects, such as razor blades, knives, and broken glass. The edges of a smooth cut appear straight, with no apparent tears or jagged areas. Deep incisions can cause severe tissue damage and life-threatening bleeding.

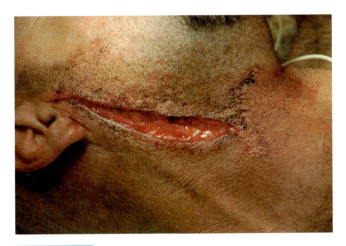

Figure 17.16 • The edges of a smooth cut (incision) are straight.

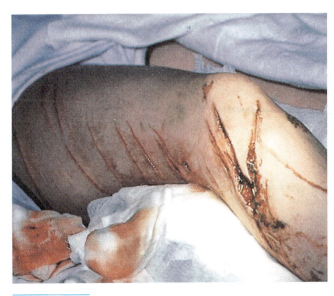

Figure 17.17 • Tissues along the edges of a jagged cut (laceration) will be torn and rough.

- Jagged cuts are tears with rough edges (Figure 17.17). Sometimes jagged cuts can be produced from the impact of a blunt object. Usually, they occur when the skin is cut by an object that does not have a very sharp edge.
- *Punctures.* Objects such as knives, nails, and ice picks can produce puncture wounds. An object puncturing the body will tear through the skin and usually proceed in a straight line, damaging tissues in its path. A puncture wound can range from shallow to deep (Figure 17.18). It also may have both an entrance and an exit wound, after the object, such as a bullet, passes through the body. Often, the exit wound is the larger and more serious of the two wounds (Figure 17.19).
- *Avulsions.* These wounds most frequently involve the tearing loose or the tearing off of large flaps of skin (Figure 17.20). A torn ear, an eyeball removed from its socket, and the loss of a tooth are also examples of **avulsions**.

avulsion ▶ the tearing loose of skin or other soft tissues.

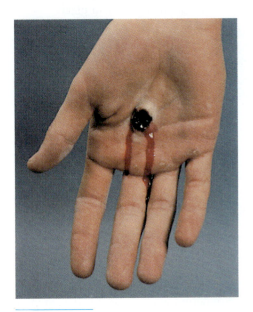

Figure 17.18 • Puncture wound.

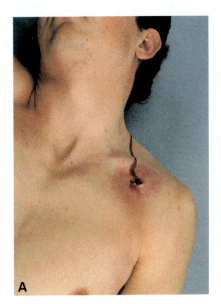

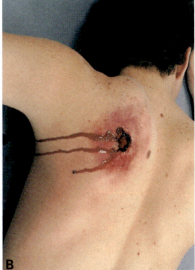

Figure 17.19 • A penetrating wound can have both (A) an entrance wound and (B) an exit wound. Often the exit wound is the more serious of the two.

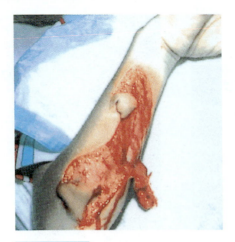

Figure 17.20 • Avulsions are open wounds.

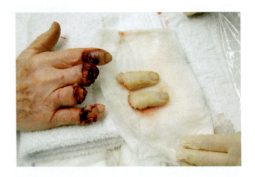

Figure 17.21 • Amputation.

amputation ▶ the cutting or tearing off of a body part.

- *Amputations.* These wounds involve the cutting or tearing off of the fingers, toes, hands, feet, arms, or legs (Figure 17.21). Because an **amputation** can be a surgical procedure, this injury is often called a *traumatic amputation.*
- *Crush injuries.* Crush injuries occur when a body part is pressed between two surfaces, the greater the force the greater the damage. Soft tissues and internal organs may also be crushed, often rupturing (Figure 17.22). Both external and internal bleeding can be profuse.

Emergency Care of Open Wounds

To provide emergency care for open wounds, follow these steps:

1. Expose the wound. Cut away clothing over and around an open wound.
2. Remove superficial foreign matter from the surface of the wound with a sterile gauze pad.
3. Control bleeding with direct pressure and elevation. Do not elevate a limb if there is the possibility of a fracture. A tourniquet should be used if direct pressure and elevation do not control the bleeding. Administer oxygen as per local protocols.
4. Prevent further contamination by using a sterile dressing or clean cloth to cover the wound. After the bleeding has been controlled, bandage the dressing in place.
5. Keep the patient lying still, as any activity will increase circulation. Keep the patient lying flat, using a blanket or other form of covering to provide protection from the elements.
6. Reassure the patient. This will reduce patient movement and may help lower the patient's blood pressure toward a normal level.
7. Care for shock. This applies to all but the simplest of wounds.

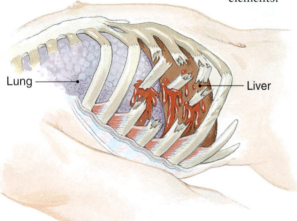

Figure 17.22 • Both soft tissues and internal organs are damaged in crush injuries.

When cutting away clothing to expose an open wound, avoid cutting directly through holes made by knives or bullets. They may serve as valuable evidence if the patient is a victim of a crime.

Emergency Care of Specific Injuries

Puncture Wounds

When dealing with any puncture wound, assume that there is extensive internal injury and internal bleeding. Always check for an exit wound, realizing that exit wounds can be more

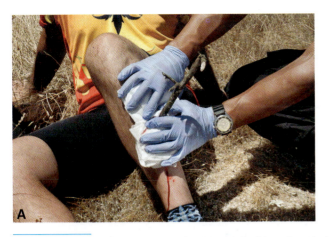
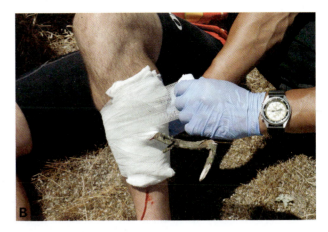

Figure 17.23 • Emergency care for a wound with an impaled object. (A) Stabilize the object with bulky dressings. (B) Secure the dressings with an appropriate bandage.

serious than entrance wounds (in the case of gunshot injury). Care for entrance and exit wounds as you would any open wound.

If a puncture wound contains an impaled object (such as glass, a knife, wood, metal, or plastic), do the following (Figures 17.23 and 17.24):

1. Take appropriate BSI precautions.
2. Expose the wound, without disturbing the impaled object.
3. Do not remove an impaled object.
4. Control bleeding. Administer oxygen as per local protocols.
5. Stabilize the impaled object by using bulky dressings. An alternative approach is to cut a hole in the center of a bulky dressing, making the cut slightly larger than the impaled object. Gently pass the dressing over the object. Bandaging these dressings in place will improve stability.
6. Keep the patient at rest and provide care for shock.

You may find that adhesive tape does not stick to the skin around an impaled object wound site. (Blood and sweat on the skin may cause the tape to slip.) Cravats can be used

OBJECTIVE

9. Explain the proper care for a patient with an impaled object.

KEY POINT ▼

Take special care not to cut your gloves or hands on an impaled object. Spread your fingers around the object and apply pressure to the wound site. Do not put any pressure on the object or the tissues that are up against the edge of a sharp impaled object.

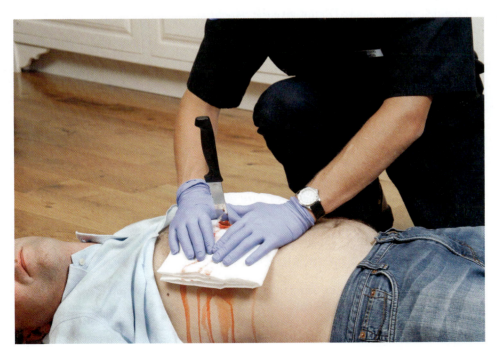

Figure 17.24 • Stabilizing an impaled object in the chest.

instead to tie the dressings in place. The cravats should be made from folded triangular bandages. Once folded, the cravats should be at least two inches wide. If the object is impaled in the chest or abdomen, a thin splint or coat hanger can be used to push the cravats under the natural void created by the curvature of the patient's back, so that the cravat can be tied around the patient's trunk.

Avulsions and Amputations

OBJECTIVE

10. Explain the proper care for an amputation injury.

Emergency care for avulsions and amputations are the same. If skin or another body part is torn from the body, or if a flap of skin has been torn loose, care for the wound with bulky dressings and direct pressure. Follow these steps:

1. Take appropriate BSI precautions.
2. Expose the wound.
3. Control bleeding and provide care as you would for any open wound.
4. If an avulsion, gently fold the skin back to its normal position prior to applying direct pressure. Follow local protocols.
5. Provide care for shock. Administer oxygen per local protocols.

Save and preserve an avulsed or amputated part. This is best done by wrapping the body part in a sterile dressing and placing it into a plastic bag or wrapping it in plastic wrap. If possible, keep the part cool (not cold; avoid freezing). Do not place the avulsed or amputated part in water or in direct contact with ice. Be certain that the bag with the part in it gets transported with the patient. Label the bag with the patient's name.

In most cases of avulsion or amputation, bleeding can be controlled by direct pressure, elevation, and a pressure bandage secured firmly over the stump or area of avulsion. Apply a tourniquet if the bleeding continues.

Protruding Organs

A deep open wound to the abdomen can cause organs such as the intestines to protrude through the wound opening. This is known as an *evisceration*. Follow these guidelines when caring for an open abdominal wound:

- Do not try to push protruding organ(s) back into the body cavity.
- Place a plastic covering over the exposed organs. If possible, apply a thick dressing over the top of this covering to help conserve heat.
- Provide care for shock. Do not give the patient anything by mouth.

Scalp Injuries

Injuries to the scalp can be difficult to care for because of the numerous blood vessels found there. Many of these vessels are close to the surface of the skin, producing profuse bleeding even from minor wounds. Additional problems arise if the bones of the skull are involved.

Injuries to the scalp (and face) require an extra effort on the part of the Emergency Medical Responder to provide emotional support for patients. The injuries tend to be very painful, produce bleeding that frightens many patients, and are in a body region where people have concern for their appearance.

The procedures for the emergency care of soft-tissue injuries covered previously in this chapter apply to the care you should provide for injuries to the soft tissues of the scalp. Use caution when applying direct pressure to a scalp wound. If there is the possibility of a skull fracture, you do not want to push the broken pieces into the skull.

Emergency care of scalp wounds includes the following:

- Control bleeding with a dressing held in place with gentle pressure. Avoid exerting excessive pressure if there are signs of a fractured skull or the injury site feels spongy.
- A roller bandage or gauze can be wrapped around the patient's head to hold dressings in place once bleeding has been controlled. If there is any indication of neck or

spine injuries, use caution to keep the patient's head immobilized when applying the bandage.

- If there are no signs of skull fracture or injuries to the spine, neck, or chest, you may position the patient so that the head and shoulders are elevated.

Facial Wounds

The first concern when caring for facial injuries is to make certain that the patient's airway is open and breathing is adequate. Even though bleeding may appear to be external only, check the airway and ensure that blood is not causing an obstruction. Continue to watch the patient to be sure that the airway remains open and clear of fluids and obstructions (tongue, teeth, blood clots).

When caring for patients with facial injuries, you should do the following:

1. Ensure an open and clear airway, being careful to note and properly care for neck and spine injuries.

2. Control bleeding by direct pressure, being careful not to press too hard because many facial fractures are not obvious.

3. Apply a dressing and bandage.

▶ GERIATRIC FOCUS ◀

Facial injuries generally bleed profusely in any patient, but in the elderly, who may be taking "blood thinners" such as Coumadin or aspirin, the bleeding may be life threatening. Be prepared to treat the wounds aggressively with bandages and direct pressure.

If you find the patient has an object that has passed through the cheek wall and is sticking into the mouth, you may have to remove it. This is the only time that an impaled object can be removed. Do so only if the object blocks the airway or is loose and could fall into the airway. To remove an impaled object from the cheek, follow these steps (Figure 17.25):

1. Look into the mouth to see if the object has passed through the cheek wall.

2. If you find penetration, carefully pull or push the object out of the cheek wall, back in the direction from which the object entered. Avoid cutting your gloves and yourself. If the object has not penetrated the cheek wall or if you cannot easily remove the object, stabilize it with dressings applied to the outer surface of the cheek.

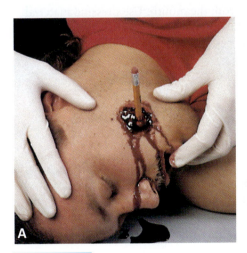 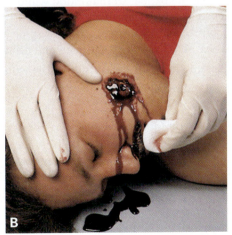

Figure 17.25 • Removing an object impaled in the cheek. (A) Look into the mouth and probe to see if the object has passed through the cheek wall. If it has, remove it. (B) Use dressing material packed against the inside wound to control the flow of blood.

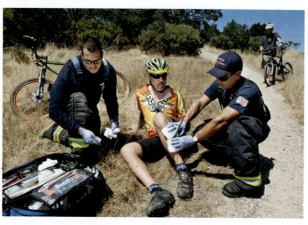

17.3.1 | Control bleeding.

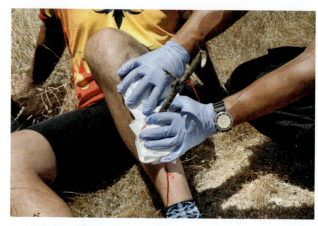

17.3.2 | Stabilize object in place.

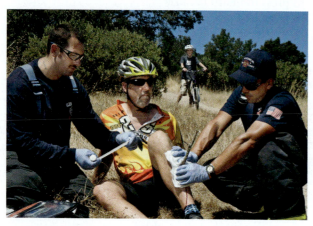

17.3.3 | Add bulky dressings.

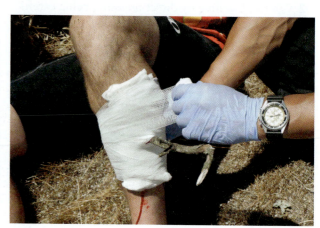

17.3.4 | Bandage.

3. If you remove an impaled object, place the dressing material between the wound and the patient's teeth, leaving some of the dressing outside the mouth so that it can be held to prevent swallowing it. Watch closely to be sure that the dressing does not work its way loose and into the airway.

4. Position the patient so that blood will drain from the mouth. Use dressing material packed against the inside wound to control the flow of blood. If bleeding is difficult to control and you suspect neck or spine injuries, roll the patient while maintaining manual stabilization of the head and neck.

5. Dress and bandage the outside of the wound.

6. Provide care for shock.

Impaled Objects

An impaled object must be left in place. Even though it created the wound, the impaled object also is sealing the wound. If it is removed, the patient may bleed profusely. The object must be stabilized with bulky dressings or pads. Begin by placing these materials on opposite sides of the object. Use tape or cravats to hold all dressings and pads in place (Scan 17.3).

Eye Injuries

Injuries to the eyes are rarely life threatening, but they can be emotionally traumatic. The prospect of losing one's sight can be overwhelming. The following are a few important points that must be emphasized when caring for an injury to the eye: Do not remove any

OBJECTIVE

12. Explain the proper care for an injury to the eye.

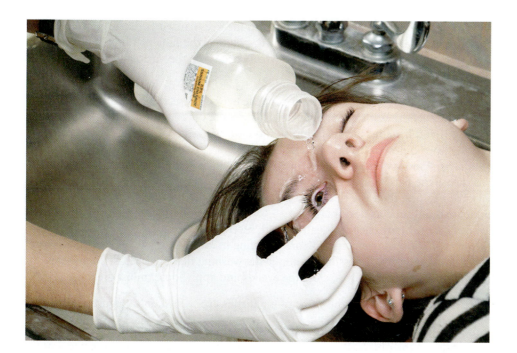

Figure 17.26 • Foreign objects can be washed from the eye. Flush with water from a medial to a lateral direction.

IS IT SAFE?

In some instances, it may be appropriate to secure the hands of an unresponsive patient who has eye injuries. If the patient becomes responsive, he may attempt to remove the bandages. Do this only if allowed by your local protocols.

impaled objects. Do not try to put the eye back into its socket. Do not apply pressure directly to an injured eyeball.

Problems resulting from foreign objects in the eyes are common. These problems can range from minor irritations to permanent injury. If the patient's own tears do not wash away a foreign object, use running water to remove it (Figure 17.26). *Do not apply the wash if there are impaled objects or cuts in the eye.* Apply the flow of water at the corner of the eye socket closest to the patient's nose. You may have to help the patient hold open the eyelids. As you pour the water, direct the patient to look from side to side and up and down. Before completing the wash, have the patient blink several times. When possible, continue the wash for at least 20 minutes or for the time recommended by medical direction.

If there are sharp objects in the patient's eye, do not direct the patient to move the eyes during the wash. After the wash, cover both eyes with dry dressings (Figure 17.27).

Whenever you are caring for a patient with eye injuries, you will have to cover both of the patient's eyes. In most cases, only one eye will actually be injured. However, when one eye moves, the other eye also will move (sympathetic movement). If you cover the injured eye and leave the uninjured eye uncovered, the uninjured eye will continue to react to activities and movement. Each time the uninjured eye moves, so will the injured one. Having both eyes covered reduces eye movements.

Having both eyes covered can cause fear and anxiety in the patient. Tell him why you are covering the uninjured eye. Keep close to him or have someone else stay close. Try to maintain contact with him through conversation and touch.

Always remember to close the eyelids of unresponsive patients. Because unresponsive people do not blink, moisture is quickly lost from the eye surface, damaging the eye. If you notice that the patient is wearing contact lenses, be sure to point this out to the EMTs who take over the care of the patient.

Burns to the eye must always be considered serious, requiring special in-hospital care. As an Emergency Medical Responder, you

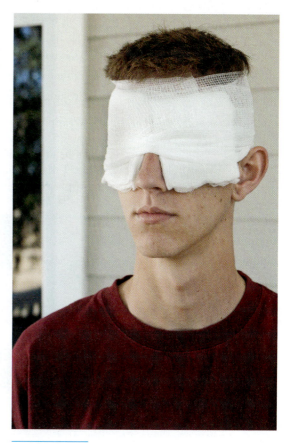

Figure 17.27 • Use bulky dressing to help secure and stabilize an impaled object.

may have to provide emergency care for burns to the eyes caused by heat, light, or chemicals. Your actions can make the difference as to whether the patient's sight can be saved.

The following are guidelines to follow when caring for the various types of burns to the eyes:

- *Thermal (heat) burns.* Do not try to inspect the eyes if there are signs of thermal burns to the eyelids. With the patient's eyelids closed, cover the eyes with loose, moist dressings. If you have no means to moisten the dressings, apply dry dressings. Do not apply any burn ointment to the eyelids.
- *Light burns.* "Snow blindness" and "welder's blindness" are two examples of light burns. Close the patient's eyelids and apply dark patches over both eyes. If you do not have dark patches, then use thick dressings or dressings followed with a layer of an opaque material such as dark plastic.
- *Chemical burns.* Many chemicals cause rapid, severe damage to the eyes. Flush the eyes with water. Do not delay emergency care by trying to locate sterile water. Use any source of clean drinking water. If possible, continue the washing flow for at least 20 minutes. After washing the patient's eyes, close the eyelids and apply loose, moist dressings.

If you find an object impaled in the globe of a patient's eye, you should (Figure 17.28):

1. Use several layers of dressing or small rolls of gauze to make thick pads. Place them on the sides of the object. If you have only enough material for one thick pad, cut a hole, equal to the size of the eye opening, in the center of this pad. Set the pad over the patient's eye, allowing the impaled object to stick out through the opening cut into the pad.
2. Fit a disposable cardboard drinking cup or paper cone over the impaled object. This will serve as a protective shield. Rest the cup or cone onto the thick dressing pad, but do not allow this protective shield to come into contact with the impaled object.
3. Hold the pad and protective shield in place with a roller bandage or with a wrapping of gauze or other cloth material.
4. Use dressing material to cover the uninjured eye, and bandage this dressing in place. This will reduce sympathetic eye movements.
5. Provide care for shock.
6. Provide emotional support to the patient.

Wrapping a paper cup or cone with gauze is tricky and cannot be done easily unless you practice. Ideally, you should wrap around the cup and then continue around the patient's head and wrap around the cup again. This procedure is repeated until the cup is stable. Take great care not to push the cup down onto the impaled object or pull the cup out of place.

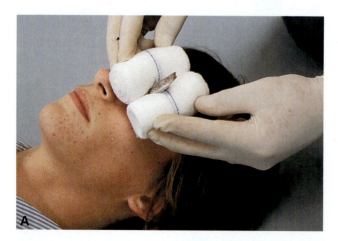 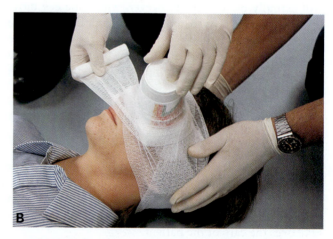

Figure 17.28 • Emergency care for a patient with an object impaled in the globe of the eye includes (A) stabilizing the object and (B) securing it in place.

If the eye is pulled out of the socket (avulsed eye), the care provided is the same as for an object impaled in the eye.

Ear Injuries

Emergency care for external ear injuries includes the following:

- *Cuts.* Apply dressings and bandage in place.
- *Tears.* Apply bulky dressings, beginning with several layers behind the torn tissue.
- *Avulsions.* Use bulky dressings bandaged into place. Save the avulsed part in a plastic bag or plastic wrap. Keep the part dry and cool. If no plastic is available, then wrap in dressing material. Be certain to label the bag, wrap, or dressing with the patient's name.

Internal ear injuries may appear as bleeding from the ears. Any such bleeding must be considered a sign of serious head injury. Bloody or clear fluids draining from the ear may indicate the presence of skull fracture. For such cases, assume there is serious injury and provide the necessary care. (For more about head injuries, see Chapter 20.)

Do not pack the external ear canal. If there is bleeding or clear fluid leaking from the ears, apply external dressings, sterile if possible, and hold them in place with bandages. Report this bleeding to the EMTs.

Do not attempt to remove foreign objects from inside the ear. Apply external dressings, if necessary, and provide emotional support to the patient.

If the patient tells you that it feels like his ears are "clogged" or "stopped up," suspect possible damage to the eardrum, fluids in the middle ear, or objects in the ear canal. Those conditions must be treated in a medical facility.

Nose Injuries

When dealing with injuries to the nose—when there are no suspected skull fractures or spine injuries—you will have two duties: maintain an open airway and control bleeding.

For a nosebleed in a responsive patient, maintain an open airway. Have the patient assume a seated position, leaning slightly forward. This position will help prevent blood and mucus from obstructing the airway or draining down the throat and into the stomach, which can cause nausea and vomiting. Next, have the patient pinch the nostrils. Bleeding is usually controlled when the nostrils are pinched shut. If the patient cannot pinch them shut, you will have to do so. Do not pack the patient's nostrils. Do not allow the patient to blow his nose (Figure 17.29).

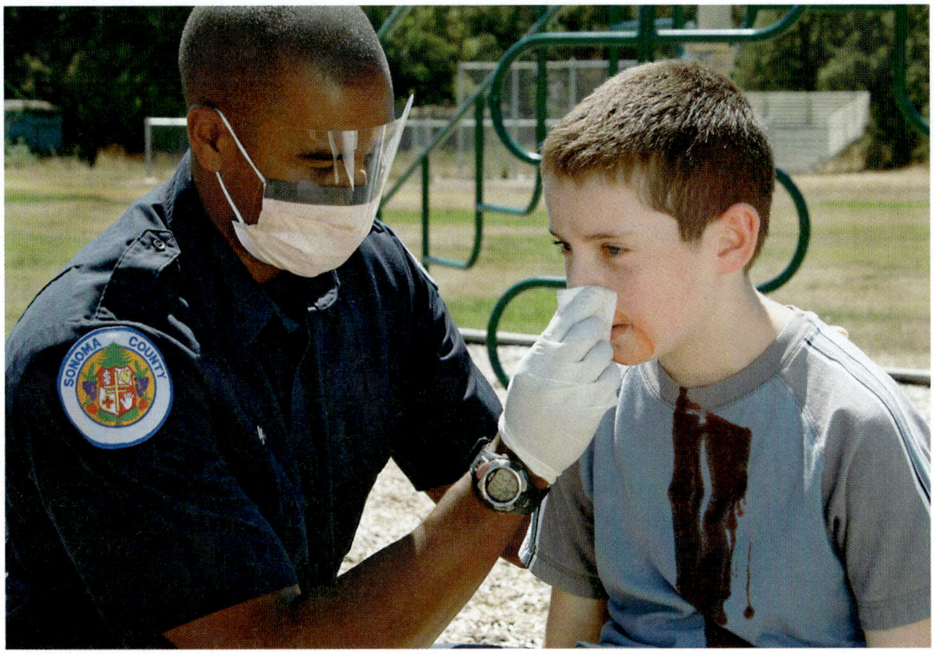

OBJECTIVE

11. Explain the proper care for nosebleed.

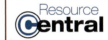

Learn more about nosebleeds.

Figure 17.29 • For a nosebleed, if the patient cannot pinch the nostrils shut, you should do so. Remember to position the patient for drainage.

For a nosebleed in an unresponsive patient or in a patient injured in such a way that he cannot be placed in a seated position, place him on one side with the head turned to provide drainage from the nose and mouth. Attempt to control bleeding by pinching the nostrils shut. Do not pack the nose. Do not remove objects or probe into the nose.

For an avulsion of the nose, apply a pressure bandage to the site. Save the avulsed part in plastic or a sterile or clean dressing. Keep the body part cool.

Injury to the Mouth

As with all injuries that occur in or around the airway, your first concern will be to ensure an open airway. If there are no suspected skull, neck, or spine injuries, position the patient in a seated position with the head tilted slightly forward to allow for drainage. If the patient cannot be placed in a seated position, position him on one side with the head turned slightly downward to provide some drainage for blood and other fluids.

For cut lips, use a rolled or folded dressing. Place the dressing between the patient's lip and gum. Take great care that the patient does not swallow this dressing.

For avulsed lips, apply a pressure bandage to the site of injury. Save the avulsed part in plastic or a sterile or clean dressing. Keep the avulsed part cool.

For cuts to the internal cheek, position a dressing between the patient's cheek and gum. (Do not pack the mouth with dressings.) Hold the dressing in place with a gloved hand. Always leave three to four inches of dressing material outside the patient's mouth to allow for quick removal. This is necessary to prevent the patient from swallowing the dressing. If possible, position the patient's head to allow drainage.

Neck Wounds

As an Emergency Medical Responder, be aware of the following signs that indicate soft-tissue wounds to the neck:

- Difficulty speaking, loss of voice
- Airway obstruction when the mouth and nose are clear and no object can be dislodged from the airway. This is often due to swollen tissues
- Obvious swelling or bruising of the neck
- Pain on swallowing or speaking
- Trachea pushed off to one side (tracheal deviation)
- Obvious cuts or puncture wounds

Follow these steps when caring for an open wound to the neck (Figure 17.30):

1. Immediately apply direct pressure to the wound, using the palm of your gloved hand.
2. Apply an occlusive dressing or some type of plastic over the wound. Use tape to seal this dressing on all sides. This will minimize the possibility that air can be drawn into the wound, causing an air embolism.
3. Care for shock and provide oxygen if allowed. Follow local protocols.

An alternative method of securing a dressing to the neck is as follows. This method uses the same procedure for both arterial and venous bleeding of the neck:

1. Place a roll of gauze dressing or dressing materials over the occlusive dressing and continue to apply pressure.
2. While maintaining pressure, secure the entire dressing with a figure-eight wrap of roller bandage. This eliminates the problem of trying to make adhesive tape stick to a bloody surface.
3. Place the patient on his left side for transport, with the body slightly slanted in a head-down position.
4. Care for shock and provide oxygen if allowed. Follow local protocols.

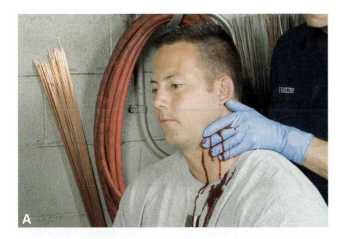

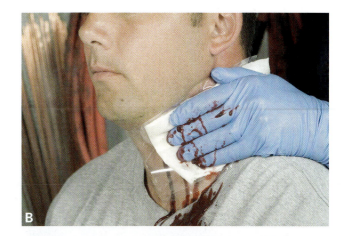

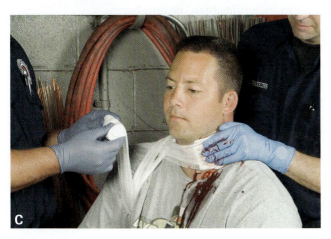

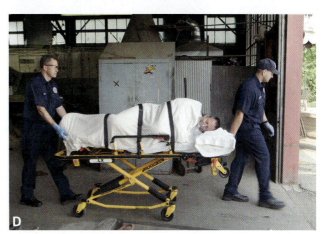

Figure 17.30 • Use a gloved hand or an occlusive dressing to help control bleeding from the neck. (A) Apply direct pressure. (B) The dressing should extend beyond all sides of the wound. (C) Secure the dressing with a figure-eight wrap, using a roller bandage. (D) If no spine injury is suspected, place the patient on his left side and care for shock.

Injury to the Genitalia

Because of the location, external reproductive organs are not common sites of injury. The pelvis and the thighs usually prevent injury to these organs, which are known as the external *genitalia*. When injury does occur, two types of soft-tissue injury are commonly seen:

- *Blunt trauma*. Such an injury is very painful, but little can be done by the Emergency Medical Responder. An ice pack, if available, can help.
- *Cuts*. Bleeding should be controlled by direct pressure. A sterile dressing or a sanitary pad should be used. If either is not available, then use any clean, bulky dressing.

The emergency care for all soft-tissue injuries applies when caring for injuries to the genitalia: Do not remove impaled objects. Save avulsed parts, wrapping them in plastic, sterile dressings, or any clean dressing.

Emergency Medical Responders are a part of the professional health-care team. As such, you must carry out your role in a manner that will reduce embarrassment for the patient. Tell the patient what you are going to do. Tell him why you must examine and care for the genitalia. Protect him from the sight of onlookers by having them leave the scene. Conduct all procedures in the same manner as you would care for an injury to any other part of the body.

Genital injury may be the result of rape. Maintain the patient's privacy, and remain professional in your conversation and care. Inform the patient not to wash, urinate, or change clothing. The patient should be transported by EMS to the emergency department.

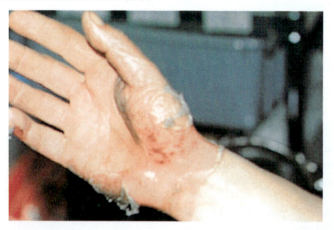

Superficial   Partial   Full
               thickness   thickness

Epidermis

Dermis

Fat
Muscle

Skin reddened   Blisters   Charring

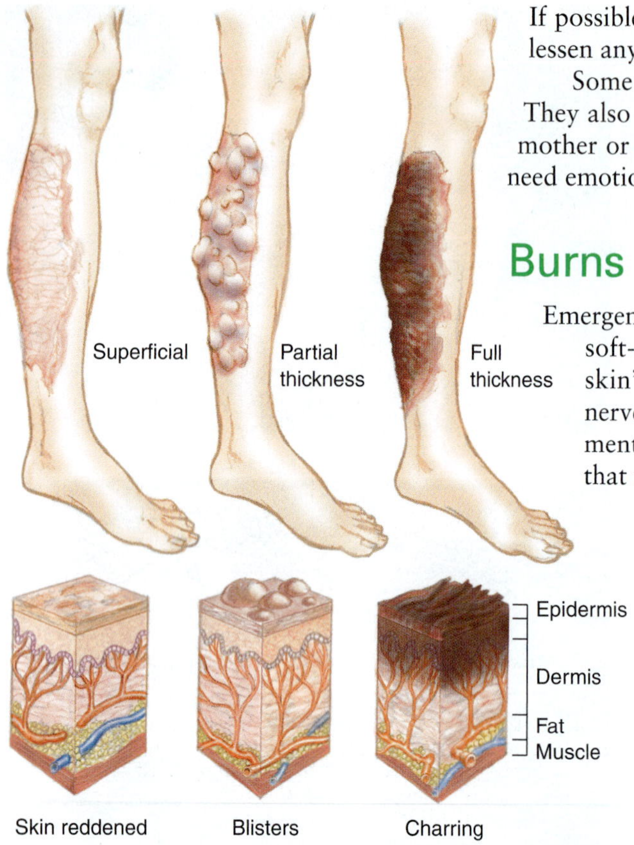

Figure 17.31 • Burns are classified by depth.

OBJECTIVE

13. Differentiate superficial, partial-thickness, and full-thickness burns.

KEY POINT ▼

Even though the nerves have been damaged by full-thickness burns and may not be painful, the areas surrounding the burns will be very painful.

Figure 17.32 • Partial-thickness burn.

If possible, the caregiver should be of the same gender as the patient to lessen any fears that the patient may have.

Some genital injuries are self-inflicted or are the result of abuse. They also may be caused by an attempt to abort an unborn fetus by the mother or other unlicensed person. Whatever the cause, the patient will need emotional support and understanding.

Burns

Emergency Medical Responders should consider burns to be complex soft-tissue injuries that can range from a superficial burn to the skin's surface (epidermis) to a serious deep injury that involves nerves, blood vessels, muscles, and bones. Careful patient assessment is necessary to avoid missing injuries or medical problems that may be far more serious than obvious burns.

Classification of Burns

Burns are classified in a number of ways. One way is to categorize burns based on the agent that caused the injury (source of the burn). This information should be gathered and forwarded to more highly trained personnel during transfer of care. Categories of burns based on source include:

- *Heat (thermal) burns,* which may be caused by fire, steam, or hot objects
- *Chemical burns,* which may be caused by caustics, such as acids and alkalis
- *Electrical burns,* which originate from outlets, frayed wires, and faulty circuits
- *Lightning burns,* which occur during electrical storms
- *Light burns,* which occur with intense light. Light from the arc welder or industrial laser will damage unprotected eyes. Also, ultraviolet light (including sunlight) can burn the eyes and skin.
- *Radiation burns,* which usually result from nuclear sources

Most often burns are categorized according to the depth of the burn (Figure 17.31). *Superficial burns* involve the top layer of skin known as the *epidermis.* Signs and symptoms include reddening of the skin and pain at the site. A common example is sunburn. *Partial-thickness burns* involve both the epidermis and the dermis (the top two layers of skin) (Figure 17.32) and present with intense pain, white to red skin that is moist and mottled (in light-skinned patients), and blisters. A classic example is a steam burn. *Full-thickness burns* extend through all dermal layers and may involve subcutaneous layers, muscle, bone, or organs (Figure 17.33). Full-thickness burns can be dry and leathery and may appear white, dark brown, or charred. Because there is often nerve damage present, there may be little to no sensation of pain present.

Severity of Burns

An important aspect of emergency care is being able to assess the severity of a burn, or extent of the damage. Defining the severity of a burn will involve evaluating the depth of burn as well as the total body surface area affected. A superficial or partial-thickness burn that involves less than 9% of the patient's total body surface area is considered a minor burn. The exceptions are if the burn involves the respiratory system, face, hands, feet, groin, buttocks, or major joint.

Any burn to the face (other than sunburn) should be considered a serious burn. Other serious burns include any partial-thickness burns covering a large area of the body or burns involving the feet, hands, groin, buttocks, or major joints.

One system used for estimating the amount of body surface area burned is called the *rule of nines* (Figure 17.34). For adults, the head and neck, chest, abdomen, each arm, the front of each leg, the back of each leg, the upper back, and the lower back and buttocks are each considered equal to 9% of the total body surface area. This gives a total of 99%. The remaining 1% is assigned to the genital area.

For infants and children, a simple approach assigns 18% to the head and neck, 9% to each upper limb, 18% to the chest and abdomen, 18% to the entire back, 14% to each lower limb, and 1% to the genital area. This method adds up to a total of 101% but provides an easy way to make approximate determinations.

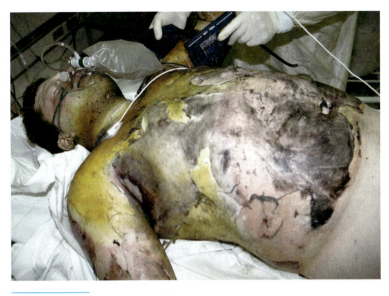

Figure 17.33 • Full-thickness burns.

OBJECTIVE

14. Explain the process for determining percentage of body surface area (BSA) affected by a burn.

By using the rule of nines, you can add up the areas affected by burns to determine how much of the patient's body has been injured. For example, if an adult patient has full-thickness thermal burns to the chest and front of one leg, this 9% plus 9% means that 18% of the total body surface area has been burned. Note that burns often overlap different body regions. So, when in doubt, always estimate to the higher percentage.

Emergency Care of Burns

Regardless of the system used to evaluate burns, follow these guidelines:

- Always perform a scene size-up and primary assessment, and support the ABCs as needed.
- Provide care for all burns, even the most minor or superficial ones.
- The following partial- or full-thickness burns should be considered serious and should be evaluated by a physician:
  - Burns to the hands, feet, face, groin, buttocks, thighs, and major joints

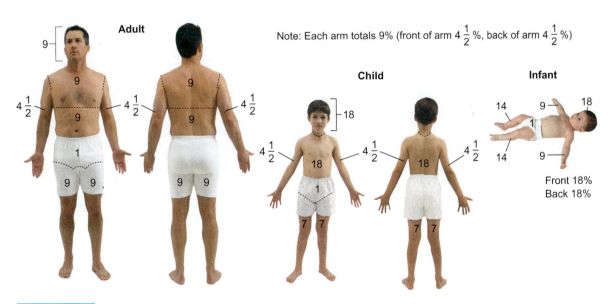

Figure 17.34 • Rule of nines.

- Any burn that encircles a body part
- Burns estimated at greater than 15% of the patient's body
- Burns that include respiratory involvement
- When in doubt, over-classify.
- Always consider the effects of a burn to be more serious if the patient is a child, elderly, the victim of other injuries, or someone with a medical condition (e.g., respiratory disease).

For emergency care of a patient with burns, take BSI precautions. For the contents of a typical burn kit. Then follow these steps:

1. Stop the burning process immediately. This may require the patient to stop, drop, and roll to extinguish the flames. You might also have to smother the flames and wet down or remove smoldering clothing.

2. Flush minor burns with cool or running water (or saline) for several minutes. For serious burns, do not flush burns with cool water unless they involve an area of less than 9% of the total body surface area. Follow local protocol. Flushing large burn areas may chill the patient and increase the risk of developing shock and infection.

3. Remove smoldering clothing and jewelry. Do not remove any clothing that is melted onto the skin.

4. Continually monitor the airway. Any burns to the face or exposure to smoke may cause airway problems. Administer oxygen as per local protocols.

5. Prevent further contamination. Keep the burned area clean by covering it with a dressing. Infection is common with burns.

6. Cover the burn area with dry, clean dressing. In some EMS systems, you may be instructed to moisten dressings before placing them on the patient. Otherwise, place dry, sterile dressings onto the burned area. Follow local protocols.

7. Give special care to the eyes. If the eyes or eyelids have been burned, place clean dressings or pads over them. Moisten these pads with sterile water if possible.

8. Give special care to the fingers and toes. If a serious burn involves the hands or feet, always place a clean pad between toes or fingers before completing the dressing.

9. Provide oxygen and care for shock.

Thermal Burns

See Scan 17.4 for a summary of caring for thermal burns.

Chemical Burns

Many chemicals are harmless if they are used properly or remain contained. However, if those chemicals come in contact with the human body, they can cause harm. Some irritate the skin and create burns very quickly. Others create a slow, painful burning process. In either case, it is crucial to stop the burning process and remove the irritant (Figure 17.35).

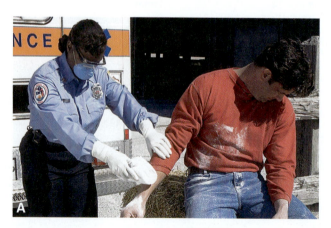
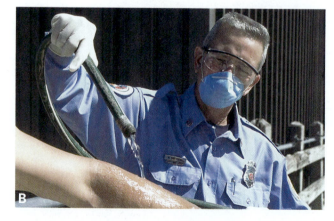

Figure 17.35 • Chemical burns: (A) Brush away dried powders and then (B) flush the skin with water.

TYPE OF BURN	TISSUE BURNED					
	OUTER LAYER OF SKIN	SECOND LAYER OF SKIN	TISSUES BELOW SKIN	COLOR CHANGES	PAIN	BLISTERS
Superficial	Yes	No	No	Red	Yes	No
Partial-thickness	Yes	Yes	No	Deep red	Yes	Yes
Full-thickness	Yes	Yes	Yes	Charred black or white	Yes	Yes

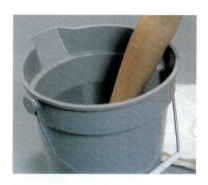

MINOR: Superficial and Partial thickness

- Cool the burn, if possible.
- Cover entire burn with dry, clean dressing.
- Moisten dressing only if burn is less than 9% of skin surface. Follow local protocol.

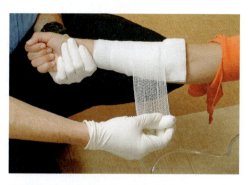

SERIOUS BURNS: Partial-thickness and any full-thickness burns

- Stop the burning process.
- Support the ABCs.
- Wrap area with dry, clean dressing.
- Provide care for shock.
- Moisten dressing only if burn is less than 9% of skin surface. Follow local protocol.

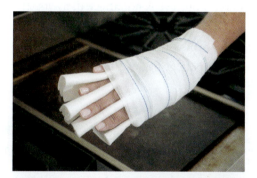

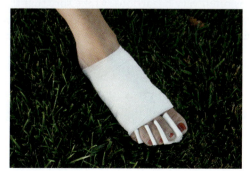

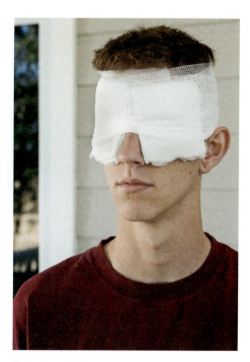

If hands or toes are burned:
- Separate digits with clean gauze pads.
- When appropriate, elevate the extremity.

Burns to the eyes:
- Do not open eyelids if burned.
- Be certain burn is thermal, not chemical.
- Apply moist, clean gauze pads to both eyes.

Scenes involving patients with chemical burns can be very dangerous. Thus, completing a scene size-up and ensuring scene safety is important. If you believe there are hazards at the scene that will place you in danger, do not attempt a rescue unless you have been trained to do so and have the necessary equipment.

The primary method of caring for chemical burns is to wash away the chemical with water. A simple wetting of the burned area is not enough. Flush the area of the patient's body that has been exposed. Continue to flush the area for at least 20 minutes. Be sure to remove all contaminated clothing, shoes, socks, and jewelry from the patient during the wash.

Once you have flushed the area for at least 20 minutes, apply a dry, clean dressing, care for shock, and make sure EMS has been notified. If the patient begins to complain of increased burning or irritation once a dressing is in place, remove the dressing and flush the burned area with water for several minutes more. Then apply a new dry dressing.

Remember, when providing emergency care for chemical burns:

1. Flush the burned area for at least 20 minutes. If possible and if it can be done quickly, try to identify any chemical powders before applying water. Water could cause a reaction that will produce heat and increase burning of the skin.
2. Apply a dry, clean dressing.
3. If burning continues, remove dressing and flush again.

If dry lime is the agent causing the burn, *do not* begin by flushing with water. Instead, use a *dry* dressing to *brush* the substance off the patient's skin, hair, and clothing. Also have the patient remove any contaminated clothing or jewelry. Once this is done, you may flush the area with water.

Chemical burns to the eyes require immediate attention. Assume that both eyes are involved. When caring for chemical burns to the eyes, you should:

1. Taking appropriate BSI precautions.
2. Perform a primary assessment and support the ABCs as necessary.
3. Immediately flush the eyes with clean water.
4. Keep the water flowing from a faucet, bucket, or other source into the eye. Use caution not to contaminate the good eye, if one eye is not affected, as you flush.
5. Continue flushing for at least 20 minutes.
6. After flushing the eyes, cover both of them with moistened pads.
7. Remove the pads and flush again if the patient begins to complain about increased burning sensations or irritation.

Electrical Burns

On the scene of an electrical injury, burns are not usually the most serious problem a patient sustains. Cardiac arrest, nervous system damage, fractures, and injury to internal organs may occur with these incidents (Figure 17.36).

The scene of an electrical injury is often very hazardous. Make sure that the source of electricity has been turned off before caring for the victim. If the electricity is still active, do not attempt a rescue unless you have been trained to do so and have the necessary equipment.

To provide emergency care to a patient with an electrical burn, you should:

1. Perform scene size-up and take appropriate BSI precautions.
2. Perform a primary assessment. Electricity passing through a patient's body will cause cardiac arrest. Even if the patient appears stable, be prepared for complications involving the airway and heart. Administer oxygen as per local protocols.
3. Evaluate the burn. Look for two burn sites—an entrance and an exit wound. The entrance wound (often the hand) is where the electricity entered the body. The exit wound is where the electricity came into contact with a ground (often a foot). The entrance wound may be small, and you may need to look very carefully for it. The exit wound may be large and obvious.

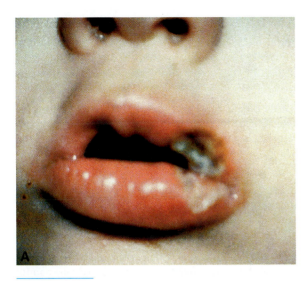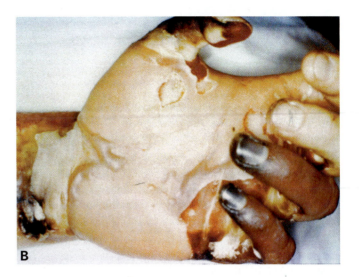

Figure 17.36 • Injuries due to electrical incidents. (A) Electrical burns caused by chewing on a power cord. (B) Burns associated with lightening injury.

4. Apply dry, clean dressings to the burn sites. You may apply moistened dressings if transport is delayed, the burn involves less than 9% of the body, and the patient will not be in a cold environment.

5. Provide oxygen and care for shock.

Infants and Children

Children are frequently the victims of accidental burns, but it is all too common that burns are used as a form of discipline or punishment by adults. As an advocate for the patient, carefully evaluate the injuries and the story provided by the caregivers. Remain objective and focus on caring for the child. Consider the possibility of child abuse when the injuries and the explanation provided are not consistent. If the burns are suspicious, document your findings carefully. Report your suspicion to the appropriate authorities.

WRAP-UP

FIRST ON SCENE

Gina has just finished dressing and bandaging Casey's finger when an ambulance arrives in the parking lot with sirens blaring. Casey has regained some of his color and says the nausea is pretty much gone but that the pain is understandably still "10 out of 10."

The EMTs thank Taine for activating the EMS system and Gina for recognizing and caring for Casey appropriately when he started to go into shock.

As the ambulance pulls out of the parking lot to transport Casey to the nearest trauma center, Gina takes a deep breath, smiles, and walks back into the convenience store with a new bounce in her step.

Summary

- To prevent possible exposure to infectious diseases while caring for patients who are bleeding, the use of BSI precautions and personal protective equipment (PPE) such as gloves and eye protection should be used.

- Arterial bleeding is characterized by blood that spurts or sprays from a wound. Venous bleeding can be heavy but flows steadily from a wound. Capillary bleeding will slowly ooze from a wound.

- If a patient is bleeding from an open wound, you should apply direct pressure, apply a pressure bandage, and elevate the injury site if necessary. If none of those techniques works, consider applying a tourniquet.

- Bruising, swelling, abdominal rigidity or guarding, vomiting blood, bleeding from the rectum or vagina, or the onset of shock following blunt trauma can all indicate internal bleeding. Emergency care for internal bleeding involves recognition, activating the EMS system, keeping the patient still and comfortable, being alert for vomiting, and treating for shock.

- External soft-tissue injuries include abrasions, lacerations, avulsions, punctures, and amputations.

- Impaled objects should be stabilized in place using bulky dressings or improvised materials. Never remove an impaled object unless it is interfering with the patient's airway.

- Multisystem trauma occurs when a patient has suffered a significant mechanism of injury that has caused trauma to numerous body systems, such as the skin, muscles, circulation, and nerves. It is often characterized by the signs and symptoms of internal and external bleeding, pain in numerous locations, altered levels of consciousness, and the rapid onset of shock.

- Amputations should initially be cared for with direct pressure or tourniquets to control bleeding. The patient should then be treated for shock and transported by ambulance (with the amputated part) as soon as possible.

- Nosebleeds should be cared for by pinching the nostrils together and having the patient lean forward. Activate the EMS system if the bleeding cannot be controlled or grows worse.

- Eye injuries can be very serious and must be treated carefully to prevent permanent damage and blindness. Although it is important to cover the uninjured eye to prevent movement of the injured eye, this can be frightening to the patient. Constantly reassure these patients by speaking to them and touching them.

- The three burn classifications are superficial, partial-thickness, and full-thickness. Superficial burns can be red and painful but are not generally serious because they only affect the top layer of the skin. Partial-thickness burns are more severe, with the damage reaching into the dermis and presenting with pain, swelling, and blisters. Full-thickness burns cause damage down to the bone, killing affected nerves and tissues and presenting with white, rigid skin and very little pain.

- Burns are treated by first stopping the burning process and removing any affected clothing or jewelry. For chemical burns, the chemicals should be flushed thoroughly with large amounts of water (after first brushing off any dry chemicals). For electrical burns, the source must be determined and shut off immediately. Burned areas should then be covered with dry, sterile gauze while awaiting the arrival of EMS personnel. For severe burns, you should constantly monitor the patient's airway and treat for shock.

- The "rule of nines" is a simple, widely accepted method of determining the body surface area affected by a burn. It divides the body into quadrants valued in 9% increments and allows for easy estimation of burned area.

- Dressings are made of clean or sterile cloth. They help to control bleeding and protect wounds from contamination. Bandages are used to hold dressings in place.

Take Action

THE SPILL DRILL

This activity will help you to become better at estimating external blood loss. Like any other skill that you will learn as an Emergency Medical Responder, it will take practice to acquire and to remain proficient at it. You will need a fellow student, a metric measuring cup, and some red food coloring.

1. Without letting your partner know the amount, add water to the measuring cup and put in a few drops of red food coloring to simulate blood.

2. Find a suitable hard floor surface that you can pour the water onto without creating a hazard or a stain.

3. Have your partner examine the spill and estimate the amount of liquid spilled onto the floor.

Take turns and use different amounts of water and see how closely you each can come to estimating the fluid amounts. Once you and your partner get more proficient at guessing, try putting the water onto some old clothing. Since clothing absorbs fluid, it becomes much more of a challenge to guess the amount.

GUESS THE BSA

This is an easy yet practical way to quickly learn the skill of estimating body surface area (BSA). Estimating BSA is most commonly done for burn patients, as some facilities can only manage small burns and some patients may need to be transported to burn centers for immediate care.

1. Working in groups of three or four students, have one student determine a body part or area to be affected and then verbally describe it to the others.

2. Keeping their answers confidential, the other students must then estimate the percentage of BSA affected according to the verbal description given.

3. Everyone then compares answers to see if they all agree. If they do not, find out why.

The activity should continue until all of the students have had the opportunity to be the host.

First on Scene Run Review

Recall the events of the "First on Scene" scenario in this chapter and answer the following questions, which are related to the call. Rationales are offered in the Answer Key at the back of the book.

1. What information should the dispatcher give the responders about the call?

2. Why did Gina ask permission if she could help him?

3. Could the skin from the finger be reattached, and how would you transport it?

4. What would the treatment be for Casey?

Quick Quiz

To check your understanding of the chapter, answer the following questions. Then compare your answers to those in the Answer Key at the back of the book.

1. Which one of the following is NOT a typical characteristic of arterial bleeding?
   a. Blood spurts from the wound.
   b. Blood flows steadily from the wound.
   c. The color of the blood is bright red.
   d. Blood loss is often profuse in a short period of time.

2. When attempting to control bleeding, which one of the following procedures will follow direct pressure?
   a. Indirect pressure
   b. Tourniquet
   c. Elevation combined with direct pressure
   d. Pressure points

3. Most cases of external bleeding can be controlled by:
   a. applying direct pressure.
   b. using a tourniquet.
   c. securing a pressure bandage.
   d. applying a clotting agent.

4. The material placed directly over a wound to help control bleeding is called a(n):
   a. bandage.
   b. elastic bandage.
   c. occlusive dressing.
   d. dressing.

5. The tearing loose or the tearing off of a large flap of skin describes which one of the following types of wound?
   a. Abrasion
   b. Amputation
   c. Laceration
   d. Avulsion

6. You are caring for a patient with a severe soft-tissue injury to the lower leg. You have exposed the wound. What should you do next?
   a. Apply direct pressure.
   b. Remove debris from the wound.
   c. Care for shock.
   d. Elevate the extremity.

7. When providing care for an open injury to the cheek in which the object has entered through the skin into the mouth, you must ensure an open airway and:
   a. remove the impaled object.
   b. turn the patient's head to one side.
   c. dress and bandage the outside of the wound.
   d. place dressings into the mouth.

8. When providing care for an open injury to the external ear:
   a. pack the ear canal.
   b. use a cotton swab to clear the ear canal.
   c. wash out the ear canal.
   d. apply dressings and bandage in place.

9. Which one of the following patients is most at risk for multisystem trauma?
   a. 16-year-old who fell four feet from a ladder
   b. 66-year-old female ejected from a vehicle rollover
   c. 44-year-old male whose foot was crushed by a forklift
   d. 27-year-old struck in the head by a baseball bat

10. When caring for a patient with severe burns, you must take BSI precautions and then:
   a. stop the burning process.
   b. prevent further contamination.
   c. flush only large burn areas.
   d. remove jewelry.

11. All of the following are signs or symptoms of internal bleeding EXCEPT:

    a. increased pulse rate.
    b. decreasing blood pressure.
    c. decreasing pulse rate.
    d. pale skin color.

12. Your patient has a large open wound to his neck. You have controlled bleeding with direct pressure, so you should then:

    a. pack the inside of the wound with clean dressings.
    b. pour sterile saline over the wound.
    c. cover the wound with a dry, clean dressing.
    d. cover the wound with an occlusive dressing.

13. Which one of the following best describes the appropriate care for an amputated body part?

    a. Wrap it with clean gauze and place it on ice.
    b. Apply a tourniquet to the exposed end of the part.
    c. Bandage the part back onto the body.
    d. Place the part in sterile water.

14. A bandage that is applied too tightly is at risk for:

    a. restricting circulation to the distal extremity.
    b. pushing the dressings too far into the wound.
    c. restricting blood flow to the proximal extremity.
    d. causing a blood clot.

15. A 23-year-old female has been kicked in the abdomen by a horse. She is alert and oriented and complaining of pain to her lower abdomen. You should suspect:

    a. a flail chest.
    b. internal bleeding.
    c. a fractured pelvis.
    d. an ectopic pregnancy.

16. Your patient has been impaled through the right thigh by a long piece of metal bar. The ABCs are intact and there is very little external bleeding. You should:

    a. carefully remove the object.
    b. tie both legs together.
    c. stabilize the object with bulky dressings.
    d. cut both ends of the bar to make it shorter.

17. You are caring for a 10-year-old boy whose eye has been pulled from the socket following a dog attack. The eye is hanging down the cheek by some tissue. The ABCs are intact and bleeding has been controlled. You should:

    a. place the injured eye back in the socket.
    b. remove the injured eye and place it on ice.
    c. cover the uninjured eye.
    d. cover both eyes with bulky dressings.

18. You arrive on the scene to find a young girl with an active nosebleed. She is crying and the sight of the blood is scaring her. You should:

    a. position her on her side while holding pressure on the nose.
    b. have her lean forward while you pinch the nostrils.
    c. have her lean backward as far as possible while holding the nose.
    d. pack both nostrils with sterile gauze.

19. You are caring for a burn victim who has partial-thickness burns covering his entire right arm and the front of his torso. What is the estimated BSA affected?

    a. 18%
    b. 25%
    c. 27%
    d. 36%

20. You are caring for a burn victim with both partial- and full-thickness burns over 40% of her body. The ABCs are intact and you have her on high-flow oxygen. You should:

    a. cover her with sterile burn sheets.
    b. apply cool water over the burns.
    c. apply moist dressings over the burns.
    d. not cover the burns, but you should arrange transport.

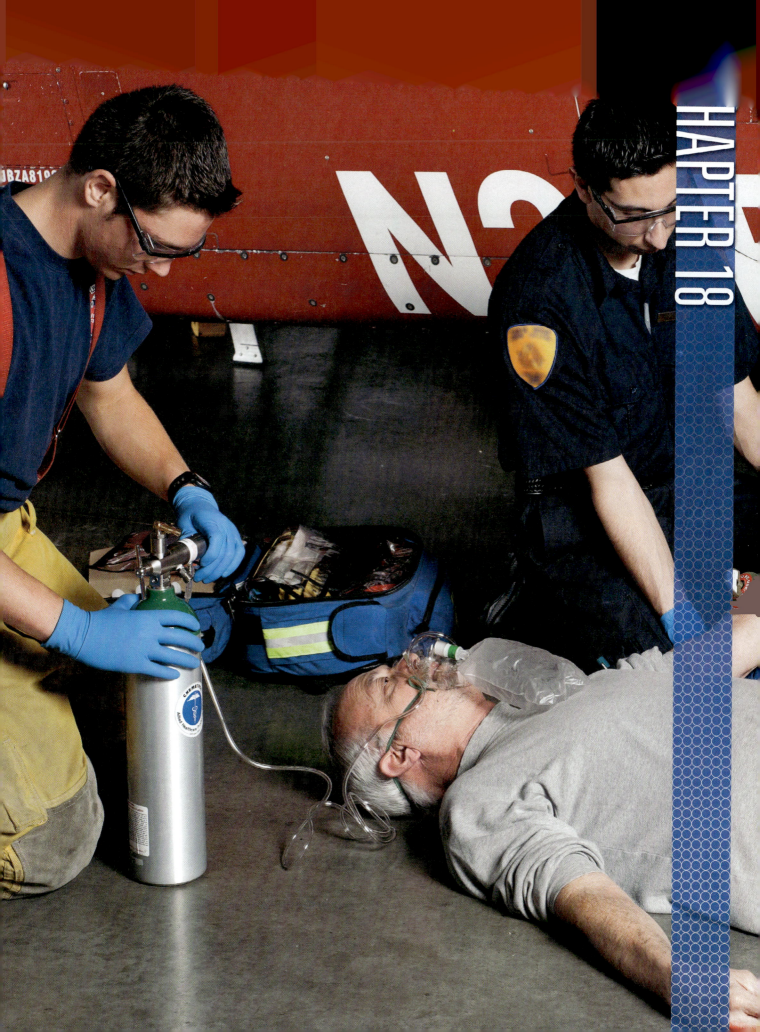

Recognition and Care of Shock

CHAPTER OVERVIEW

According to the Centers for Disease Control and Prevention (CDC), trauma is the fourth leading cause of death in the United States. Many of those deaths can be directly attributed to the shock that almost always develops secondary to injury. This is the reason that it is so critical for Emergency Medical Responders not only to understand the process called shock, or hypoperfusion, but also how to anticipate it, recognize it, and, most important, care for it. Inevitably, you will be called upon to provide emergency care to victims of shock. Early identification, appropriate care, and coordinating rapid transport contribute greatly to the patient's chance of survival. Understanding the signs, symptoms, and management of shock is a vital part of good prehospital care.

This chapter covers the four primary categories of shock and the common types of shock, and how you, as an Emergency Medical Responder, will be able to recognize and care for patients experiencing this life-threatening condition.

OBJECTIVES

Upon successful completion of this chapter, the student should be able to:

COGNITIVE

PSYCHOMOTOR

7. Demonstrate the proper techniques for caring for a patient at risk for shock.

AFFECTIVE

8. Value the importance of proper body substance isolation (BSI) precautions when caring for a patient with suspected shock.

Jordan, an Emergency Medical Responder and firefighter, has just finished washing the engine parked in the driveway of Station Four when the radio buzzes to life.

"Engine Four, trauma activation." The dispatcher pauses for a moment and then continues. "You're going to 9-1-4-4 Founders Parkway, the Smith Cabinet Shop, for a power saw injury."

"Engine Four responding from the station." Jordan keys the portable radio. Another firefighter appears in the truck bay, followed closely by one more, and they all climb up into the glistening red truck while Jordan starts the engine.

"Wow," Cass, the last one into the truck, says as he bounces into the passenger seat. "I hope it's not like that last call we had out there. Remember? That guy with the amputated hand."

"I remember." Jordan frowns. The road dust that the tires are kicking up is already settling on the still wet truck.

Perfusion and Shock

Simply stated, **perfusion** is the adequate supply of well-oxygenated blood and nutrients to all the vital organs. **Shock**, also known as **hypoperfusion**, is the failure of the body's circulatory system to provide enough oxygenated blood and nutrients to all vital organs. During normal perfusion, oxygen and carbon dioxide are exchanged, nutrients and waste products (CO_2) are exchanged, and fluid and salt balance is maintained between the blood and the tissues. When those processes are interrupted for any reason, hypoperfusion develops and the patient goes into shock (Figure 18.1).

Shock develops or occurs in a step-by-step progression. The development of shock can be rapid or it can come about slowly. Most new rescuers expect shock to develop rapidly. However, this is not always the case. Some patients can go into shock "a little at a time." Experienced rescuers know that often they have enough warning to be able to recognize the signs and slow down the process. They also know that if they do not continue to monitor patients, they can miss some of the subtle, early signs and symptoms. Shock is a dynamic process that if allowed to go unrecognized can be life threatening.

Care for patients with shock should not be delayed. The problem worsens with time, and early intervention is crucial. The initial problem must be corrected, and shock must be managed. Care at the Emergency Medical Responder level should begin to correct problems and stop the decline.

> ▶ **GERIATRIC FOCUS** ◀

Trauma from falling is a leading cause of injury for the geriatric population. As they age, their ability to see where they are stepping is diminished and they become less stable and therefore much more prone to falling. What would otherwise be a benign fall for you or me can be life threatening for the elderly patient.

Categories of Shock

Whenever the body is hurt, either by injury or illness, it often reacts by trying to correct the effects of the problem. If the damage is severe, one consequence is shock. There are several common types of shock, which will be discussed in some detail later in this chapter. It is important to understand that all types of shock fall into one of four categories, depending on the part of the circulatory system that is affected (Scan 18.1):

OBJECTIVE

2. Explain the pathophysiology of shock.

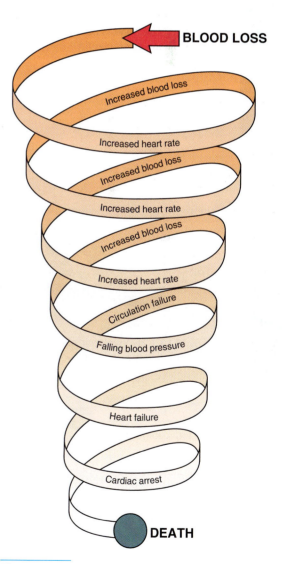

BLOOD LOSS

Increased blood loss

Increased heart rate

Increased blood loss

Increased heart rate

Increased blood loss

Increased heart rate

Circulation failure

Falling blood pressure

Heart failure

Cardiac arrest

DEATH

Figure 18.1 • If left untreated, blood loss will lead to death.

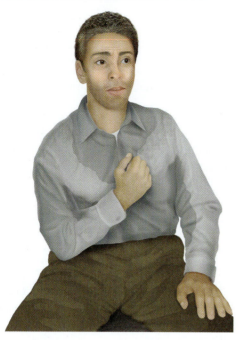

18.1.1 | Cardiogenic shock is a pump problem. The heart is not pumping the blood properly or efficiently.

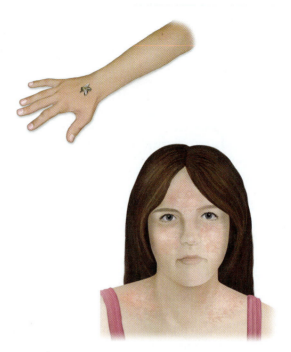

18.1.2 | Distributive shock is a vascular tone problem. The blood is not allocated properly.

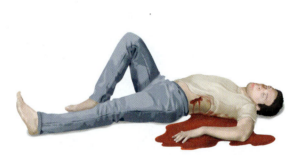

18.1.3 | Hypovolemic shock is related to extreme blood loss or too little volume.

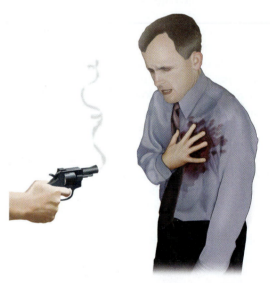

18.1.4 | Obstructive shock can develop when an obstruction of a vessel causes less blood to be pumped by the heart.

OBJECTIVE

3. Describe the four categories of shock.

perfusion ▶ the adequate supply of well-oxygenated blood and nutrients to all vital organs.

shock ▶ the failure of the body's circulatory system to provide an adequate supply of well-oxygenated blood and nutrients to all vital organs. Also known as *hypoperfusion*.

From the Medical Director

Shock

To understand the types of shock, you need merely to think of the human body as a fluid-filled (blood) container with a pump (heart) and tubing (vessels). Shock occurs when there is not enough fluid, the pump fails, or the vessels dilate.

• *Cardiogenic shock.* The heart (pump) is at the center of the circulatory system and must be functioning properly to maintain a proper blood pressure to circulate blood adequately. If the heart fails to pump an adequate volume of oxygenated blood, the

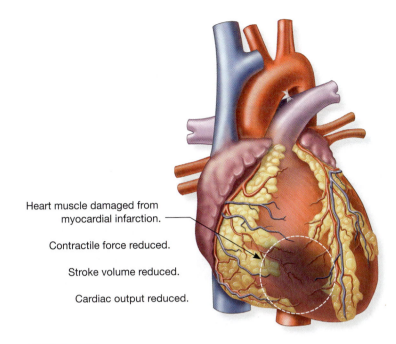

hypoperfusion ▶ a condition in which the organs and cells are not receiving an adequate supply of well-oxygenated blood and nutrients. Also known as *shock*.

Heart muscle damaged from myocardial infarction.

Contractile force reduced.

Stroke volume reduced.

Cardiac output reduced.

Figure 18.2 • Heart attack as a cause of cardiogenic shock: Damaged heart muscle results in reduced force of contractions and reduced cardiac output.

KEY POINT ▼

Any patient who is showing signs and symptoms of shock must be considered unstable and requires immediate care and transport to a hospital. Keeping patients from going into shock and helping stabilize patients who are in shock are two of the most important responsibilities of Emergency Medical Responders. If nothing is done for the patient who is in shock, death will almost always result.

blood pressure can fall, resulting in hypotension. This category of shock is sometimes referred to as *pump failure* (Figure 18.2).

- *Distributive shock*. Blood circulates throughout the body by way of a closed system of vessels. The vessels are made up of smooth muscle and can dilate and constrict, depending on the needs of the body. Certain conditions can cause the vessels to dilate excessively, resulting in a much larger space than the available blood supply can fill. When there is more space within the system than blood to fill it, blood pressure drops and shock results (Figure 18.3).
- *Hypovolemic shock*. The term *hypovolemic* means low fluid volume. **Hypovolemic shock** includes all types of shock caused by fluid loss, such as bleeding, burns,

hypotension ▶ abnormally low blood pressure.

hypovolemic shock ▶ a category of shock caused by an abnormally low fluid volume (blood or plasma) in the body.

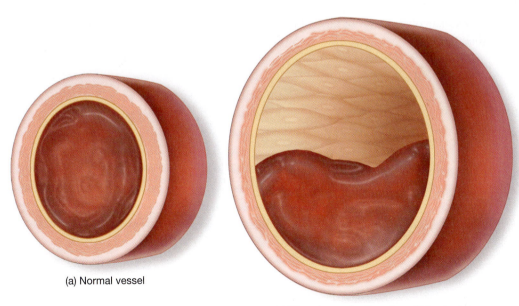

(a) Normal vessel

(b) Dilated vessel with reduced blood volume

Figure 18.3 • Uncontrolled dilation of the blood vessels.

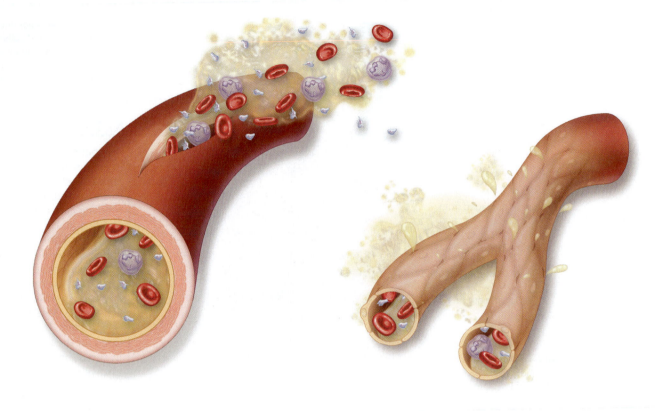

(a) Hemorrhagic hypovolemia: loss of whole
blood (plasma and formed elements)

(b) Nonhemorrhagic hypovolemia:
loss of plasma

Figure 18.4 • (A) Hemorrhagic hypovolemia: loss of whole blood; (B) nonhemorrhagic hypovolemia: loss of plasma

vomiting, diarrhea, and severe dehydration. There must be an adequate amount of fluid within the body and circulatory system at all times. If there is loss of fluid volume, blood pressure will drop and shock results (Figure 18.4).

• *Obstructive shock.* The adequate flow of blood can be disrupted due to a variety of obstructions to the heart, lungs, and great vessels. Damage to the heart from trauma and blockages in the vessels that connect the heart and lungs are causes of obstructive shock. The obstruction of blood flow reduces perfusion, which can lead to shock (Figure 18.5).

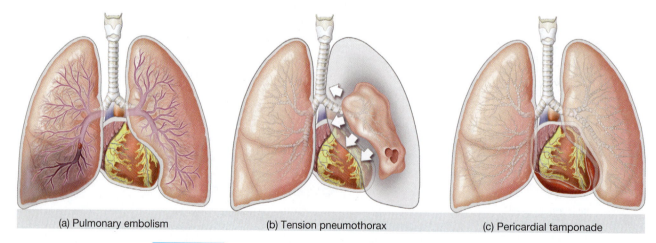

(a) Pulmonary embolism

(b) Tension pneumothorax

(c) Pericardial tamponade

Figure 18.5 • Causes of obstructive shock: (A) pulmonary embolism; (B) tension pneumothorax; (C) pericardial tamponade.

As the fire engine pulls up to the large roll-up door leading to the main cabinet workshop, the crew is greeted by a very nervous-looking man with blood soaking the front of his denim apron.

"He's just inside," the man says a little too loudly. "A broken saw blade hit his arm and he's bleedin' like a stuck pig."

The patient, a 28-year-old carpenter named Parker, is holding a blood-soaked towel tightly around his left forearm and leaning unsteadily against a workbench. Cass immedi-

ately notices that the man's clothes are soaked with blood and that he is very pale.

"Tell you what," Jordan says as he helps to stabilize the swaying man. "Let's get you down on the floor and more comfortable."

"I was . . . um . . . I was working on a hinge cutout . . . and . . . and . . ." The man's voice trails off and sweat begins to accumulate on his forehead.

"Quick," Cass says. "Lay him down. Someone get me a blanket or some jackets."

Types of Shock

There are several types of shock to which a patient can fall victim. Each one falls into one of the four categories mentioned above. A patient in shock may experience one or more of the following:

- *Hemorrhagic shock.* **Hemorrhagic shock** is a form of hypovolemic shock, which occurs when the body loses a significant amount of whole blood from the circulatory system. It can be caused by uncontrolled internal or external bleeding. When the body loses significant amounts of blood, it can no longer maintain an adequate blood pressure or carry oxygen to the vital organs.
- *Cardiogenic shock.* **Cardiogenic shock** is both a category and specific type of shock that results when the heart is unable to pump enough blood at a consistent pressure to all the vital organs. The heart can become damaged due to injury or from a heart attack, making it unable to pump blood efficiently.
- *Neurogenic shock.* A form of distributive shock, **neurogenic shock** is caused when the spinal cord is damaged and is unable to control the tone of the blood vessels by way of the sympathetic nervous system. The vessels are then allowed to dilate uncontrollably. The dilation of the blood vessels causes an increase in the space within the circulatory system, causing a drop in blood pressure resulting in inadequate perfusion and shock.
- *Anaphylactic shock.* Another form of distributive shock also known as allergy shock, **anaphylactic shock** is caused when the body experiences a severe allergic reaction. That reaction causes the blood vessels to dilate uncontrollably, resulting in a loss of blood pressure and thus perfusion.
- *Respiratory/metabolic shock.* **Respiratory/metabolic shock** is typically caused by a disruption of the transfer of oxygen into the cells or the ability of the cells to utilize the available oxygen. Certain poisons such as cyanide and carbon monoxide can disrupt the body's ability to utilize oxygen, resulting in a lack of oxygen to the vital organs.
- *Psychogenic shock.* Another form of distributive shock, **psychogenic shock** often causes fainting and usually occurs when some factor, such as fear, causes the nervous system to react and rapidly dilate the blood vessels. This rapid dilation of the vessels is followed by a sudden drop in blood pressure, which disrupts the flow of blood to the brain. In most cases, this is a self-correcting form of shock. Once the patient lies down, the situation will correct itself and the patient should return to normal.
- *Septic shock.* **Septic shock** is another form of distributive shock and is caused by a widespread infection of the blood. Poisons are released that cause the blood vessels to dilate. As in other cases of shock, the blood volume is too low to fill the circulatory system. This type of shock is seldom seen by Emergency Medical Responders.

OBJECTIVE

4. List the seven main types of shock and their causes.

hemorrhagic shock ▶ a form of hypovolemic shock that occurs when the body loses a significant amount of blood.

cardiogenic shock ▶ a form of shock caused when the heart is unable to pump blood efficiently.

neurogenic shock ▶ a form of distributive shock, resulting from spinal-cord injury.

anaphylactic shock ▶ a form of distributive shock caused by a severe allergic reaction.

respiratory/metabolic shock ▶ a form of shock caused by the disruption of the transfer of oxygen into the cells or the ability of the cells to utilize oxygen.

psychogenic shock ▶ a form of distributive shock that results in a sudden, temporary dilation of blood vessels.

septic shock ▶ a form of distributive shock caused by a widespread infection of the blood.

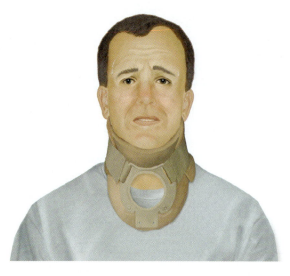

18.2.1 | The patient will experience anxiety and mental status changes. The brain begins to feel the effect of decreased oxygen.

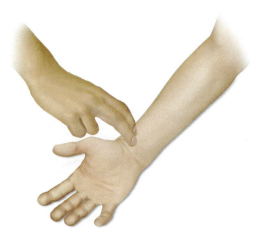

18.2.2 | The patient will have cool, pale, sweaty skin and an increased pulse and respirations. Blood is shunted from the skin the vital areas. Pulse and respirations increase to compensate for shock.

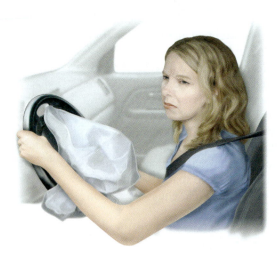

18.2.3 | In addition to sweating, the patient also may experience nausea and vomiting as blood is shunted from the abdomen to more vital areas.

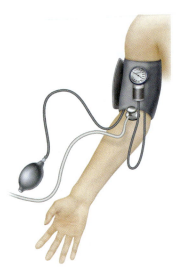

18.2.4 | Late signs of shock include a drop in blood pressure.

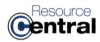

Find out more about the stages of shock.

compensated shock ▶ the condition in which the body is using specific mechanisms, such as increased pulse rate and increased breathing rate, to compensate for a lack of adequate perfusion.

The Body's Response During Shock

The human body has an amazing ability to adjust and compensate when things go wrong. In the case of shock, there are sophisticated pressure receptors throughout the circulatory system that can detect the slightest change in blood pressure. Those receptors can detect changes in blood pressure long before there are any outward signs of shock. In the early stages of shock, the sympathetic nervous system is activated and causes such things as increased heart rate, constriction of the blood vessels, and increased contraction of the heart. All of these things work together to help maintain an adequate blood pressure, which is necessary for perfusion. The changes are all a part of what is commonly referred to as **compensated shock**, because they are attempting to compensate for a drop in blood pressure (Scan 18.2).

The geriatric patient experiences many physical changes with age. Many of the body's systems become less effective and do not function as well as they did when the person was younger. This includes many of the body's mechanisms that help defend against the loss of blood and the onset of shock. Geriatric patients may need more aggressive care when presenting with signs and symptoms of shock.

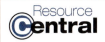

Resource Central

Learn more about the types of shock and then learn ways to control bleeding.

As the body detects the slightest drop in pressure within the circulatory system, it releases hormones such as epinephrine that will increase heart rate in an attempt to maintain blood pressure. If the increase in heart rate alone is not enough to maintain a good blood pressure, additional hormones are released that will constrict the blood vessels in the nonessential areas, such as the skin and intestinal tract. The constriction will redirect the blood to the vital organs where it is needed.

If the root cause of the shock is not corrected soon enough, the body's compensatory mechanisms will begin to fail because they, too, are not receiving adequate perfusion. When this happens, the heart rate begins to slow, breathing slows, and blood pressure drops to a dangerous level. This failure of the normal compensatory mechanisms is referred to as **decompensated shock**. If the root cause of the shock is not cared for soon enough, the patient will eventually enter a condition called irreversible shock and will die.

decompensated shock ► the condition in which the body is no longer able to compensate for a lack of adequate perfusion.

Signs and Symptoms of Shock

As we mentioned earlier, shock is a progressive process that the body uses to compensate for poor perfusion, and the signs and symptoms typically develop over time. Depending on the severity of the situation, the signs of shock can appear over several minutes to several hours.

The early signs and symptoms of shock are restlessness, altered mental status, increased heart rate, normal to slight low blood pressure, mildly increased breathing rate, skin that is pale, cool, and moist, sluggish pupils, and nausea and vomiting.

Those signs and symptoms follow the order in which they may be detected during the primary assessment of the patient. However, all signs and symptoms of shock may not be present at once, and they do not necessarily occur in the order listed above. Shock is progressive (becoming worse with time). Look for the following patterns:

OBJECTIVE

5. Describe the signs and symptoms of shock.

- *Increased pulse rate.* The body is trying to adjust to the drop in blood pressure and poor perfusion.
- *Increased breathing rate.* When the body is not receiving enough oxygen and the level of carbon dioxide increases, the body tries to compensate by increasing the breathing rate.
- *Restlessness or combativeness.* The patient is reacting to the body's attempt to adjust to the loss of proper circulatory function. The patient feels that something is wrong and may look afraid. In some cases, this behavioral change may be the first sign of developing shock.

From the Medical Director

Signs and Symptoms

The signs and symptoms of shock may be difficult to identify. In some patients with shock, the signs may be absent. Lack of perfusion results in shock, and the organ that depends most on perfusion is the brain. That is why an altered mental status is the most sensitive indicator for the presence of shock.

- *Pale, cool, moist skin.* As blood is redirected to the vital organs from the skin, the skin will become pale and feel cool to the touch. Stimulation from the sympathetic nervous system also causes sweating.
- *Changes in mental status.* As adequate circulation to the brain continues to fail, the patient will become confused, disoriented, sleepy, or unresponsive.
- *Respiratory and cardiac arrest* can develop.

In a younger person, the heart rate will increase steadily in an attempt to maintain an adequate blood pressure. In the geriatric patient, the heart is limited in its ability to beat faster due to the effects of aging. Many geriatric patients take medications that are designed to keep their heart rate low and thus may counteract the body's normal compensatory mechanisms.

KEY POINT ▼

Provide care for all injured patients as if shock will develop. Do the same for all patients with problems involving the heart, breathing, abdominal pain, diabetes, drug abuse, poisoning, and abnormal childbirth. Carefully monitor all patients for the early signs of shock.

If the cause of the shock is not stopped, the normal compensatory mechanisms mentioned above will begin to fail, resulting in decompensated shock. The following are the late signs and symptoms of shock, the ones that appear as the patient enters decompensated shock: unresponsiveness, decreasing heart rate, very low blood pressure, slow and shallow respirations, skin that is pale, cool, and moist, and dilated, sluggish pupils.

Mechanism of Injury and Shock

One of the keys to the successful care of shock is early detection. Do not want to wait for signs and symptoms to develop before you begin caring for shock. In cases of trauma or injury, examine and consider the mechanism of injury carefully. If there is any chance that the patient may have suffered blunt trauma to the head, chest, abdomen, or pelvis, suspect that internal bleeding exists and care for the patient accordingly. Of course, you also must identify and stop all external bleeding immediately upon discovery.

Caring for Shock

OBJECTIVE

6. Explain the proper care of a patient presenting with signs and symptoms of shock.

In most cases the patient will require more advanced care both in the field and in the hospital. However, if recognized early, the Emergency Medical Responder can provide care that will minimize the progression of shock and ensure prompt transport to the hospital.

Help delay the progression of shock by doing the following (Figure 18.6):

1. Perform a primary assessment and ensure the ABCs are properly supported.
2. Control external bleeding.
3. Administer oxygen per local protocol.
4. Keep the patient in a supine position.
5. Calm and reassure the patient, and maintain a normal body temperature.
6. Monitor and support the ABCs.

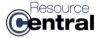

Learn more about bleeding.

From the Medical Director

Hypothermia

Even after finding success with tourniquets for bleeding injuries, the military continued to lose patients to shock. Research found that complications with hypothermia was the cause. Keep the victims warm because they are unable to maintain normal body temperature.

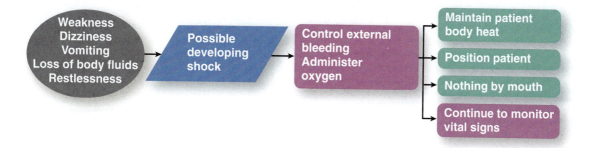

Figure 18.6 • Algorithm for emergency care of patients with developing shock.

7. Do not give the patient anything by mouth. Even if the patient expresses serious thirst, do not give any fluids or food, and be alert for vomiting.

8. Monitor the patient's vital signs. This must be done at least every five minutes.

You will not be able to reverse shock, but you may be able to delay the onset of shock or keep it from worsening by following the procedures mentioned above.

If you are trained to do so and if your state laws allow, oxygen can be significant in the care of shock patients. Administer oxygen as per local protocols.

Fainting (Syncope)

Fainting, also known as syncope, is usually a self-correcting form of mild shock, also called psychogenic shock. However, the patient may have been injured in a fall due to fainting. Be certain to examine the patient for injury. Even if no other problems are apparent, keep the patient lying down and at rest for several minutes.

Fainting can also be a warning of a serious underlying condition such as a brain tumor, heart disease, or diabetes. Always recommend that the patient see a physician as soon as possible if he experiences a fainting spell.

WRAP-UP

The patient is carefully lowered to the floor in a supine position and covered with a blanket. Jordan places a nonrebreather mask on him and administers 15 LPM of oxygen. Within a few minutes, an ambulance arrives and rapidly transports Parker to the trauma center, where he is treated for shock, blood loss, and a deep five-centimeter laceration on his left forearm.

Parker is released from the hospital the next morning and, except for some weakness in one finger, makes a full recovery. He has since returned to work and is proudly working on a new set of cabinets that his company is donating to the Station Four kitchen.

FIRST ON SCENE

Summary

- Perfusion is the adequate supply of well-oxygenated blood and the removal of waste products from the body's tissues, especially the vital organs.

- Shock, also known as hypoperfusion, is the failure of the body's circulatory system to provide enough oxygenated blood and nutrients to all vital organs.

- The signs and symptoms of shock include increased pulse, increased breathing rate, restlessness or combativeness, pale, cool and moist skin, thirst, weakness, nausea and vomiting, and loss of responsiveness.

- There are several types of shock, and each type falls into one of four main categories. They are cardiogenic shock, hypovolemic shock, distributive shock, and obstructive shock.

- It is important to begin caring for shock if the mechanism of injury suggests internal injury or bleeding.

- Do not wait for the signs and symptoms to appear before caring for shock.

- Care for shock includes supporting the ABCs, keeping the patient lying flat, controlling all external bleeding, administering oxygen if allowed, maintaining a normal body temperature, and expediting transport.

Take Action

YOU CAN RUN, BUT YOU CANNOT HIDE

This activity will help you become better at taking repeated sets of vital signs, an important skill when monitoring patients for shock. You will need a blood pressure cuff, a stethoscope, and another student to act as your patient. Then, follow these steps:

1. To begin, take a complete set of baseline vital signs on your partner and record them on a piece of paper.

2. Now have your partner run a predetermined course. It can be several hundred yards or up and down several flights of stairs. The goal is to get the pulse well above the resting rate.

3. Once your partner returns, have him immediately lie down and obtain his blood pressure, pulse, and respirations. Record them on the same paper.

4. Wait five minutes (as your "patient" relaxes) and repeat the vitals.

5. Obtain the vital signs at least three times or until they have returned to normal.

This activity will allow you to get practice taking vital signs on someone other than a resting simulated "patient." It will also give you more practice taking vitals quickly and comparing each set with the previous set—just as you would do when monitoring a potentially hypoperfusing patient.

First on Scene Run Review

Recall the events of the "First on Scene" scenario in this chapter and answer the following questions, which are related to the call. Rationales are offered in the Answer Key at the back of the book.

1. What information would you want from dispatch en route to the call?

2. Why did Jordan place him down on the floor?

3. How would you control the bleeding?

Quick Quiz

To check your understanding of the chapter, answer the following questions. Then compare your answers to those in the Answer Key at the back of the book.

1. All of the following are signs of shock EXCEPT:
   a. increased pulse rate.
   b. decreasing blood pressure.
   c. pink, warm, moist skin.
   d. altered mental status.

2. When the body suffers a significant loss of blood, which type of shock is most likely to occur?
   a. Anaphylactic
   b. Cardiogenic
   c. Hemorrhagic
   d. Septic

3. Burns most often result in _____ shock.

   a. hypovolemic

   b. septic

   c. respiratory

   d. neurogenic

4. Psychogenic shock is commonly known as:

   a. hyperperfusion.

   b. stress reaction shock.

   c. decompensation.

   d. fainting.

5. Which one of the following is NOT one of the primary causes of shock?

   a. Dilated blood vessels

   b. Restricted movement

   c. Severe fluid loss

   d. Low levels of oxygen in the blood

6. You arrive at the scene of an unresponsive male patient who crashed his motorcycle into a tree at a high rate of speed. His respirations are 8 and shallow, pulse is 44 and weak, and you are unable to obtain a blood pressure. This patient is most likely experiencing _____ shock.

   a. psychogenic

   b. compensated

   c. decompensated

   d. respiratory

7. Decompensated shock is very serious and can quickly become:

   a. irreversible.

   b. hypoperfusion.

   c. compensated.

   d. anaphylaxis.

8. You are caring for a patient who was thrown from a horse and landed on her head. She is complaining of severe pain to the posterior neck. This patient is at risk for _____ shock.

   a. psychogenic

   b. hemorrhagic

   c. compensated

   d. neurogenic

9. You arrive at the scene of a small child who fell 15 feet. She is conscious and alert and complaining only of pain in her right arm, which has some deformity. Which one of the following best describes the appropriate care for this person?

   a. Splint the arm and suggest that her parents take her to the hospital.

   b. Assume she has internal injuries and treat for shock.

   c. Provide oxygen and splint the arm.

   d. Place her on a long backboard and transport.

10. Why does a patient's pulse rate increase as shock develops?

   a. To force oxygenated blood out of the patient's body core

   b. To counteract the high blood pressure

   c. To maintain adequate perfusion

   d. To create more blood to compensate for fluid loss

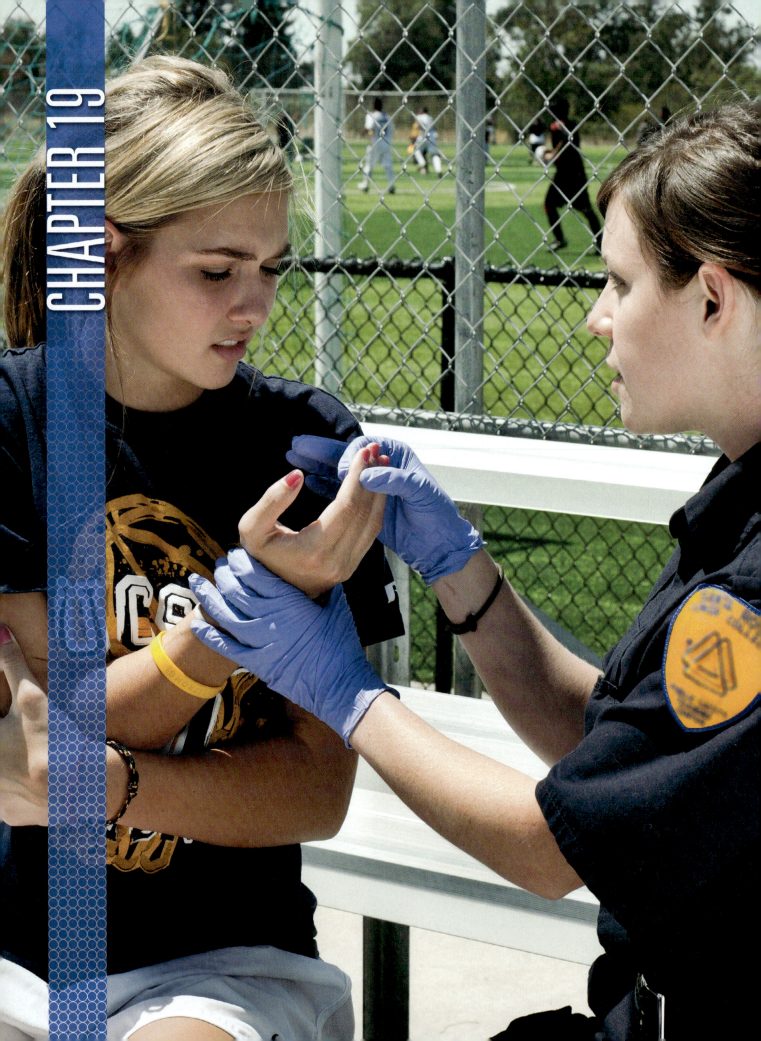

CHAPTER 19

Caring for Muscle and Bone Injuries

EDUCATION STANDARDS
- Trauma—Orthopedic Trauma

COMPETENCIES
- Uses simple knowledge to recognize and manage life threats based on assessment findings for an acutely injured patient while awaiting additional emergency medical response.

OVERVIEW

Bones are the foundation of the body. Like the steel girders that provide the strength and structure for buildings, bones provide the tough, internal structure and support for the demanding activities we put our bodies through on a daily basis. Unlike steel girders, bones are made of living tissue, able to move and bend by the actions of muscles and other tissues and by the messages received from a system of nerves controlled by the brain.

In your career as an Emergency Medical Responder, you will manage many patients with muscle and bone injuries. Such injuries are fairly common. To help you learn to assess and care for them, this chapter covers the general causes, types, and signs and symptoms of muscle and bone injuries, as well as the care that should be provided by Emergency Medical Responders.

OBJECTIVES

Upon successful completion of this chapter, the student should be able to:

COGNITIVE

1. Define the following terms:

   a. anatomical position *(p. 420)*

   b. angulated *(p. 413)*

   c. blunt trauma *(p. 415)*

   d. closed fracture *(p. 438)*

   e. cravat *(p. 427)*

   f. dislocation *(p. 413)*

   g. manual stabilization *(p. 418)*

   h. open fracture *(p. 415)*

   i. position of function *(p. 427)*

   j. sling *(p. 422)*

   k. splint *(p. 422)*

   l. sprain *(p. 413)*

   m. strain *(p. 413)*

   n. swathe *(p. 422)*

2. Describe the components that make up the musculoskeletal system. *(p. 408)*

3. Explain the functions of the musculoskeletal system. *(p. 408)*

4. Describe the major bones of the skeletal system. *(p. 409)*

5. Describe the signs and symptoms of a musculoskeletal injury. *(p. 415)*

6. Differentiate between a strain, sprain, fracture, and dislocation. *(p. 413)*

7. Differentiate between an open and closed skeletal injury. *(p. 413)*

8. Explain the appropriate care for a patient with a skeletal injury. *(p. 417)*

9. Explain the importance of an appropriate assessment of the distal extremity. *(p. 415)*

10. Differentiate between direct and indirect forces and the injuries they cause. *(p. 412)*

11. Explain the criteria for placing an angulated extremity injury into an anatomical position. *(p. 421)*

12. Explain the purpose and methods for manual stabilization of a skeletal injury. *(p. 421)*

13. Explain the priority of care for a patient with a suspected open skeletal injury. *(p. 417)*

14. Explain the priority of care for patient with multisystem trauma. *(p. 417)*

PSYCHOMOTOR

15. Demonstrate the appropriate assessment of a skeletal injury.

16. Demonstrate the appropriate care for a patient with a long-bone injury.

17. Demonstrate the appropriate care for a patient with a joint injury.

18. Demonstrate the appropriate technique for manual stabilization of a skeletal injury.

19. Demonstrate the proper placement of an angulated extremity injury into an anatomical position.

20. Demonstrate the proper placement of an arm sling.

21. Demonstrate the ability to place the hand/foot in the position of function during immobilization of an extremity.

AFFECTIVE

22. Value the importance of proper body substance isolation (BSI) precautions when caring for patients with musculoskeletal injuries.

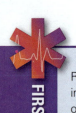

Ron Sloan reaches down, pushes a brightly colored golf tee into the soft ground facing the fairway, and balances his ball on it. "Okay," he says to his wife, Annie, after standing back up. "I'll bet you lunch that I get a birdie on this hole."

"You're on," she says, smiling from her seat in the golf cart. He repositions his feet several times, draws the club back over his shoulder, and swings it in surprisingly good form, considering how the rest of his game has been going. The ball flies high and straight, moving in sharp contrast to the royal blue of the early morning sky. Annie steps from the cart, mouth agape, and using the scorecard to shield her eyes, she follows the ball's descent to the distant green.

"Annie! The cart!" Ron yells, forgetting about the nearly perfect drive.

Annie turns and sees the golf cart rolling slowly backward, gaining speed as it heads for a nearby sand trap. She jogs over to it and tries to step back into the driver's seat, but just as she reaches it, there is a loud snap and her right leg folds underneath her.

She falls to the ground, clutching her badly bent leg. The cart continues down the slope and overturns into the trap, sending a spray of sand up onto the dark green fairway.

Musculoskeletal System

The *musculoskeletal system* is made up of many muscles, bones, joints, connective tissues, blood vessels, and nerves. Trauma, whether minor or major, can cause a variety of injuries to the muscles, bones, and other tissues that make up the musculoskeletal system. When assessing those injuries, Emergency Medical Responders are not expected to determine whether an injury is a fractured bone, a dislocated joint, a ligament sprain, or a muscle strain. Instead, the Emergency Medical Responder's job is to carefully assess the patient, looking for signs and symptoms of injury such as pain, swelling, deformity, and discoloration. Sometimes injuries can be easily identified as fractures, dislocations, or both, simply due to the amount of deformity. However, most musculoskeletal injuries are not that obvious, and often pain is the only symptom.

The extremities include the many bones and joints of the arms and legs. Surrounding the bones and joints are muscles and other soft tissues such as ligaments, tendons, blood vessels, and nerves. The tissues work with the skeletal system to nourish, support, and move those structures. Figure 19.1 shows the major blood vessels and a few of the major nerves found in the arms and legs. You do not need to remember every vessel and nerve, but you must remember that a large network of both are woven throughout the body. Injuries to the blood vessels and nerves can cause swelling, loss of movement or function, and significant pain. Careful assessment and management is important for minimizing pain, further damage to vessels and nerves, and blood loss. Your actions can minimize further injury to the extremity, promote healing, and help restore the function of the musculoskeletal system.

The musculoskeletal system has four major functions:

- *Support.* Bones support the soft tissues of the body, acting as a framework to give the body form and to provide a rigid structure for the attachment of muscles and other body parts.

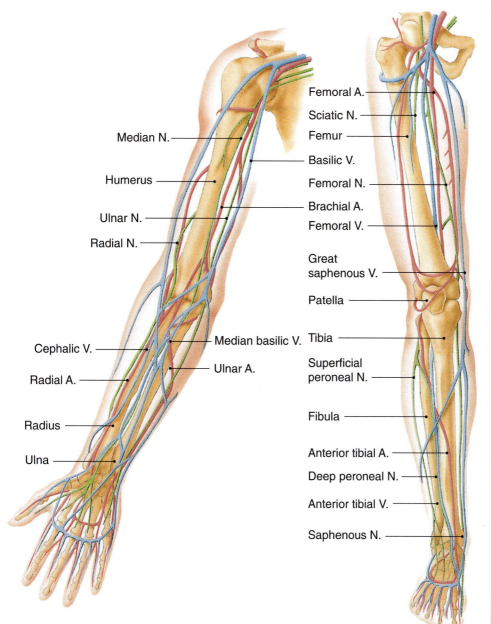

Figure 19.1 • Anatomy of the extremities. (A = artery. N = nerve. V = vein.)

Median N.

Humerus

Ulnar N.

Radial N.

Cephalic V.

Radial A.

Radius

Ulna

Median basilic V.

Ulnar A.

Femoral A.

Sciatic N.

Femur

Basilic V.

Femoral N.

Brachial A.

Femoral V.

Great saphenous V.

Patella

Tibia

Superficial peroneal N.

Fibula

Anterior tibial A.

Deep peroneal N.

Anterior tibial V.

Saphenous N.

KEY POINT ▼

This chapter uses terms such as *fracture, dislocation, strain,* and *sprain* for educational purposes only. That in no way suggests you as an Emergency Medical Responder will be diagnosing those injuries in the field. That is not the job of an Emergency Medical Responder. Most of those injuries will appear to be the same anyway. So instead, use an assessment-based approach, which means assess the patient, identify signs and symptoms, and provide care based on the signs and symptoms. For that reason, anyone with pain associated with a mechanism of injury that suggests a possible musculoskeletal injury should be cared for as though he has a fracture until proven otherwise.

- *Movement.* Muscles, bones, and joints act together to allow for movement.
- *Protection.* Many of the bones in the body provide protection for vital organs: the skull protects the brain; the spine protects the spinal cord; the ribs protect the heart, lungs, liver, stomach, and spleen; and the pelvis protects the urinary bladder and internal reproductive organs.
- *Cell production.* Some bones have the special function of producing blood cells.

The bones and joints of the body are what make up the *skeletal system*. Its two major divisions are (Figure 19.2):

- *Axial skeleton.* All the bones that form the upright axis of the body, including the skull, spinal column, sternum (breastbone), and ribs.
- *Appendicular skeleton.* All the bones that form the upper and lower extremities, including the collarbones, shoulder blades, arms, wrists, hands, hips, legs, ankles, and feet.

OBJECTIVE

4. Describe the major bones of the skeletal system.

Figure 19.2 • Two major divisions of the skeletal system are the appendicular skeleton (shown in the first figure in yellow) and the axial skeleton (shown in the second figure in yellow).

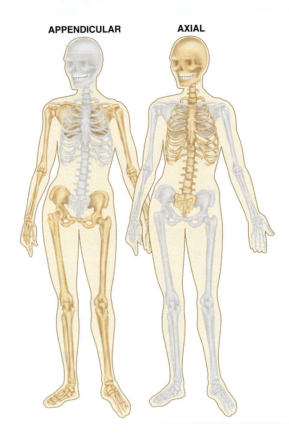

Appendicular Skeleton

As stated above, the appendicular skeleton is made up of the bones that form the upper and lower extremities. The upper extremities are made up of the shoulder girdle and both arms, down to and including the fingers (Figure 19.3). Table 19.1 lists the bones of the upper extremities and the number of bones that form each structure.

Figure 19.3 • Bones of the upper extremities.

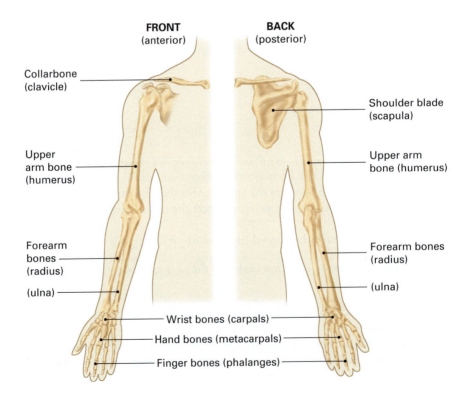

FRONT (anterior)   BACK (posterior)

Collarbone (clavicle)

Shoulder blade (scapula)

Upper arm bone (humerus)

Upper arm bone (humerus)

Forearm bones (radius)

Forearm bones (radius)

(ulna)

(ulna)

Wrist bones (carpals)

Hand bones (metacarpals)

Finger bones (phalanges)

TABLE 19.1 | Bones of the Upper Extremities

COMMON NAMES	MEDICAL NAMES
Shoulder girdle	
• Collarbone (1/side)	Clavicle
• Shoulder blade (1/side)	Scapula
Upper arm bone (1/arm, from shoulder to elbow)	Humerus
Forearm bones (2/arm, from elbow to wrist: 1 medial and 1 lateral)	Ulna (medial) Radius (lateral)
Wrist bones (8/wrist)	Carpals
Hand bones (5/palm)	Metacarpals
Finger bones (14/hand)	Phalanges

The lower extremities are made up of the pelvis and both legs, down to and including the toes (Figure 19.4). Table 19.2 lists the bones of the lower extremities and the number of bones that form each structure.

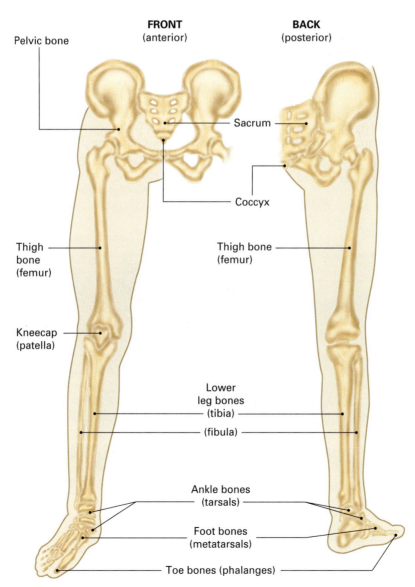

FRONT (anterior) **BACK** (posterior)

Pelvic bone
Sacrum
Coccyx
Thigh bone (femur)
Thigh bone (femur)
Kneecap (patella)
Lower leg bones (tibia)
(fibula)
Ankle bones (tarsals)
Foot bones (metatarsals)
Toe bones (phalanges)

Figure 19.4 • Bones of the lower extremities.

TABLE 19.2 | Bones of the Lower Extremities

COMMON NAMES	MEDICAL NAMES
Pelvic girdle (pelvis and hips)	Innominate or os coxae
Thigh bone (1/leg)	Femur
Kneecap (1/leg)	Patella
Lower leg bones (2/leg: 1 medial and 1 lateral)	Tibia (medial) Fibula (lateral)
Ankle bones (7/foot)	Tarsals
Foot bones (5/foot)	Metatarsals
Toe bones (14–15/foot)	Phalanges

▶ **GERIATRIC FOCUS** ◀

Aging and disease are leading contributors to skeletal injuries. As people age, the bones can become weak and brittle and break more easily. People with certain medical conditions such as bone cancer, kidney disease, or osteoporosis have very fragile bones, and the slightest force can result in a fracture.

Causes of Extremity Injuries

OBJECTIVE

10. Differentiate between direct and indirect forces and the injuries they cause.

There are three primary forces that cause musculoskeletal injuries. They are *direct force*, *indirect force*, and *twisting force* (Figure 19.5). Extremities often are injured because of the direct force applied to a bone when a person falls and strikes an object or when a person is struck by an object. Sometimes the energy of a force may be transferred up or down the extremity, which can result in an injury farther along the extremity. Such indirect-force injuries can occur, for instance, when one puts out the hand to break a fall and dislocates the shoulder instead of breaking the wrist.

Figure 19.5 • There are three basic types of mechanism of injury.

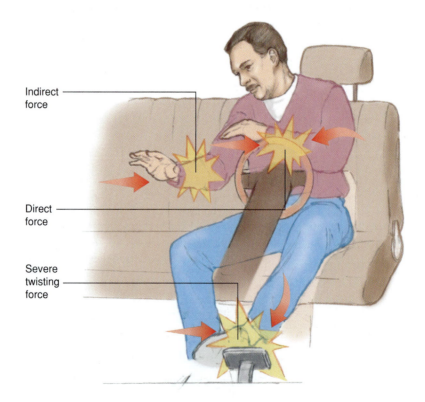

Indirect force

Direct force

Severe twisting force

An example of an injury caused by a twisting force is when someone gets a hand or foot caught in a wheel or gear. The body remains stationary while the hand or foot turns in the wheel. Twisting injuries can also be caused when the body keeps moving forward while the hand or foot remains trapped.

Types of Injuries

Skeletal injuries can be categorized into one of two basic types: *closed injuries* or *open injuries* (Figure 19.6). An injury is considered closed when there is no break in the skin. In some cases, the bones and surrounding soft tissue can be damaged extensively even though the skin is unbroken.

There is an exception to the term *closed injury* when referring to injuries to the head. A closed head injury may indeed have an open wound to the scalp but because the *cranium* remains intact, it is referred to as a closed injury.

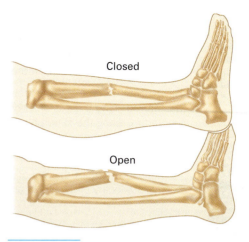

Figure 19.6 • Closed and open injuries.

An injury is considered to be *open* when the soft tissues adjacent to an injury are damaged and open. The mechanism of injury causes the bone ends or pieces of bone to tear through the skin from inside out or, in some cases, something enters and opens the skin from the outside and also breaks the bone underneath (e.g., a gunshot wound).

Any strong force to the extremities (such as a blunt force trauma) can cause damage to bones and surrounding tissues (Scan 19.1). At the very least, most musculoskeletal injuries will present with pain. In more severe injuries, swelling, discoloration, and deformity also may be present. Do not try to diagnose the injury as a fracture, dislocation, sprain, or strain. In most cases, the true extent of the injury cannot be determined until X-rays are taken and examined by a physician. Instead, you should assess the mechanism of injury and provide care for the injury based on the signs and symptoms.

Although you will not diagnose specific types of musculoskeletal injury, you should know something about each one:

- *Fracture.* Any time a bone is broken, chipped, cracked, or splintered, it results in what is commonly referred to as a *fracture*.
- *Dislocation.* This occurs when one end of a bone that is part of a joint is pulled or pushed out of place. **Dislocations** often result in serious damage to tendons, ligaments, nerves, and blood vessels because of the way they hold a joint together or weave in and around a joint. Sometimes the force that caused a dislocation of a bone will also cause it or an adjoining bone to fracture, resulting in what is referred to as a fracture-dislocation.
- *Sprain.* The tough, fibrous tissues called *ligaments* hold together the bones that make up a joint. Tendons attach muscle to bones. Excessive twisting forces can cause ligaments and tendons to stretch or tear, resulting in a **sprain** injury.
- *Strain.* A **strain** is caused by overexerting, overworking, overstretching, or tearing of a muscle.

A sign common to many serious bone injuries is angulation or deformity. **Angulated** (deformed) injuries occur when an extremity is bulging, bent, or angulated where it normally should be straight. These injuries may be slight, which means that the vessels and nerves that serve the extremity likely will still be intact. In those cases, you will most likely be able to feel a distal pulse, and the patient will have normal *sensation* (able to feel your touch) and *motor function* (able to move the limb). If angulated injuries are extreme, you may not feel a distal pulse, and the patient may experience a change in sensation and/or motor function. Deformed injuries may be open or closed.

Signs and Symptoms of Extremity Injuries

The main signs and symptoms to look for in an extremity injury include:

- *Pain.* Pain occurs when nerves surrounding the injury have been injured and are being pressed by swelling tissue or broken bone ends. Tissues near the injury site will be

OBJECTIVE

7. Differentiate between an open and closed skeletal injury.

IS IT SAFE?

Scene safety is especially important at emergency scenes that involve injuries and trauma. The conditions that caused the injury for the patient may still exist even after you arrive on the scene. Pay close attention to the dispatch, and keep a close eye for both obvious and not so obvious hazards. Once you make patient contact, it will be difficult to keep an eye out for hazards. Do your best to identify and correct hazards before they affect you.

OBJECTIVE

6. Differentiate between a strain, sprain, fracture, and dislocation.

dislocation ▶ the pulling or pushing of a bone end partially or completely free of a joint.

sprain ▶ a partial or complete tearing of the ligaments and tendons that support a joint.

strain ▶ the overstretching or tearing of a muscle.

angulated ▶ refers to an injured limb that is deformed and out of normal alignment.

MECHANISM OF INJURY the force or forces that may have caused the patient's injury.

DIRECT FORCE energy that is transmitted directly to an extremity, causing an injury at the site of impact.

INDIRECT FORCE energy from a direct force blow that is transferred along the axis of a bone and causes an injury farther along the extremity.

TWISTING FORCE the forces caused when an extremity or part of an extremity is caught in a twisting or circular mechanism, while the rest of the extremity or the body is stationary or moving in another direction.

DOWNWARD BLOW Clavicle and scapula

LATERAL BLOW Clavicle, scapula, and humerus

LATERAL BLOW Knee, hip, femur (very forceful)

INDIRECT FORCE Pelvis, hip, knee, leg bones, shoulder, humerus, elbow, forearm bones

TWISTING FORCE Hip, femur, knee, leg bones, ankle, shoulder, elbow, forearm, wrist

FORCED FLEXION OR HYPEREXTENSION Elbow, wrist, fingers, femur, knee, foot

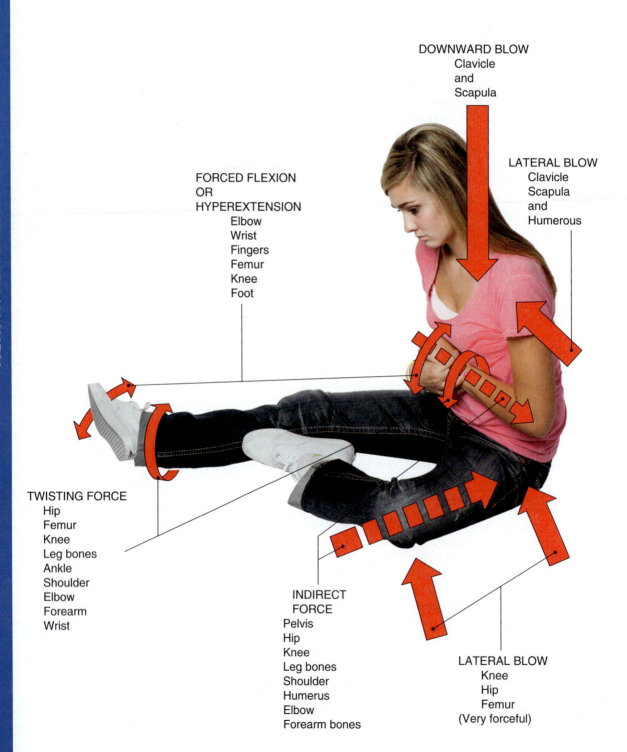

DOWNWARD BLOW
Clavicle
and
Scapula

LATERAL BLOW
Clavicle
Scapula
and
Humerous

FORCED FLEXION
OR
HYPEREXTENSION
Elbow
Wrist
Fingers
Femur
Knee
Foot

TWISTING FORCE
Hip
Femur
Knee
Leg bones
Ankle
Shoulder
Elbow
Forearm
Wrist

INDIRECT
FORCE
Pelvis
Hip
Knee
Leg bones
Shoulder
Humerus
Elbow
Forearm bones

LATERAL BLOW
Knee
Hip
Femur
(Very forceful)

very tender. The patient can usually tell you where it hurts. As part of your secondary assessment, gently palpate the areas above and below the injury site to help determine the extent of the pain.

- *Swelling.* The area around the injury will begin to swell because blood from ruptured blood vessels is collecting inside the tissues.
- *Discoloration.* Blood trapped under the skin may cause it to look reddish or discolored. Later, as these blood cells die, they cause the typical black-and-blue bruising, which may take 24 hours or longer to develop.
- *Deformity.* When this occurs, a part of a limb appears different in size or shape than the same part on the opposite side of the patient's body. (Always compare both arms and legs to one another.) If a bone appears to have an unusual angle, bulge, or swelling, consider this deformity to be a sign of possible fracture or dislocation. Feel gently along the patient's limbs, noting any lumps, swelling, discoloration, or ends of bones through the skin.

Other common signs and symptoms of an extremity injury include:

- *Inability to move a joint or limb.* Sometimes movement is possible but very painful. If the patient can move an arm but not the fingers, or if a patient can move a leg but not the toes, a fracture may have caused severe damage to nerves and blood vessels. The patient will often cradle, or guard, an injured arm or hold it close to the body to stabilize it in a comfortable position. An injured person will often ask you not to touch or move the injured extremity.
- *Numbness or tingling sensation.* This can be from pressure on nerves or blood vessels caused by swelling or broken bones.
- *Loss of distal pulse.* Bone ends or bone fragments may be pressing against or cutting through an artery. Swelling from internal bleeding may be pressing against an artery. The extremity may be pale and cold because of restricted blood flow and then turn bluish (cyanotic) because of lack of oxygen.
- *Slow capillary refill.* A decrease in perfusion may be indicated by an increase in capillary refill time. (This will be explained later in this chapter.)
- *Grating.* When the patient moves, the ends of fractured bones rub together, making a grating sound referred to as *crepitus*. Do not ask a patient to move in order to confirm or reproduce this sound.
- *Sound of breaking at the time of injury.* If the patient or bystanders tell you they heard this sound, suspect a fracture has occurred.
- *Exposed bone.* In cases of **open fracture**, the fragments or ends of broken bones may be visible where they break through the skin.

▶ GERIATRIC FOCUS ◀

Pain perception is often blunted in the elderly; therefore, they may not always complain of pain at the site of injury. Also, it is not uncommon for geriatric patients to have referred pain. For example, they may complain of knee pain when in fact they have a broken hip. Thus, it is important to examine the entire extremity of the elderly patient to determine more precisely what is injured.

All injured extremities should be assessed for adequate circulation, sensation, and motor function (CSM) before and after immobilization. Check circulation by assessing distal pulses and capillary refill. In the absence of a pulse, good color can be interpreted as good circulation. If possible, compare the injured side to the uninjured side. To assess for normal sensation of the distal extremity, squeeze the fingers or toes of the injured extremity and ask the patient to tell you if he can feel your touch and where you are touching. Ask him if your touch feels normal or if it feels numb or tingly. You can further evaluate sensation by squeezing just one finger or two and then asking the patient if he can tell which finger or toe you are squeezing.

To evaluate motor function, begin by asking the patient to wiggle his fingers or toes. Next, you can check the strength of the extremity by placing your thumbs in each hand

OBJECTIVES

5. Describe the signs and symptoms of a musculoskeletal injury.

9. Explain the importance of an appropriate assessment of the distal extremity.

blunt trauma ▶ an injury that is caused by the impact with a blunt surface such as the ground or a large object.

IS IT SAFE?

As an Emergency Medical Responder, you may be called on to help lift or move a patient with a musculoskeletal injury. Doing so can put great stress on your back if you do not use good body mechanics. Use caution when lifting patients or heavy objects, and do not attempt a lift unless you have enough people to assist. Back injuries are a common cause of disability for EMS personnel. It is important to use care whenever participating in a lift.

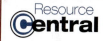

Resource Central

Learn more about fractures by viewing images of fractures and by taking an interactive tutorial about fractures and sprains.

open fracture ▶ a broken bone with an associated break in the outer layers of the skin.

KEY POINT ▼

When assessing the motor function of the extremity by having the patient grasp or push against your hands, be sure to assess both extremities simultaneously. This will allow for a more accurate assessment of strength between the injured and uninjured side.

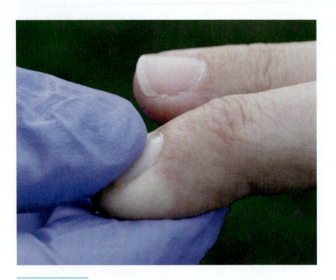

Figure 19.7 • Assessing capillary refill in the fingers.
(© Dan Limmer)

and asking him to squeeze. For the feet, place your hands at the bottom of his feet and ask him to press down on your hands. In either case, note the strength and compare the good side with the injured side. In most instances you will notice a weakness on the injured side, which is usually due to pain. Ask the patient if it causes pain when he squeezes or presses on your hands.

Checking for sensation and motor function gives you information about the status of the nerves that supply the injured extremity. A lack of feeling or the inability to move may indicate that there is pressure on or damage to a nerve. This nerve damage may be the result of injury to the spinal cord and not just an injury to the extremity.

Several important signs will tell you the state of circulation to the extremity:

- If the injury site is swollen and discolored, there is bleeding in the tissues.
- If there is no distal pulse and the extremity is pale and cool, circulation to the extremity may be compromised.
- If the extremity is blue, there is lack of circulation and thus a lack of oxygen in the limb.

Another tool for assessing the circulation or perfusion status of a distal extremity is called *capillary refill time*. To assess capillary refill time, press the nail bed or pad of the finger or toe on the injured extremity between your finger and thumb. When you press the skin, it forces blood out of the tissues, causing them to blanch, or turn white. When you release pressure, the blood should flow back into the tissues in less than two seconds. If it takes longer than two seconds for the tissues to refill with blood, it may be a sign of compromised circulation to the extremity. Capillary refill time also may be affected by factors such as temperature, medications, and preexisting medical conditions. When possible, capillary refill should be assessed on both the injured and uninjured extremities for comparison (Figure 19.7).

Patient Assessment

In the scene size-up, quickly determine scene safety and don all appropriate personal protective equipment. Note the mechanism of injury and the total number of patients. Then determine what additional assistance you may need. If the mechanism of injury suggests a possible spine injury and the scene is safe to enter, immediately stabilize your patient's head and neck. (More on this in Chapter 20.)

During your primary assessment, get an impression of the environment and the patient, and determine how quickly the patient needs to be moved and transported. Do not focus on obvious injuries. Instead, assess the ABCs and mental status. Detect and correct life-threatening problems as quickly as possible. Look for and control all major bleeding.

From the Medical Director

Patient Assessment

You should make every attempt to preserve your patient's dignity while examining him for injuries. If you must expose a woman's chest or remove anyone's pants, delegate rescuers to hold up a sheet or form a "human shield" from onlookers. Only rarely is it necessary to completely undress a patient.

There is a certain order to caring for injuries. If there is time after correcting and stabilizing life-threatening injuries to the ABCs, checking for and stabilizing neck and spine injuries, and providing care for shock, then you can focus on any extremity injuries. Always be sure to note the mechanism of injury, because this will give you an idea of the possible extent, type, and location of injuries.

When caring for skeletal injuries, the first priority is given to possible injury to the spine. Next is care for possible injuries to the following:

- *Skull*. It protects the brain and contains a portion of the airway.
- *Rib cage*. It protects the heart and lungs. Broken sections may damage the function of these organs as well as prevent adequate breathing.
- *Pelvis*. It protects reproductive and urinary organs, major nerves, and blood vessels.
- *Thighs*. It takes major trauma to injure the largest, sturdiest bone (femur) in the body, which is surrounded by major nerves and blood vessels. Blood loss from a thigh injury can be life threatening.
- Any extremity injury where no distal pulse is detected during the primary assessment.

Always evaluate the mechanism of injury, and be concerned with major bleeding and possible shock whenever there are injuries to the chest, pelvis, or thighs. A significant amount of blood can be lost internally in those areas. Monitor the patient's signs and symptoms carefully. A rapid, weak pulse; pale or blue skin color; an altered mental status; and cold extremities are signs and symptoms that should alert you to manage and transport this patient as soon as possible.

Remember the following emergency care steps when caring for a patient with musculoskeletal injuries (Figure 19.8):

1. Always take proper BSI precautions and perform a primary assessment before focusing on a particular injury.
   - Assess and provide support for the ABCs.
   - Manage life-threatening problems first.
   - Prioritize and manage other injuries second.

OBJECTIVES

8. Explain the appropriate care for a patient with a skeletal injury.

14. Explain the priority of care for patient with multisystem trauma.

OBJECTIVE

13. Explain the priority of care for a patient with a suspected open skeletal injury.

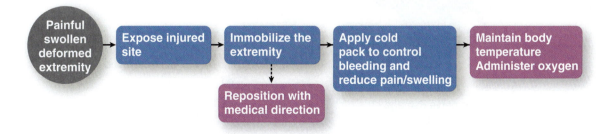

Figure 19.8 • Algorithm for emergency care of patients with musculoskeletal injuries.

2. Carefully cut away clothing to expose the injury site. Control bleeding if there is an open wound. Check for distal circulation, sensation, and motor function in the affected extremity.

3. Immobilize the extremity using manual stabilization or splints, if available.
   - Immobilize the suspected fracture site.
   - Immobilize the joints above and below the suspected fracture site. Use a sling and swathe for an arm to keep it elevated across the chest. Splinted, immobilized legs may be propped up on a folded blanket or pillow if there is no indication of spine injury.
   - Recheck distal circulation, sensation, and motor function often.

4. Apply a cold pack or ice pack to the injury site to help reduce the pain and swelling. Never put a cold pack directly on the skin. Wrap it in gauze or a towel first. Then place it gently over the injury site. If the patient experiences pain from this extra pressure on the injury, place the cold pack just above the site.

5. Administer oxygen as soon as possible per local protocol.

6. Assess the patient's vital signs. Maintain a comfortable body temperature to help minimize the effects of shock.

Emotional support is important when caring for a patient with musculoskeletal injuries. Tell the patient what you suspect may be wrong, how you will manage it, and what will be done by other emergency care providers on scene and at the hospital. You may need to remind the patient that fractures can be set at the hospital and bones will heal. Talking with the patient gives him confidence and relieves anxiety. It may also help lower blood pressure, pulse rate, and breathing rate.

Splinting

Splinting is the process of immobilizing an injury, using a device such as a piece of wood, cardboard, or folded blanket. Any object that can be used to restrict the movement of an injury is called a splint. **Manual stabilization** is the process of using your hands to restrict the movement of an injured person or body part.

manual stabilization ▶ the process of restricting the movement of an injured person or limb with one's hands.

Why Splint?

The application of splints allows emergency care providers to reposition and transfer the patient while minimizing movement of the injury. Moving a patient who has musculoskeletal injuries prior to splinting can cause damage to soft tissues, leading to complications and even prolonging recovery (Figure 19.9). Complications include:

- *Pain*. A splint can reduce much of the patient's pain because it secures the broken or dislocated bones in place and prevents them from compressing or damaging surrounding nerves and tissues.

Figure 19.9 • Complications associated with extremity injuries can be prevented or decreased with splinting.

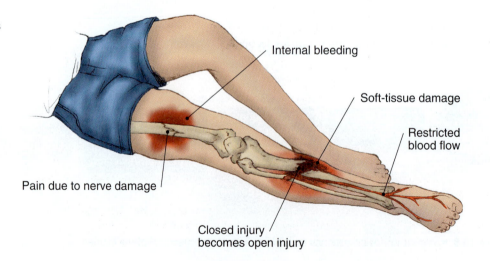

Internal bleeding

Soft-tissue damage

Restricted blood flow

Pain due to nerve damage

Closed injury becomes open injury

- *Damage to soft tissues.* The movement of an injured extremity may cause blood vessels, nerves, and muscles to be crushed, ruptured, pinched, or compressed. Splinting reduces movement of the injured part, the possibility of further damage to soft tissues, and the accompanying pain, internal bleeding, and swelling.
- *Bleeding.* The initial force of injury may have caused bone ends to damage soft tissues and blood vessels. Splinting will stabilize the injury and apply a steady pressure that can reduce and control bleeding.
- *Restricted blood flow.* Dislocated joints and fractured bones and fragments also can press against blood vessels and shut off blood flow. Splinting can help relieve the pressure against blood vessels.
- *Closed injuries become open injuries.* The sharp edge of a broken bone can rip through skin to produce an open wound. Immobilizing the injured extremity by splinting it will minimize movement of the broken part and help prevent a closed wound from becoming an open wound.

▶ GERIATRIC FOCUS ◀

Although padding is always important when splinting, it is particularly important for the elderly patient. Pressure from a hard splint could interrupt blood supply to the skin or limb and result in long-term problems well after the simple injury is healed. Be sure to add extra padding to any splint applied to an elderly patient.

Emergency Medical Responder Responsibilities

The primary duty of an Emergency Medical Responder is to detect and control life-threatening problems. Then, during the secondary assessment, attempt to find all injuries and care for the worst ones first. Most bleeding will be controlled with direct pressure and elevation, and once potential neck or spine injuries are stabilized, care for suspected extremity injuries. Shock is managed with proper positioning, oxygen administration, and maintaining the patient's body temperature. In the case of major trauma, EMTs will likely arrive before you have an opportunity to apply splints.

Some patients may have indications of neck or spine injuries, and you will not be able to splint extremities until you have additional help or equipment from more advanced providers. In the meantime, this patient must not be moved but should be kept still while you stabilize his head and neck with your hands. (That is explained in more detail in Chapter 20.)

General Rules for Splinting

For all cases of splinting, you will (Scan 19.2):

- Assess and reassure the patient, and explain what you plan to do.
- Expose the injury site. Cut away clothing if it cannot be easily removed or folded back. Remove jewelry from the injured limb if it can be done without using force, causing pain, or repositioning the patient or the limb.
- Control all major bleeding. If necessary, use direct pressure. Avoid applying pressure directly over exposed bone ends. To control major bleeding, use bulky dressings secured snugly with a bandage.
- Dress open wounds. Do not push bone ends back into the wound. Do not try to pick bone fragments from the wound. If the bone ends withdraw into the wound as you care for it, report this to personnel who take over patient care so they can take steps to prevent infection in the patient.
- Check distal circulation, sensation, and motor function before and after splinting.
- Splint injuries before moving the patient. Move the patient before splinting only if another injury or the environment is life threatening.

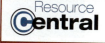

Read more about long-bone injuries and splints.

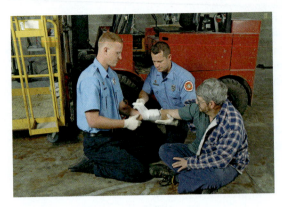

19.2.1 | After controlling bleeding, dress and bandage open wounds to the injured extremity.

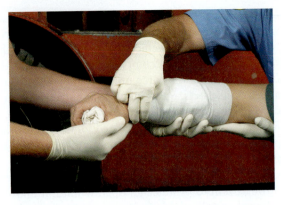

19.2.2 | Check distal circulation, sensation, and motor function before splinting.

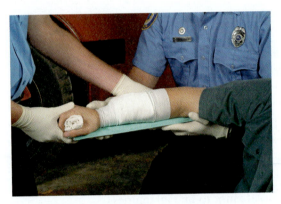

19.2.3 | Select an appropriate size splint for the injury and pad the splint thoroughly.

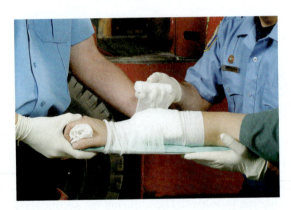

19.2.4 | Firmly secure the splint, leaving fingertips (or toes) exposed so you can monitor circulation.

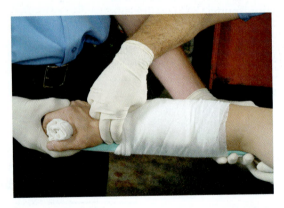

19.2.5 | After immobilization, reassess distal circulation, sensation, and motor function.

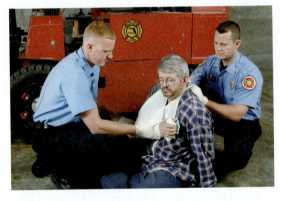

19.2.6 | Elevate the extremity. For an arm, use the sling to immobilize it against the chest. For a leg, prop it on a pillow or rolled blanket (if there is no indication of spine injury).

anatomical position ▶ the standard reference position for the body in the study of anatomy; the body is standing erect, facing the observer with arms down at the sides, palms forward.

- Have all materials ready and at hand before splinting. Use padded splints for patient comfort and improved contact between limb and splint. Wrap unpadded splints in dressings before applying them.
- If distal circulation is absent and local protocols allow, gently attempt to realign an angulated limb in the **anatomical position** before splinting. Attempt to reposition the limb to regain a pulse if the limb is cold, blue, and has no pulse.
- Immobilize the suspected fracture site and the joints above and below the injury site. Secure upper extremities to the torso with a sling and swathe. Secure lower

extremities to each other. Assist the EMTs in transferring the patient to a spine board or similar device.

- Secure splints with cravats or roller gauze, starting at the distal end of the extremity. Leave fingertips and toes exposed so you can monitor circulation, sensation, and motor function.
- Elevate the extremity. For an arm, use a sling and swathe. For a leg, prop it on a pillow or rolled blanket if there is no indication of spine injury. If there is an indication of a spine injury, leave the patient lying flat (supine).
- Minimize the effects of shock by maintaining body temperature and providing oxygen if local protocols allow.

Manual Stabilization

Manual stabilization involves using your hands to keep an injured extremity from moving. In most instances the patient will be holding manual stabilization of their own injury when you arrive. It may be appropriate to take over manual stabilization of the injury from the patient so that he can assume a more comfortable position, such as lying down. In the case of arm injuries, the patient may be holding the arm tight against the body to keep it from moving. This may be the best position for him, so do not be in too much of a hurry to take control of the extremity. You can still evaluate distal circulation, sensation, and motor function while he is holding the arm secure (Figure 19.10).

When caring for leg injuries, it is best to take over manual stabilization for the patient. Assign one person for this purpose and have him maintain manual stabilization throughout the splinting process. You may find that even the slightest amount of movement is very painful for the patient. In those instances, consider just holding manual stabilization until the ambulance arrives.

OBJECTIVE

12. Explain the purpose and methods for manual stabilization of a skeletal injury.

Managing Angulated Injuries

Some EMS systems do not allow Emergency Medical Responders to straighten deformed injuries. Do only what you have been trained to do and what is allowed in your EMS system. Check your local protocols to find out what you are allowed to do if there is angulation of an extremity with no distal circulation. If you find no distal pulse, and the skin in the distal extremity is pale or blue and cold, take action immediately to minimize potential permanent damage. You may be directed to gently align the limb in an attempt to restore a distal pulse. Do not force the limb if you meet resistance or if the patient complains of too much pain. Apply a soft splint and elevate the limb by propping it on a blanket roll or pillow. Provide oxygen (if allowed) and other appropriate emergency care interventions until the EMTs arrive.

OBJECTIVE

11. Explain the criteria for placing an angulated extremity injury into an anatomical position.

Follow these steps when attempting to straighten an injured limb when a pulse cannot be detected:

1. Carefully explain to the patient what you plan to do and why.

2. Support the extremity with both hands to minimize movement of the injury site. Use additional rescuers if needed.

3. While supporting the limb, gently pull traction from the distal end as you carefully straighten the extremity.

4. Move slowly until you bring the extremity into a natural position similar to the uninjured limb.

5. Reassure the patient as best you can.

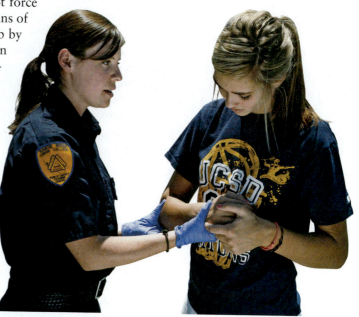

Figure 19.10 • Manual stabilization of an injured limb.

The main reason for straightening closed deformed injuries is to restore circulation, but straight limbs also make it easier for you to apply a rigid splint. If the limb cannot be straightened or if you are not allowed to straighten it, immobilize the limb in the position found. The procedure for straightening closed deformed injuries is as follows:

- Attempt to straighten closed deformed injuries only if there is no distal circulation.
- Make only one attempt to straighten the angulation.
- Stop if you meet resistance or if the patient complains of severe pain.

Some jurisdictions only allow for straightening angulated injuries under certain conditions or for certain extremities. Always follow your local protocols.

Types of Splints

There are many types of splints on the market today. As an Emergency Medical Responder you should be familiar with those commonly used by your agency or in your region.

Soft Splints

splint ▶ any device that is used to immobilize an injured extremity.

There are two main types of splints: soft and rigid. When properly applied, **soft splints** such as pillows, blankets, towels, cravats, and dressings may be very effective in stabilizing injuries. Soft splints can provide support and help decrease both pain and swelling. A commonly used soft splint is the *triangular bandage*. It can be folded to any width to fit any part of the body, to secure arms to the torso and legs to each other, or to secure extremities to rigid splints. A triangular bandage is frequently used for a sling and swathe.

sling ▶ a large triangular bandage or other cloth device that is used to immobilize an elbow and support the forearm.

A **sling** is a triangular bandage used to stabilize an upper extremity. A properly placed sling will adequately immobilize an injured elbow and provide support to the lower arm. Once the arm is placed in a sling, a **swathe** is used to hold the arm against the side of the chest and restrict movement of the shoulder. A swathe is made from a triangular bandage, which is folded to about a two-inch to four-inch width so it fits the area of the arm between the shoulder and elbow. Together, the sling and swathe work well to immobilize both the elbow and shoulder joints, which is necessary when caring for suspected fractures of the arm.

swathe ▶ a large cravat used to secure a sling or splint to the body.

The sling and swathe are generally effective for injuries to the shoulder, upper arm, elbow, lower arm, and wrist. To make and apply a sling and swathe, you should (Scan 19.3):

1. Use a commercial sling, or make one from a piece of cloth or sheet. Fold or cut this material so that it is in the shape of a triangle. The ideal sling should be about 50 to 60 inches long at its base and 36 to 40 inches long on each of its sides.

2. Position the triangular material over the patient's chest. The top of the triangle should point toward the patient's injured arm and extend beyond the elbow. The top end should be draped over the opposite shoulder. Have the patient position his arm so the hand is above the elbow. If he cannot hold his arm, have your partner or a bystander support the arm while you prepare and secure the sling.

3. Take the bottom end of the triangle and bring it up and over the patient's arm and shoulder on the injured side.

4. Draw up on the ends of the sling so that the patient's hand on the injured side is about four inches above the elbow. Tie the two ends together. Be sure to position the knot so it does not rest on the back of the patient's neck. Place a flat layer of cloth (gauze pads or handkerchief) under the knot for comfort. Leave the patient's fingertips exposed so you can check for circulation, sensation, and motor function. If circulation is absent following immobilization, support the arm while the sling is removed and, if local protocols allow, gently reposition it until you can feel the pulse. Replace the sling.

5. Take the point of the sling at the patient's elbow and fold it forward. Then tuck it in or pin it in place, or twist and tie the point. It may be easier to tie the point before the sling is placed on the patient. This will form a pocket for the patient's elbow.

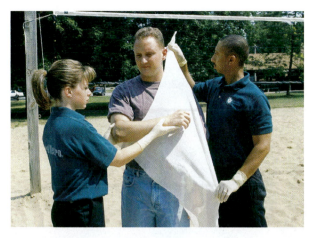

19.3.1 | Place one end of the base of the triangular bandage over the uninjured shoulder. Ensure that the apex is pointed toward the injured arm.

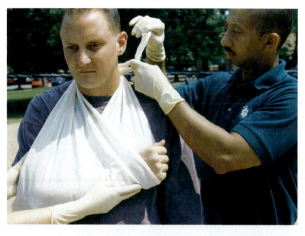

19.3.2 | Bring the lower end of the bandage up and over the shoulder on the injured side. Tie a knot at the side of the neck.

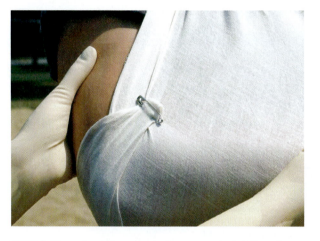

19.3.3 | Pin or tape the apex to form a pocket at the elbow.

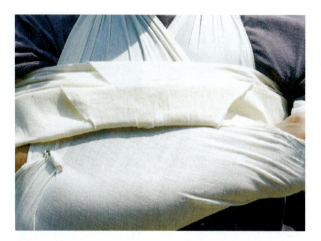

19.3.4 | Secure the arm to the body with a swathe.

6. Take a second piece of triangular cloth and fold it to a two- or four-inch width. Center it on the widest part of the patient's injured arm. Take one end across the patient's back and one end across the chest and tie on the opposite side under the other arm. Be sure that the swathe is placed as low over the injured arm as possible. This will ensure that it stays close to the body and minimize movement of the shoulder.

Rigid Splints

Rigid splints can be made of plastic, metal, wood, or compressed cardboard and have very little give or flexibility. They are applied along an injured extremity to immobilize the suspected fracture site and, if possible, the joints directly above and below the injury site as well.

From the Medical Director

Rigid Splints

When applying a rigid splint to an extremity, fill the space between the patient and the splint with soft cushions or bandages. Do this whether or not the injury is angulated.

Warning: Air splints may leak. When applied in cold weather, an air splint will expand when the patient is moved to a warmer place. Pressure also will change at different altitudes. Monitor the pressure in the splint by pressing with your fingertip. These splints may stick to the patient's skin in hot weather.

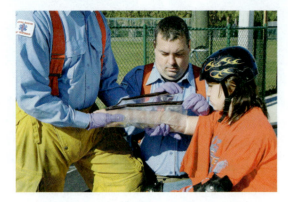

19.4.1 | Partially inflate the splint and slide it over the patient's extremity. Allow the fingers or toes to remain exposed at the end of the splint.

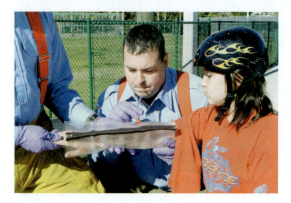

19.4.2 | Maintain manual stabilization of the extremity while your partner inflates the splint. Inflate so that you leave a slight dent when the splint is pressed with one finger.

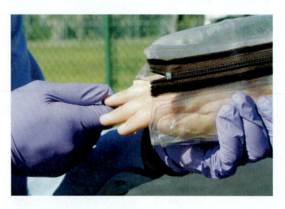

19.4.3 | Reassess circulation, sensation, and motor function, and monitor the pressure of the splint. Add air if necessary.

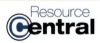

Resource **Central**

Learn about the Sagar splint.

Commercial Splints

A wide variety of commercial splints are available for emergency care. They are made of wood, aluminum, cardboard, foam, wire, or plastic. Some come with their own washable pads and others require padding to be applied before being secured. Most splints are either solid rigid pieces or inflatable plastic splints. They include air splints, vacuum splints, board-and-wire ladder splints, heavy-duty cardboard splints, and flexible aluminum splints. All EMTs and many Emergency Medical Responders carry traction splints for splinting and stabilizing isolated femur injuries.

Local protocols may provide guidelines for using a pneumatic antishock garment (PASG), a special device for suspected pelvic and femur fractures. You must receive training and use the PASG only as allowed by local protocols.

Inflatable Splints

Inflatable splints, or air splints, are not carried by all Emergency Medical Responder units. If you carry them and your jurisdiction allows you to use them, your instructor will teach you their application. Typically, air splints are used for patients with injuries to the arm or lower leg bones. When using an air splint, slip it uninflated over your forearm. Then grasp the patient's hand or foot and pull gentle traction while you slip the air splint onto the patient's limb. Smooth out the splint and inflate it. The splint is fully inflated and effective when you can make a slight surface indentation with your fingertip (Scan 19.4).

After inflating the splint, you must monitor the limb for changes in circulation, sensation, and motor function. Monitor the splint for changes in pressure. If the patient is moved to a warmer or colder location, the air in the splint will expand or contract with the temperature change. You will have to recheck the pressure in the splint. You may have to remove increased pressure by deflating the splint slightly. The pressure in the splint also will change if the patient is moved to a different altitude, which can be a concern when patients are flown, or transported down from mountain accident scenes. Always monitor the pressure in the splint.

Once an air splint is applied, you may not be able to assess the distal pulse. Instead, evaluate capillary refill, skin color, sensation, and motor function.

Improvised Splints

Emergency Medical Responders may arrive at the scene of an emergency without any splints, or they may use their supply of splints on one patient and have none for another patient. So it is helpful to know how to make splints from materials found at the scene. Such an improvised splint may be soft or rigid and may be made from a variety of materials.

Rigid splints can be made from pieces of lumber, plywood, compressed wood products, cardboard, rolled newspapers or magazines, umbrellas, canes, broom or shovel handles, sporting equipment (shin guards are an example), and tongue depressors for fingers. Soft splints can be made from towels, blankets, pillows, and bulky clothing such as sweaters and sweat suits. Most of the items can be found at the scene of a typical incident.

Management of Specific Extremity Injuries

Usually, the mechanism of injury and the patient's signs and symptoms indicate possible injuries that require splints. In general, apply rigid splints for injuries to the forearm and the lower leg. Rigid splints also may be used for injuries to the thigh, but traction splints are more effective. (Follow local protocols.) Use soft splints (blanket, towel, pillow, sling and swathe) if rigid splints are not available, and provide further rigid support by securing upper extremities to the torso with a swathe and lower extremities to each other. Use soft or rigid splints for injuries to the arm, elbow, wrist, or hand. Use soft splints for injuries to the ankle or foot.

For an algorithm of assessment and care of patients with specific extremity injuries, see Figure 19.11.

Upper Extremity Injuries

Methods for splinting each type of upper extremity injury are summarized in Scan 19.5. For injuries to the upper extremities, be sure to place the hand in a

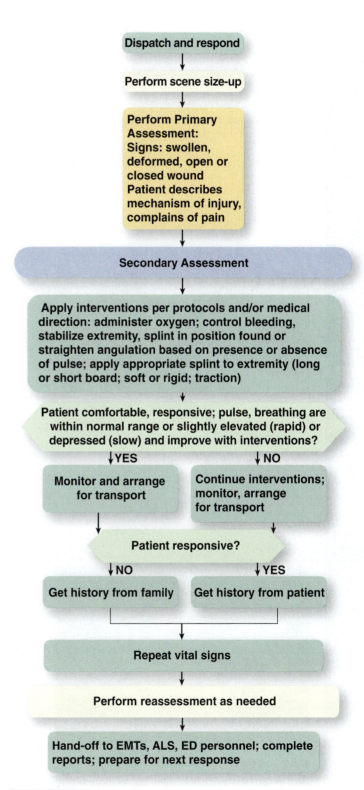

Figure 19.11 • Algorithm for the assessment and emergency care of patients with extremity injuries.

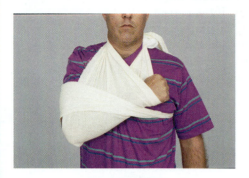

19.5.1 | Shoulder. Apply a sling and swathe. Elevate the wrist above the elbow and support it with the swathe.

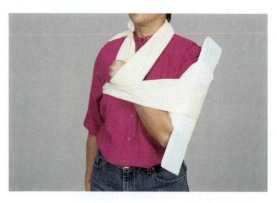

19.5.2 | Upper arm. Immobilize with a rigid splint from the shoulder to the elbow. Apply a sling and swathe that will elevate and support the limb.

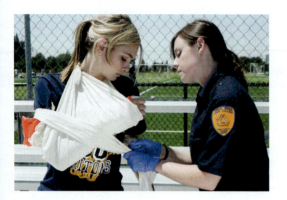

19.5.3 | Elbow (bent). Apply a sling and swathe to elevate and support the limb.

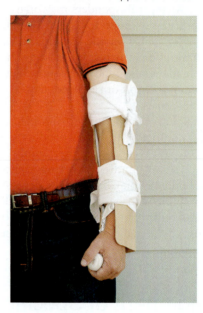

19.5.4 | Elbow (straight). Pad the armpit. Splint should extend from the armpit beyond the fingertips. Use roller bandages to secure the splint to the arm starting at the distal end. Secure the arm to the body with cravats.

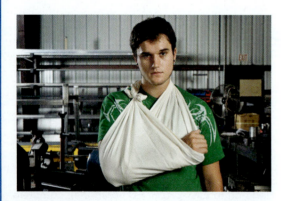

19.5.5 | Forearm, wrist, hand. The splint should extend from the elbow to beyond the fingertips. Use a sling and swathe for elevation and support.

Note: Place a roll of dressing in the hand to maintain position of function.

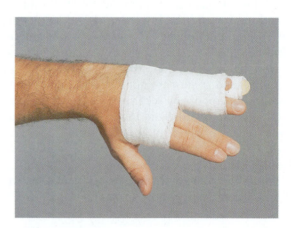

19.5.6 | Finger. Use a tongue depressor as a splint or tape the finger to an uninjured finger.

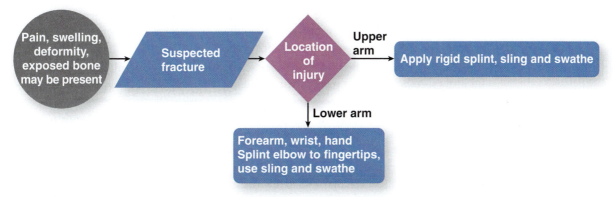

Figure 19.12 • Algorithm for the emergency care of patients with upper extremity injuries.

position of function, in which the fingers are slightly flexed and the wrist is cocked slightly upward. The position of function is a normal and comfortable position for the patient, especially if the extremity from forearm to hand is secured against a rigid splint. You may easily secure the hand in its position of function by placing a roll of gauze in the patient's hand before immobilizing or simply by allowing the fingers of the hand to extend over the end of the splint. (For upper extremity care, see Figure 19.12.)

position of function ▶ refers to a hand or foot; the natural position of the body at rest.

▶ GERIATRIC FOCUS ◀

Elderly patients often have less soft tissue covering their bodies. Their skin is also much thinner and easily damaged. Use extra caution when applying rigid splints, and use plenty of padding to ensure their comfort for as long as the splint may be in place.

Injuries to the Shoulder

A common sign of shoulder injury is a condition known as *knocked-down shoulder*, or *dropped shoulder* (Figure 19.13). The patient's injured shoulder will appear to droop. The patient usually holds the arm up against the side of the chest.

Injuries to the shoulder joint often produce what is known as an *anterior* (to the front) *dislocation*. The end of the upper arm bone that forms the shoulder joint can be felt, or even seen, bulging or protruding under the skin at the front of the shoulder.

It is not practical to use a rigid splint for injuries to the collarbone, shoulder blade, or shoulder joint. Place padding between the patient's injured arm and chest, use a cravat to secure the padding in place, and use a sling and swathe to secure the arm to the chest. Remember to check for distal circulation, sensation, and motor function before and after splinting. If there is no pulse, attempt to reposition to regain a pulse, but do not force the arm. Do not attempt to straighten injuries that involve the joint. Joint injuries should be immobilized in the position in which they are found.

When you provide care for patients with shoulder injuries, you will:

1. Take appropriate BSI precautions.
2. Assess and provide support for the ABCs.
3. Check distal circulation. If there is no pulse, notify the responding EMTs or notify the hospital and arrange to transport as soon as possible. Note the time that you observed the absence of the distal pulse.

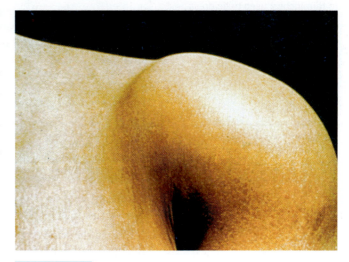

Figure 19.13 • Deformity caused by dislocation of the shoulder joint.

4. Check for sensation and motor function of the fingers on the injured arm. If the patient has no feeling or cannot move, then there is pressure on a nerve and the patient will need transport as soon as possible.

5. Apply a sling and swathe. If necessary, place padding (pillow, blanket, or towel) to fill any space between the patient's arm and chest on the injured side before applying the sling and swathe.

6. Reassess the distal pulse. If the pulse is absent, you may have to gently reposition the injured arm and reapply the sling and swathe. In such cases, follow your local protocols or contact the emergency department physician for directions before repositioning the limb. Sometimes a dislocated shoulder will correct (reduce) itself. If this happens, check the distal circulation, sensation, and motor function, and apply a sling and swathe. This patient still must see a physician. Arrange for transport, and make certain you tell the EMTs that the dislocation apparently corrected itself and the time it took place.

Injuries to the Upper Arm

Injury to the upper arm (humerus) can be at its upper end (proximal end) where the shoulder joint is formed, along the midshaft of the bone, or at the lower end (distal end) where the elbow joint is formed. Care for a patient with upper arm injuries is usually the same as for all injury locations. Deformity is often a key sign of injury to this bone, but if you see no deformity, the patient will tell you the site is tender and painful when you examine it.

Emergency Medical Responders may use a soft splint (sling and swathe) or a rigid splint to immobilize an upper arm injury. If you use a sling and swathe on an injury that seems very close to the elbow, modify the full sling to minimize pressure on the elbow.

If the upper arm is angulated, check for a distal pulse. If it is present and the patient can tolerate movement, gently move the arm to the splinting position (bend the elbow with the hand elevated above the level of the elbow) and splint it. Do not force the arm to this position, and do not try to straighten the angulation. Recheck for a distal pulse.

If you do not feel a pulse, attempt to straighten the angulation in the upper arm bone, if your EMS system allows you to do so. Do not force the arm. You should attempt to straighten the angulation only once and stop if there is resistance or severe pain. If straightening the limb fails to restore a distal pulse, arrange to transport the patient as soon as possible. If the pulse is restored, splint the arm and recheck the distal pulse.

If you use a rigid splint, secure it to the lateral (outside) part of the arm with roller gauze or cravats. A **cravat** is simply a triangular bandage that has been folded in such a way that it creates a long tie approximately two inches wide. Next, apply a sling and swathe. The swathe will secure the injured arm to the body and immobilize the joints above and below the injury site.

When you apply a splint to an upper arm injury, work with a partner. One of you will maintain manual stabilization, while the other applies the splint and the sling and swathe. To apply a splint for injuries to the upper arm bone:

1. Check for distal circulation, sensation, and motor function.

2. Select a padded splint long enough for the area between shoulder and elbow.

3. Apply manual stabilization to the injured extremity. If there is angulation or no distal pulse, gently realign and recheck for pulse.

4. Place the splint against the injured extremity.

5. Secure the splint to the patient with a roller bandage, handkerchiefs, cravats, or cloth strips. Begin securing at the distal end of the splint.

6. Maintain the hand in the position of function, and apply a sling and swathe. Recheck distal circulation, sensation, and motor function.

7. Provide oxygen as soon as possible, and maintain body temperature to prevent the effects of developing shock.

cravat ▶ a triangular bandage that is folded to a width of three to four inches; used to tie dressings and splints in place.

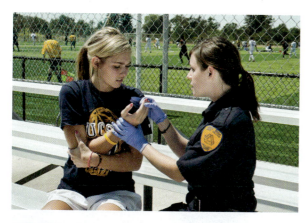

19.6.1 | Check circulation, sensation, and motor function (CSM) prior to splinting.

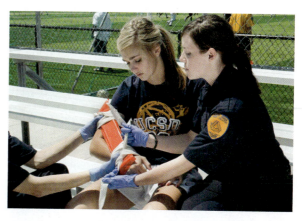

19.6.2 | Secure a rigid splint to the arm.

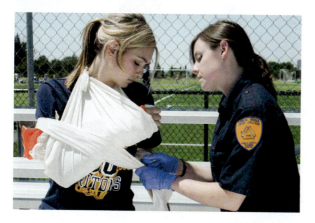

19.6.3 | Apply a sling and swathe.

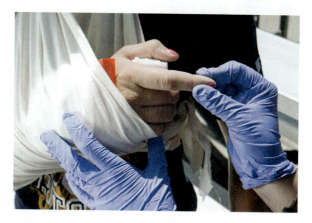

19.6.4 | Recheck circulation, sensation, and motor function (CSM).

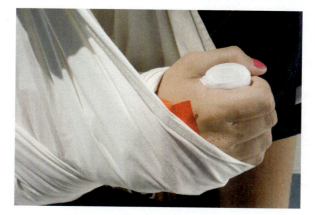

19.6.5 | Ensure the hand is in the position of function.

Injuries to the Elbow

The elbow is a joint formed by the lower, or distal, end of the upper arm bone (humerus) and the upper, or proximal, end of the forearm bones (radius and ulna).

When caring for elbow injuries, immobilize the elbow in the position in which it is found. Have your partner stabilize the arm while you apply and secure the splint. Check circulation, sensation, and motor function before and after splinting.

The following methods can be used in caring for a patient with an elbow injury (Scan 19.6):

- If the elbow is found in a flexed (bent) position natural for the joint, rigid splinting is preferred. However, a simple sling and a swathe may be effective. Apply a splint.

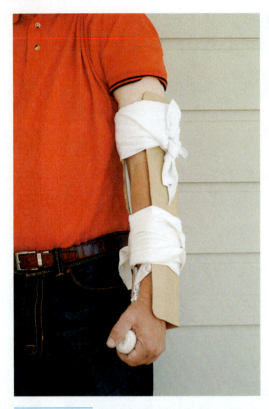

Figure 19.14 • Splinting an injured elbow in a straight position.

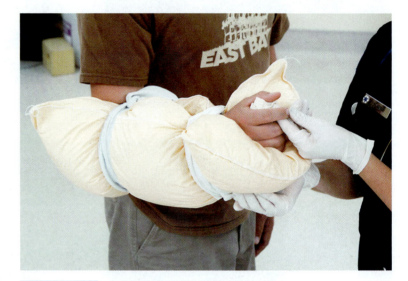

Figure 19.15 • Soft splint for wrist and hand injuries.

- If the elbow is found in the straight position and cannot be placed in the natural flexed position, immobilize it in the straight position. Rigid splinting is preferred, but body splinting is effective. This is done by tying the injured arm along the side of the patient's torso. If you use a rigid splint, select a padded splint that will extend from the patient's armpit past the fingertips. Place a roll of dressing in the patient's hand to maintain it in the position of function and secure the splint with roller gauze or folded cravats starting at the distal end of the arm (fingertips) (Figure 19.14).
- If the elbow appears to be dislocated and it is in an unnatural or awkward position and cannot be repositioned, place padding around the arm and between the arm and chest, if necessary. If possible, secure the arm to the body with a sling and swathe.

Injuries to the Forearm, Wrist, and Hand

The most effective splint for an injured forearm, wrist, or hand is a rigid one. However, the patient can be made comfortable with a pillow splint (Figure 19.15) and a sling and swathe. A sling and swathe used alone is also effective for a forearm. Be sure to check distal circulation, sensation, and motor function before and after splinting.

To use a rigid splint for any injury to the forearm, wrist, or hand, select a padded rigid splint that extends from beyond the elbow to past the fingertips. Place a roll of dressing in the patient's hand to maintain the hand in the position of function. The steps for splinting the forearm, wrist, and hand are the same as steps 3–7 listed above for the upper arm. An alternative method for maintaining the position of function in the hand is to allow the fingers to curve over the end of the rigid splint (Figure 19.16).

Rolled newspapers, magazines, and creased cardboard make effective rigid splints for injuries to the forearm or wrist, but they still should be padded. Apply a sling after splinting to keep the forearm elevated. Add a swathe to secure the forearm to the chest, and immobilize the joint above and below the injury site. (See Scan 19.7.)

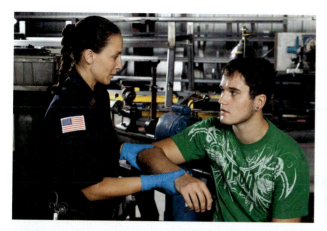

19.7.1 | Manually stabilize the limb prior to splinting.

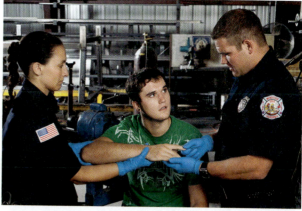

19.7.2 | Check circulation, sensation, and motor function (CSM).

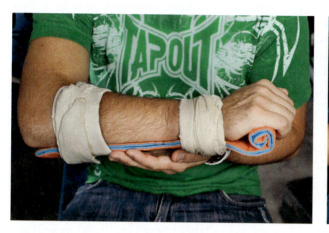

19.7.3 | Apply a rigid splint to the limb.

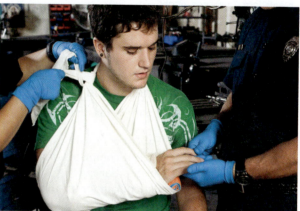

19.7.4 | Place the limb in a sling and recheck circulation, sensation, and motor function (CSM).

Injuries to the Fingers

Not all injuries to the fingers require rigid splinting. You can immobilize an injured finger by taping the finger to an adjacent, uninjured finger (Figure 19.17). You can tape the finger to a tongue depressor, an aluminum splint, or a pen or pencil. You can also make a soft splint by placing a roll of gauze in the patient's hand and wrapping more gauze around the hand

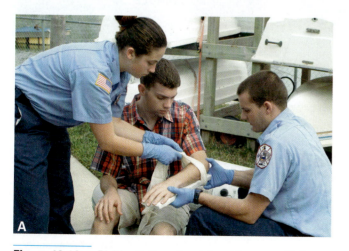

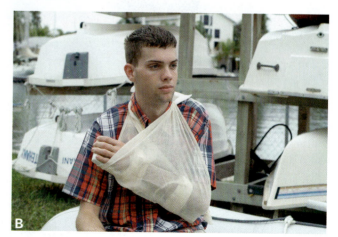

Figure 19.16 • Rigid splinting of an injured forearm. (A) Secure rigid splint to the limb. (B) Place the arm in a sling.

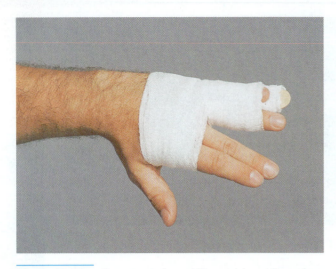

Figure 19.17 • One way to immobilize an injured finger is to tape it to an adjacent, uninjured finger.

and dressing. This soft-splint method immobilizes the hand and fingers and keeps them in the position of function.

Apply a sling to keep the forearm elevated. Apply a swathe to immobilize the joints above the injury site, as well as to improve circulation and patient comfort.

Do not attempt to "pop" dislocated fingers back into place. Immobilize dislocated fingers as you would an injured hand.

Lower Extremity Injuries

When the patient has multiple injuries or has suffered multisystem trauma, it usually is best to totally immobilize him on a long spine board or a scoop (orthopedic) stretcher rather than to try to immobilize each individual injury. Valuable time can be lost trying to immobilize individual injuries. If you suspect multisystem trauma, immobilization on a long board and rapid transport are essential.

Before moving or rolling a patient with suspected spine injury or with lower extremity injuries, be sure you have the proper equipment ready and a sufficient number of rescue personnel on hand to assist. For lower extremity care, see Figure 19.18.

Injuries to the Pelvic Girdle

The patient may have injuries to the pelvic girdle (pelvis and hip joints) if:

- Patient complains of pain in the pelvis, hips, or groin.
- Patient complains of pain when gentle pressure is applied to the sides of the hips or to the hip bones.
- Patient cannot lift the legs while lying face up (supine). The patient will usually tell you that "it hurts" or "I can't move my legs."
- The foot on the injured side turns outward (laterally) or inward (medially) more than the uninjured side.
- Injured extremity appears shorter than the uninjured side.
- Pelvis or the hip joint has noticeable deformity.

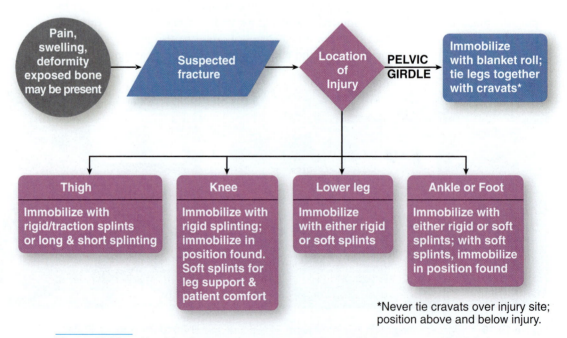

Figure 19.18 • Algorithm for emergency care of patients with lower extremities injuries.

Pelvic Girdle

Pelvic fractures result in significant bleeding because the arteries that supply the legs with blood are tightly bound to the pelvic bones. When a fracture occurs, the arteries could be torn. Applying pressure to hold the pelvic bones together reduces both pain and bleeding. There are commercial devices called pelvic slings that can be tightened around the pelvis to serve as a splint.

Pelvic injuries are serious because they can damage major blood vessels and internal organs. Injuries to these soft tissues can cause profuse internal bleeding and sterility, and the force that caused the pelvic injury may also have caused spinal injuries. Because of all these critical factors, it may be best to wait for more advanced care to arrive before attempting to immobilize a patient with a pelvic injury. In the meantime, provide oxygen as soon as possible and maintain body temperature to delay the onset of shock. Note the mechanism of injury so you can report it to the responding EMTs.

Pelvic girdle injuries may be managed at the scene with a specialized splint. One such splint is a pressure garment called a *pneumatic antishock garment (PASG)*. Your instructor will advise you if Emergency Medical Responders are trained and allowed to use or assist more advanced providers with PASGs in your area. Follow your local protocols or medical direction when considering the use of a PASG. Other devices and materials that are effective for immobilizing injuries to the pelvic girdle include pelvic splints (Figure 19.19), long spine boards, scoop stretchers, and blankets. If you do not carry this equipment, you may continue patient assessment while you are waiting for more advanced care to arrive.

As an Emergency Medical Responder, you can care for patients with suspected fractures to the pelvic girdle by using a soft splint. Place a blanket roll between the patient's legs and tie them together with cravats. This simple and quick immobilization method will stabilize the injury and provide patient comfort before more advanced care arrives.

To immobilize a pelvic injury with a blanket roll, do the following:

1. Complete a thorough assessment of the injury site.

2. Assess circulation, sensation, and motor function in both distal extremities.

3. Provide oxygen to the patient as soon as possible.

4. Place a folded blanket, large towel, or other thick padding material between the patient's legs from groin to feet.

5. Prepare four cravats (folded triangular bandages) or other strips of material.

6. Use a short splint or coat hanger and drape the ends of all four cravats over the splint or hanger. Slide them under the space behind the knees.

7. Gently slide two cravats above the knees and two below the knees.

8. Starting at the feet (distal end), tie one cravat at the ankles, one just below the knees, one just above the knees, and one just below the hips. Do not tie a cravat over or too near the injury site.

When the EMTs arrive, you can help them place the stabilized patient on a scoop stretcher or spine board. Remember to provide oxygen to the patient as soon as possible and cover the patient to maintain body temperature and to help reduce the chance of developing shock. If you suspect spine injury, do not attempt to move the patient until the EMTs arrive with additional help. In the meantime, stabilize the patient's head and neck and continue to reassure him.

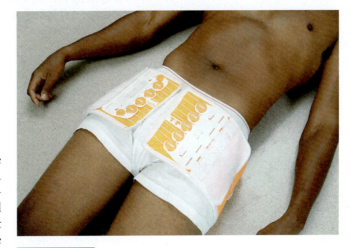

Figure 19.19 • The application of a commercial pelvic splint helps to stabilize the pelvis and minimize bleeding.

Because the signs and symptoms of musculoskeletal injuries are similar, you will not be trying to determine which type of injury the patient has. Even so, there are certain signs that indicate a possible hip dislocation. Look for them, because you do not want to attempt to move an injured leg if there is a possible hip dislocation. If you suspect a hip dislocation, there also may be injury to the thigh bone (femur). Do not try to straighten an angulated femur if the hip appears to be dislocated.

The following points describe two types of hip dislocation. Suspect the patient has a dislocated hip if you find:

- *Anterior hip dislocation.* The leg from hip to foot is rotated outward (laterally) farther than the uninjured side. Leg rotation also may be an indication of hip fracture. With hip fracture, the injured leg may appear to be shorter than the other leg. You will probably see or feel the bony end of the femur under the skin at the front or side of the leg where it joins the torso.
- *Posterior hip dislocation (most common).* The leg is rotated inward (medially) and the knee is usually bent. You may see or feel the bony end of the femur under the skin at the back of the leg where it joins the buttocks.

If you suspect the hip is dislocated, wait for more advanced care to arrive. While waiting, provide oxygen as soon as possible, and cover the patient to maintain body temperature and help prevent shock. You can immobilize the injured leg by placing and securing pillows or folded blankets or towels around the injured leg, which will support the leg and provide comfort to the patient. Do not reposition or move the patient's leg when you place or secure pillows or blankets.

Injuries to the Upper Leg

Injuries to the upper leg or thigh bone (femur) can be life threatening even when the injury is closed, because bleeding inside the tissues can be severe. There may be a severe and obvious deformity with femur fractures. The leg below the injury site may be bent where there is no joint, or it will appear twisted.

Consider the use of a rigid splint or a special device called a *traction splint* for injuries to the femur. Traction splints are mechanical devices that allow for the application of constant traction of the injured extremity. This is helpful to reduce pain, swelling, and movement of the injury. Traction splints should be considered only for suspected isolated mid-shaft femur fractures when the injury does not involve the knee or the hip/pelvis. They should also not be used if there are injuries to the lower leg or ankle.

Emergency Medical Responder units may carry traction splints, and you may be trained and allowed to use them. (Your instructor will advise you if tractions splints are part of your local protocols.) Soft splints are not as effective as rigid or traction splints, but they will stabilize the injury and provide some pain relief.

While waiting for the EMTs to arrive, provide the patient some relief from pain by securing a blanket roll between the legs in the same way you would for injuries to the pelvic girdle. This is effective once the patient is secured to a spine board or scoop stretcher, a form of rigid splinting. Provide oxygen as soon as possible, and cover the patient to maintain body warmth to help prevent shock.

An alternative approach is to immobilize the leg using a long rigid splint that extends from the patient's buttocks to past the foot. Use cravats to secure the splint. Use a splint or coat hanger to push the cravats under the patient's trunk and legs at the natural voids (lower back and knees). Do not place a tie over the injury site, but instead place one tie above and one tie below the injury.

Injuries to the Knee

In most cases, you will not be able to tell if the knee is fractured, dislocated, or both. Because of the many nerves and blood vessels and the possibility that soft tissues were damaged, immobilize an injured knee in the position in which it is found. Do not attempt to reposition or straighten the injured knee. Some EMS systems allow Emergency Medical Responders to make one attempt at straightening the limb if there is no distal pulse. Your instructor will let you know the requirements of your local protocols.

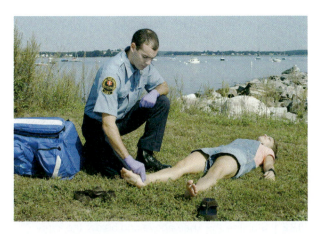

19.8.1 | Assess distal circulation, sensation, and motor function (CSM).

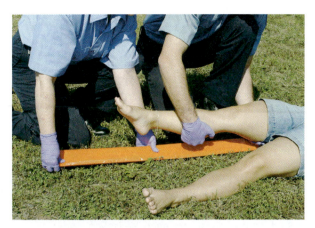

19.8.2 | Place rigid splint below the limb.

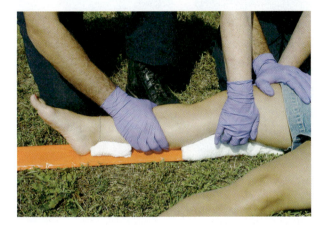

19.8.3 | Pad the voids.

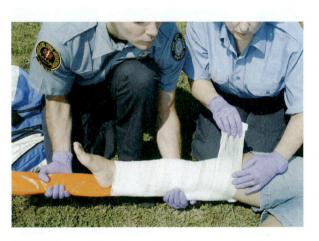

19.8.4 | Secure the splint to the limb and recheck circulation, sensation, and motor function (CSM).

Rigid splinting is the most effective method to use when immobilizing an injured knee, but you can provide support to the leg and comfort to the patient with soft splints. Place and secure pillows or folded blankets around the knee, especially if it is found in the bent position. Do not reposition or move the patient's legs to place or secure pillows or blankets. If the injured knee is found in the straight position, you can effectively immobilize it with a blanket placed between both legs and secured with cravats, just as you would for a femur injury.

To immobilize an injured knee in the straight position, secure a long splint behind the leg from the patient's buttocks to beyond the foot (Scan 19.8). You also may use the method described below for splinting the lower leg. In cases where the patient's leg will remain flexed at the knee, you may secure one or two shorter splints at an angle across the thigh and lower leg (A-frame) with cravats (Scan 19.9).

continued

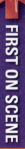

After carefully straightening Annie's leg, Ron is able to find a strong pulse in her foot. "Now we need to splint it in this position," he says, looking at a stand of small trees that line the course. Perhaps the branches are strong enough for a splint.

"Why don't you use the golf clubs," Annie whispers as she tries to breathe deeply through the pain. Ron grins and shakes his head slightly, imagining his buddies at the volunteer fire station finding out that he was prepared to break down a tree to make a splint when he was surrounded by golf clubs.

"That's a great idea," he says and jogs over to the overturned golf cart and grabs several clubs and the shoulder straps from both bags.

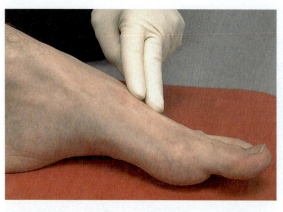

19.9.1 | Assess distal circulation, sensation, and motor function (CSM).

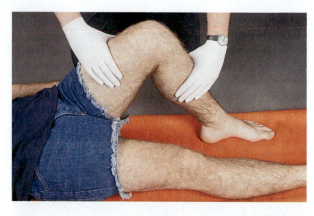

19.9.2 | Stabilize the knee above and below the injury site.

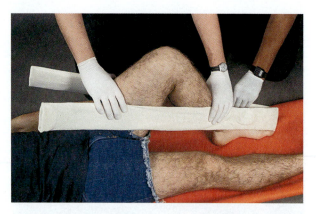

19.9.3 | Place the padded side of the splints next to the injured extremity. Note that they should be equal in length and extend 6–12 inches beyond the midthigh and midcalf.

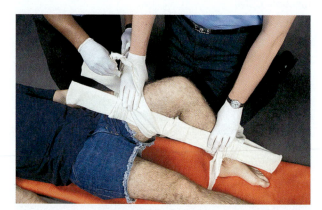

19.9.4 | Secure splints at both ends, using cravats or similar material.

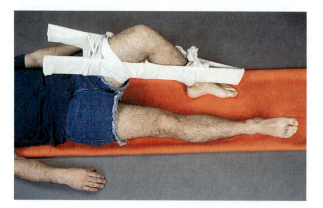

19.9.5 | Using a figure-eight configuration, secure one cravat to the ankle and the boards and the second cravat to the thigh and the boards. Reassess distal circulation, sensation, and motor function (CSM).

Injuries to the Lower Leg

You can provide care for injuries to the lower leg with either rigid or soft splints. A blanket roll between the legs is an effective soft splint. Secure it as you did for pelvic, thigh, and knee injuries described previously. Once you assist the EMTs in placing the patient on the spine board or scoop (orthopedic) stretcher, a form of rigid splinting, you have completed immobilizing all joints above and below the injury site (Scan 19.10).

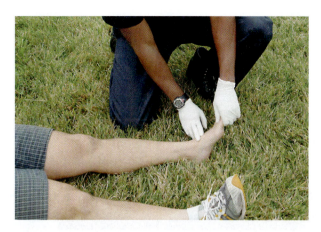

19.10.1 | Access circulation, sensation, and motor function (CSM) prior to splinting the extremity.

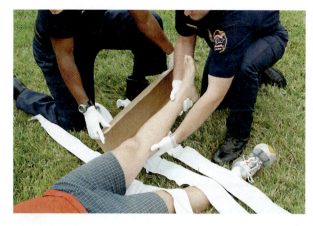

19.10.2 | Choose a splint that extends from the heel to well above the knee.

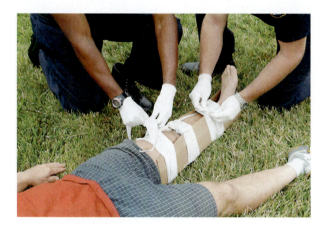

19.10.3 | Secure the splint above and below the knee and at the ankle.

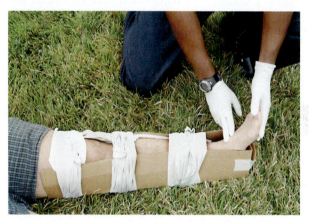

19.10.4 | Reassess circulation, sensation, and motor function after the splint is secure.

If you use a rigid splint, you will need assistance. One person must maintain manual stabilization while you apply the splint. A single-splint method also may be used to immobilize lower leg injuries.

Before and after splinting, check for distal circulation, sensation, and motor function. If you live in an area where skiing is a popular sport, you may have to care for a certain kind of injury called the *boot-top injury* (Figure 19.20). This is an injury to the tibia and/or fibula (usually both) that typically occurs when a skier falls forward of the ski tips. The leg bends hard over the top of the ski boot, causing a *transverse fracture* (a break in the bone that is at a right angle to the long part of the bone) of one or both bones. The leg below the fracture is often angulated or rotated, and the fracture is quite painful.

Follow these guidelines when caring for an injured skier: Notify the ski patrol immediately. (Send another skier to an emergency phone or lift shack.) Keep the patient warm with others' coats, and place something between the skier and the snow. Remove the ski from the boot of the injured extremity while manually stabilizing the injury. Leave the leg alone or in the position found until the ski patrol arrives, or gently align the injury to see if that will reduce the patient's pain. Manually stabilize or splint the injury. A ski or ski pole will work, or use splints. Secure with scarves, handkerchiefs, or cravats.

Do not apply snow to the injury site. Swelling is due to bleeding from the damaged soft tissues; thus, applying cold will only hasten the development of frostbite and/or hypothermia.

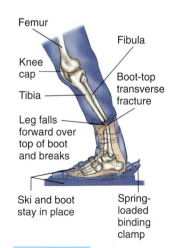

Figure 19.20 • Boot top injury common to skiers.

Figure 19.21 •
Immobilization of the
lower leg using a towel.

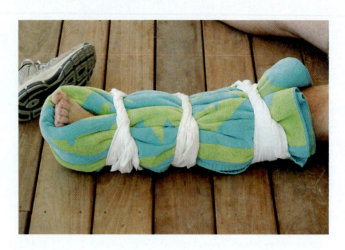

closed fracture ▶ a broken
bone that does not have an
associated break in the outer
layers of the skin.

Injuries to the Ankle or Foot

Rigid splints may be used for injuries to the ankle or foot, but the soft splint is probably the most comfortable for the patient and the quickest for the Emergency Medical Responder to apply. If you apply a rigid splint, use one that extends from above the patient's knee to beyond the foot as described for the single-splint method for the lower leg.

When soft-splinting an injury to the foot or ankle, immobilize it in the position found with a pillow or folded blanket. Secure the soft splint around the foot and ankle with several cravats or with roller gauze (Figure 19.21), and then elevate it by propping it on a blanket roll or pillow.

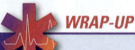

WRAP-UP

FIRST ON SCENE

Ron has just finished splinting Annie's leg with a putter and a sand wedge when the ambulance approaches them, moving slowly across the grass. The EMTs compliment Ron on straightening and splinting Annie's injured leg and decide to transport her with the makeshift splint. Just before the ambulance crew shuts the doors, Ron pats Annie's uninjured leg and says, "Let me just get this golf cart figured out, and I'll meet you over at the E.D."

"Ron!" She looks at him sternly, her voice muffled by the oxygen mask. "Don't you dare finish the game without me!"

CHAPTER REVIEW

Summary

- The musculoskeletal system is made up of muscles, bones, joints, connective tissues, blood vessels, and nerves.

- Support, movement, protection, and cell production are the primary functions of the musculoskeletal system.

- The bones of the axial skeleton (skull, spine, ribs, and sternum) and appendicular skeleton (upper and lower extremities) make up the skeletal system.

- The signs and symptoms of musculoskeletal injury include pain, swelling, discoloration, and deformity.

- A strain is the stretching or tearing of a muscle, whereas a sprain is the partial or complete tearing of a ligament. A fracture is the cracking or breaking of a bone, and a dislocation is when the end of a bone is pulled partially or completely away from a joint.

- An open skeletal injury is when a broken bone end or bone fragments tear through the skin.

- Proper care for a musculoskeletal injury includes assessment and monitoring the patient's ABCs and appropriate immobilization of the injury.

- It is critical to assess the circulation, sensation, and motor function of extremities distal to an injury to determine if blood vessels or nerves may have been damaged.

- Direct force causes injury at the point where it actually impacts the body, but an indirect-force injury is caused when energy is transmitted from the point of contact to a different area of the body where it causes injury.

- If an injured extremity is angulated, it should be splinted in place unless there is no distal circulation and the limb can be placed back into correct anatomical position with ease and without causing pain for the patient.

- Skeletal injuries should be stabilized to prevent them from worsening, such a **closed fracture** becoming an open fracture.

- When caring for a patient with an open skeletal injury, it is important to begin with a primary assessment to evaluate for life threats and determine if other injuries are present. It is important to expose the injury site and control excessive bleeding. The injury also should be properly immobilized and splinted. Administer oxygen, if allowed, and monitor the patient's vital signs until transport.

- When caring for a multisystem trauma patient, it is critical to assess and monitor ABCs, assume and care for spine injury, control any severe bleeding, and treat for shock while coordinating rapid transport.

Take Action

PRACTICE MAKES PERFECT

When it comes to developing long-bone and joint-splinting skills, there is nothing better than good old-fashioned practice. This activity will have you practicing those skills using only the most basic of materials. You will need a small assortment of supplies that should be easy to gather. Some newspaper, a couple of magazines, some short and long pieces of cardboard, and several triangular bandages should do the trick. You will need another student to play the role of patient.

Using the following four "rules," take turns with your partner splinting various simulated injuries. Alternate back and forth and change the injury from upper to lower extremity and from long-bone to joint injuries.

1. Check circulation, sensation, and motor function before moving the injury.

2. Immobilize the suspected fracture site.

3. Immobilize the joints above and below the suspected fracture site.

4. Reevaluate circulation, sensation, and motor function.

Refer to these "rules" as you progress through the splinting process. Carefully evaluate each step of the way to see if what you are doing is really meeting the objective. Since bone injuries are relatively low in the priority list of a busy emergency department, be sure to make comfort a high priority as you apply the splints. Pad all potential pressure points and fill all voids. If you are playing patient, be sure to let the "Emergency Medical Responder" know whether he touches or moves your injury in a way that might cause pain.

First on Scene Run Review

Recall the events of the "First on Scene" scenario in this chapter and answer the following questions, which are related to the call. Rationales are offered in the Answer Key at the back of the book.

1. Should you have straightened out the leg? Why or why not?

2. Did Ron do the right thing by splinting the leg? Explain your reasoning.

3. What information should Ron give the ambulance crew?

Quick Quiz

To check your understanding of the chapter, answer the following questions. Then compare your answers to those in the Answer Key at the back of the book.

1. All of the following are functions of the musculoskeletal system EXCEPT:
   a. strength.
   b. support.
   c. protection.
   d. cell production.

2. An injury that is characterized by broken bone ends protruding through the skin is commonly described as a(n) _____ wound.
   a. open
   b. closed
   c. complex
   d. superficial

3. Which one of the following would NOT be considered appropriate when caring for a suspected fracture?
   a. Cut away clothing to expose the injury site.
   b. "Pop" possible dislocations back into place.
   c. Assess circulation, sensation, and motor function.
   d. Immobilize the joint above and below the injury site.

4. When caring for patients who have sustained a significant mechanism of injury, the Emergency Medical Responder must:
   a. place in the recovery position.
   b. identify the medical problem.
   c. provide low-flow oxygen.
   d. suspect spine injury.

5. A _____ occurs when one end of a bone that is part of a joint is pulled or pushed out of place.
   a. fracture
   b. dislocation
   c. concussion
   d. rotation

6. A thorough assessment of an extremity injury includes an evaluation of distal CSM. What does CSM stand for?
   a. circulation, sensation, motor function
   b. color, sensation, motor function
   c. color, strength, manual movement
   d. circulation, strength, motor function

7. All of the following are common signs and symptoms of an extremity injury EXCEPT:
   a. pain.
   b. swelling.
   c. deformity.
   d. lengthening.

8. The process of immobilizing an injury using a device such as a piece of wood, cardboard, or folded blanket is called:
   a. immobilization.
   b. traction.
   c. splinting.
   d. manual stabilization.

9. You are caring for a patient who has an injury characterized by an open wound, severe deformity, and bleeding. Your highest priority is:
   a. straightening the deformity.
   b. covering the open wound.
   c. splinting the extremity.
   d. controlling bleeding.

10. The straightening of an angulated injury is indicated when:
    a. the distal pulse is absent.
    b. there is an open wound.
    c. a splint is unavailable.
    d. directed by your partner.

11. A triangular bandage used to stabilize the elbow and arm is called a:
    a. cravat.
    b. dressing.
    c. bandage.
    d. sling.

12. When properly applied, a sling and swathe will adequately immobilize a:
    a. wrist.
    b. forearm.
    c. shoulder.
    d. knee.

13. It is important to maintain the hand and foot of an injured extremity in a normal and comfortable position during splinting. This position is called the:
    a. recumbent position.
    b. position of function.
    c. position of comfort.
    d. resting position.

14. The energy from a blunt force that is transferred along the axis of a bone and causes an injury farther along the extremity is called:
    a. direct force.
    b. twisting force.
    c. indirect force.
    d. referred pain.

15. When caring for a patient with multiple injuries, it may be best to:
    a. splint all injuries before moving.
    b. splint only deformed injuries.
    c. immobilize on a long spine board.
    d. immobilize using a soft stretcher.

16. You are caring for a patient who has one leg that is shortened with the foot rotated to one side. These are likely signs of a possible:

a. spine injury.
b. dislocated hip.
c. dislocated knee.
d. sprained ankle.

17. Which one of the following is the most efficient method of immobilizing an injured ankle?

a. Short spine board
b. Traction splint
c. Cardboard splint
d. Folded blanket

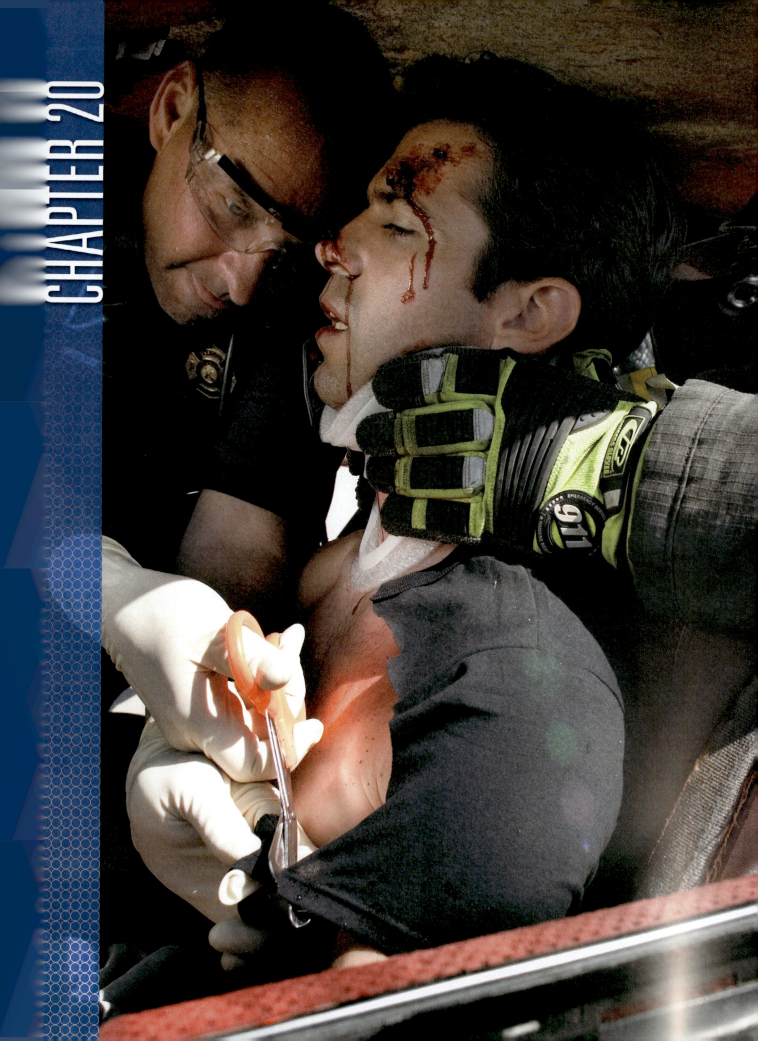

CHAPTER 20

Caring for Head and Spine Injuries

EDUCATION STANDARDS
- Trauma—Head, Facial, Neck, and Spine Trauma

COMPETENCIES
- Uses simple knowledge to recognize and manage life threats based on assessment findings for an acutely injured patient while awaiting additional emergency medical response.

CHAPTER OVERVIEW

Injuries to the head and spine are very common and can lead to significant disability and even death if not identified and managed appropriately. This chapter describes the common causes of head and spine injury as well as the proper techniques for assessment and care of someone you suspect may have a head or spine injury.

OBJECTIVES

Upon successful completion of this chapter, the student should be able to:

COGNITIVE

1. Define the following terms:
   a. central nervous system *(p. 444)*
   b. cranium *(p. 444)*
   c. paralysis *(p. 449)*
   d. peripheral nervous system *(p. 445)*

2. Describe the major components of the spinal column. *(p. 445)*

3. Describe the major components of the nervous system. *(p. 444)*

4. Describe the major components of the cranium. *(p. 444)*

5. Explain the relationship of mechanism of injury to the potential for spine injury. *(p. 445)*

6. Describe the signs and symptoms of a head injury. *(p. 448)*

7. Differentiate between an open and closed head injury. *(p. 448)*

8. Explain the appropriate assessment and care for a patient with a head injury. *(p. 448)*

9. Describe the signs and symptoms of a spine injury. *(p. 450)*

10. Explain the appropriate assessment and care for a patient with a suspected spine injury. *(p. 452)*

11. Explain the special considerations of airway management for a patient with suspected cervical-spine injury. *(p. 452)*

PSYCHOMOTOR

12. Demonstrate the appropriate assessment and care of a patient with a head injury.

13. Demonstrate the appropriate assessment and care for a patient with a suspected spine injury.

14. Demonstrate the appropriate airway management for a patient with suspected cervical-spine injury.

15. Demonstrate the appropriate technique for manual stabilization of the cervical spine.

16. Demonstrate the appropriate sizing and application of a cervical collar.

17. Demonstrate the proper technique for log-rolling a patient.

18. Demonstrate the proper technique for immobilization of a supine patient.

19. Demonstrate the proper technique for immobilization of a seated patient.

AFFECTIVE

20. Value the importance of proper body substance isolation (BSI) precautions when caring for patients with head and spine injuries.

"Safety officer to the ground stage." Shelby hears the call as she makes her way to the center of the auditorium where the stage is being set for the concert that night. A small crowd has gathered at the west side of the stage.

"He fell!" a booming voice says as Shelby enters the scene. It is the stage manager. "Marc did exactly what I told him not to do, and he fell!"

"Marc," Shelby says, setting her equipment down beside a young man who is lying on the ground beside the 10-foot-tall stage. Another young stage technician is holding his head still and straight. "My name is Shelby, and I'm going to help you until the medics arrive, okay?"

"Okay," Marc says softly, his eyes moving back and forth among the faces huddled nearby. "I'm so sorry. I didn't think I was that close to the edge. I should be fine, boss," he says as he starts to move his arms to get up.

"Don't move just yet," Shelby says, noticing a small stream of blood dripping from his scalp. "You fell from a pretty decent height onto this concrete, and I don't want you compromising your neck or spine."

"Oh my God," Marc says, panicked. "I don't think I can move my legs."

OBJECTIVES

3. Describe the major components of the nervous system.

4. Describe the major components of the cranium.

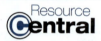
Resource Central

Complete an interactive exercise called "Label the Skull."

cranium ▶ the skull.

central nervous system ▶ a bodily system that is responsible for many of the body's involuntary functions such as heartbeat, respirations, and temperature regulation; composed of the brain and the spinal cord.

Anatomy of the Head and Spine

The **cranium** or skull is comprised of several bones that are fused together to form the cranial vault and face (Figure 20.1). The cranial vault is the area inside the skull where the brain is located. The cranium sits at the top of the spinal column and is able to twist and move in many directions. It is this position and ability to move in all directions that makes the head and neck so susceptible to injury. The face is made up of strong, irregularly shaped bones. The face bones include part of the eye sockets, the cheeks, the upper part of the nose, the upper jaw, and the lower jaw. These bones are fused into immovable joints except for the lower jaw bone, or *mandible*, which is the only movable joint in the head.

The brain and the spinal cord each make up one half of the **central nervous system**, which is responsible for many of the body's involuntary functions such as heartbeat, respirations, and temperature regulation.

The **peripheral nervous system** comprises the many nerves that extend from the spinal cord throughout the body. These nerves carry messages from the brain to the body and from the body back to the brain. Injury to the spine could damage the spinal cord and prevent it from carrying messages to or from a part of the body. That part of the body would no longer have contact with the brain and would be unable to function. The damage could be temporary, caused by pressure or swelling that may be corrected with proper care, or the damage could be permanent. In addition, the spinal cord is the site of many reflexes, which allow us to react quickly to such things as pain and heat.

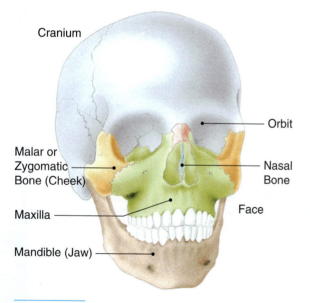

Cranium

Orbit

Malar or Zygomatic Bone (Cheek)

Nasal Bone

Maxilla

Face

Mandible (Jaw)

Figure 20.1 • The bones of the human skull.

▶ GERIATRIC FOCUS ◀

As we age, our spine loses much of its flexibility due to the loss of water content in the intervertebral disks and calcification of the supporting ligaments. Sometimes the calcification can cause narrowing of the spinal canal where the spinal cord runs. What may appear to be an insignificant mechanism of injury can cause fractures to the vertebral bodies or to the calcified ligaments, resulting in compression on the spinal cord. You should always have a high index of suspicion for spine injury in the elderly and take appropriate stabilization measures.

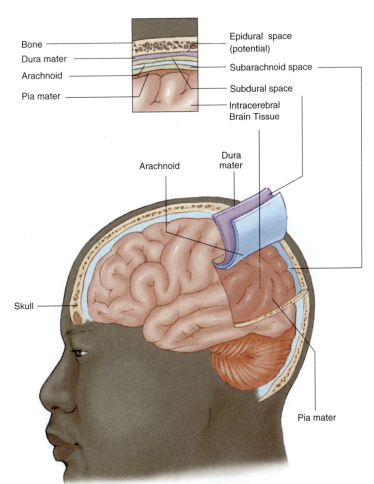

Bone
Dura mater
Arachnoid
Pia mater

Epidural space (potential)
Subarachnoid space
Subdural space
Intracerebral Brain Tissue

Arachnoid
Dura mater

Skull

Pia mater

Figure 20.2 • The brain is protected by several layers of tissue called meninges.

peripheral nervous system ▶ a bodily system that connects the CNS to the limbs and organs by way of nerves; composed of all the nerves and nerve endings that extend from the spinal cord throughout the body.

OBJECTIVES

2. Describe the major components of the spinal column.

5. Explain the relationship of mechanism of injury to the potential for spine injury.

The brain is surrounded by three protective layers called meninges (Figure 20.2). In addition, the brain and spinal cord are surrounded by a clear fluid called *cerebrospinal fluid*. This fluid serves as a protective cushion in the event of injury. When the brain becomes injured, some or all of these structures and functions can be compromised.

The spinal column begins at the base of the skull and extends down into the pelvis. It comprises approximately 33 individual bones called vertebrae (Figure 20.3). Down the center of these bones is the spinal cord.

Mechanisms of Injury

Injuries to the head and spine may not always be obvious. It is essential that you carefully evaluate and reevaluate the mechanism of injury (Scan 20.1). If the mechanism suggests that an injury to the head, neck, or spine could exist, then you must care for your patient accordingly. If the patient is unable to provide an account of what happened, then you must check with witnesses or bystanders for this information. When in doubt, provide care as if an injury exists. Be highly suspicious of injury if the mechanism of injury includes any of the following:

- Falls
- Forces that caused excessive flexion (bending) or extension (stretching) of the neck or spine
- Pulling or hanging forces that caused spinal stretching
- Motor-vehicle crashes
- Contact sports
- Significant blunt trauma

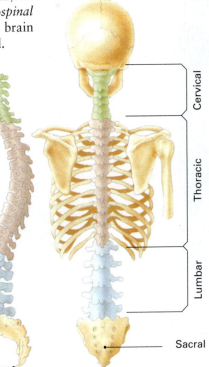

Cervical
Thoracic
Lumbar
Sacral
Coccyx

Figure 20.3 • The segments of the spinal column.

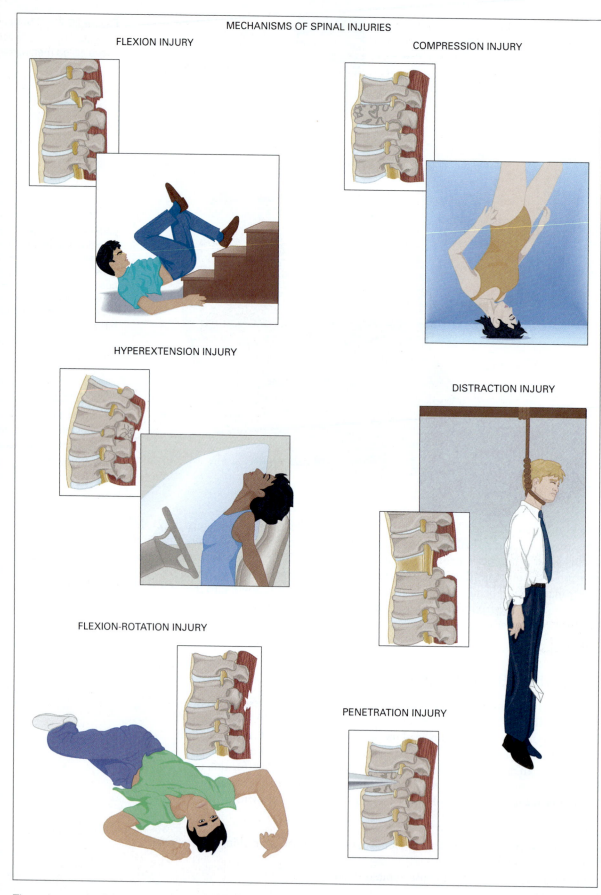

MECHANISMS OF SPINAL INJURIES

FLEXION INJURY

COMPRESSION INJURY

HYPEREXTENSION INJURY

DISTRACTION INJURY

FLEXION-ROTATION INJURY

PENETRATION INJURY

The spine can be injured by a variety of different mechanisms.

- Penetrating trauma such as that caused by gunshots or stabbings
- Blows by assault-and-battery or abuse incidents
- Any trauma situation where the patient is unresponsive

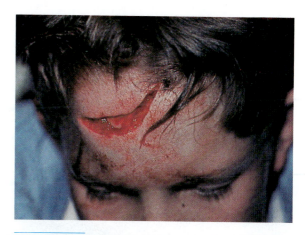

Figure 20.4 • A scalp laceration is often an indication of a closed head injury.

Injuries to the Head and Face

Injuries to the Head

Injuries to the head are commonly caused by blunt trauma. Blunt trauma can occur when an object strikes the head or when the head strikes a hard object such as the ground after a fall or the inside of a vehicle during a traffic collision.

Head injuries can be either closed or open. Closed injuries occur when the cranium remains intact (Figure 20.4). In a closed head injury, the skull is not damaged or cracked, but the brain can still be injured by the force of something striking the skull. Such a force can cause the brain to bounce off the inside of the skull. The resulting injuries to the brain include:

- *Concussion.* A *concussion* occurs when a blow to the head does not cause an open head injury but does cause damage to the brain. The injury may be so minor it does not cause a loss of consciousness; or it may be mild, causing a headache after a brief loss of consciousness; or it may be severe, causing a prolonged loss of consciousness and abnormal vital signs. Sometimes short-term memory is lost. Any signs and symptoms of concussion are an indication of brain injury.
- *Contusion (bruising).* A *contusion* occurs when the force of a blow is great enough to rupture blood vessels on the surface or deep within the brain. In a closed head injury, the blood has no opening from which to drain. The blood builds up inside the skull, presses on the brain, and affects or impairs its function or ability to send messages to the body.

Open injuries occur when the cranium and overlying soft tissue are broken, exposing the brain and other soft tissues inside the skull (Figure 20.5). It is often difficult to determine if a head injury is open or closed because the soft tissues of the scalp can be damaged and bleeding without significant injury to the cranium. It is always best to assume that a head injury is open and to care for it accordingly.

KEY POINT ▼

Young children are very prone to head injuries. One reason is that in children the head is proportionally large compared to the size of the body. This makes the head more difficult to support and protect during falls.

KEY POINT ▼

When controlling bleeding with direct pressure, be careful not to apply too much pressure against the skull. This could put pressure on the brain if the person has suffered a significant skull fracture.

Injuries to the Face

Injuries to the face can be very serious because of the potential for airway obstruction (Figure 20.6). Blood and other fluids, blood clots, bone, and teeth may cause partial or complete airway obstruction. If the force is great enough, it can fracture the cranial vault and you may see cerebrospinal fluid (CSF) leaking from the ears and nose.

Consider the possibility of face injuries when you find any of the following signs:

- Blood in the airway (nose or mouth)
- Deformities or depression of any part of the face
- Swelling and discoloration around the eyes
- Swelling or discoloration of any part of the face
- Poor function of or inability to move the jaw
- Teeth that are loose or have been knocked out, broken dentures

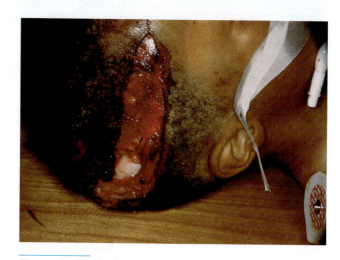

Figure 20.5 • An open head injury.

Figure 20.6 • The patient with facial injuries is at risk for airway compromise.

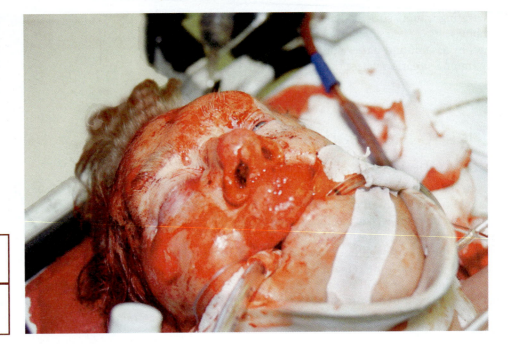

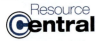

Resource **Central**

View a 3D animation of the skull.

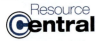

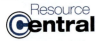

IS IT SAFE?

Always wear appropriate personal protective equipment including eye protection when caring for someone with a suspected head injury. Injuries to the head often cause significant vomiting, exposing you to the person's body fluids.

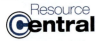

OBJECTIVES

6. Describe the signs and symptoms of a head injury.

7. Differentiate between an open and closed head injury.

8. Explain the appropriate assessment and care for a patient with a head injury.

Signs and Symptoms of Head Injury

Injuries to the head can range from minor lacerations to the scalp to severe skull fractures and significant injury to the brain. While it is difficult to know the true extent of damage when the head is injured, one of the best immediate indicators is the mental status of the injured person. A person who is alert and oriented following a head injury is likely to have less damage than a person who is unresponsive and bleeding.

The following is a list of common signs and symptoms of a head injury:

- Bleeding of the scalp
- Deformity of the cranium
- Altered mental status, unresponsiveness
- Nausea and vomiting
- Convulsions
- Abnormal vital signs
- Abnormal breathing patterns
- Combative behavior
- Repetitive questions

It is important to always consider the possibility of spine injury when caring for a person with a head injury. The force sustained by the head also could have caused injury to the vertebrae of the neck.

Caring for Head Injuries

When caring for someone with a head injury, it is important to suspect that he also may have suffered an injury to the vertebrae of the neck. Whenever possible, maintain manual stabilization of the head and neck when providing care. Remember that the control center for breathing is located deep within the brain. Any injury to the brain can disrupt normal breathing and cause the patient to become hypoxic. Constantly monitor the adequacy of breathing for all patients with a head injury.

Follow these steps when caring for an injured person with a suspected head injury:

1. Perform a primary assessment and ensure the ABCs are intact. If the person is unresponsive, open the airway with the jaw-thrust maneuver first. If this is unsuccessful, use the head-tilt/chin-lift method.

2. If necessary, provide rescue breaths using an appropriate barrier device.

3. Control any obvious bleeding. Be careful not to apply too much pressure to a head wound because you may put pressure on the brain if the skull has been fractured.

4. Keep the person still and lying flat. Maintain manual stabilization of the head and neck.

5. Administer supplemental oxygen if available. Follow local protocols.

6. Have suction prepared in case the person vomits. If no suction is available, consider rolling the patient onto his side while maintaining alignment of the head and neck.

7. Monitor vital signs, including mental status.

Care for Injuries to the Face

In all cases of injury to the face, make certain that the patient has an open airway.

Injuries to the face can damage teeth and dentures. Always look for and remove avulsed (dislodged) teeth and parts of broken dental appliances. Be careful not to inadvertently push these down the patient's airway. When a tooth is avulsed, there may be bleeding from the socket. Have the responsive patient bite down on a pad of gauze placed over the socket, but leave several inches of gauze outside the mouth for quick removal. For the unresponsive patient, hold the gauze over the socket. This will control the bleeding and prevent the airway from becoming obstructed with blood.

Wrap the avulsed tooth in a dressing. If you have a source of clean water, keep the dressing moist. (Milk can also be used.) Do not attempt to clean the tooth.

Injuries to the Spine

Injuries to the cervical spine can cause **paralysis**, impair breathing, and even cause death. Injuries along the rest of the spinal column also can cause paralysis and reduce normal body movement and function.

Spine injuries are caused by forces to the head, neck, back, chest, pelvis, or legs. Often, you will find patients with he1ad injuries who also have cervical-spine injuries. Injuries to the upper leg bones or to the pelvic bones also may cause spine injury through indirect force. Motor-vehicle crashes (including those causing whiplash), falls, diving, and skiing mishaps are common causes of spine injuries.

If a patient has numbness, loss of feeling, or paralysis in the legs with no problems in the arms, the injury to the spine is probably below the neck. If numbness, loss of feeling, or paralysis involves the arms and the legs, the injury is probably in the neck. Numbness, loss of feeling, and paralysis may be limited to only one side of the body, but usually both sides are involved.

Injuries to the spine can include fractured or displaced spinal bones (vertebrae) or swelling that presses on nerves. These injuries can produce the same signs and symptoms. In some cases, the loss of function associated with spine injuries may be temporary if the loss is caused by pressure or swelling that may eventually go away.

KEY POINT ▼

Your first attempt at opening the airway of an unresponsive person with a head injury should be with the jaw-thrust maneuver. If the jaw-thrust does not open the airway, use the head-tilt/chin-lift maneuver. Maintaining an open airway and providing adequate ventilations are critical priorities.

paralysis ▶ the loss of mobility and feeling.

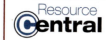

Complete an informative tutorial on spinal-cord injuries. Then learn some surprising facts and figures about spinal-cord injuries.

From the Medical Director

Spine Injuries

Most victims of spinal trauma will have suffered their neurologic injury before you arrive at their side. They will have either cut or bruised the spinal cord and/or the nerves leaving the spinal column. If they are awake, they will have signs and symptoms that help you determine the presence of injury. However, if they have an altered mental status, you must assume based on the mechanism of injury that they have a spine injury and take appropriate precautions.

Figure 20.7 • Algorithm for the assessment of a patient with suspected spine injury.

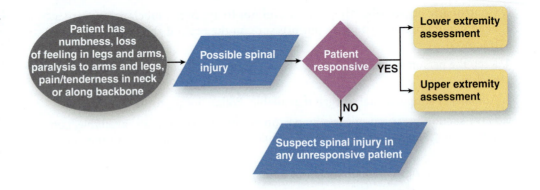

Patient has numbness, loss of feeling in legs and arms, paralysis to arms and legs, pain/tenderness in neck or along backbone → Possible spinal injury → Patient responsive — **YES** → Lower extremity assessment / Upper extremity assessment

NO ↓

Suspect spinal injury in any unresponsive patient

From the Medical Director

Assessing for Injury

In some cases there may be a loss of sensation but not movement or loss of movement but not sensation. For this reason, you should check both sensation and motor function of all extremities.

OBJECTIVE

9. Describe the signs and symptoms of a spine injury.

Signs and Symptoms of Suspected Spine Injury

Conduct a thorough patient history during your assessment of a responsive patient (Figure 20.7). Utilize the following guidelines when assessing a patient with suspected spine injury:

- Do his arms or legs feel numb? Can the patient feel you touch his hands and feet? Can he squeeze your hand or push your hand with his foot?
- Look and feel gently for injuries and deformities.
- See if the patient can move his arms and legs. Do not do this if you have noted any mechanism of injury or other signs that indicate possible injury to the spine.

For the unresponsive patient, remember to ask bystanders for information on the emergency and what they saw happen to the patient. This may help you determine the mechanism of injury. Also, look and feel for injuries and deformities. See if the patient responds to pressure on or pinching of the feet and hands. Never probe palms and soles with sharp objects.

The following is a list of the most common signs and symptoms of a spine injury:

- Pain over the spine
- Deformity over the spine
- Numbness, weakness, or tingling in the extremities
- Loss of sensation
- Paralysis
- Incontinence (bladder or bowel)
- Priapism (erection of the penis)

In extreme cases you may see a patient with abnormal flexion or extension of the arms (Figure 20.8). This is referred to as "posturing" and is a sign of significant head and/or spine injury.

Carefully check all extremities for circulation, sensation, and movement (CSM). Any problems with CSM can be an indication of a possible spine injury (Scan 20.2). Not all

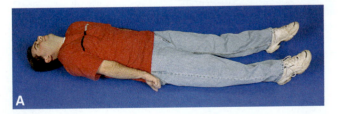
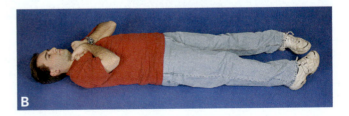

Figure 20.8 • Abnormal posturing is a sign of significant head and/or spine injury. (A) Abnormal extension (decerebrate posture). (B) Abnormal flexion (decorticate posture).

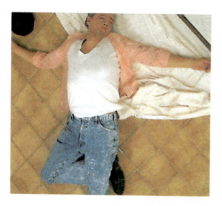

20.2.1 | Falls are common causes of spinal injury.

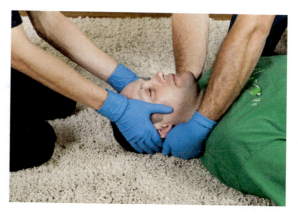

20.2.2 | Palpate the neck anterior and posterior for pain and deformity.

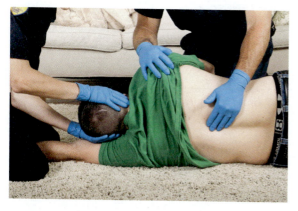

20.2.3 | Palpate the spine for pain and deformity.

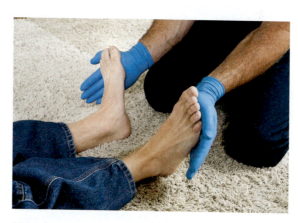

20.2.4 | Assess motor function of both feet simultaneously.

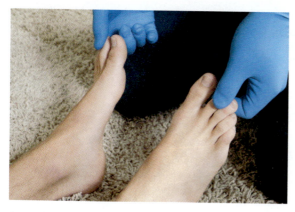

20.2.5 | Assess sensation of both feet by checking for numbness and tingling.

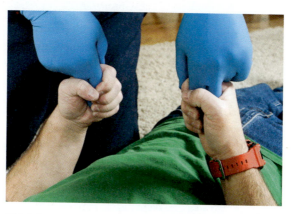

20.2.6 | Assess motor function of both hands simultaneously.

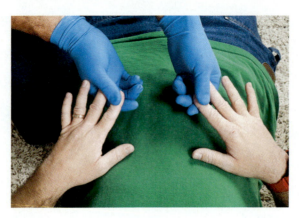

20.2.7 | Assess sensation of both hands by checking for numbness and tingling.

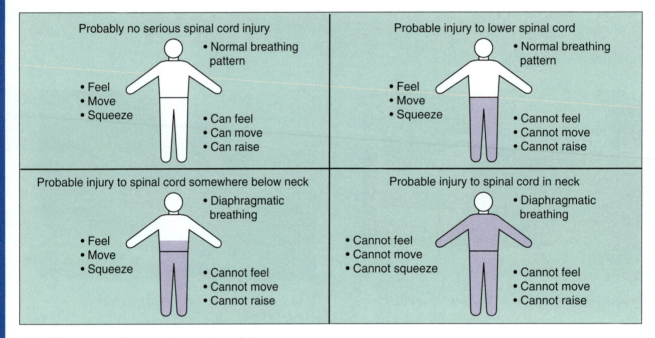

Probably no serious spinal cord injury
- Normal breathing pattern
- Feel
- Move
- Squeeze
- Can feel
- Can move
- Can raise

Probable injury to lower spinal cord
- Normal breathing pattern
- Feel
- Move
- Squeeze
- Cannot feel
- Cannot move
- Cannot raise

Probable injury to spinal cord somewhere below neck
- Diaphragmatic breathing
- Feel
- Move
- Squeeze
- Cannot feel
- Cannot move
- Cannot raise

Probable injury to spinal cord in neck
- Diaphragmatic breathing
- Cannot feel
- Cannot move
- Cannot squeeze
- Cannot feel
- Cannot move
- Cannot raise

20.2.8 | Summary of observations and conclusions.

spine injuries are immediate or permanent. The spinal cord can be damaged by direct injury or by swelling that occurs hours after the injury. Damage also can occur during care and transport of the injured person. Be especially careful when assessing an injured person with suspected spine injury.

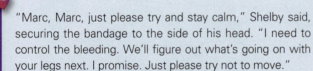

continued

"Marc, Marc, just please try and stay calm," Shelby said, securing the bandage to the side of his head. "I need to control the bleeding. We'll figure out what's going on with your legs next. I promise. Just please try not to move."

The stage manager had been beside himself with rage until Marc shouted that he couldn't feel his legs, and his demeanor changed as he ordered the small crowd away and made a path for the medics who would arrive soon.

"Can you feel my hands?" Shelby asked as she grabbed hold of Marcs quivering fingers. He nodded and she gripped onto both of his pointer fingers, which he readily identified as being held. He also squeezed pretty tightly with both hands.

"Alright, now the legs," Shelby thought as she carefully palpated both of Marc's legs down to his feet, careful not to jostle him. "I'm going to check your lower extremities. Let me know what you feel."

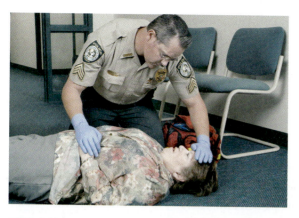

20.3.1 | Using one hand to provide manual stabilization of the head when you are at the side of the injured person.

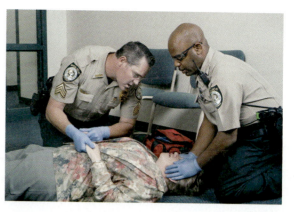

20.3.2 | Using two hands to provide manual stabilization of the injured person's head and neck.

Caring for a Suspected Spine Injury

Injuries to the spine can result in a wide range of severity. Do not be fooled by the absence of obvious signs and symptoms during your assessment. These injuries often will worsen as time passes, so be very diligent with your assessment.

When caring for an injured person with a suspected spine injury, perform a primary assessment and ensure the ABCs are intact. If you must manage the airway, attempt the jaw-thrust maneuver first, before the head-tilt/chin-lift maneuver. Then manually stabilize the head so that the head, neck, and spine do not move and are kept in line (Scan 20.3).

Perform a secondary assessment including all extremities. Obtain and monitor vital signs. Provide supplemental oxygen, if available, following local protocols.

You should be aware that not all injured people will present with obvious signs and symptoms of a spine injury. Those with altered mental status and those who appear intoxicated are not able to reliably report pain. Sometimes signs and symptoms do not appear for hours. So, any injured person who appears intoxicated, has an altered mental status, or is found unresponsive should be cared for as though he has a spine injury.

Manual Stabilization

Manual stabilization of the head and neck is an important step in caring for an injured person with a suspected spine injury. There are two basic approaches to an injured person who is supine. The first is to approach the person from the side and place your hand on his forehead to minimize movement. The second is to kneel at the top of the person's head and use both hands to grasp the head from the sides.

To perform manual stabilization of the head and neck of a supine person, follow these steps:

1. Kneel at the top or side of the injured person's head.

2. Introduce yourself and explain to the person what you are going to do.

3. Grasp the person's head by placing your hands on each side of the head, and hold firmly.

OBJECTIVES

10. Explain the appropriate assessment and care for a patient with a suspected spine injury.

11. Explain the special considerations of airway management for a patient with suspected cervical-spine injury.

KEY POINT ▼

Any person who is found unresponsive, and you are unable to determine an exact mechanism of injury or nature of illness, should be cared for as though he has a spine injury.

KEY POINT ▼

Children have a very large posterior skull. This can cause the head to tilt forward when they are placed in a supine position (flat on the back, face up). Carefully slipping a folded towel under the shoulders will help keep the head and neck in a more neutral position.

4. Instruct the person to remain still and provide reassurance.

5. Monitor the ABCs by talking to the person and listening to how he responds.

Follow the steps for performing manual stabilization of the head and neck of a seated person (Figure 20.9):

1. Stand or sit directly behind the injured person.

2. Introduce yourself and explain to the person what you are going to do.

3. Grasp the person's head by placing your hands on each side of the head, and hold firmly.

4. Instruct the person to remain still and provide reassurance.

5. Monitor the ABCs by talking to the person and listening to how he responds.

There are some instances when you might arrive at the scene to find one or more of the patients walking around. You must be sure to consider the walking wounded as patients and care for them accordingly. If you find a patient who is standing and you have reason to suspect he might have a neck or back injury, you must provide proper spinal immobilization. You can begin by standing behind him and holding manual stabilization of his head. Carefully explain to him why you are concerned for him and request his cooperation. With the assistance of other rescuers you will want to place him onto a long board and fully immobilize him for transport.

Rules for Care of Spine Injury

Always follow these rules for Emergency Medical Responder care of patients with possible spine injuries:

- Make certain the airway is open. Assist ventilations or perform CPR as needed, even though the patient may have spine injuries. Use the jaw-thrust maneuver when ventilating the patient.
- Attempt to control serious bleeding. Avoid moving the injured part of the patient and any of the limbs when applying dressings.
- Always conclude that an unresponsive trauma patient has spine injuries.
- Do not attempt to splint long-bone injuries if there are indications of spine injuries until you have appropriate help.
- Never move a patient with suspected spine injuries unless you must do so to provide CPR or assist ventilations, need to reach and control life-threatening bleeding, or must protect yourself and the patient from immediate danger at the scene.
- Keep the patient still. Tell him not to move. Position yourself to stabilize the patient's head, neck, and as much of the body as possible.
- Continuously monitor patients with possible spine injury.

Figure 20.9 • Establish manual stabilization of the head while your partner selects a collar.

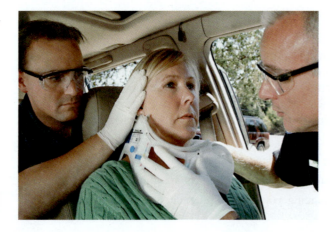

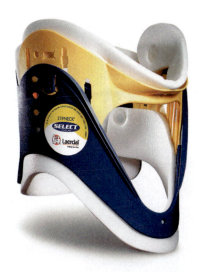

20.4.1 | A typical adjustable cervical collar.

Cervical Collars

When you package a patient on an immobilization device, you must first stabilize the head and neck by selecting and applying a cervical collar that is a size appropriate for your patient (Scans 20.4 and 20.5). Also called *extrication collars*, rigid cervical collars are applied to help maintain stability and alignment with the body in patients who have suspected neck and spine injuries (Scans 20.6 and 20.7).

Whether or not you learn to size and place cervical collars during your training, it is vital to understand one very important concept: Cervical collars will only minimize movement of the neck of a cooperative patient. A patient who is combative or otherwise uncooperative can still move his or her neck even with a cervical collar in place. Therefore, it is important to maintain manual stabilization of the head even after placement of a cervical collar.

There are many different makes and models of cervical collars on the market today. Some brands offer many sizes, while others offer a "one size fits all" adjustable collar. More than likely you will not have a choice in the matter. Instead, you will be expected to utilize whatever collars are currently in use in your agency or region. Whatever the case, it is best to follow the manufacturer's suggested method for sizing and application.

Regardless of the brand or type of collar, the following guidelines can be used to ensure a proper fit for your patient:

- Once in place, check to see that the sides of the collar do not ride too far above or below the earlobes.
- Confirm the chin fits properly on the collar. The bony part of the chin should be well supported by the collar.
- The collar should be snug on all sides and not too tight or too loose.
- Consider using a different size or adjusting the collar if it does not fit properly.

Helmet Removal

Helmets are designed to absorb energy forces and prevent injury to the head. However, well fitting helmets—even the most modern ones—cannot prevent the brain from striking the interior of the skull in extreme or high-speed crash forces.

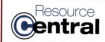

Read more about cervical injuries and application of a cervical collar.

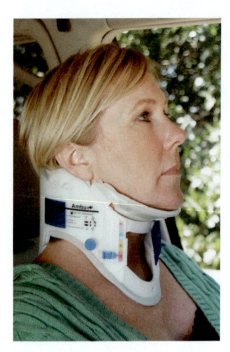

20.5.1 | When properly fitted, the sides of the collar should come very close to or slightly overlap the earlobe.

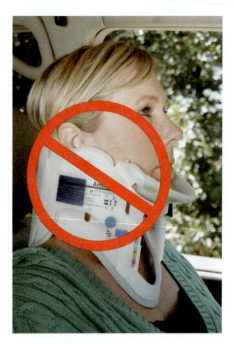

20.5.2 | A collar that is too big will extend way above the earlobes. Consider readjusting or selecting a smaller size collar.

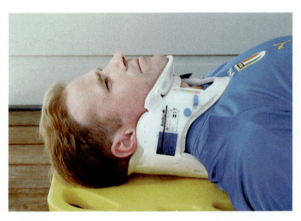

20.5.3 | When properly fitted, the patient's chin will fit completely and snugly within the saddle of the collar.

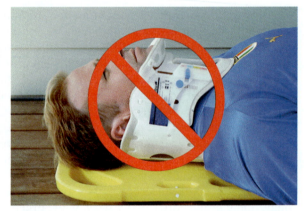

20.5.4 | A collar that is too big will extend well beyond the chin, allowing for excessive movement. Consider readjusting or selecting a smaller size collar.

The helmet should be removed immediately if there are any issues with the ABCs, such as airway obstruction or inadequate breathing. For an unresponsive patient wearing a helmet, always suspect a spine injury. Monitor the patient's ABCs and properly immobilize the spine.

For football players who are wearing shoulder pads, the helmet left in place keeps the cervical spine in a midline position. Removing the helmet but keeping the shoulder pads in place causes the head to fall back in an overextended position, which pulls the spinal column out of alignment.

There are many types of helmets. They are made in half-size, three-quarter size, and full-size. Full-size helmets cover the mouth and sometimes part of the nose and usually have a face shield. Bicycle helmets are usually half-size and open in the front and have no face shield or face guard. Football helmets are full-size and have face guards. Motorcycle helmets are available in all three sizes, with the full-size helmets having a clear face shield or visor that moves up and down and is easy to remove. Motorcyclists who wear the half-size or three-fourths size helmets will usually wear glasses or goggles to protect their eyes.

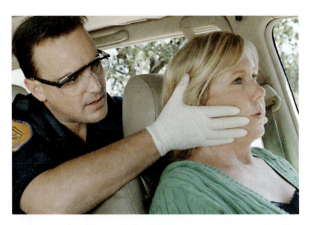

20.6.1 | Establish manual stabilization of the head while your partner selects a collar.

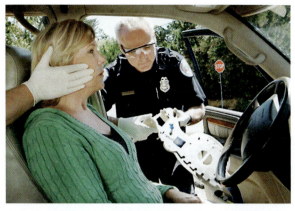

20.6.2 | Select an appropriately sized collar or adjust the collar based on the patient's size. Follow the manufacturer's guidelines for size and adjustment selection.

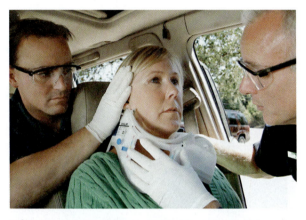

20.6.3 | Place the collar beneath the patient's chin and firmly against the lower jaw. The chin should fit well within the chin saddle of the collar.

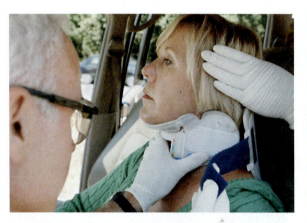

20.6.4 | Secure the collar in place by overlapping the Velcro closer at the side of the patient's neck. Confirm fit by looking at ears and chin.

If the helmet has a face guard or face shield, remove it to gain access to the patient's airway. If any patient who is not breathing is wearing a helmet with a face guard or face shield that cannot be removed, remove the helmet to gain access to the airway. If a helmet is removed, it must be done cautiously and by two people.

Before removing a helmet, perform the following steps:

1. Remove the face piece or face shield while your partner stabilizes the head. Do not cut the chin strap. Remove glasses or goggles.
2. Check to see if the patient is breathing.
3. If the patient is breathing, check the helmet for fit. A well-fitting helmet can stay in place as long as the patient is breathing.
4. If you must clear the airway or assist the patient with breathing, remove the helmet. If the patient is wearing shoulder pads (such as football pads), leave them in place.

Provide care to any unresponsive patient as if there is a spine injury. When you find any helmeted patient face down or on one side, log roll him onto his back (supine). Leave the helmet in place if you find the following:

• Helmet fits well, and the patient's head does not move (or moves very little) inside of it. A well-fitting helmet keeps the head from moving, and it should be left on if there are no airway or breathing problems and the helmet does not interfere with assessment and management of the airway and breathing.

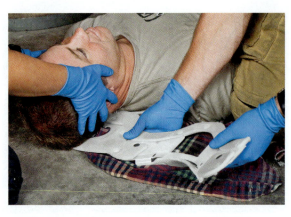

20.7.1 | Slide the back portion of the cervical-spine immobilization collar behind the patient's neck. Fold the loop Velcro inward on the foam padding.

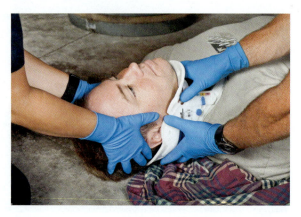

20.7.2 | Position the collar so that the chin fits properly. Secure the collar by attaching the Velcro.

ALTERNATIVE METHOD

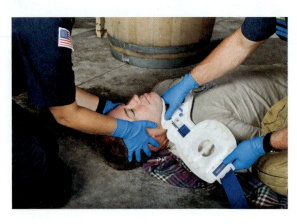

20.7.3 | An alternative method of applying the collar to a supine patient is to start by positioning the chin piece and then sliding the back portion of the collar behind the patient's neck.

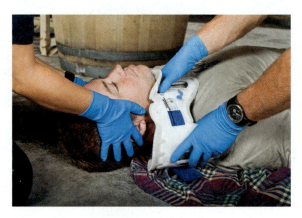

20.7.4 | Hold the collar in place by grasping the trachea hole. Attach the loop Velcro so it mates with (and is parallel to) the hook Velcro.

- Patient is breathing adequately and has no airway problems (fluids, obstructions).
- Patient can be placed in a neutral, in-line position for immobilization on a spine board.
- Helmet does not interfere with your ability to reassess and maintain the patient's airway or assist breathing.
- Patient is wearing shoulder pads. If the helmet is removed, place a similar amount of padding under the head.

Remove the helmet if you find the following:

- Helmet interferes with your ability to assess or manage the patient's airway and breathing.
- Helmet does not fit snugly, and the patient's head moves inside the helmet.
- Helmet interferes with placing the patient on a spine board in a neutral, in-line position. When the helmet rests on the spine board, its size may force the patient's head forward (hyperflexion) and close the airway. Padding can be placed under the patient's shoulders to prevent hyperflexion and maintain an in-line position.
- Patient is in cardiac or respiratory arrest. Quickly remove the helmet while a partner stabilizes the head. Proceed with CPR steps, using the jaw-thrust maneuver.

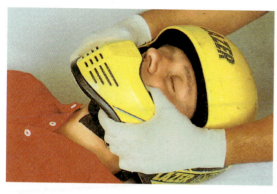

20.8.1 | Rescuer 1: Kneel at the head of the patient. Stabilize the patient's head.

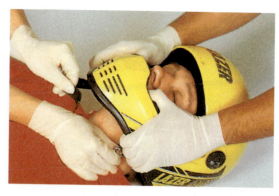

20.8.2 | Rescuer 2: Kneel at the side of the patient's shoulders. Unfasten the chin strap. Remove the face guard, face shield, goggles, or glasses if present.

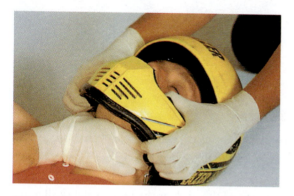

20.8.3 | Rescuer 2: Place one hand on the mandible at the angle of the jaw and the other hand behind the neck at the base of the skull to stabilize the patient's head.

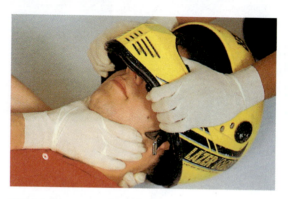

20.8.4 | Rescuer 1: Pull sides of helmet apart and carefully slip helmet halfway off.

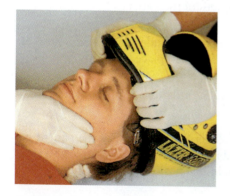

20.8.5 | Rescuer 2: Maintain position of hand stabilizing the jaw. Reposition at the back of the neck slightly higher on the back of the head to maintain in-line stabilization.

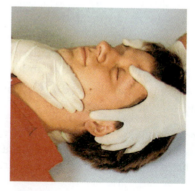

20.8.6 | Rescuer 1: Finish removing the helmet and then place hands on either side of the patient's head to take over in-line stabilization.

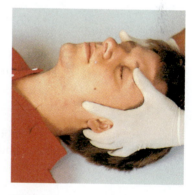

20.8.7 | Rescuer 2: Check and clear airway, provide ventilations, and apply a collar.

If you must remove the helmet, remove it according to local protocol. The steps listed below provide general directions for removal of full-size helmets (Scans 20.8 and 20.9).

1. Rescuer 1 will kneel at the head of the patient and stabilize the patient's head by placing his hands on each side of the helmet.

2. Rescuer 2 will kneel on one side of the patient at the patient's shoulders, unfasten the chin strap, remove the face guard or face shield (if not yet done), and remove the patient's glasses or goggles if present.

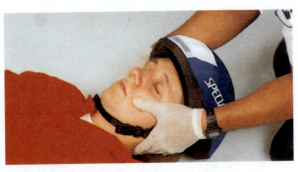

20.9.1 | Apply steady stabilization to the neck in neutral position.

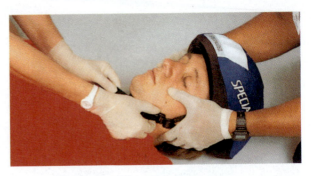

20.9.2 | Remove the chin strap.

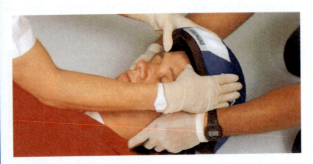

20.9.3 | Remove helmet by pulling the sides apart (laterally).

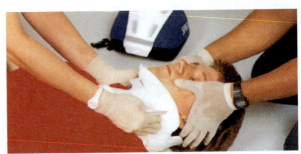

20.9.4 | Apply a suitable cervical-spine immobilization collar and secure the patient to a long board.

3. Rescuer 2 will place one hand on either side of the neck at the base of the skull and stabilize the head while rescuer 1 removes the helmet.

4. Rescuer 1 will pull the sides of the helmet apart using the straps and slowly and carefully slip the helmet off the patient's head.

5. Rescuer 2 will slowly slide his hands along the sides of the patient's head and neck to support it as the helmet is removed.

6. Rescuer 1 will finish removing the helmet, place padding under the patient's head as needed (if the patient is wearing shoulder pads), and then place his hands on either side of the patient's head to take over in-line stabilization.

7. Rescuer 2 will check and clear the airway, provide ventilations with supplemental oxygen, and apply a collar.

Remember that you do not have to remove a helmet from a patient if the patient has an airway and is breathing, if the helmet is snug, and if the patient can be secured to a spine board with the helmet on and the head in a neutral, in-line position with the spine.

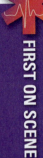

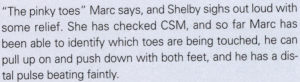

WRAP-UP

"The pinky toes" Marc says, and Shelby sighs out loud with some relief. She has checked CSM, and so far Marc has been able to identify which toes are being touched, he can pull up on and push down with both feet, and he has a distal pulse beating faintly.

"The medics are here!" comes the loud, booming voice of the stage manager.

"Hear that, Marc?" Shelby says as she rechecks his ABCs. "We're going to hold your head still while the medics get over here, and they're going to get you to the hospital immediately."

"Thank you," comes the stage director's voice. "He's a good kid. I'll ride with him to the hospital."

"Unfortunately," Shelby says, sternly, "you will be helping me set up the safety ropes I required you to have around the stage, and we'll fill out an incident report. I'm calling a safety meeting tonight." She winks at Marc and he smiles, wiggling his toes in relief.

Summary

- Open head injuries are those that result in a break in the bone and the overlying soft tissue. A closed head injury involves no opening of the skull; however, there may be soft-tissue damage of the scalp.

- Head injuries can range from a very mild concussion to significant open fractures of the skull. A person with a head injury often will have signs and symptoms ranging from a mild headache to bleeding of the scalp, altered mental status, deformity of the cranium, unresponsiveness, convulsions, and vomiting. Someone with a head injury also may display aggressive behavior and ask repetitive questions.

- Your first concern when caring for a person with a suspected head injury is to manage and monitor the ABCs. Consider the possibility of a neck injury and provide care accordingly. Control bleeding as appropriate.

- Management of the airway in an unresponsive person with a suspected neck injury can be challenging, but it is important to remember that the airway is always the top priority. If you must open the airway of an unresponsive injured person with a suspected neck injury, begin with the jaw-thrust maneuver. If the jaw-thrust maneuver is unsuccessful, use the head-tilt/chin-lift maneuver.

- When caring for a person with a suspected spine injury, you must first try to identify the mechanism of injury. Always assume there is a spine injury if the mechanism suggests it, even if the injured person has no obvious signs or symptoms.

- A person with a spine injury may have pain and/or deformity over the injury site. He also may present with numbness, tingling, and weakness of the extremities, loss of sensation, paralysis, and incontinence.

- Once you have confirmed that the ABCs are intact, your primary concern becomes stabilization of the head, neck, and spine. Provide manual stabilization of the head and neck until EMS arrives and is able to place the patient onto a long spine board.

Take Action

ON A ROLL

Our jobs would be much easier if every patient we came across was found lying supine and in perfect alignment. Of course this is not the case. There will be times when it is necessary to carefully roll a patient into a position that will allow you to assess the ABCs or control bleeding. It also becomes necessary to roll a patient when he needs to be immobilized to a long backboard. This activity will allow you to practice this valuable skill and develop the confidence necessary to facilitate a log roll when necessary.

Begin by gathering at least two and preferably three of your friends or fellow classmates. Have one of them play patient and lie on the floor as if he were injured. Start by having the patient lying supine. The rest of you will take your positions next to the patient in preparation for a log roll. The point of this activity is to allow you to experiment with various techniques for holding on to the patient and rolling him. You should change positions each time and get a feel for what must be done by each person in different positions. Your goal is to keep the spine in alignment as much as possible throughout each roll.

After a few simple rolls from the supine position, have the patient lie prone or in a more challenging position. Notice how difficult it gets trying to keep the head in alignment with the spine in these different positions. Remember to always make the move on the count of the person at the head. The more you practice these moves, the more confident and efficient you will become.

First on Scene Run Review

Recall the events of the "First on Scene" scenario in this chapter and answer the following questions, which are related to the call. Rationales are offered in the Answer Key at the back of the book.

1. What information should Shelby obtain?

2. Why did Shelby ask permission to help?

3. Why is it important to hold the C-spine?

Quick Quiz

To check your understanding of the chapter, answer the following questions. Then compare your answers to those in the Answer Key at the back of the book.

1. What is the most important initial step that you can take when caring for a person with a suspected spine injury?

   a. Assess the patient for circulation, sensation, and movement.
   b. Determine the mechanism of injury.
   c. Transport the patient to the nearest trauma center.
   d. Manually stabilize the patient's head and neck.

2. Which one of the following mechanisms of injury would cause you to suspect spine injury?

   a. Circular saw amputation of fingers
   b. Fall from an anchored speedboat
   c. Bicycle crash
   d. Self-inflicted gunshot wound to the hip

3. You are requested to assist with an unresponsive person who was found facedown on a hotel lobby floor. How would you choose to move the patient into the recovery position?

   a. Two-person extremity lift
   b. Three-person log roll
   c. With a stair chair
   d. It would be better to wait for EMS.

4. Your patient is unresponsive following a motorcycle crash on the interstate. You find that he is not breathing and you try to open his airway with the jaw-thrust maneuver but are not successful. What should you do next?

   a. Maintain manual stabilization and wait for EMS to arrive.
   b. Attempt the head-tilt/chin-lift maneuver.
   c. Attempt to ventilate the patient anyway.
   d. Begin chest compressions.

5. Combative behavior, abnormal breathing patterns, and repetitive questions are all signs of a(n):

   a. cervical-spine injury.
   b. unresponsive person.
   c. peripheral nervous system trauma.
   d. injury to the head.

6. You witness a low-speed ATV collision at a local recreational area that knocks both riders from their vehicles. Neither of the men is wearing a helmet but both quickly get back to their feet. You notice one of them is walking oddly as he retrieves his vehicle. You ask if he is okay and he tells you that his legs "just feel really heavy." You should suspect:

   a. head injury.
   b. internal bleeding.
   c. spine injury.
   d. hip dislocation.

7. What are the two main components of the central nervous system?

   a. Peripheral and central nerves
   b. Discs and vertebrae
   c. Brain and spine
   d. Spine and nerves

8. You are caring for a motorcycle rider who was ejected from his vehicle. You are the only rescuer at the scene. He is responsive and breathing adequately. You should:

   a. remove the helmet and clear the airway.
   b. maintain manual stabilization of the head and helmet.
   c. roll him onto his side to inspect his back.
   d. ask him to remove his own helmet.

9. The purpose of a properly sized cervical collar is to:

   a. completely immobilize the head and neck.
   b. completely immobilize the neck only.
   c. maintain an open airway.
   d. remind the cooperative patient not to move her neck.

10. You are caring for a patient with a suspected open skull injury. When attempting to control bleeding, you should:

   a. apply firm fingertip pressure on the open wound.
   b. use gentle pressure with the palm of one hand.
   c. tightly wrap a pressure bandage around the skull.
   d. keep the patient in a head-down position while holding pressure.

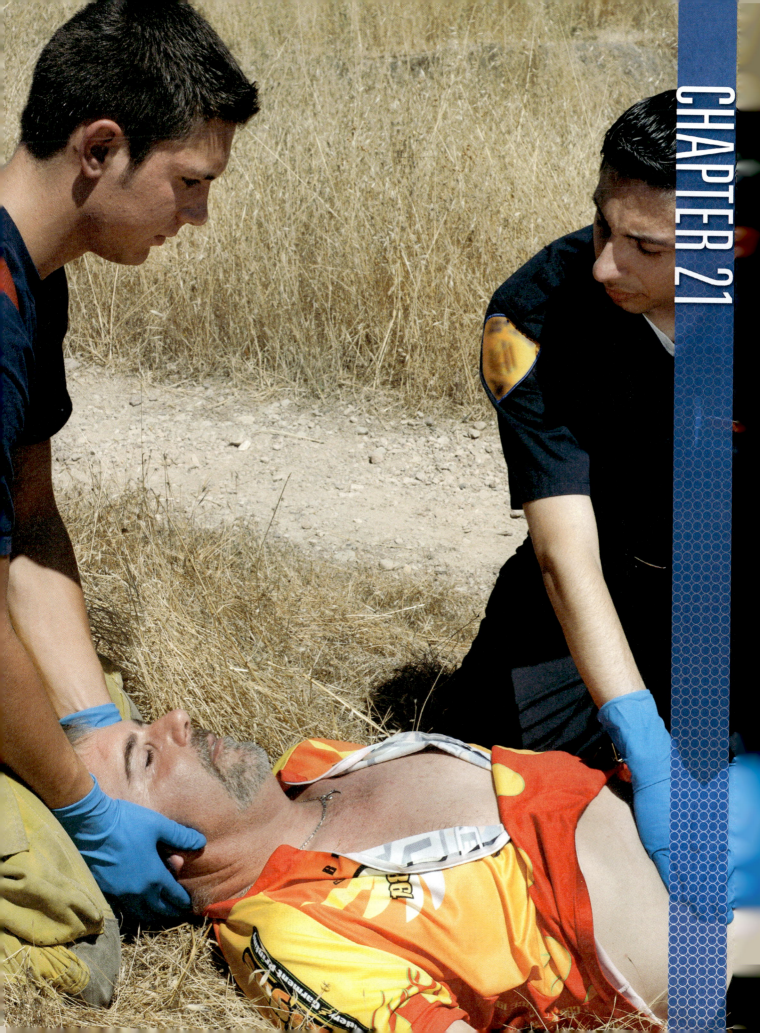

CHAPTER 21

Caring for Chest and Abdominal Emergencies

EDUCATION STANDARDS
- Trauma—Chest Trauma, Abdominal, and Genitourinary Trauma
- Medicine—Abdominal and Gastrointestinal Disorders

COMPETENCIES
- Uses simple knowledge to recognize and manage life threats based on assessment findings for an acutely injured patient while awaiting additional emergency medical response.

CHAPTER OVERVIEW
Injuries to the chest and abdomen are very common simply due to the large part of the body that the two areas make up. Chest and abdominal injuries also pose great risk to the patient, as the majority of the body's vital organs are contained within these two cavities. This chapter discusses some of the more common injuries associated with the chest and abdomen as well as how to properly assess and care for these injuries.

OBJECTIVES

Upon successful completion of this chapter, the student should be able to:

COGNITIVE

1. Review the anatomy of the chest and abdomen from Chapter 4.
2. Define the following terms:
   a. closed chest injury *(p. 467)*
   b. crepitus *(p. 468)*
   c. diaphragm *(p. 471)*
   d. distention *(p. 473)*
   e. evisceration *(p. 474)*
   f. flail chest *(p. 468)*
   g. guarding *(p. 473)*
   h. hemothorax *(p. 468)*
   i. mediastinum *(p. 465)*
   j. occlusive dressing *(p. 470)*
   k. open chest injury *(p. 467)*
   l. paradoxical movement *(p. 468)*
   m. penetrating injury *(p. 466)*
   n. pleura *(p. 466)*
   o. pleural space *(p. 466)*
   p. pneumothorax *(p. 468)*
   q. quadrant *(p. 472)*
   r. retroperitoneal cavity *(p. 472)*
   s. spontaneous pneumothorax *(p. 468)*
   t. sucking chest wound *(p. 467)*
   u. tension pneumothorax *(p. 470)*
3. Describe the major structures of the thoracic cavity. *(p. 465)*
4. Explain the relationship between chest injury and perfusion. *(p. 467)*
5. Differentiate between an open and closed chest injury. *(p. 466)*
6. Describe the signs and symptoms of a closed chest injury. *(p. 469)*
7. Explain the appropriate assessment of a patient with a chest injury. *(p. 469)*
8. Explain the appropriate care of a patient with a closed chest injury. *(p. 470)*
9. Explain the appropriate care of a patient with an open chest injury. *(p. 471)*
10. Describe the major structures of the abdominal and pelvic cavities. *(p. 473)*
11. Describe the signs and symptoms of internal bleeding. *(p. 473)*
12. Explain the appropriate assessment and care of a patient with abdominal pain. *(p. 473)*
13. Explain the appropriate assessment and care of a patient with an open abdominal injury. *(p. 474)*

PSYCHOMOTOR

14. Demonstrate the appropriate assessment and care of a patient with a chest injury.

15. Demonstrate the appropriate assessment and care of a patient with abdominal pain.

16. Demonstrate the appropriate assessment and care of an open abdominal injury.

17. Value the importance of proper body substance isolation (BSI) precautions when assisting with chest and abdominal injuries.

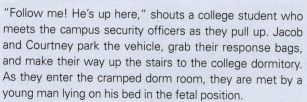

"Follow me! He's up here," shouts a college student who meets the campus security officers as they pull up. Jacob and Courtney park the vehicle, grab their response bags, and make their way up the stairs to the college dormitory. As they enter the cramped dorm room, they are met by a young man lying on his bed in the fetal position.

"Hi," Jacob says as he sets his bag down and kneels beside the bed. "My name is Jacob. I'm trained as an Emergency Medical Responder. I'm here to here to help you. Okay? Can you tell me your name?"

"It's Nico," he says, wincing. "My stomach is killing me! You've got to make it stop!" He winces again and draws his legs closer to his body.

"Courtney," Jacob says as he begins looking for any immediate life threats or bleeding, "go ahead and administer some oxygen while I get some vitals."

Anatomy of the Chest

The chest cavity, also known as the *thoracic cavity*, makes up approximately half of the torso. The boundaries of the chest cavity include the clavicles at the top, the diaphragm muscle at the bottom, the sternum on the anterior side, and the spinal column at the posterior side (Figure 21.1). The chest gets most of its shape from the 12 pairs of ribs that begin at the spine and continue around to the anterior side of the chest.

The major organs contained within the chest are the heart and lungs. There also are major vessels such as the aorta and the vena cava that either originate or terminate in the chest. The heart and lungs are well protected by the ribs that make up the chest.

Deep within the center of the chest is a space called the mediastinum. The **mediastinum** houses the trachea, esophagus, heart, vena cava, and aorta. The left and right

OBJECTIVE

3. Describe the major structures of the thoracic cavity.

mediastinum ▶ the structure that divides the two halves of the chest cavity.

CHEST CAVITY

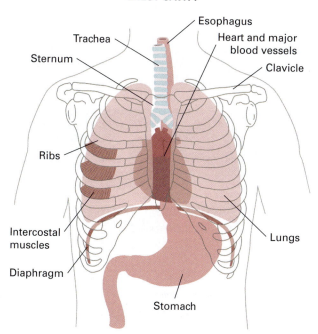

Figure 21.1 • The chest contains the heart and lungs and is separated from the abdominal cavity by the diaphragm muscle.

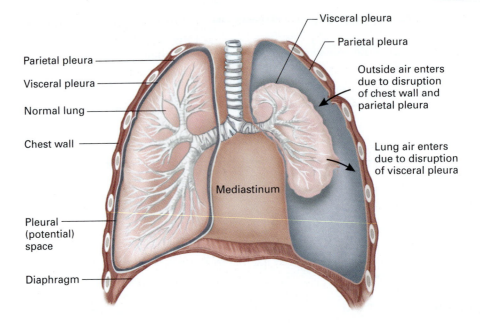

Parietal pleura

Visceral pleura

Normal lung

Chest wall

Visceral pleura

Parietal pleura

Outside air enters due to disruption of chest wall and parietal pleura

Lung air enters due to disruption of visceral pleura

Mediastinum

Pleural (potential) space

Diaphragm

sides of the chest are occupied by the lungs. Each lung is surrounded by a thin saclike structure called the pleura (Figure 21.2). There are actually two layers to the pleura. The *visceral pleura*, which is in direct contact with each lung, and the *parietal pleura*, which lines the inner wall of the chest. The space between the visceral and parietal pleura is called the *pleural space*. When the lungs are functioning normally, the two pleural layers remain in close contact with one another. They are lubricated by a specialized fluid that allows for smooth movement between the two layers each time the person breathes in and out.

pleura ▶ the thin saclike structure that surrounds each lung.

pleural space ▶ the potential space that exists between the visceral and parietal pleura in the chest.

Chest Injuries

Much like soft-tissue or head injuries, chest injuries fall into two major categories: open and closed (Figure 21.3). Most closed chest injuries are the result of blunt force trauma. Falls, contact sports, vehicle collisions, and blasts are common causes of closed chest injuries. Open chest injuries are often the result of a **penetrating injury** such as from a bullet, knife, or similar projectile.

The chest can be injured in a number of ways, including blunt trauma, penetrating objects, and compression:

- *Blunt trauma.* A blow to the chest can fracture the ribs, the sternum, and the rib cartilages. Whole sections of the chest can collapse. With severe blunt trauma, the lungs and airway can be damaged and the heart may be seriously injured.

Figure 21.3 • An open chest injury.

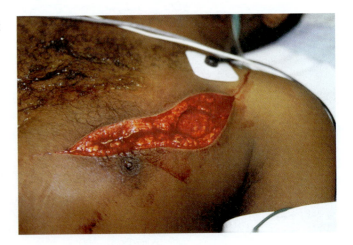

- *Penetrating objects*. Bullets, knives, pieces of metal or glass, steel rods, pipes, and various other objects can penetrate the chest wall, damaging internal organs and impairing respiration.
- *Compression*. This results from severe blunt trauma in which the chest is rapidly compressed, as when a driver in a motor-vehicle collision strikes his chest on the steering column. The heart can be severely squeezed, the lungs can be ruptured, and the sternum and ribs can be fractured.

Closed Chest Injuries

Closed chest injuries are most often caused by blunt force trauma to the chest or back and are not associated with an open wound. Closed chest injuries can cause a variety of complications, from minor to life threatening. One of the most common types of closed chest injuries is damage to the ribs. While not usually life threatening, broken ribs can cause enough pain to keep the patient from breathing adequately. Because the chest wall moves in and out with each breath, even shallow breaths can cause pain. The patient will try to minimize the pain by taking breaths that are much more shallow than usual. Over time, this could make the patient hypoxic. In many cases, the care for injured ribs is simply to splint the injured area with bulky dressings (Figure 21.4). If the injury is on the anterior or lateral chest, the patient will often self-splint by holding an arm tightly against the chest wall. It is appropriate to allow these patients to assume a position of comfort and provide high flow oxygen if local protocols allow.

Pneumothorax

A common result of injury to the chest involves the chest cavity filling with air from a ruptured lung. This is called a **pneumothorax**. A pneumothorax can occur secondary to injury or it can occur spontaneously. In other words, it can happen without any outside force. This is often caused when a thin spot on the lung ruptures. A **spontaneous pneumothorax** is rarely life threatening, and often presents with a sudden onset of sharp pain and shortness of breath.

A pneumothorax that is caused by trauma can result in complications. Trauma to the chest will often damage ribs, muscle tissue, and internal organs. Blood from damaged soft tissues and vessels also can enter the chest cavity. This is referred to as a **hemothorax**.

The most obvious sign of an injured lung in the responsive patient is difficulty breathing. Due to the decrease in available lung capacity, the patient will attempt to compensate by breathing faster. Injuries to the lungs will also result in sharp pain during inhalation or exhalation.

Flail Chest

One of the signs of a serious closed chest injury is a flail chest. A flail chest is most often the result of significant blunt force trauma. A **flail chest** results when two or more ribs are broken in two or more places (Figure 21.5). Depending on the size of the patient, a flail chest may be difficult to discover in the field. If you suspect chest trauma, you must expose the patient's chest and palpate carefully for patches that feel soft and spongy. There may be a sound caused when the bones are rubbing together. This is heard as a grating sound and is called **crepitus**. There will be significant pain on palpation, and you may see the flail segment move in the opposite direction as the rest of the chest as the patient breathes. This opposite movement of the flail segment is known as **paradoxical movement** and may be very difficult to see in the field.

A flail chest can be life threatening for the patient because it can greatly decrease the patient's tidal volume. If you discover what appears to be a flail chest, you must attempt to splint the flail segment using bulky dressings or folded towels. Depending on the

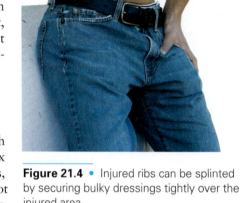

Figure 21.4 • Injured ribs can be splinted by securing bulky dressings tightly over the injured area.

OBJECTIVE

4. Explain the relationship between chest injury and perfusion.

KEY POINT ▼

Injuries to the ribs and muscles between the ribs should not be taken lightly. While these injuries are rarely life threatening, they can lead to hypoxia.

closed chest injury ► an injury to the chest that is not associated with an open wound.

KEY POINT ▼

People between the ages of 20 and 40 who are tall and underweight are at greater risk for a spontaneous pneumothorax.

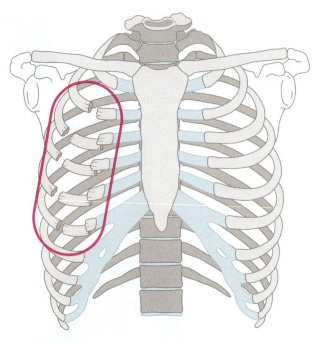

Figure 21.5 • A flail segment results when two or more ribs are fractured in two or more places.

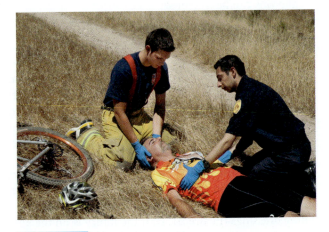

Figure 21.6 • Use both hands to carefully and thoroughly palpate the chest for pain and deformity.

OBJECTIVE

6. Describe the signs and symptoms of a closed chest injury.

pneumothorax ▶ air in the chest cavity.

spontaneous pneumothorax ▶ a sudden collapse of one or more lobes of a lung; not typically associated with trauma.

hemothorax ▶ blood in the chest cavity.

flail chest ▶ a chest injury characterized by two or more ribs that are broken in two or more places.

crepitus ▶ a grating noise or the sensation felt when broken bone ends rub together.

paradoxical movement ▶ the abnormal movement of the chest wall commonly associated with a flail chest.

KEY POINT ▼

When assessing the patient who has suffered blunt force trauma to the chest, you must expose the chest and palpate carefully for signs of a flail segment.

patient's condition, you may have to hold the dressings in place manually or secure them using cravats.

If the patient has suffered a blunt impact to the chest or torso and presents with any of the following signs or symptoms, suspect closed chest injuries:

- Pain on breathing
- Increased difficulty breathing
- Accessory muscle use
- Uneven chest wall movement during breathing
- Signs and symptoms of shock

Assessment of the Patient with a Chest Injury

Your assessment of a chest injury will begin with exposing the chest. You must remove or cut away clothing over any area where there is a complaint of pain. If the patient is unresponsive, you will want to expose the entire chest.

You must observe and palpate for any signs of deformity (Figure 21.6). Use your hands to press firmly across all areas of the chest wall. Be sure to palpate the anterior, lateral, and posterior sides of the chest wall. Note any signs of bruising or discoloration. Pay particular attention to any areas that feel soft or spongy. These could be signs of a flail chest.

The care that an Emergency Medical Responder provides for closed chest injuries is as follows:

1. Perform a primary assessment and ensure the ABCs are intact.
2. Provide positive pressure ventilations, if breathing is inadequate.
3. Administer oxygen, if allowed to do so. (Follow local protocols.)
4. Splint the chest using bulky dressings or towels.
5. Place the patient in a position of comfort, if there is no suspected spine injury.
6. Care for shock.
7. Ensure that advanced medical care is summoned to transport the patient.

"Jacob," Courtney says, removing her stethoscope and jotting something down in her notes, "Nico's blood pressure is 130 over 78."

"Okay Nico, so your pulse is a little high, but your breathing rate and blood pressure are in the normal range. Tell me again about the pain that you said started about 45 minutes ago."

Nico remains still on his right side, guarding his abdomen. "I just thought I was having stomach cramps. My mom suggested mint tea, but the pain just keeps getting worse and I feel like I need to throw up, but I haven't."

Jacob looks toward the hallway, where Courtney was on the phone with Nico's very worried mother. "Well, I'm going to check your abdomen now, all right?" Nico covers his abdomen at the very mention of it, and Jacob adds, "But I'm going to be very careful and I'll stop if it starts to hurt, okay?" Nico seems to consider this for a moment before he moves his hands to his side.

Open Chest Injuries

Injuries that penetrate the chest wall are considered **open chest injuries** and can result in a variety of specific problems that must be identified and properly cared for.

Open Pneumothorax

When the mechanism of injury causes the chest wall to be penetrated, there is great risk for both air and blood to enter the chest cavity (Figure 21.7). Common mechanisms of injury include bullets, knives, and other penetrating objects. It is common for the lung beneath the injury to be punctured, collapse, and allow air to enter the chest cavity. Blood from the damaged tissues also will begin to fill this space. If the hole in the chest wall is large enough, it will allow air to pass through into the chest cavity with each inspiration by the patient. This is referred to as a **sucking chest wound** because air can be heard as it is being sucked through the wound when the patient breathes in. If a sucking chest wound is not identified and promptly cared for, it can result in the development of a **tension pneumothorax**. A tension pneumothorax occurs when air is allowed to build up inside the chest cavity, causing excessive pressure on one side of the chest. If left untreated, this pressure will cause the collapse of the remaining lobes of the lung. In the worst case scenario, the pressure also may increase to the point where it pushes across the chest, putting pressure on the heart and remaining lung. An early sign that pressure may be building up inside the chest is an increasing work of breathing. A late sign of this pressure is a shift in the trachea to the opposite side. This is called *tracheal deviation*. Be sure to assess the trachea by palpating it with your fingers for normal alignment. This should be done for all patients with a chest injury.

OBJECTIVES

6. Describe the signs and symptoms of a closed chest injury.

7. Explain the appropriate assessment of a patient with a chest injury.

open chest injury ▶ an injury to the chest that is associated with an open wound.

IS IT SAFE?

Be sure to wear gloves and eye protection when caring for patients with open chest injuries. It is common for blood to be coughed up or spray out of an open wound.

sucking chest wound ▶ an open chest wound that is characterized by a sucking sound each time the patient inhales.

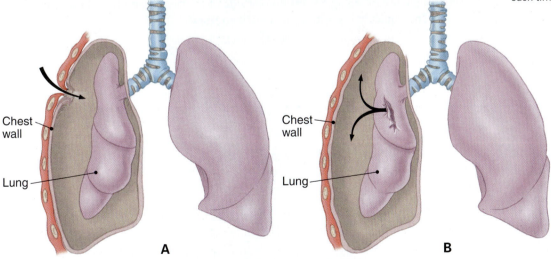

Chest wall

Lung

A

Chest wall

Lung

B

Figure 21.7 • (A) Penetrating chest injuries can allow air and blood to enter the chest cavity. (B) A collapsed lung (spontaneous pneumothorax) can occur without outside trauma.

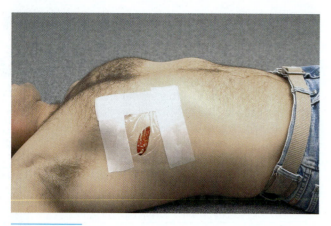

Figure 21.8 • Place an occlusive dressing over an open chest wound and tape in either three or four sides. Follow local protocol.

tension pneumothorax ▶ an abnormal buildup of pressure in the chest cavity.

KEY POINT ▼

Monitor the breathing status of your patient carefully. Any sign of increased work of breathing could mean a developing tension pneumothorax.

occlusive dressing ▶ a dressing that is nonpermeable and will not allow air to pass through.

OBJECTIVE

8. Explain the appropriate care of a patient with a closed chest injury.

Caring for an Open Chest Injury

You must always inspect the torso on all sides for wounds, depending on the mechanism of injury. In the case of gunshot wounds, it is quite common for there to be an exit wound on the opposite side of the body from the entrance wound. Both wounds must be cared for equally.

Open chest wounds should be immediately sealed with something that will prevent air from entering the wound when the patient breathes in. In most instances you will want to immediately cover the wound with your gloved hand. This will be temporary until you can secure a more permanent dressing. Anything such as a glove or plastic bag that does not allow air to pass through can serve as an occlusive dressing. A commercial **occlusive dressing** is the best choice for open chest wounds. It consists of sterile gauze that is saturated with petroleum jelly. The occlusive dressing should extend two or more inches beyond the edges of the wound. It is helpful to place a gauze dressing or piece of plastic over the occlusive dressing because the tape will not stick well to the petroleum jelly.

If blood or perspiration prevents the tape from sticking to the patient's skin, you may have to hold the dressing in place with your hands. You must monitor the patient's breathing status very closely. It is possible that pressure will build up despite the wound being sealed from the outside. If difficulty breathing continues to worsen, release the occlusive dressing momentarily to see of air will escape through the wound.

The following steps should be followed when caring for an open chest wound. If the wound is a sucking chest wound, this method will allow for the release of air trapped in the chest:

1. Take appropriate BSI precautions. Seal the wound with the palm of your gloved hand. Be sure to inspect the patient front and back for exit wounds.

2. Place an occlusive dressing directly over the wound and hold it in place.
   - *Tape three sides:* Have someone seal it by placing tape on three sides (Figure 21.8). This will produce a flutter valve effect. That is, when the patient inhales, the free edge will seal against the skin. When the patient exhales, the free edge will break loose from the skin and allow any buildup of air in the chest cavity to escape.
   - *Tape four sides:* Some EMS systems prefer that all four sides be taped. The last side is taped as the patient exhales. Your instructor will inform you of local protocol.

   With either taping method, the patient must be monitored. If the patient begins to have trouble breathing again, lift up one side of the plastic and have him forcefully exhale. Then quickly reposition the plastic to reseal.

3. Provide high-flow oxygen and care for shock.

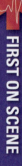

continued

"Ow! Stop!" Nico cries out, instantly knocking Jacob's hands away. "I'm sorry," Nico says through clenched teeth, "that's where it hurts most. It's so sharp, like a jabbing knife."

Jacob notes that the pain is restricted mostly to the lower right quadrant of the abdomen, but the area is free of any trauma, distention, or swelling.

The responding ALS unit enters the room just then and Courtney relays Nico's vitals to the lead medic. "Were

there any other findings besides the abdominal pain?" he asks.

"No," Jacob responds, "There were no remarkable findings from his secondary assessment or medical history. The onset and progression of pain were pretty rapid."

"Nico," the medic says as he positions himself beside the bed. "I'm thinking you may be experiencing appendicitis, which as you know by now is pretty painful. We need to get you to a hospital, and quick!"

Impaled Chest Wounds

Injuries to the chest may result in an object becoming impaled in the chest. Impaled objects must be stabilized as soon as possible to minimize further injury to internal structures.

An impaled object must be left in place. Even though it created the wound, the impaled object also is sealing the wound. If it is removed, the patient may bleed profusely. The object must be stabilized with bulky dressings or pads (Figure 21.9). Begin by placing bulky dressings around the object. You also may cut a hole in a large trauma dressing and slip it over the object. Place several layers to build up support around the object. You may use tape or cravats to hold all dressings and pads in place. You may find it more effective to have someone simply hold the dressings in place with his hands.

Follow these steps when caring for a patient with an impaled object in the chest:

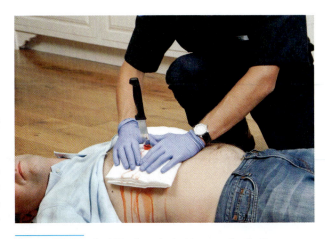

Figure 21.9 • Stabilize impaled objects using bulky dressings.

1. Take appropriate BSI precautions.
2. Perform a primary assessment and ensure the ABCs are intact. Assist ventilations as appropriate.
3. Immediately stabilize the object.
4. Provide high-flow oxygen, if allowed by local protocol.
5. Provide care for shock.
6. Initiate immediate transport.

Abdominal Emergencies

Much like injuries to the chest, the abdominal and pelvic areas are susceptible to the same types of forces and injuries. In addition to injury, abdominal emergencies include a variety of non-traumatic problems as well. A sudden or gradual onset of pain in the abdomen or pelvis can be a symptom of a serious problem. Due to the fact that the abdomen and pelvis contain so many organs, it is often difficult to determine the exact cause of the pain. Abdominal pain without a history of injury, as well as trauma to the abdomen, are all considered serious medical emergencies. This is due to the variety of organs and structures contained within the abdomen and the fact that serious bleeding can go undetected, leading to shock and death.

Anatomy of the Abdomen and Pelvis

The abdominal cavity is separated from the chest cavity by the **diaphragm** muscle at the top and extends down into the pelvis. The abdomen and pelvis contain many organs including the liver, stomach, pancreas, gallbladder, spleen, bladder, and intestines. These organs can be categorized as solid and hollow organs (Table 21.1). Solid organs generally contain a richer

OBJECTIVE

9. Explain the appropriate care of a patient with an open chest injury.

diaphragm ▶ the primary muscle of respiration; divides the chest cavity from the abdominal cavity.

TABLE 21.1	Solid and Hollow Organs	
SOLID ORGANS	**HOLLOW ORGANS**
Liver	Stomach
Spleen	Gallbladder
Kidneys	Urinary bladder
Pancreas	Intestines
	Uterus and fallopian tubes (females)

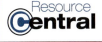

Resource Central

View a 3D animation of the digestive system and complete an interactive review that asks you to label the parts of the digestive system.

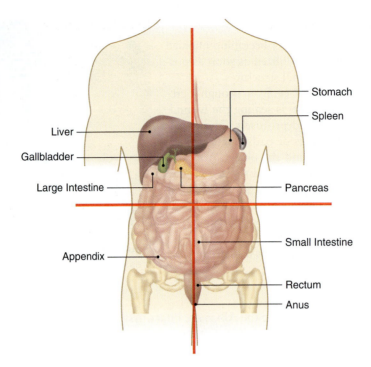

Figure 21.10 • For assessment purposes, the abdomen is divided into four quadrants.

Stomach

Spleen

Liver

Gallbladder

Large Intestine

Pancreas

Small Intestine

Appendix

Rectum

Anus

quadrant ▶ an area of the abdomen; used to identify the location of pain during palpation.

retroperitoneal cavity ▶ the area behind the abdominal cavity that contains the kidneys and ureters.

KEY POINT ▼

There are many potentially life-threatening conditions that are manifested by a sudden or gradual onset of abdominal pain. These patients should be considered unstable and receive immediate care from advanced providers.

blood supply and may result in significant blood loss when damaged. Hollow organs often contain fluids that when allowed to spill out into the abdomen will cause pain.

For assessment purposes, the abdomen is commonly divided up into four **quadrants**, with the navel being at the center of all four quadrants (Figure 21.10). Organs may be contained in one or more quadrants depending on their size.

Similar to the lungs, the internal organs of the abdomen are lined by two thin layers of tissue called the *peritoneum*. It is important to point out that the kidneys are not contained inside the same space as the other abdominal organs. They lie in a space directly behind the peritoneum on either side of the body. This space is called the **retroperitoneal cavity**.

Generalized Abdominal Pain

As mentioned earlier, a sudden or gradual onset of abdominal pain can occur for many reasons and must be cared for as a true emergency. Because there are so many potential causes, it is not important or possible for the Emergency Medical Responder to determine the exact cause. Common causes of acute abdominal pain include:

- Bleeding
- Infection
- Ulcers
- Indigestion
- Constipation
- Food poisoning
- Menstrual cramps
- Diabetic emergencies
- Kidney stones
- Gallstones
- Appendicitis
- Ectopic pregnancy

Signs and Symptoms of Acute Abdominal Pain

Abdominal pain can present suddenly (acute) or slowly over many hours or days. The pain can be described as either sharp or dull, depending on the underlying cause. In most cases the pain can be localized to a specific location or locations within the abdomen. It is best to start out by asking the patient if he is able to point with one finger where it hurts the most. Patients with abdominal pain will often attempt to protect the abdomen by curling up in the fetal position and by holding their hands over the painful area (Figure 21.11). These behaviors are referred to as **guarding**.

Common signs and symptoms of acute abdominal pain include:

- Pain that is either sharp or dull
- Pain on palpation
- Rigid or tight abdomen
- Bloating, or **distention**
- Nausea/vomiting
- Cramping
- Pain that radiates to other areas
- Guarding (protecting the abdomen)

Bleeding within the gastrointestinal system is a common problem for many people and can occur with or without injury or pain. A patient who vomits bright red blood or has bright red blood in his stool likely has an active internal bleed and should be considered unstable. Blood that is old and digested will appear like dark coffee grounds when it is vomited up. Blood that has passed through the intestines and makes its way out in the feces will appear very dark, like tar. It is always appropriate to ask a patient about recent bowel movements and if they appeared normal.

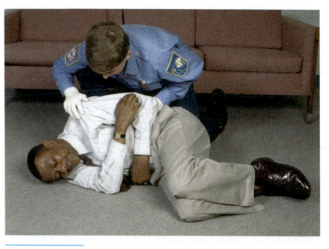

Figure 21.11 • A patient experiencing acute abdominal pain will often lie on his side and guard his abdomen.

Assessing the Patient with Acute Abdominal Pain

Your assessment of the patient with acute abdominal pain must begin by ruling out any history of trauma. Ask the patient if he sustained any blunt force trauma to the upper body within the past few hours or days. Many times the patient forgets about a recent fall or injury and will not associate it with the current complaint. Injuries to the abdomen can cause bleeding that is very slow. Signs and symptoms can be delayed for hours and sometimes days.

Your assessment will center on a thorough medical history. The following are questions you will want to include in your secondary assessment of the patient with acute abdominal pain:

- When did the pain begin?
- Can you point with one finger where the pain is most?
- Did you experience any injury or trauma?
- When did you last eat/drink? What did you eat/drink?
- Are you experiencing nausea or vomiting?
- Does anything make the pain better or worse?
- Is there any chance you could be pregnant?
- When was your last menstrual period?
- Has there been any blood in your vomit or stool?

OBJECTIVES

10. Describe the major structures of the abdominal and pelvic cavities.

11. Describe the signs and symptoms of internal bleeding.

guarding ▶ the protection of an area of injury or pain by the patient.

distention ▶ swelling of the abdomen.

Abdominal Injuries

Injury to the abdomen can produce life-threatening emergencies that must be cared for immediately. Damage to internal organs can cause them to stop functioning normally. In addition to organ failure, bleeding from damage to organs and soft tissues can result in hemorrhagic shock and death if not identified and cared for promptly.

OBJECTIVE

12. Explain the appropriate assessment and care of a patient with abdominal pain.

From the Medical Director

Assessing the Patient

Always assume that abdominal pain is a potentially life-threatening emergency despite the fact that there are many causes. In addition, the patient with abdominal pain should be assessed closely for the presence of shock.

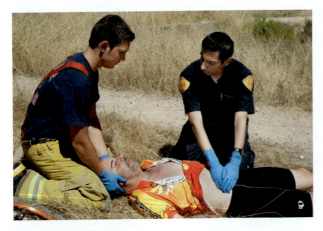

Figure 21.12 • Use both hands to palpate the abdomen one quadrant at a time.

evisceration ▶ an open wound of the abdomen characterized by protrusion of the intestines through the abdominal wall.

OBJECTIVE

13. Explain the appropriate assessment and care of a patient with an open abdominal injury.

As an Emergency Medical Responder, you should be aware of the following signs and symptoms, which may indicate injury to organs of the abdomen and pelvis:

- Deep cut or puncture wound to the abdomen, pelvis, or lower back
- Indications of blunt trauma to the abdomen or pelvis
- Pain or cramps in the abdominal or pelvic region
- Guarding (protecting the abdomen)
- Lying still with legs drawn up
- Rapid, shallow breathing and a rapid pulse
- Rigid, distended, and/or tender abdomen

Injuries to the abdomen and pelvis can be either open or closed. Closed injuries are most often caused by blunt trauma and may have little to no obvious signs of injury. In those cases you will have to rely on the mechanism of injury and maintain a high index of suspicion for internal injuries if the mechanism suggests it. Your most common symptom of a closed injury will be pain over one or more quadrants of the abdomen.

Caring for a Closed Abdominal Injury

Caring for a patient with a closed abdominal injury is simple. You must perform a thorough assessment of the abdomen and palpate all quadrants to determine precisely where the pain is and where it is not (Figure 21.12). Always expose the abdomen to observe for any signs of injury, such as abrasions (seat-belt injury) or bruising. If there is no reason to suspect a spine injury, allow the patient to maintain a position of comfort. This will likely be lying down either on his back with the knees raised or on his side with knees bent.

Open Abdominal Injuries

Open injuries to the abdomen are most often caused by sharp objects such as knives and sharp metal. The abdomen is also susceptible to penetrating injury, such as from a gunshot wound. Regardless of the mechanism, the likelihood of damage to internal organs and severe bleeding is high, so you must always consider these patients as unstable and in need of immediate transport.

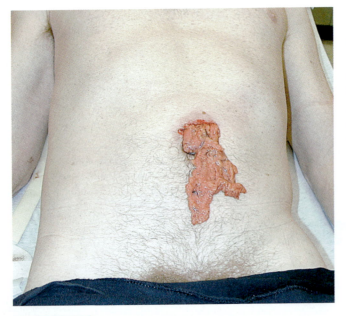

Figure 21.13 • An abdominal evisceration.

Abdominal Evisceration

A common type of open abdominal injury is called an evisceration. An **evisceration** occurs when the abdominal wall is penetrated by a sharp object and the contents of the abdomen are allowed to spill out (Figure 21.13). Never attempt to place spilled abdominal contents back into an open wound. This could cause many complications as well as introduce infection into the wound.

Care for a person with an abdominal evisceration should include the following (Scan 21.1):

1. Expose the wound and any organs that may have spilled out.
2. Position the patient on his back. If no spine injury is suspected, have the patient bend his knees. This will put less tension on the abdominal muscles.
3. Open a large sterile trauma dressing and soak with sterile water or saline.

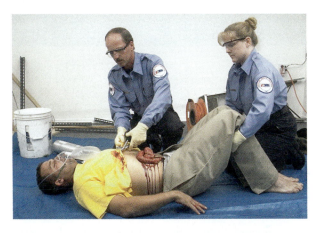

21.1.1 | Cut away clothing to expose the entire injury.

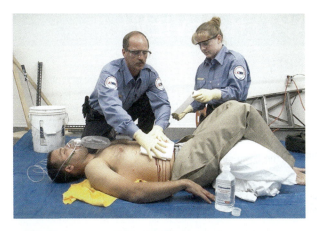

21.1.2 | Place a large sterile dressing moistened with sterile water or saline over the exposed abdominal contents.

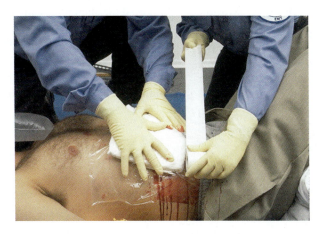

21.1.3 | Place a plastic sheet over the dressing and secure in place.

4. Place the moist dressing over the spilled contents. Do your best to contain as much of the contents under the dressing as possible.

5. Cover the moist dressing with plastic. This will help contain the moisture and keep the exposed tissue from drying out.

6. Provide high-flow oxygen if allowed by local protocols.

7. Care for shock and initiate transport as soon as possible.

WRAP-UP

"I thought for sure he was going to pass out," Courtney says as soon as the doors to the ambulance close.

"I know," Jacob says as he sets the oxygen bottle into its case. "He just about cried out with every lift, bump, or shift of the gurney. It's a shame he wasn't on the ground level of these dorms."

"Well, we did a pretty good job I guess," Courtney says, reviewing her notes. "The medic was able to get Nico in the rig pretty quick by confirming our impression and assessment."

"I have to admit, though," Jacob says, scratching his head. "I think I better review the abdominal cavity again so I know for sure where the organs are for our future calls."

CHAPTER REVIEW

Summary

- Injuries to the chest can affect the ability of the patient to breathe adequately as well as cause damage to internal organs such as the heart and lungs.

- Injuries to the chest can be classified as either open or closed.

- Common types of closed injuries are broken ribs and collapse of a lung (pneumothorax) and blood in the chest cavity (hemothorax).

- Signs and symptoms of closed chest injuries include pain on breathing, difficulty breathing, discoloration, deformity, and paradoxical movement.

- A flail chest is caused when two or more ribs are broken in two or more places. This compromises the integrity of the chest wall and makes it very difficult for the patient to breathe adequately.

- When assessing a patient with a chest injury, be sure to expose all areas and palpate thoroughly with both hands. Consider high-flow oxygen when local protocols indicate.

- Open chest injuries can result in a sucking chest wound and must be covered immediately with an occlusive dressing.

- Stabilize all impaled objects and do your best to secure the object in place. Do not attempt to remove an impaled object.

- The abdomen and pelvis contain many organs that are both hollow and solid. Injuries to those organs can cause organ failure as well as severe internal bleeding.

- Signs and symptoms of an abdominal emergency include pain, rigidity, distention, blood in the vomit, or feces.

- Abdominal injuries can be classified as either closed or open. Closed injuries can result in organ damage and/or severe bleeding.

- An abdominal evisceration is an open wound that has allowed the abdominal contents to spill out. These should be covered with a sterile moist dressing and covered with plastic to minimize the chances that the exposed organs will dry out.

- Impaled objects should be stabilized in place and secured for transport. Do not attempt to remove an impaled object.

Take Action

HIDE AND SEEK

The cornerstone to a good assessment of the patient with chest or abdominal pain is the physical exam. You must be as thorough as possible and palpate all areas. This activity will help you become better at performing a physical assessment of the chest and or abdomen.

To begin you will need a fellow student or willing family member to serve as patient. Next, take several objects such as a large paperclip, large coins, erasers, or similar objects. The person who will play patient must go into another room and carefully tape several items to different areas around his torso or abdomen.

When he is done, he must return and lie down on the floor. Begin by having him lie supine. Now perform your usual assessment of both the chest and abdomen, attempting to locate all the items.

To make this a bit more challenging you can tape different-size coins to the volunteer's body. Of course the smaller the coin the more difficult it will be to palpate beneath the clothing.

First on Scene Run Review

Recall the events of the "First on Scene" scenario in this chapter and answer the following questions, which are related to the call. Rationales are offered in the Answer Key at the back of the book.

1. What medical history would you want to get from Nico?

2. As an Emergency Medical Responder, how would you treat this person?

3. What information would you like to get from his mother, and what information would you give to his mother?

Quick Quiz

To check your understanding of the chapter, answer the following questions. Then compare your answers to those in the Answer Key at the back of the book.

1. You are caring for a patient who was struck in the lateral chest by a blunt object. You palpate a flail segment on the right lateral chest area. This type of injury is most likely to affect the:
   a. patient's ability to breathe normally.
   b. heart and lungs.
   c. patient's pulse rate.
   d. patient's ability to cough.

2. In the case of an open chest wound, place an occlusive dressing over the open wound and then:
   a. cover it loosely with a cloth bandage.
   b. tape it on three or four sides.
   c. hold it in place with a gloved hand.
   d. pack the opening with clean gauze.

3. A 29-year-old male has been stabbed once in the posterior chest. How would you describe this injury when completing your documentation?
   a. Evisceration
   b. Closed chest injury
   c. Open chest injury
   d. Flail chest

4. You are caring for a patient who was shot in the right lower chest. Which one of the following signs would indicate this patient is developing a tension pneumothorax?
   a. Unequal chest rise
   b. Tracheal deviation
   c. Rapid breathing
   d. Rapid pulse

5. The purpose of placing an occlusive dressing over an open chest wound is to:
   a. control the bleeding.
   b. keep chest contents from spilling out.
   c. keep air from entering the chest cavity.
   d. make it easier for the patient to breathe.

6. You are caring for a patient with an open chest wound and have covered the wound with an occlusive dressing. The patient becomes increasingly short of breath. You should:
   a. add another dressing to the wound.
   b. release the dressing to allow air to escape.
   c. apply more pressure to the wound.
   d. remove the dressing altogether.

7. You are caring for a patient who appears to have only injured a rib or two. There is no flail segment and the patient is alert and oriented. What is the most likely potential complication from a simple rib injury?
   a. Hypoxia from shallow respirations
   b. Puncture of the heart or lung
   c. Internal bleeding
   d. Pneumothorax

8. Which one of the following is the most appropriate care for an open abdominal injury?
   a. Pack the inside of the wound with clean dressings.
   b. Pour sterile saline over the wound.
   c. Cover the wound with a dry, clean dressing.
   d. Cover the wound with moist, sterile dressing.

9. You are caring for a patient with abdominal pain for the past two days. She states that she had a bowel movement this morning that was very dark and tarry. Those signs and symptoms are consistent with:
   a. internal bleeding that is old.
   b. internal bleeding that is fresh.
   c. appendicitis.
   d. an evisceration.

10. A patient has been shot in the right upper quadrant of the abdomen. You should assume which one of the following organs may have been injured?
    a. Stomach
    b. Liver
    c. Spleen
    d. Pancreas

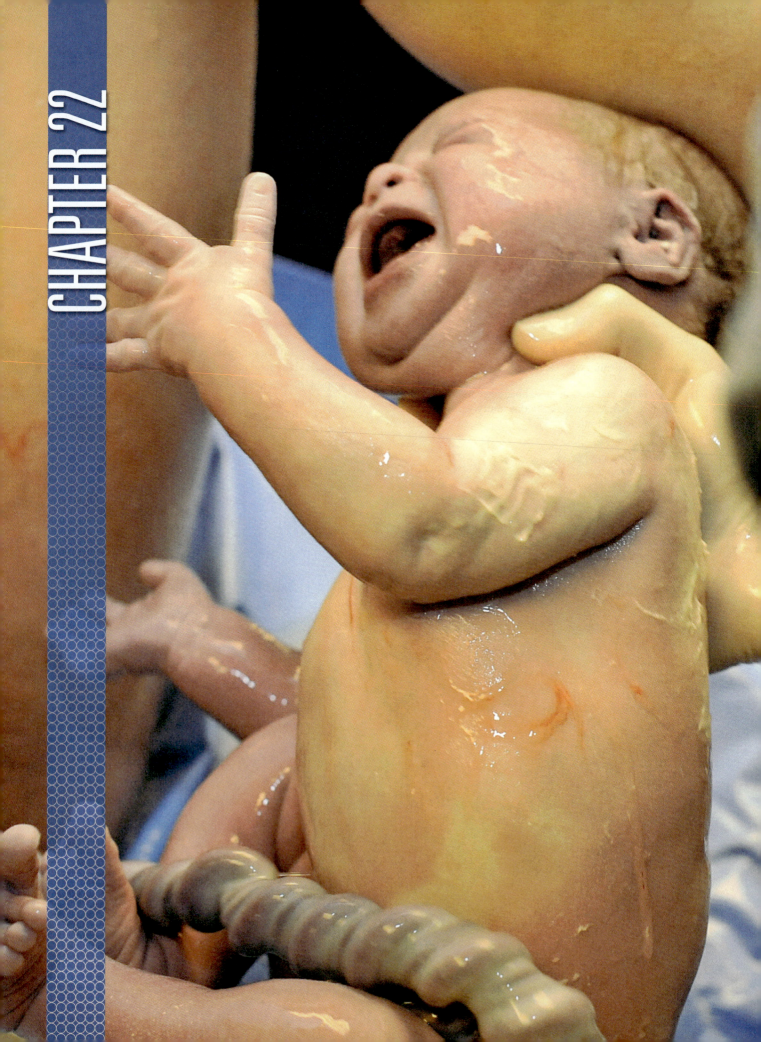

Care During Pregnancy and Childbirth

Care During Pregnancy and Childbirth

- Medicine—Gynecology
- Special Patient Populations—Obstetrics

EDUCATION STANDARDS

COMPETENCIES
- Recognizes and manages life threats based on assessment findings of a patient with a medical emergency while awaiting additional emergency response.

CHAPTER OVERVIEW
Most expectant mothers know that they need to care for themselves and their unborn infants during pregnancy. They usually do not have to call for emergency services to assist with a delivery. Sometimes, though, a situation can cause a birth to occur unexpectedly or with complications. A trauma to the mother, for example, could affect the fetus. Because EMS might be called for those situations, this chapter introduces you to the terminology and processes involved with a normal pregnancy and childbirth. It also introduces some of the more common complications related to pregnancy and childbirth and how to care for the mother and baby during and after delivery.

OBJECTIVES

Upon successful completion of this chapter, the student should be able to:

COGNITIVE

1. Define the following terms:
   a. amniotic fluid *(p. 482)*
   b. amniotic sac *(p. 482)*
   c. birth canal *(p. 482)*
   d. bloody show *(p. 481)*
   e. breech birth *(p. 498)*
   f. cervix *(p. 481)*
   g. crowning *(p. 482)*
   h. eclampsia *(p. 501)*
   i. ectopic pregnancy *(p. 497)*
   j. fallopian tube *(p. 497)*
   k. fontanel *(p. 489)*
   l. full term *(p. 481)*
   m. imminent delivery *(p. 482)*
   n. labor *(p. 481)*
   o. meconium *(p. 498)*
   p. miscarriage *(p. 496)*
   q. newborn *(p. 491)*
   r. nuchal cord *(p. 490)*
   s. ovary *(p. 497)*
   t. ovum *(p. 481)*
   u. placenta *(p. 482)*
   v. placenta previa *(p. 502)*
   w. preeclampsia *(p. 501)*
   x. prenatal care *(p. 484)*
   y. prolapsed cord *(p. 499)*
   z. spotting *(p. 496)*
   aa. supine hypotensive syndrome *(p. 501)*
   bb. trimester *(p. 481)*
   cc. umbilical cord *(p. 482)*
   dd. uterus *(p. 481)*
   ee. vagina *(p. 481)*

2. Describe the function of the following anatomy related to childbirth: amniotic sac, birth canal, cervix, placenta, umbilical cord, and uterus. *(p. 481)*

3. Describe the three stages of labor and when each begins and ends. *(p. 482)*

4. Describe the signs of an imminent delivery. *(p. 485)*

5. Explain the steps for preparing for a field delivery. *(p. 485)*

6. Explain the steps for assisting with a field delivery. *(p. 486)*

7. Explain the purpose of each of the items in a typical field obstetrics (OB) kit. *(p. 484)*

8. Explain the priorities of care for the newborn following a field delivery. *(p. 490)*

9. Explain the priorities of care for the mother following a field delivery. *(p. 494)*

10. Explain the common causes of vaginal bleeding during the first trimester. *(p. 496)*

11. Explain the common causes of vaginal bleeding during the third trimester. *(p. 496)*

12. Explain the appropriate care for a pregnant patient with vaginal bleeding. *(p. 496)*

13. Describe the signs and symptoms of supine hypotensive syndrome. *(p. 501)*

14. Explain the appropriate care for a patient with signs and symptoms of supine hypotensive syndrome. *(p. 501)*

15. Describe the signs and symptoms of preeclampsia. *(p. 501)*

16. Explain the appropriate care for a patient with signs and symptoms of preeclampsia. *(p. 501)*

17. Explain the common complications related to a field delivery and how to properly care for each. *(p. 497)*

PSYCHOMOTOR

18. Demonstrate the ability to identify the signs of an imminent delivery.

19. Demonstrate the steps for preparing for and assisting with a field delivery.

20. Demonstrate the proper care of the infant following a field delivery.

21. Demonstrate the proper care of the mother following a field delivery.

22. Demonstrate the ability to identify a complicated delivery.

23. Demonstrate the proper assessment and care for a complicated field delivery.

AFFECTIVE

24. Value the importance of proper body substance isolation (BSI) precautions when assisting with a field delivery.

FIRST ON SCENE

The first thing that Lucas sees other than the blinding white of the snow swirling across the hood of his truck is the red and blue flashing lights of a state trooper's car. The heavily bundled officer has blocked both lanes with his patrol car and is waving traffic toward the snow-packed off ramp. Lucas rolls his window down and a wave of cold air instantly fills the cab, numbing his face and arms. "What's going on?" he shouts above the howling afternoon wind.

"Interstate's closed!" the trooper shouts back, his voice blurred by the mask that he wears. "Pull off here and find a place to park."

Lucas sits for a moment, trying to quickly calculate another route to Denver, and then sighs, rolls the window up, and follows the officer's order.

The end of the off ramp opens up into the parking lot of a small, crowded travel stop. As he creeps up and down each aisle of the lot, looking for a space where his pickup will fit in the field of car-shaped snow mounds, he begins to regret not flying to the MERT conference.

He is just backing into a slim opening between an overflowing garbage dumpster and an idling semi when he hears a man yelling for help. The man is sparsely dressed for the extreme weather and running up and down between vehicles, shouting for help and knocking on snow-blinded windows.

"My wife!" the man shouts in a heavy foreign accent, his breath exploding out in thick white clouds. "I think she's having her baby! Somebody please help!"

KEY POINT ▼

In a normal delivery, mothers do the majority of the work. Emergency Medical Responders assist. Your role will be to assist the mother as she delivers her child and to identify and care for complications that may occur.

Understanding Childbirth

You may have noticed that this chapter's title refers to "childbirth" and not "emergency childbirth." As a culture, many people consider a birth that occurs away from a hospital delivery room as an emergency. That is just not true. In many parts of the world, babies are born away from medical facilities each and every day. The anatomy of the female, the unborn child, and the structures formed during pregnancy enable the birth process to occur with few problems.

Sometimes complications do occur. At the scene of a birth away from a medical facility, an Emergency Medical Responder can be the key factor in a baby's survival if something should go wrong. The mother may need his or her skills during the birth process to

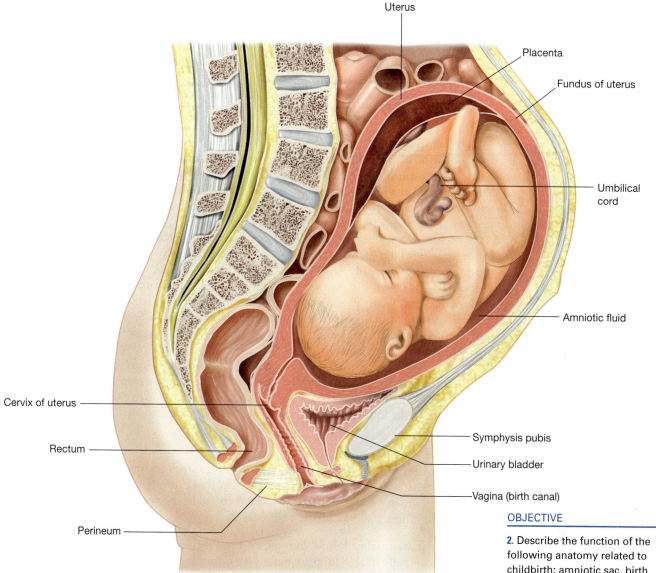

Uterus

Placenta

Fundus of uterus

Umbilical cord

Amniotic fluid

Cervix of uterus

Rectum

Symphysis pubis

Urinary bladder

Vagina (birth canal)

Perineum

Figure 22.1 • Anatomy of pregnancy.

ensure safe delivery if there are complications. The care provided after delivery is just as important. The first hour of life after birth can be a difficult time for some babies and mothers. Your assistance can make a difference.

Anatomy of Pregnancy

An unborn baby is called a *fetus* as it develops and grows inside of the mother. The fetus begins as an unfertilized egg, called an **ovum**. The fetus develops inside a muscular organ called the womb, or **uterus** (Figure 22.1). The average period of development is between 38 to 40 weeks, or approximately nine months. A baby that reaches the 38th week of development prior to delivery is referred to as **full term**. The gestational period is divided into three-month segments called **trimesters**.

Labor is the process the body goes through to deliver a fetus. During labor, the muscles of the uterus contract and push the baby down through the opening of the uterus, which is called the **cervix**. As the cervix expands to allow the head of the fetus through, the mother may notice a slight staining of blood or blood-tinged mucus. This is called **bloody show** and is normal. The fetus passes through the cervix and enters the birth canal, or **vagina**, through which it moves to the outside world to be born.

OBJECTIVE

2. Describe the function of the following anatomy related to childbirth: amniotic sac, birth canal, cervix, placenta, umbilical cord, and uterus.

ovum ▶ the unfertilized egg produced by the mother.

uterus ▶ the muscular structure that holds the baby during pregnancy.

full term ▶ a pregnancy that has achieved a complete gestation of between 38 and 40 weeks.

trimester ▶ three months of pregnancy.

labor ▶ the process the body goes through to deliver a baby.

cervix ▶ the opening of the uterus.

bloody show ▶ the normal discharge of blood prior to delivery.

vagina ▶ the birth canal.

crowning ▶ the bulging out of the vagina caused by the baby's head during delivery.

imminent delivery ▶ a delivery that is likely to occur within the next few minutes.

amniotic sac ▶ the fluid-filled sac that surrounds the developing fetus.

amniotic fluid ▶ the fluid surrounding the baby contained within the amniotic sac.

birth canal ▶ the interior aspect of the vagina.

placenta ▶ the organ of pregnancy that serves as the filter between the mother and developing fetus.

umbilical cord ▶ the structure that connects the baby to the placenta.

OBJECTIVE

3. Describe the three stages of labor and when each begins and ends.

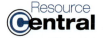
Protect Yourself

While childbirth is a beautiful event, it is often messy. Appropriate BSI includes gloves, gown, mask, and eye protection. When the membrane ruptures, amniotic fluid can easily shower you. In addition, it is not uncommon for the woman to unexpectedly urinate and defecate.

During your assessment of the mother, you must examine her for crowning. **Crowning** is the showing of the baby's head at the opening of the vagina. However, any part of the baby may present first, including the buttocks or feet. Once the baby passes into the birth canal, more of the head (or other presenting part) will show, or appear to grow larger, with each contraction. This means that delivery is *imminent*. An **imminent delivery** is a delivery that is likely to occur within a few minutes.

The fetus grows inside a special sac called the **amniotic sac**. It is filled with fluid, called (**amniotic fluid**), which surrounds and protects the baby. Although the sac may have ruptured earlier, it usually breaks during labor, and the fluid, or water, flows out of the vagina. This is called the *rupture of membranes* and is an important milestone in the birthing process. When you are assessing the mother, you will ask her if her "water has broken." She will usually know and be able to tell you if it has or not. Sometimes the sac will break very early in the labor process. Sometimes it will break much later. The fluids help lubricate the **birth canal** for the passage of the baby.

During pregnancy, a special organ called the **placenta** develops in the womb. Oxygen and nourishment from the mother's blood pass through the placenta and enter fetal circulation through the **umbilical cord**. Fetal wastes pass back through the umbilical cord and the placenta to the mother's circulation to be eliminated.

Stages of Labor

On average, the process of labor lasts about 16 hours for the first-time mother. In some cases, labor may take longer, or it can be much shorter. The time can vary with each patient and with each delivery. It is quite common for the labor process to be shorter with each successive birth.

There are three stages of labor (Figure 22.2):

- The first stage of labor begins with the onset of regular contractions and ends when the cervix is fully dilated (approximately 10 centimeters) allowing the baby to enter the birth canal.
- The second stage of labor begins when the baby enters the birth canal and ends when he is born.
- The third stage of labor begins when the baby is born. It ends when the placenta, commonly referred to as the *afterbirth*, is delivered.

It is normal to have vaginal discharges throughout labor. During the first stage of labor, the first type of discharge to appear should be a watery, bloody mucus. Later, the discharge will appear as a watery, bloody fluid. This is normal and not the same as bleeding. If there is bleeding from the vagina prior to delivery, rather than the normal blood-tinged fluids, then something may be wrong. This could be a serious problem that requires assistance from a higher level of EMS provider. Arrange transport for the mother as soon as possible.

Contractions of the uterus cause labor pains, and they occur in cycles of contraction and relaxation. At first, contractions are mild and spaced far apart. However, as the fetus is pushed into the birth canal and the time of birth gets closer, the time between contractions becomes shorter. The first contractions are about 30 minutes apart and become closer and closer until they are three minutes or less apart. Pain during labor is normal and usually starts as an ache in the lower back. Then, as labor progresses, the pain is felt in the lower abdomen. As the muscles of the uterus contract, the pain begins. When the muscles relax, the pain is usually relieved. Labor pains normally come at regular intervals and last for about 30 seconds to one minute. It is not unusual for the pains to start, stop for a period of time, and then start again.

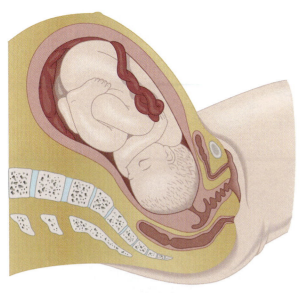

FIRST STAGE:
First uterine contraction to dilation of cervix

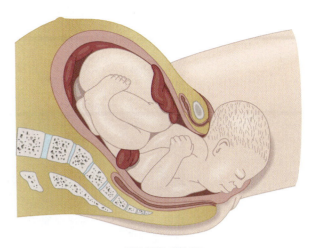

SECOND STAGE:
Birth of baby or expulsion

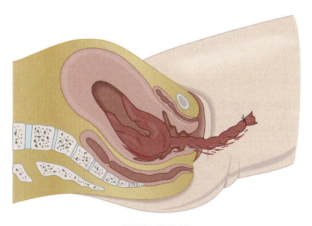

THIRD STAGE:
Delivery of placenta

Figure 22.2 • Stages of labor.

Emergency Medical Responders can time labor pains in two ways (Figure 22.3):

- *Contraction time.* The span of time from the beginning of a contraction until it relaxes is called the contraction time.
- *Interval time.* This is the span of time from the start of one contraction to the beginning of the next contraction. As labor progresses, the interval time will become shorter. This is the time that is referred to when discussing the frequency of contractions.

Throughout pregnancy the mother might experience light, painless, irregular contractions, which may increase gradually in intensity and frequency during the third trimester. This is known as *false labor,* also referred to as *Braxton Hicks contractions.* False labor pains are not as regular and rhythmic as true labor contractions.

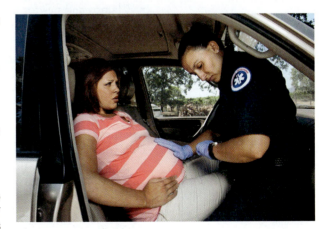

Figure 22.3 • Measure the contraction intervals by counting the beginning of one contraction to the beginning of the next contraction.

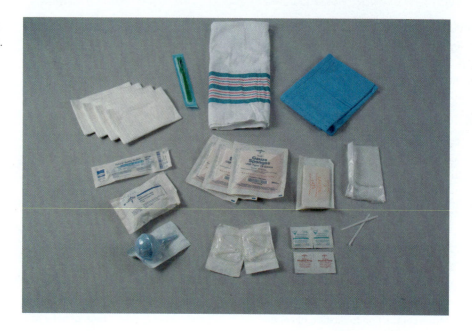

Figure 22.4 • Contents of a commercial obstetric (OB) kit. All items are disposable.

It may be difficult for you and the mother to distinguish false labor pains from true labor. Any pregnant woman who is having contractions should be evaluated by her doctor.

Remember that your primary role is to help the mother deliver the baby when birth is imminent. You will need to make sure that you have the necessary supplies and materials to do this.

Supplies and Materials

OBJECTIVE

7. Explain the purpose of each of the items in a typical field obstetrics (OB) kit.

The items you will need for preparing the mother for delivery and initial care are provided in a commercial *obstetric (OB) kit* (Figure 22.4). If your response unit does not carry a commercial OB kit, assemble and store the required items in a special kit and keep it on your unit. Some of these items may be available at the patient's home, but during delivery is not the time to find supplies. The items that you will need include the following:

- Personal protective equipment such as protective gloves, face masks, eye shields, and gowns
- Towels, sheets, and blankets for draping the mother, for placement under the mother, and for drying and wrapping the baby
- Gauze pads for wiping mucus from the baby's mouth and nose
- Rubber bulb syringe
- Clamps and ties for use on the umbilical cord before cutting
- Sterile scissors or a single-edged razor for cutting the cord
- Sanitary pads or bulky dressings for vaginal bleeding
- A basin and plastic bags for collecting and transporting the placenta
- Red, plastic biohazard bags for storing and disposing soiled linens and dressings

Your primary and secondary assessments will help you determine if the mother is ready to deliver. If birth appears likely before EMTs can transport her to the hospital, follow these steps: Place supplies so they are within your reach during the delivery process. Don your personal protective equipment. Then prepare the mother for delivery. It may be helpful to ask the mother if she has been receiving **prenatal care**. This is the regular care and monitoring of the fetus by a physician or other caregiver throughout the pregnancy.

prenatal care ▶ the routine medical care provided to a mother during her pregnancy.

Delivery

The delivery of a baby is one of the most exciting calls for any EMS provider. Knowing what to expect and being properly prepared will go a long way for making this a successful event.

Preparing for Delivery

Due to the nature of childbirth, it is important for you to wear appropriate face and eye protection and a gown, in addition to protective gloves, to minimize exposure to the mother's body fluids during delivery. Make sure that EMS has been activated. Let the mother know that you have called for additional assistance and that you will stay with her to help if she starts to deliver the baby. Provide emotional support throughout the entire process of birth. Talk with the mother to help her remain calm.

If the expectant mother complains that she feels as if she needs to go to the bathroom, tell her that this is normal and that it is caused by pressure on her bladder and rectum. Encourage her to remain lying down. Explain that her body is reacting normally to all the changes taking place. It is important that you keep her calm and begin assessing her status as soon as possible. Place clean sheets or towels under her buttocks. If she does have a bowel movement or urinates, tell her that this is normal. Remove soiled linens and replace them with fresh ones.

Begin to evaluate the mother by asking for the following information (Figure 22.5):

- Her name, age, and expected due date
- If she has been seeing a doctor during her pregnancy. If so, ask for the contact phone number
- If this is her first delivery, labor will typically last about 16 hours. Labor time is usually shorter for subsequent deliveries.
- If she has any known complications, particularly a multiple birth
- If she has discharged any watery or bloody mucus
- How long she has been having labor pains
- How frequent her contractions are
- If her water has broken, when, and what color (clear, which is normal; or cloudy or green, which indicates a stressed fetus and requires immediate transport)
- If she feels strain in her pelvis or lower abdomen, if she feels as if she needs to move her bowels, and if she can feel the baby beginning to move into her vaginal opening
- If she has any significant medical information such as a history of seizures, diabetes, or vaginal bleeding during the pregnancy

If the mother says she feels the baby trying to be born or that she has the urge to bear down, birth may be imminent. If the mother is having contractions two minutes apart or less, delivery is imminent. Should she also be straining, crying out, and complaining about having to go to the bathroom, prepare to deliver very shortly. Even a first-time mother will have some understanding of what is going on. When she says she feels the baby coming, believe her.

Find out if she has taken a childbirth preparation class or natural childbirth classes. In those classes, the expectant mother works with someone she chooses to be her coach. Use her coach if this person is present or tell her that you will work with her to help her follow

OBJECTIVE

5. Explain the steps for preparing for a field delivery.

IS IT SAFE?

The delivery of an infant in the field setting presents a significant risk of exposure to blood and other potentially infectious materials to the Emergency Medical Responder. This is one of the rare occasions when you would actually take full BSI precautions, including gloves, face mask, and gown.

IS IT SAFE?

It is important to understand that when the baby enters the birth canal, he is causing downward pressure on the rectum. This pressure will feel to the mother as if she needs to have a bowel movement. She may insist on using the bathroom during the delivery process. Be prepared for this, and never allow a mother in active labor to use the restroom.

OBJECTIVE

4. Describe the signs of an imminent delivery.

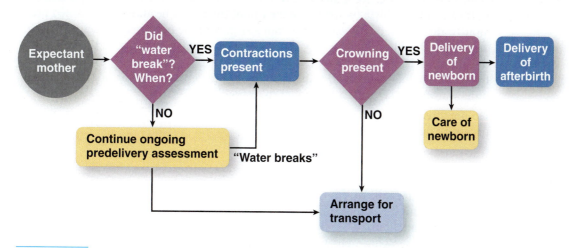

Figure 22.5 • Algorithm for assisting a mother in a normal delivery.

the procedures she learned in her class with her coach or partner. Although you must follow standard EMS system practices for assisting with the delivery and for providing care afterward, you or her coach can help the mother with breathing exercises as she was taught in her classes. In addition, you or her coach also can offer the encouragement and support she will need throughout labor. You or her coach can make suggestions on how she can breathe and when to push or relax. Following are a few simple coaching steps: During delivery as each contraction begins, have the mother take a deep breath and encourage her to gently bear down, or push. She can push with several breaths during each contraction. The mother should rest until the next contraction. As the baby's head emerges, ask the mother to stop pushing and to start panting so that the baby's head can slide slowly out of the birth canal.

After evaluating and examining the mother and finding that birth may occur shortly, immediately prepare her for delivery:

1. Take BSI precautions. Put on your personal protective equipment (gloves, mask with eye shield, gown), if you have not already done so.

2. Control the scene so that the mother will have privacy. Ask unneeded bystanders to leave. You may have to carry her a short distance to a more private place. Do not allow the mother to walk. If she appears to be in early labor and this is her first child, her labor pains typically will have long contraction and interval times.

3. Position the mother on her back with her knees bent, feet flat, and legs spread wide apart. If this position causes her to feel dizzy and faint, it is because the weight of the baby is pressing on the inferior vena cava, the vessel that returns blood from the lower part of the body to the heart, and restricting blood flow back to the heart. If the mother feels dizzy and faint, position her slightly on her left side with one knee bent and foot flat, the other leg extended, and her legs spread wide apart. Place pillows or blankets under her right side to support the pelvis in the raised position.

4. Feel the abdomen for contractions when the patient says she is having labor pains. Explain what you are going to do and place the palm of your hand on her abdomen above the navel. It is not necessary to remove any of the patient's clothing to feel for contractions. If the mother says that she can feel the baby coming, skip this step. Feel for and time several contractions to help determine if birth is near. As birth nears, the interval time will decrease, and you will feel the uterus and the abdomen become more rigid. If the interval time between contractions is three minutes or less, consider that birth may be imminent.

5. Prepare the mother for examination. Tell her that you need to see if her baby has entered the birth canal. Help her remove clothing or underclothing that obstructs your exam of her vaginal opening. Use clean sheets or towels to cover the mother. If you have a commercial obstetrical (OB) kit, use the materials provided. Make sure you have enough light to see what you are doing.

6. Check for crowning. See if any part of the baby is visible at the vaginal opening. In a normal head-first birth, you will see the top of the baby's head. As you learned previously, this is called *crowning*, although any part of the baby may present first. The area of the head that you see on your first inspection may be less than the size of a dollar coin. The mother is now in the second stage of labor because the baby is in the birth canal. Do not try to transport the mother yourself in your first response unit. Wait for EMT or ALS personnel to respond.

7. Do not attempt any type of internal or vaginal exam. Touch the vaginal area only as necessary during the delivery process.

Normal Delivery

During the delivery, talk to the mother. Ask her to relax between contractions. If her water breaks, remind her that this is normal. Consider the delivery to be normal if the baby's head appears first.

Perform the following steps when assisting the mother in a normal delivery (Figure 22.6 and Scan 22.1):

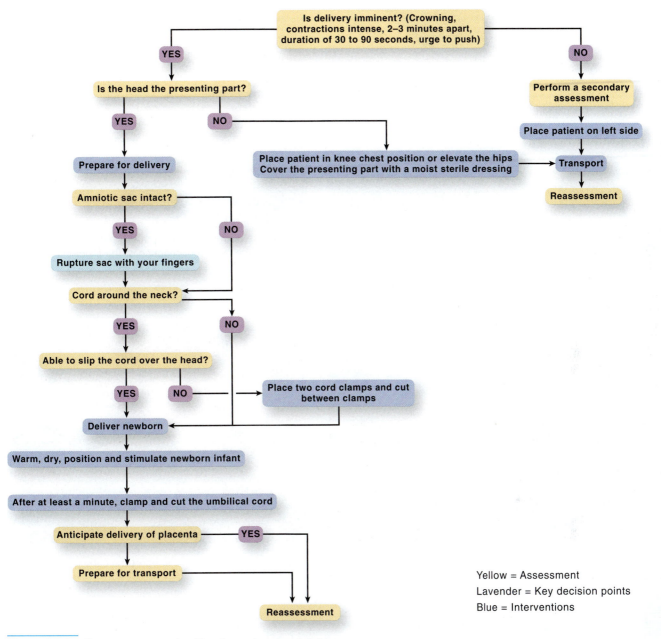

Figure 22.6 • Emergency care algorithm for an imminent delivery.

Yellow = Assessment
Lavender = Key decision points
Blue = Interventions

continued

"Hey! Buddy!" Lucas pushes his door open, scraping it on the dumpster next to him. "Where is she?"

The man, drawn by a response to his cries for help, begins running toward Lucas, shaking his clasped hands in front of him as if begging. "She is in my car." The man breathes heavily. Sparkling strands of ice hang from his mustache and beard. "Please help her. I do not know what to do."

"Well, for starters, we've got to get her inside," Lucas says as he pulls on his heavy jacket and wool gloves. "Take me to your car." The man quickly shakes Lucas's hand with

both of his, turns, and jogs back through the cars, continually looking back over his shoulder to make sure that Lucas is following.

Like many of the other vehicles in the lot, the man's car looks like a snow sculpture. The rising exhaust smoke and the dull red glow of the buried taillights are the only clues that there is actually a vehicle there. The man knocks a clump of white powder from the handle and pulls the door open wide, exposing the warm interior of the car and his very pregnant, very terrified wife.

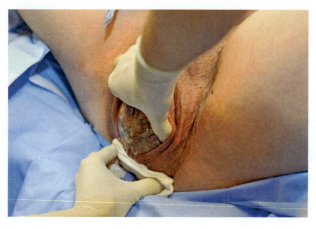

22.1.1 | Crowning is evident as the head emerges from the vagina.

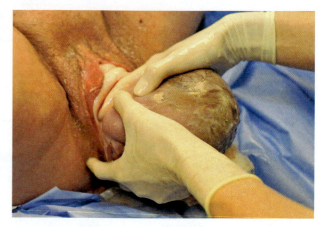

22.1.2 | Use both hands to support the head as it delivers and check the neck for presence of the umbilical (nuchal) cord.

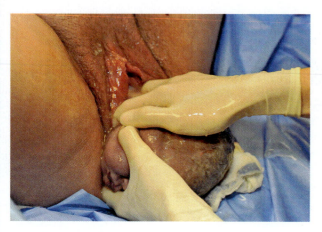

22.1.3 | Guide the baby's head downward to facilitate delivery of the top shoulder.

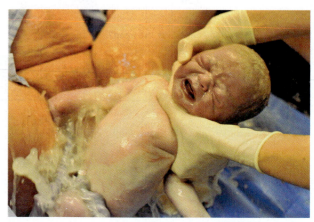

22.1.4 | Use both hands to support the baby following delivery.

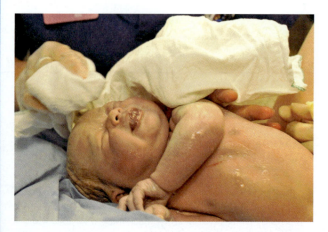

22.1.5 | Carefully dry the baby and cover him to conserve heat.

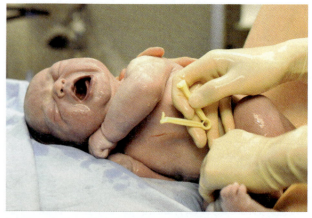

22.1.6 | Once the cord has stopped pulsating, clamp it in preparation for cutting.

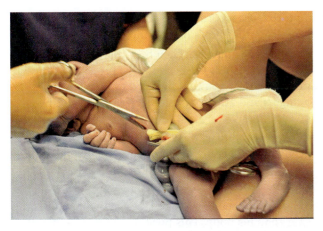

22.1.7 | Cut the cord between the clamps.

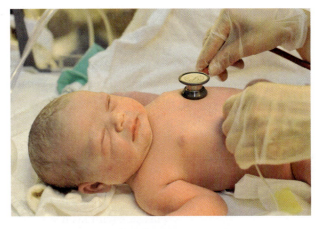

22.1.8 | Assess breathing and pulse rate for the newborn.

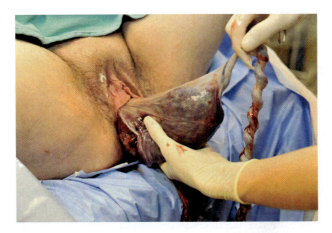

22.1.9 | Expect delivery of the placenta within 20 to 30 minutes following the delivery of the baby.

1. Wash your hands with soap and water, or use a commercial hand wash. Don personal protective equipment (gloves, mask with eye shield, gown), if you have not already done so.

2. Drape the mother and place her on top of clean sheets or towels. Place a folded blanket, towels, or sheets under her buttocks to lift her pelvis about two inches. You may place a pillow under her head and shoulders for comfort.

3. Place someone near the mother's head or use the mother's coach to reassure and offer her encouragement and to turn her head in case she vomits. If no one is on hand to help, talk with the patient during the delivery process and be alert for vomiting.

4. Place one hand below the baby's head as he delivers. Spread your fingers evenly around the head to support the baby but avoid pressing the soft areas known as **fontanels**, at the top of the baby's skull. They are areas where the skull bones have not completely closed together. Apply a slight pressure on the baby's head as it emerges to control the delivery speed. Sometimes the head can "pop out" too quickly from the birth canal, which can badly tear the skin at the vaginal opening. (Some stretching and tearing is normal.) Use your other hand to help cradle the baby's head. Do not pull on the baby.

   As the baby's head emerges, you may notice that it has caused the skin area between the vaginal and rectal openings (called the *perineum*) to tear. This is normal and will be treated at the hospital. After the delivery, place a sanitary pad at the vaginal opening, which will help control bleeding from torn tissues. Replace sanitary pads as needed.

KEY POINT ▼

Newborn babies are very slippery. Make certain you have a good but gentle grip on the baby and provide proper support throughout the delivery process.

fontanel ▶ an area on the infant's skull where the bones have not yet fused together, leaving a soft spot.

5. If the amniotic sac has not yet ruptured, use a cord clamp or your gloved fingers to tear the membrane and pull it away from the baby's mouth and nose.
6. Most babies are born facedown as the head emerges. Then they rotate to the right or left. Once the head is delivered, you must inspect the neck for the presence of the umbilical cord. This is called a **nuchal cord.** If you find the cord to be wrapped around the baby's neck, use two fingers and attempt to slip it over the baby's head or shoulders.

nuchal cord ▶ a condition where the umbilical cord is around the baby's neck during delivery.

7. The upper shoulder usually delivers next, followed quickly by the lower shoulder. Continue to support the baby throughout the entire birth process. Gently guide the baby's head downward, which will assist the mother in delivering the baby's upper shoulder. Scan 22.1 illustrates hand placement during delivery.
8. Once the baby's feet deliver (the end of the second stage of labor), lay the baby on his side with his head slightly lower than his body. This position will enable blood, other fluids, and mucus to drain from the mouth and nose. Wipe the baby's mouth and nose with gauze pads.
9. Note the exact time of birth. In many systems, the normal procedure is to notify dispatch or medical direction, where time of birth is recorded.
10. Keep the baby at the level of the vagina until the cord is cut.
11. Wait at least one minute following delivery and clamp or tie the umbilical cord. The first clamp should be placed approximately six inches from the baby's abdomen. The second clamp should be placed approximately two to three inches away from the first (further from the baby). Then cut the cord between the clamps. If you do not have sterile equipment, do not cut the cord. Simply clamp it. Some jurisdictions may not allow Emergency Medical Responders to cut the cord. Follow local protocol.
12. Monitor and record the baby's and mother's vital signs. Support the ABCs as necessary.
13. Watch for more contractions, which may signal the delivery of the placenta. It is important to save the placenta for examination. If any part of it remains attached inside the uterus, it can cause bleeding and an infection. Place the placenta in a plastic biohazard bag, and give it to EMT or ALS personnel to transport to the hospital.
14. Place a sanitary pad over the mother's vaginal opening. Lower her legs, and place them together. Label the bag with the mother's name.

Caring for the Baby

OBJECTIVE

8. Explain the priorities of care for the newborn following a field delivery.

As you assist the mother with the delivery of her baby (Figure 22.7):

1. Clear the baby's airway. Position the baby on his side with head slightly lower than his body to allow for drainage. Keep the baby's body at the level of the vagina until the cord is clamped. Use a sterile gauze pad or a clean handkerchief to clear mucus

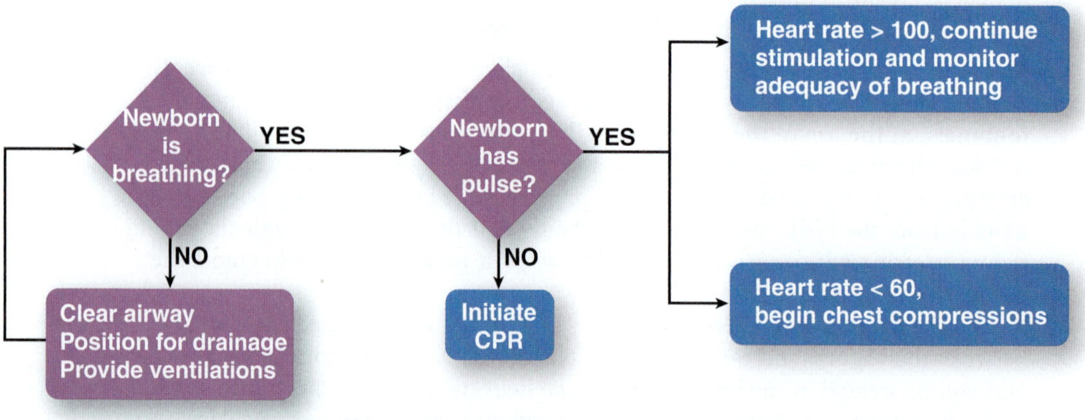

Figure 22.7 • Algorithm for assessment of the newborn.

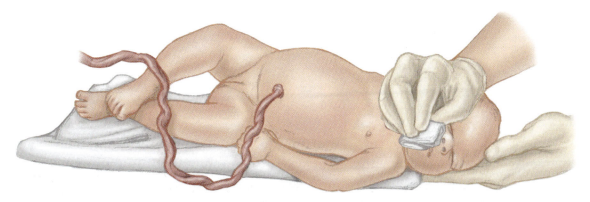

Figure 22.8 • Use a sterile pad or clean handkerchief to wipe blood and mucus from around the baby's mouth and nose.

and blood from around the baby's nose and mouth (Figure 22.8). Throughout the rest of your care steps, be sure that the baby's nose remains clear. Babies are nose breathers. Plugged nostrils may prevent adequate breathing.

Following delivery, if the baby is not breathing adequately or appears to be experiencing respiratory distress, it may be helpful to suction the airway. The correct steps for using the bulb syringe for that purpose are as follows:

- Squeeze the bulb first.
- Insert the tip about one inch into the baby's nose or mouth.
- Gently release the pressure to allow the syringe to take up fluids.
- Remove the tip of the filled syringe from the baby and squeeze out any fluids onto a towel or gauze pad.
- Repeat this process two or three times for the mouth and for each nostril.

2. Make certain that the baby is breathing. Usually the baby will be breathing on his own by the time you clear the airway, which will take about 30 seconds.

   If the baby is not breathing, then you must encourage him to do so. Begin by vigorously but gently rubbing the baby's back. If this fails to stimulate breathing, snap one of your index fingers against the soles of the baby's feet (Figure 22.9). (Care for the nonbreathing **newborn** is covered later in this chapter.)

3. Once you are sure the baby is breathing, perform a quick assessment. Note skin color (blue, normal, pale), any deformities, the strength of his cry (strong or weak), and whether he moves on his own or just lies still. After a few minutes, note if there are any changes in those conditions. It is important to give this information to the transport personnel for relay to the hospital physician, who will base the baby's subsequent exam on the original assessment.

4. Clamp or tie off the cord, if protocols allow.

5. Keep the baby warm. Dry the baby and discard the wet material in a biohazard bag. Wrap the baby in a clean, dry towel, sheet, or baby blanket and place him on the mother's abdomen. Keep the baby's head covered to help reduce heat loss.

   The mother may want to nurse the baby. You may suggest and encourage the mother to do so because it helps contract the uterus and control bleeding.

6. If tape is available, write on a long piece of it the mother's last name and the delivery time. Place a slightly shorter piece of tape on the back of the first one so the adhesive does not come in contact with the baby's skin. Leave an end exposed so that you can tape them together in a loop. Place the paper bracelet loosely around the baby's wrist.

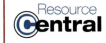

Resource Central

Watch a video on assessment of the newborn.

newborn ▶ a baby that is less than 28 days old. Also called *neonate*.

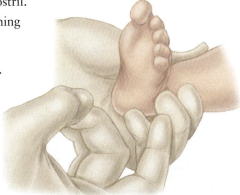

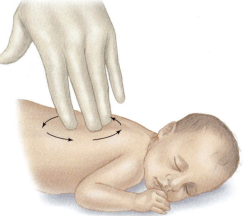

Figure 22.9 • It may be necessary to stimulate the newly born baby to breathe.

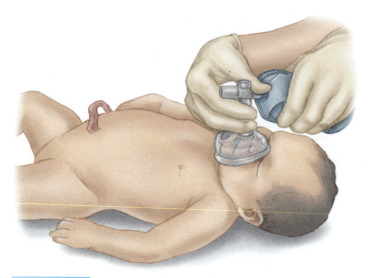

Figure 22.10 • Resuscitate the newly born baby with a bag-mask resuscitator that is an appropriate size.

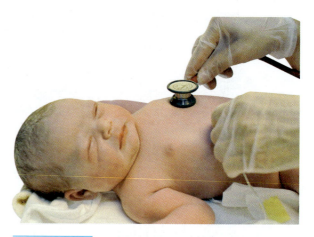

Figure 22.11 • Sometimes it is easier to use a stethoscope to access a newborn's pulse.

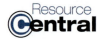
Resource Central

Learn more information about newborn resuscitation.

Caring for the Nonbreathing Newborn

If the baby is not breathing you must provide rescue breaths. Begin with two gentle but adequate breaths using the mouth-to-barrier or bag-mask technique (Figure 22.10). Then assess breathing and heartbeat. To check the heartbeat of a newborn, listen at the chest with your stethoscope (Figure 22.11) or feel for a pulse by lightly grasping the base of the umbilical cord.

Do not use a bag-mask device or airway adjuncts designed for older children or adults to resuscitate a newborn. Do not use any device unless you have been trained and your jurisdiction allows Emergency Medical Responders to use it. Be careful not to hyperextend the head and neck of the baby, which would close off the airway.

Provide ventilations if breaths are shallow, slow, or absent. Ventilate at 40 to 60 breaths per minute (about one breath every second). Watch for the chest to rise, which is the best indication of adequate ventilation. Reassess breathing after 30 seconds of assisted ventilations. The next step depends on the heart rate (Table 22.1):

- If the heart rate is 100 beats per minute or greater and the infant is breathing adequately, stop ventilations but continue to provide gentle stimulation (rub the back) to help maintain and improve the baby's breathing. Continue to provide oxygen.
- If the baby's heart rate is below 100 beats per minute and respirations are inadequate, continue to assist ventilations with a bag-mask device.
- If the heart rate is less than 60 beats per minute, continue to assist ventilations and begin chest compressions. Perform CPR with either your fingertips or your thumbs

TABLE 22.1	Care for the Nonbreathing Newborn	
IF THERE IS A PULSE, BUT YOU SEE THIS	**THEN DO THIS**
Breathing rate is inadequate.	Ventilate at 40 to 60 breaths per minute for 30 seconds and reassess breathing.
Heart rate is at least 100 beats per minute and spontaneous breathing is present.	Stop ventilations but continue to gently stimulate the baby by rubbing the skin.
Heart rate is less than 60 beats per minute.	Continue to assist ventilations. Start chest compressions.

with your hands encircling the chest, not the heels of your hands. Continue resuscitation until the baby is able to maintain adequate breathing and a pulse, or when a higher level of EMS provider relieves you. For the newborn, perform CPR using a compression/ventilation ratio of 3 to 1.

If you are allowed to provide oxygen to the baby, do not blow a stream of oxygen directly into the baby's face. This might cause him to react by holding his breath. In addition, the rich oxygen supply can cause other medical problems. Instead, direct a stream of oxygen toward the baby's face, either through a face mask or by passing an oxygen tube through the bottom of a paper cup. Hold the mask or cup several inches from the baby's face and allow the oxygen to blow by the face as the baby breathes (Figure 22.12). This is referred to as "blow-by" oxygen and is a good technique when a traditional mask or cannula is not appropriate.

Research has found that withholding oxygen may be more damaging than delivering too much. Follow local protocols for delivering oxygen, but never withhold oxygen from a sick baby or one who is struggling to breathe in the prehospital setting. The above ventilation and chest compression steps will usually revive the baby, but it is still important to have him and the mother transported as quickly as possible to the hospital.

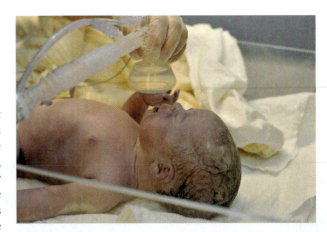

Figure 22.12 • Use an oxygen face mask or similar object attached to oxygen and hold it near the baby's face to supply blow-by oxygen.

Umbilical Cord

Your instructor will tell you if local protocol allows Emergency Medical Responders to clamp and cut the umbilical cord. If you are allowed to do so, remember that the baby can get an infection through the cord, so cut it only if you have sterile conditions. If you must cut the cord, you will need a sterile pair of scissors, a single-edged razor blade, or a sharp-edged knife.

Cutting the umbilical cord is usually a low priority, and Emergency Medical Responders may provide other care until EMT or ALS personnel arrive. In most cases, if dispatch has alerted EMT or ALS personnel, they should arrive before the cord needs to be clamped or tied.

Usually, it is not necessary to tie and cut the cord until the afterbirth is delivered and the cord is empty of blood and stops pulsating. If you see or feel the cord pulsating, it is still delivering oxygen to the baby from the mother. The baby will benefit from this oxygen.

However, if during the delivery you see that the umbilical cord is around the baby's neck, you must either slip one or two fingers under the cord and try to slip it back over the infant's head or you must cut it. If the cord cannot be slipped over the head, then quickly place clamps or ties on it and cut it. If this is not done and the infant delivers, the cord may strangle him.

If you are allowed, take the following steps in a normal delivery when the cord has stopped pulsating (Figure 22.13):

1. Use sterile clamps or umbilical ties found in the OB kit.

2. Apply one tie or clamp to the cord about six inches from the baby's abdomen.

3. Place a second tie or clamp about two inches farther from the baby.

4. Cut between the two ties or clamps. Never untie or unclamp the cord once it has been cut. Examine the cut ends of the cord. After trapped blood drains, bleeding should stop if the clamps or ties are secure. If bleeding continues, apply another tie or clamp as close to the original as possible.

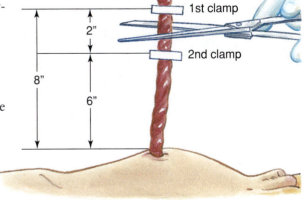

Figure 22.13 • Cutting the umbilical cord.

The loud talking at the travel stop's small restaurant grows silent. The crowd instinctively parts as Lucas and the other man crash through the doors, carrying the pregnant woman.

"What's wrong with her?" an elderly woman holding a steaming cup of coffee with both hands asks, peering over the tops of her glasses.

"She's having a baby," Lucas grunts as he grabbed a tablecloth from an empty table and hands it to a trucker wearing a puffy down vest. "Lay that out flat on the floor, please. Quick." The trucker complies, and within moments the crying woman is resting on the floor with her head propped up by a hastily gathered pile of jackets.

"Could you get me some towels and a couple more table cloths?" Lucas asks a waitress, who, without thinking, scribbles his request onto a notepad and disappears into the wall of people surrounding them. "And could you all turn around and give the lady some privacy?"

"Please, do something for my wife," the husband says, grabbing at Lucas's jacket sleeves.

"I am. I am. Just stay calm," he says before turning his attention to the panting woman. "Everything's going to be okay. Just relax." He then asks the patient, "What's your name?"

"Pamela," the woman growls. As her face contorts in pain, she grabs her large stomach with both hands.

"Okay, Pamela," Lucas says, getting a handful of towels and tablecloths from the waitress. "I'm going to cover you up and then I need to look down there to see how close the baby is. Okay?"

Face now shining with sweat, the woman glances at the circle of people—all with their backs to her—and nods rapidly at Lucas before clenching her teeth with another strong contraction.

If the afterbirth delivers while you are still providing care to the baby and protocols do not allow you to cut the cord, then place the afterbirth at the same level as the baby, or slightly higher. The placenta is still the baby's blood source, and blood can continue to flow to him if the placenta is positioned as described. If the placenta is placed lower than the baby, blood can flow away from him back into the placenta.

Caring for the Mother

OBJECTIVE

9. Explain the priorities of care for the mother following a field delivery.

Care for the mother includes helping her deliver the afterbirth (the placenta and other birth tissues), controlling vaginal bleeding, making her as comfortable as possible, and providing reassurance.

Delivering the Placenta

The delivery of the placenta (afterbirth) is the third stage of labor. It delivers anywhere from a few minutes to 20 minutes or longer after the baby is born. Some women prefer to sit upright following delivery. You may have to remind them that they will have to remain at rest until they deliver the afterbirth. Make the mother as comfortable as possible and wait for the delivery. You will both know it will be soon when she begins to have more contractions. The contractions will be milder with little discomfort.

Save the placenta, all attached membranes, and all soiled sheets and towels. A physician must examine those items to ensure the entire organ and its membranes were expelled from the uterus. Try to position a basin or container at the vaginal opening so the afterbirth will deliver into it (Figure 22.14). Once you collect it, place the container in a biohazard bag. If no container is available, allow the afterbirth to deliver directly into a biohazard bag and place the bag into another biohazard bag. Always label the bag with the mother's name.

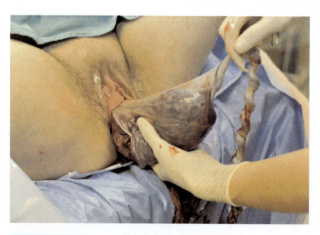

Figure 22.14 • Collect the placenta following delivery and transport to the hospital for inspection.

Controlling Vaginal Bleeding After Delivery

Bleeding from the vagina is normal after the mother has delivered the placenta. Perform the following steps to care for vaginal bleeding after delivery:

1. Place a sanitary pad or clean towel over the vaginal opening. Do not place anything in the vagina.

2. Have the mother lower her legs and keep them together. (She does not have to squeeze them.)

3. Feel the mother's abdomen until you find a grapefruit-size object. This is the uterus. Gently but firmly massage from the pubis bone at the front of the pelvis upward only and toward the naval. This will help stimulate the uterus to contract and stop bleeding. (See Figure 22.15.)

4. If bleeding continues, provide oxygen and maintain normal body temperature. Arrange transport as soon as possible. Continue to massage the uterus. If the mother wants to nurse, allow her to do so. Nursing stimulates contraction of the uterus and helps control bleeding.

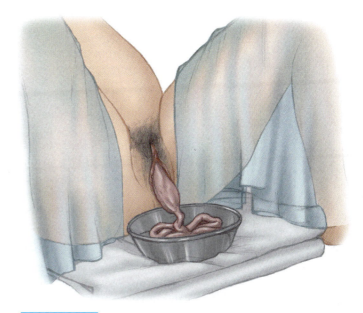

Figure 22.15 • Have the afterbirth transported with the mother and infant. A physician must examine the placenta.

Providing Comfort to the Mother

Talk with the mother throughout the entire birth process, explaining what you are doing and what is happening. She will especially want to know about the baby. Once you have completed your duties with the afterbirth, replace any soiled towels or sheets with clean, dry ones. Make sure that both she and the baby remain warm and comfortable.

Complications and Emergencies

There are a variety of complications related to pregnancy and childbirth of which you should be aware. While most of these problems are relatively uncommon, it is still possible to encounter them in the field. Complications include such things as abnormal bleeding, miscarriage, breech delivery, premature delivery, multiple births, and stillbirths. Keep in mind that most pregnancies and births are normal. Emergency Medical Responders often can care for some of the difficulties that arise. However, some severe complications must be handled by ALS personnel and require immediate transport to a medical facility.

The risk of complications before, during, and after delivery increases when the patient has one or more of the following factors:

- Younger than 18 or older than 35 years of age
- First pregnancy or more than five pregnancies
- Swollen face, feet, or abdomen from water retention
- High or low blood pressure
- Diabetes
- Illicit drug use during pregnancy
- History of seizures
- Predelivery bleeding

From the Medical Director

Controlling Vaginal Bleeding

Once you have ensured that the infant is breathing adequately, place him to the mother's breast. Allow the infant to begin nursing if that is the mother's desire. This causes a release of a hormone that contracts the uterus and reduces bleeding.

- Infections
- Alcohol dependency
- Injuries from trauma
- Premature rupture of membranes (water broke more than a few hours before delivery)

You will find out this information when you gather the patient's history during the secondary assessment. As you assess the patient, ask her the questions necessary to see if she is in a high-risk group.

Infections of the reproductive organs, especially infection by sexually transmitted diseases (STDs), can be transmitted to the baby and to you during birth. Remember to take BSI precautions and wear all personal protective equipment, which will protect you as well as the mother and the infant. Report to the hospital any information you receive from the mother about a history of infection.

Predelivery Emergencies

There are a variety of emergencies that can occur during pregnancy and prior to the delivery. While most of the emergencies are relatively rare, you should be familiar with what they are and how they present.

Prebirth Bleeding

When a pregnant woman has vaginal bleeding early in pregnancy, it may be that she is having a **miscarriage** (spontaneous **abortion**). Light, irregular discharges of blood, called **spotting**, are normal in early pregnancy but may concern the patient. If bleeding occurs late in pregnancy or while the patient is in labor, the problem may be with the placenta. Regardless of the cause of bleeding or stage of pregnancy, you must:

1. Make certain that an ambulance is on the way.
2. Take BSI precautions if you have not done so already.
3. Place the patient on her left side, but do not hold her legs together (Figure 22.16).
4. Provide care for shock, monitor the patient's airway, and administer oxygen as per local protocol.
5. Place a sanitary pad or bulky dressings over the vaginal opening.
6. Replace pads or dressings as they become soaked. Do not place anything in the vagina.

Figure 22.16 • Position the patient to control excessive prebirth bleeding.

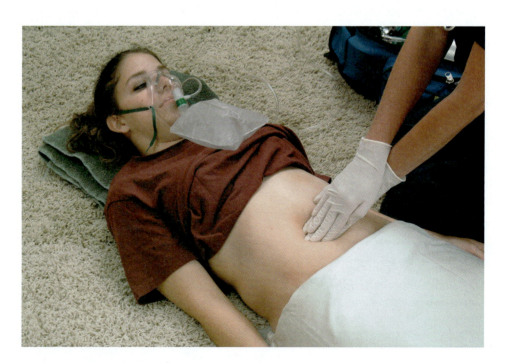

7. Save all blood-soaked pads and dressings, as well as any tissues that the mother passes. Place them in a biohazard bag for transport to the hospital and examination by a physician.

8. Monitor and reassure the patient while you wait for EMT or ALS personnel.

Miscarriage

If the fetus delivers before it can survive on its own (before the 26th week), it is considered a miscarriage. The medical term for a miscarriage is a *spontaneous abortion*. However, because the word *abortion* has other meanings in our society, never use that medical term with a woman who is having a miscarriage or premature signs of labor.

Miscarriage and abortion patients typically have abdominal cramps and pains. Vaginal bleeding is to be expected and can be mild to severe. In many cases, there will be vaginal discharges of bloody mucus and tissue particles.

When caring for a woman having a suspected miscarriage or from vaginal bleeding following an elective abortion, first get a general impression of the environment and the patient, perform a primary assessment, and then focus on the physical exam and patient history. Take the following steps to care for the patient:

1. Place the patient on her side, provide care for shock, and administer oxygen per local protocols.

2. Take a baseline set of vital signs. Then continue to take vital signs every few minutes thereafter.

3. Place a sanitary pad or bulky dressing over the vaginal opening. Do not place anything in the vagina.

4. Save all blood-soaked pads and any tissues that are passed. Place them in a biohazard bag.

5. Provide emotional support.

6. Arrange for EMT or ALS personnel to transport immediately.

Regardless of the cause of the emergency, the patient will need emotional support. Provide professional care, show concern, and reassure the patient.

Ectopic Pregnancy

A leading cause of pregnancy-related death is **ectopic pregnancy**. This occurs when the fertilized egg implants somewhere other than the uterus. Most commonly, ectopic pregnancies occur within a **fallopian tube**. Normally, just prior to conception, the unfertilized egg from the mother leaves the **ovary** and begins a journey through a fallopian tube on its way to the uterus. During conception, the sperm from the male joins up with the egg while it is still in a fallopian tube. Eventually, the fertilized egg implants along the wall of the uterus. This is normal. However, when the fertilized egg implants along the wall of the fallopian tube, it will not take long before the developing fetus outgrows the narrow space, causing it to rupture. This will always result in the loss of the fetus and is a life-threatening emergency for the mother.

The most common signs and symptoms of an ectopic pregnancy include:

- Abdominal pain
- Absence of normal menstrual cycle
- Vaginal bleeding

The care is the same for any woman with a general complaint of abdominal pain, including a thorough history and physical, oxygen if available, and transport to a hospital.

ectopic pregnancy ▶ a condition that occurs when the fertilized egg implants somewhere other than the uterus.

fallopian tube ▶ the tube-like structure that connects the ovary to the uterus.

ovary ▶ the structure that produces the ovum.

Complications During Delivery

See Figure 22.17 for the steps to take in the assessment of a mother in labor with signs of a complication of childbirth.

OBJECTIVE

17. Explain the common complications related to a field delivery and how to properly care for each.

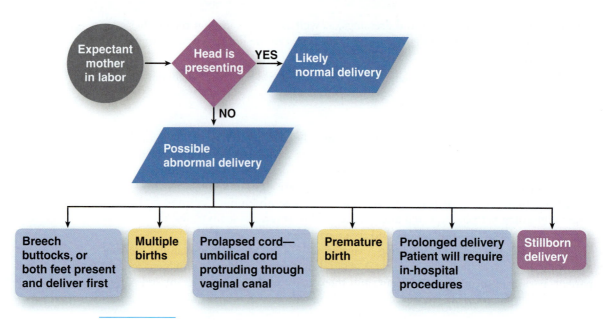

Figure 22.17 • Algorithm for complications of childbirth.

Meconium Staining

A stressful or difficult delivery affects both the mother and the baby. When the baby is stressed during delivery, he may defecate (empty the bowel). The fecal material is called **meconium**. When this material mixes with amniotic fluid, the normally clear fluid is stained green or brownish-yellow and is called *meconium staining*. If the baby inhales this fluid on his first attempt to breathe, he will develop aspiration pneumonia, a lung infection caused by aspirating (breathing in) the meconium.

Sometimes the amniotic sac will rupture many hours before delivery. You will have to rely on information from the mother to determine if the fluids were clear or stained. Ask the mother if she noticed the color of the fluid when her water broke. If you witness the rupture, look for meconium staining. Be prepared to wipe the baby's mouth and nose and to suction.

Breech Birth

In a **breech birth,** the buttocks or both feet (not just one) present and deliver first. Even in this position, the baby can be born without complications. As the buttocks and trunk deliver together, place one hand and forearm under the baby for support. Be sure to support the head as it delivers. A breech birth can be a complication if the baby's head will not deliver.

In a breech birth, when the baby's head does not deliver within three minutes after the buttocks and trunk, you must immediately notify dispatch to alert responding EMT or ALS personnel. They must transport the mother and infant as soon as possible. While waiting for them to arrive, do the following:

1. Place the mother on a high concentration of oxygen.

2. Create an airway for the baby because the umbilical cord will be compressed between the infant and vaginal wall, shutting off blood flow. Tell the mother what you must do and why. Insert your gloved hand into the vagina, with your palm toward the baby's face. Form a V by placing one finger on each side of the baby's nose (Figure 22.18). Push the wall of the birth canal away from the baby's face. If you cannot complete this process, then try to place one fingertip into the infant's mouth and push away the birth canal wall with your other fingers.

3. Maintain the airway. Once you have created an airway for the baby, keep the airway open. Do not pull on the baby. Allow delivery to take place while you continue to support the baby's body and head.

meconium ▶ the product of the baby's first bowel movement.

breech birth ▶ a birth in which the buttocks or feet deliver first.

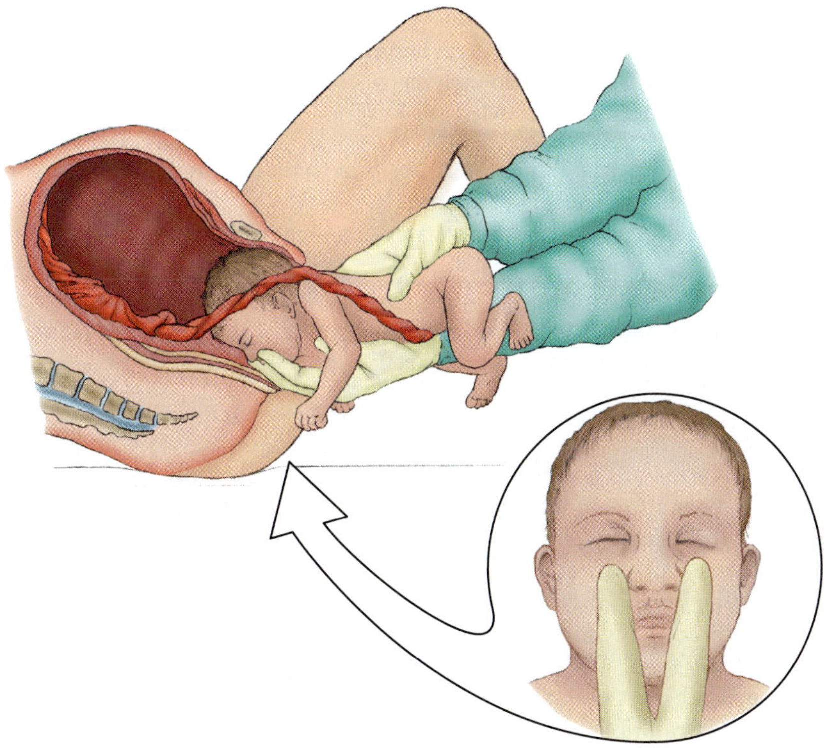

Figure 22.18 • Create and maintain an airway for the baby during a breech birth.

4. If the head does not deliver in three minutes after you have created an airway, it is necessary to have the mother and infant transported to a medical facility immediately. Maintain the airway throughout all stages of care until higher-level EMS personnel relieve you.

Limb Presentation

The presentation of an arm or a single leg is called a *limb presentation* and is an emergency requiring EMT or ALS personnel to transport the mother to a medical facility immediately. Ask dispatch to notify EMT or ALS responders of the emergency. Do not pull on the limb or try to place your gloved hand into the birth canal. Do not try to place the limb back into the vagina. Place the mother in the knee-chest position (Figure 22.19) to help reduce pressure on the fetus and the umbilical cord. Medical direction and protocols may instruct you to keep the mother in the typical delivery position. Follow your protocols.

prolapsed cord ▶ a condition resulting in the delivery of the umbilical cord prior to the delivery of the baby.

Prolapsed Cord

When you examine the mother for crowning, you may find the umbilical cord protruding from the vaginal opening. When the umbilical cord delivers first, this is called a **prolapsed cord** and is common in a breech birth. Call for EMT or ALS personnel to transport the mother with a prolapsed cord to a medical facility immediately.

A prolapsed cord endangers the life of the baby. As the baby emerges through the vaginal opening, his head presses the umbilical cord against the vaginal wall, reducing or completely cutting off blood flow and oxygen. When oxygen flow through the cord is obstructed, the baby will try to breathe. But because the baby's face is pressed against the wall of the birth canal, the mouth and nose cannot take in air. To help the baby breathe, provide an airway, using the same methods described for breech birth.

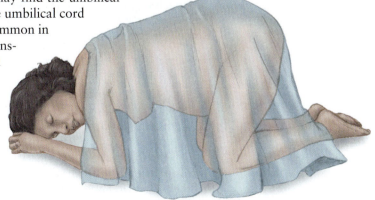

Figure 22.19 • Place the mother in the knee-chest position, which will help keep pressure off the umbilical cord in a limb presentation birth.

That is, place your fingers into the vaginal opening in front of the infant's face and make a V. Do not try to push the cord back into the birth canal.

In addition, take the following steps (check with medical direction or your protocols to find out what Emergency Medical Responders are allowed to do):

- Place the mother in a knee-chest position to reduce pressure on the cord.
- Try to maintain a pulse in the cord.
- Place wet dressings (use sterile water or saline if it is available) over the cord to keep it moist.
- Wrap the cord in a towel or dressings to keep it warm.
- Provide the mother with a high concentration of oxygen as soon as possible.
- Monitor vital signs and arrange for transport immediately.

Multiple Births

Multiple births are not necessarily abnormal, but they do frequently involve premature delivery. Premature infants may not be fully developed and often have respiratory complications. If the mother is giving birth to more than one infant, she will have contractions begin again shortly after the birth of the first baby. The contractions may deliver the afterbirth of the first or another baby.

The procedures for assisting the mother remain the same. If the umbilical cord has stopped pulsating, you will tie or clamp the cord of the first baby before the second baby is born. Check with your instructor about the protocols in your area for how to address the cords in multiple births. Once the babies are delivered and they are breathing, assess each one, noting skin color (blue, normal, pale), any deformities, strength of their cries, and whether they move on their own or just lie still. When assessing the quality of skin color on dark-skinned babies, check the nail beds, lips, and palms of the hands for signs of cyanosis. After a few minutes, note if there are any changes in those conditions. If necessary, perform resuscitation. Document the time of birth for each baby. Call for assistance as soon as possible.

Premature Births

Any baby weighing less than 5.5 pounds at birth or any baby born before the thirty-seventh week (prior to the ninth month) of pregnancy is considered a *premature baby*. If the mother tells you the baby is early by more than two weeks, play it safe and consider the baby to be premature.

In addition to the procedures for normal births, you must take special steps to keep a premature baby warm. It is important to dry the baby. Wrap him in a blanket, sheet, or towel. A blanket covered with foil is ideal. (Fold the edges of the foil to avoid cutting the baby.) There also are commercial wraps available, which your unit may carry or your department may purchase. Cover the baby's head, but keep his face uncovered. Transfer the baby to a warm environment (90°F to 100°F [32°C to 37°C]), but do not place a heat source too close to the baby. Ventilate a premature baby who needs resuscitation using a mouth-to-mask technique or an appropriately sized bag-mask device. Wipe or suction blood and mucus from the mouth and nose first before ventilating.

Stillborn Deliveries

A fetus that is delivered dead is called *stillborn*. Some die shortly after birth. Either event is very traumatic for the mother and father, family members, and care providers. Do not feel embarrassed to show your emotions, but be prepared to continue to act professionally and provide comfort to the mother, father, and other family members who are present.

If the infant shows no signs of life at birth (no attempts to breathe and move) or goes into respiratory or cardiac arrest, provide the resuscitation measures described earlier in this chapter. Do not stop resuscitation until the baby regains respirations and a heartbeat, other emergency care providers relieve you, or you are too exhausted to continue.

There are cases in which a baby has died hours or longer before birth. Do not attempt to resuscitate a stillborn infant that has large blisters and a strong unpleasant odor. There may be other indications that the infant died earlier in the uterus, such as a very soft head, swollen body parts, or obvious deformities.

Other Emergencies

There are a few other complications that you should know about that affect both the mother and the baby during pregnancy. They include supine hypotensive syndrome, preeclampsia and eclampsia, trauma, vaginal bleeding, and sexual assault.

Supine Hypotensive Syndrome

There is a condition that can occur during the last couple months of pregnancy called **supine hypotensive syndrome**. It is caused when the mother lies on her back and the weight of the fetus and other organs press on the mother's inferior vena cava, the large vessel in the abdomen that returns blood back to the heart. The pressure on the vena cava restricts blood return to the heart, causing signs of shock such as low blood pressure, increased pulse, pale skin, and in some cases an altered mental status.

Care for supine hypotensive syndrome is usually as simple as repositioning the mother to more of a seated position (semi-Fowler's) or having her lie on her left side. The weight of the fetus will shift to the left and off the vena cava, allowing better blood flow (venous return) to the heart.

Preeclampsia and Eclampsia

Another potentially dangerous condition that affects approximately 5% of all pregnant women is known as **preeclampsia**. The exact causes of preeclampsia are not well understood, but it most often occurs after the twentieth week of pregnancy and seems to favor younger women who are pregnant for the first time.

Signs and symptoms of preeclampsia include:

- Abnormally high blood pressure
- Fluid retention causing swelling of the arms, hands, and face
- Headache
- Nausea

If left untreated, preeclampsia can lead to **eclampsia**, which is characterized by seizures, coma, and eventually death of both the mother and baby.

The only treatment for preeclampsia is the delivery of the baby. If you should see signs of either condition in a pregnant woman, rapid transport to a hospital is essential. While waiting for transport, provide the following care: Support the ABCs as necessary. Provide high-flow oxygen, if protocols allow. Have suction ready, and be prepared for seizures.

Trauma

Vital signs of a pregnant woman are usually different from a woman who is not pregnant. A pregnant woman's blood volume increases up to about 45%, a natural protection and preparation for the mother who will lose blood during delivery. Her heart rate increases by about 15 beats per minute, and her blood pressure falls 10 to 15 mmHg. Do not mistake the high pulse rate and low blood pressure for signs of shock in the normal nontrauma pregnant woman. But in a trauma situation, the mother's larger blood volume allows her body to compensate for blood loss and therefore may not show early signs of shock.

A pregnant woman can lose almost 40% of her blood volume before she shows any signs of shock. In shock, the mother's body shunts blood away from the uterus first. Less blood to the uterus affects the fetus, causing harm well before the mother shows any signs. Blood loss may be internal and not obvious to the Emergency Medical Responder. Always suspect internal bleeding in any pregnant trauma patient, even if she seems to be initially unharmed and shows normal vital signs for a pregnant woman. Even if the mother is not injured, the fetus may be injured in an advanced pregnancy.

OBJECTIVES

13. Describe the signs and symptoms of supine hypotensive syndrome.

14. Explain the appropriate care for a patient with signs and symptoms of supine hypotensive syndrome.

15. Describe the signs and symptoms of preeclampsia.

16. Explain the appropriate care for a patient with signs and symptoms of preeclampsia.

supine hypotensive syndrome ▶ an abnormally low blood pressure that results when the mother is supine and the fetus puts pressure on the vena cava.

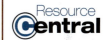

Learn more information about preeclampsia

preeclampsia ▶ a potentially life-threatening condition that affects the mother during the third trimester and is characterized by high blood pressure and fluid retention.

eclampsia ▶ a life-threatening condition characterized by seizures, coma, and eventually death of both the mother and baby.

During the scene size-up, look carefully at the environment, the patient, and the mechanism of injury. Try to determine what injuries might have been caused. Two common types of trauma that can cause significant harm to the mother and the fetus are blunt force and penetrating injuries:

- *Blunt-force injuries* are common in falls, vehicle crashes, abuse, and assaults.
- *Penetrating injuries* are usually a result of gunshot wounds and stabbings or punctures from the debris of auto wreckage.

During the early months of pregnancy when the fetus is small, the fluids in the amniotic sac provide some protection from blunt force trauma. As the fetus grows, and especially in the last two months of pregnancy, blunt force trauma can cause more damage to the fetus. As a result, Emergency Medical Responders should provide direct care for the mother and indirect care for the fetus.

The greatest danger to both the mother and the baby is bleeding and shock. First ensure an open airway and adequate breathing and look for and control external bleeding. Provide a high concentration of oxygen as soon as possible and keep the patient warm but do not overheat her. The steps that prevent or care for shock will assist the fetus also. Arrange for immediate transport, and while waiting for EMT or ALS personnel to arrive, provide appropriate care based on the mechanism of injury, such as immobilization for possible spine injuries, splinting for possible fractures, and dressing wounds.

Vaginal Bleeding

There are many reasons for excessive vaginal bleeding during pregnancy. Emergency Medical Responders must be aware of them and look carefully for the mechanism of injury that caused them, including the following:

- Blunt force and penetrating trauma
- Intercourse
- Sexual assault
- Reproductive organ problems
- Abnormal pregnancy
- Placental tears and uterine rupture

placenta previa ▶ a condition that results when the placenta grows and develops over the cervix.

There are two types of placenta tears: placenta previa and placenta abruptio. In **placenta previa**, the placenta lies low in the uterus and attaches itself over the opening of the cervix, meaning it would have to emerge before, or previous to, the fetus during birth. In this position, the placenta tears and bleeds when the cervix dilates during labor. *Placenta abruptio* can occur in a trauma situation when the force of the trauma abruptly tears the placenta partially or completely away from the wall of the uterus. The pregnant woman may have major internal blood loss because blood can be trapped between the placenta and the uterine wall. She also may lose blood vaginally.

The only indications you may have of internal blood loss and developing shock are changes in vital signs, feeling a hard uterus when examining the abdomen, and the mother's complaint that her abdomen is painful or tender. Get a set of baseline vital signs as soon as possible in your assessment, and monitor the vital signs by retaking them every few minutes. If local protocols allow, provide her with a high concentration of oxygen as soon as possible and maintain body temperature to help reduce the effects of shock. Arrange for immediate transport.

The care for controlling vaginal bleeding includes the following: Place sanitary pads or bulky dressings over the vaginal opening. Replace pads or dressings as they become soaked. Do not place anything in the vagina. Save all blood-soaked pads and dressings, and place them in a biohazard bag for transport to the hospital and examination by a physician.

Sexual Assault

Sexual assault or rape is always a psychologically and physically traumatic experience. The Emergency Medical Responder's professional manner, attitude, and emotional support are important steps in the care of the expectant mother who has been assaulted.

As the woman struggles or resists the attacker, and as the attacker uses force to make her submit, she can receive many types of injuries to the external soft tissues, the vaginal canal, and the internal organs. The fetus is also a victim in the assault. The injuries the fetus receives may be direct from blows to the abdomen, or indirect as a result of injuries to the mother.

You may have multiple roles to perform as an Emergency Medical Responder who is caring for a pregnant woman. You may have to provide care for injuries, including spine immobilization, extremity splinting, and wound dressing. In sexual assault cases, you will need to provide emotional support and protect the patient from embarrassment from on-lookers. Do not clean the vaginal area. Do not let the patient wash. Do not let her go to the bathroom. But if she insists on cleaning herself and changing clothes, you cannot stop her. You should advise her that hospital personnel may be able to collect evidence from her that will help with the investigation. Emergency Medical Responders should collect clothing and any items that were used during the assault for examination and legal needs. Transport anything that may be evidence in a paper bag or wrap it in a towel. Do not place such items in plastic, because plastic can promote the growth of bacteria.

For any emotional, violent, or traumatic injury and for complicated deliveries, provide care that will prevent or manage shock and arrange transport as soon as possible. Promote patient confidence by providing emotional support and physical comfort. Listen to your patient and talk to her throughout all procedures. You will find that some roles come easily. Other roles will take knowledge, practice, and skill.

WRAP-UP

FIRST ON SCENE

As snowflakes continue to fall in gentle arcs and swirls outside the steamed windows of the restaurant, the cries of the pregnant woman are replaced by the small wails of a newborn.

"It's a boy," Lucas says, wiping his forehead with the back of one trembling hand as the child's father stands proudly smiling down at the small, bloody infant.

"You did a great job," the waitress says, as she leans in close to see the baby. "The ambulance told me they couldn't get here for an hour or more though."

"That's fine," Lucas replies as he finishes wiping the baby down and wrapping him in several clean, warm towels. "There's absolutely nothing wrong with this little guy." He gently passes the bundled child to his parents and stands to stretch his back.

As he watches the husband and wife in their unguarded amazement at the tiny person in their arms, Lucas is suddenly very glad he didn't take that plane to Denver after all.

CHAPTER REVIEW

Summary

- The normal gestation period for a human fetus is 40 weeks or approximately nine months. An infant is considered premature if he is delivered prior to the thirty-seventh week of gestation.

- Labor is the normal process the body uses to deliver a baby. The average labor is 16 hours but can be much shorter or much longer than that.

- Labor has three stages. The first begins with the onset of labor and ends with full dilation of the cervix. The second stage begins with dilation of the cervix and ends with the delivery of the baby. The third stage begins after delivery of the baby and ends with the delivery of the placenta.

- Signs of an imminent delivery include contractions that are less than three minutes apart, the mother's feeling of needing to bear down, and crowning at the vaginal opening. When the signs of an imminent delivery are obvious, you must prepare for delivery at the scene.

- Upon delivery of the head, you must check for the presence of the umbilical cord around the neck. If present, gently slip it over the baby's head. Suction the nose and mouth prior to delivery of the baby.

- After delivery, stimulate the baby by drying him with a clean dry cloth. The baby should begin breathing on his own. If breathing or pulse is inadequate, provide the appropriate care immediately.

- Immediately call for ALS back up for any delivery that appears to be abnormal or complicated, such as a breech presentation or a prolapsed cord. Place the mother in the knee-chest position and provide high-flow oxygen if available. Follow local protocols.

Take Action

KNOW YOUR TOOLS!

As an Emergency Medical Responder you will learn many skills that cover a wide variety of emergencies. Some emergencies are more common than others, and some you may only see once or twice in your career. Delivering a child in the field is just one of those emergencies that does not come along very often. For that reason it is important to occasionally review the steps necessary to care for a mother in labor and as well as the specialized tools you will need to assist the delivery of the baby.

For this activity, borrow a commercial OB kit from your instructor and explore the contents of the kit item by item. To make it a little more engaging, invite a fellow classmate to join you. Together discuss the specific use for each item in the kit. Using 3×5 index cards, write each item on a card and on the reverse of the card write an explanation of what the item is used for. Later on the cards can be used as a great tool when reviewing the steps for caring for a woman in labor.

First on Scene Run Review

Recall the events of the "First on Scene" scenario in this chapter and answer the following questions, which are related to the call. Rationales are offered in the Answer Key at the back of the book.

1. Do you need to ask permission before treating this woman? Why or why not?

2. What are the stages of labor?

3. What information would you want from the woman about her pregnancy?

4. What information would you need to record about the baby?

Quick Quiz

To check your understanding of the chapter, answer the following questions. Then compare your answers to those in the Answer Key at the back of the book.

1. The structure that is only present during the development of a fetus is the:
   a. placenta.
   b. uterus.
   c. vagina.
   d. cervix.

2. The rupturing of membranes is an important milestone in the birthing process. It is the:
   a. first contraction of which the mother is aware.
   b. widening of the cervical opening.
   c. rupturing of the amniotic sac.
   d. detachment of the placenta.

3. The organ that delivers oxygenated blood and nourishment to the fetus and removes fetal wastes is the:
   a. pubis.
   b. placenta.
   c. vagina.
   d. cervix.

4. A vaginal discharge occurs:
   a. only during the first stage of childbirth.
   b. during the first and second stages of childbirth.
   c. throughout the different stages of childbirth.
   d. only during abnormal childbirth.

5. Which one of the following statements about labor pains is most accurate?
   a. They come at the same time intervals during all stages of labor.
   b. They come at longer time intervals as the birth of the child nears.
   c. They come at shorter time intervals as the birth of the child nears.
   d. They come at regular time intervals during all stages of labor.

6. For your personal safety during a field birth, it is best to have gloves and:
   a. face mask, eye shield, and gown.
   b. face mask, gown, and red biohazard bags.
   c. gown, red biohazard bags, and basin.
   d. face mask, red biohazard bags, and basin.

7. When evaluating the mother before delivery, all of the following information is important to have, EXCEPT:
   a. her name, age, and expected due date.
   b. if she has been under a physician's care during pregnancy.
   c. if her water has broken and, if so, when and what color.
   d. when she expected to begin labor contractions.

8. All of the following are signs that the birth of the baby is imminent EXCEPT when the mother:
   a. has the feeling that the baby is trying to be born.
   b. is experiencing labor contractions that are two minutes apart.
   c. is experiencing labor contractions at 10-minute intervals.
   d. is straining, crying out, and complaining of the urge to go to the bathroom.

9. It is essential that you take BSI precautions for your safety as well as the mother's:
   a. during both assessment and delivery.
   b. while you are assessing the patient.
   c. only if you determine as necessary.
   d. as the baby delivers only.

10. You should consider the delivery normal if the:
    a. baby's feet appear first.
    b. baby's head appears first.
    c. mother is experiencing irregular contractions.
    d. mother tells you the baby is about to be born.

11. During a normal delivery, you should do all of the following, EXCEPT:
    a. support the head, trunk, and legs.
    b. suction the baby's mouth, nose, and the cord.
    c. support the head and assist in the birth of the shoulders.
    d. keep the baby level with the vagina until the cord stops pulsating.

12. When preparing to cut the umbilical cord, place the first clamp:
    a. 6 inches from the baby's belly.
    b. 4 inches away from the baby's belly.
    c. only if your jurisdiction allows you to do so.
    d. 10 inches from the belly.

13. The placenta, or afterbirth:
    a. does not concern you because it will deliver at the hospital.
    b. needs to be delivered by you and saved for further examination at the hospital.
    c. needs to be delivered by you and discarded into a red biohazard bag.
    d. needs to be delivered and examined by you before being discarded.

14. When caring for the baby, you must do all of the following immediately after the birth, EXCEPT:
    a. clear the baby's airway.
    b. make sure the baby is breathing.
    c. perform a quick assessment of the baby.
    d. clamp off the cord and cut it.

15. During the assessment of the infant, remember that the heart rate is:
    a. slower than that of a child or an adult.
    b. the same as that of a child or an adult.
    c. faster than that of a child or an adult.
    d. dependent on the weight of the newborn.

16. You are caring for a pregnant woman who is 24 weeks along and is complaining of a headache and nausea. Her pulse is 140 strong and regular, and her blood pressure is 174/96. Her condition is most likely caused by:
    a. supine hypotensive syndrome.
    b. ectopic pregnancy.
    c. preeclampsia
    d. placenta previa.

17. You are caring for a pregnant woman who states she is 36 weeks along. Blood pressure 74/60. Her skin signs are pale and cool. You should:
    a. keep her flat on her back.
    b. roll her onto her left side.
    c. prepare for an imminent delivery.
    d. have her bear down and push.

18. You are caring for an 18-year-old female with a complaint of severe abdominal pain and vaginal bleeding. You should:
    a. apply low-flow oxygen.
    b. inspect the vagina.
    c. ask her when her last menstrual cycle was.
    d. find out what she had to eat.

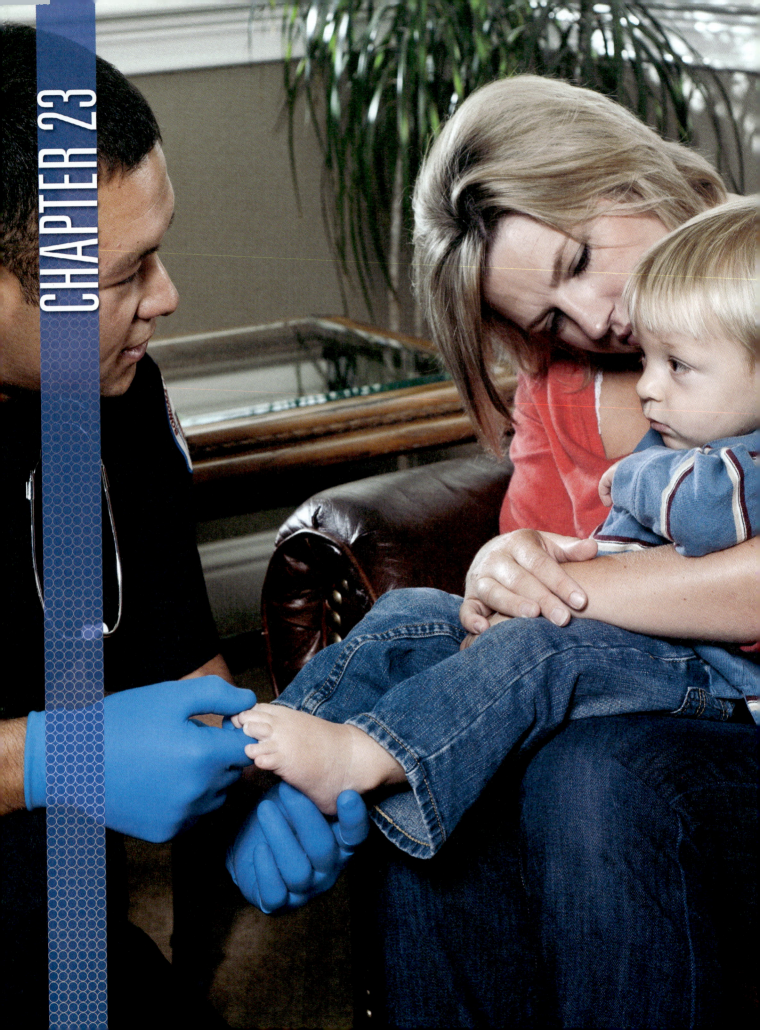

CHAPTER 23

Caring for Infants and Children

EDUCATION STANDARDS • Special Patient Populations—Pediatrics, Neonatal Care, Patients with Special Challenges

COMPETENCIES • Recognizes and manages life threats based on assessment findings of a patient with a medical emergency while awaiting additional emergency response.

CHAPTER OVERVIEW This chapter introduces methods used in providing care for medical and trauma emergencies that involve the pediatric patient. Pediatric patients must be managed and cared for differently than adults because of their age, physical and mental development, personalities, and experiences. Children respond well to familiar, normal routines. Many have difficulty handling strange situations and unfamiliar adults, including Emergency Medical Responders.

Seriously ill and injured children also provoke strong emotions in those who must provide care for them. Through proper training and practice, Emergency Medical Responders can increase their confidence and manage the pediatric emergency calmly and effectively. As a result, pediatric patients will find an empathetic care provider in the Emergency Medical Responder.

OBJECTIVES

Upon successful completion of this chapter, the student should be able to:

COGNITIVE

1. Review the major stages of lifespan development for the pediatric patient (Chapter 4).

2. Define the following terms:

   a. abuse *(p. 533)*

   b. adolescent *(p. 512)*

   c. croup *(p. 524)*

   d. epiglottitis *(p. 524)*

   e. febrile *(p. 526)*

   f. infant *(p. 512)*

   g. mandated reporter *(p. 536)*

   h. neglect *(p. 537)*

   i. pediatric assessment triangle (PAT) *(p. 517)*

   j. retractions *(p. 518)*

   k. school age *(p. 512)*

   l. shaken-baby syndrome *(p. 539)*

   m. sudden infant death syndrome (SIDS) *(p. 530)*

   n. toddler *(p. 512)*

   o. work of breathing *(p. 518)*

3. Explain various techniques that can be employed to maximize successful assessment of the pediatric patient. *(p. 517)*

4. Explain the components of the pediatric assessment triangle. *(p. 517)*

5. State the most common cause of cardiac arrest in the pediatric patient. *(p. 522)*

6. Describe the signs and symptoms of sudden infant death syndrome (SIDS). *(p. 530)*

7. Explain the appropriate steps for management of a suspected SIDS death. *(p. 530)*

8. Describe common signs and symptoms of abuse and neglect. *(p. 533)*

9. Explain the role of the Emergency Medical Responder in cases of suspected abuse and/or neglect. *(p. 533)*

10. Explain the assessment and management of the following emergencies in pediatric patients:

    a. Upper airway obstruction *(p. 522)*

    b. Lower reactive airway disease *(p. 524)*

    c. Seizures *(p. 525)*

    d. Shock *(p. 526)*

PSYCHOMOTOR

11. Demonstrate the ability to properly assess and care for a pediatric patient.

12. Demonstrate various techniques that can be employed to maximize successful assessment of the pediatric patient.

13. Demonstrate the application of the pediatric assessment triangle.

14. Demonstrate sensitivity for the feelings of the family while caring for an ill or injured pediatric patient.

15. Recognize the emotional impact that responding to pediatric patients can have on the Emergency Medical Responder.

16. Value the role of the Emergency Medical Responder with respect to patient advocacy.

FIRST ON SCENE

City police officer Bryn Moradi backs the cruiser into an empty parking space and opens her laptop, hoping to catch up on paperwork for what is turning out to be a very busy swing shift. It seems to her that as the sun sinks behind the city's well-known skyline, the streets are filling with people up to no good. "Bizarre," she thinks. "Maybe it's the full moon."

Just as she gets connected to the department's server, the radio blares to life. "Adam eight, priority call on tach three." The dispatcher's voice is monotone, bordering on mechanical.

Bryn hits the radio's channel button several times and announces that she is ready for the call. "Adam eight."

A different, just as emotionless, voice answers. "Respond priority one for shots fired at the 43rd Street subway station entrance. We're trying to clear a backup unit for you, but for now, you're it."

"Adam eight copy." Bryn slides the laptop back into its black nylon case and shifts the car into drive. Her stomach is immediately tense and nauseous, and she has to force herself to breathe evenly while maneuvering the patrol car in and out of the Friday night traffic.

As she navigates the final turn to the scene, she sees that the street is in chaos. People are crouching against buildings, laying flat on the pavement, and running hunched over in all directions. The front windows to several businesses are shattered, and large shards of broken glass hang in the frames like jagged teeth. A woman huddled next to a low concrete wall bordering the subway station stairs sees Bryn's patrol car, scrambles to her feet, and runs directly toward her. As Bryn climbs from the car, gun drawn and ready, the woman reaches her and screams about an ambulance.

"Who was shooting?" Bryn demands, looking directly into the woman's terrified eyes.

"I don't know. It was from a, a car!" The woman is bordering on losing complete control of herself.

"So the shooter drove away?" Bryn notices that blood is dripping at the feet of the crying woman.

"Yes!" She screams. "It was a green van-type thing, and they just kept shooting, and then they, they drove that way. Please! I need help for my baby!" The woman moves a dark blanket she is carrying, and Bryn's stomach drops as she sees the small, pale face spattered with bright red drops of blood.

Caring for the Pediatric Patient

Responding to a call for a child's illness or injury can be stressful for the Emergency Medical Responder. Some situations will make you feel sad or angry. You will not be able to express your emotions in front of the child or parent. When faced with the assessment and care of an infant or a child, you may at first feel that you do not know what to do or where to start. An anxious, fretful, or frightened child who cannot be comforted may further add to your stress level and reduce your confidence. Remember that many of the assessment and care techniques used for adults are similar for children, with some modifications. Those modifications take into account the child's age, physical development, and emotional response.

From the Medical Director

The Pediatric Patient

Children are very sensitive to the feelings of those around them. If you feel fear, they will sense it and their discomfort will worsen. Be aware of your feelings and take the opportunity while responding to reassure yourself and your fellow rescuers as to their responsibilities, and then make every effort to remain calm.

Emergency Medical Responders who are unsure of what to do in pediatric emergencies are likely to have a stronger emotional response during and after an incident than those who are prepared and confident in their actions. By training, practicing, and drilling to prepare for pediatric incidents, you not only will improve your confidence and decrease your stress, but you will improve patient outcome as well.

Characteristics of Infants and Children

Everyone has some fear of the unknown. Because so many things are unknown to children, it is easy to see why emergencies can be so frightening for them. A severe illness or injury is a new and unknown experience for children, and it is an experience that increases their anxiety, especially if parents are not present. For most children, security comes from their parents or primary caregivers. The desire to be with his parents may be a child's first priority, even above having you offer help, comfort, or relief of pain.

Figure 23.1 • Get down at eye level and speak directly to the child.

When you are dealing with children, you need to gain their trust. Attempt to calm and reassure them by using the following techniques:

- Approach them slowly, establish eye contact from a safe distance, and ask permission to get closer.
- Let them know that someone will call their parents.
- Get down at eye level with the child. Standing makes you appear large and frightening.
- Let them see your face and expressions. You want to appear friendly, yet concerned and willing to listen. Speak directly to them. Speak clearly and slowly so that they can hear and understand you. Keep your voice gentle and calm even when you need to be firm. Try not to raise your voice or talk loudly to a crying or screaming child. Some children are bashful or uncomfortable with strangers and may not look at you. Try to maintain eye contact (Figure 23.1).
- Pause frequently to find out if the child understands what you have said or asked. Even if you communicate easily with your own children, never assume that other children understand you. Find out by asking questions.
- Quickly determine if there are any life-threatening problems and care for them immediately (Scan 23.1). If there are no immediate life threats, continue with patient assessment at a relaxed pace. Avoid moving children, if possible. Movement may cause unexpected pain.
- Responsive, alert young children may become frightened if you start your exam with the head and face. If children show fear as you reach out to touch them, begin the physical examination at the feet and slowly work your way up to the head if there are no critical injuries. While you are performing the toe-to-head assessment, look for the same signs of illness and injury as you do when assessing the adult patient. Take time, though, to consider special assessment needs based on the anatomy of the child.
- Always tell children what you are going to do before each step of your assessment. Do not try to explain the entire procedure at once. Explain one step, do it, and then explain the next step.
- Never lie to children. Tell them if it will hurt when you are examining them. If children ask if they are sick or hurt, tell the truth, but reassure them by saying that you are there to help and other people also will be helping.
- Offer comfort to children by stroking their foreheads or holding their hands. Children will let you know if they do not want to be touched. Children will show their acceptance of you by their reactions to your touch. Do not expect rapid acceptance. Use your smile and gentle words to provide comfort.
- Do not direct all your conversation to the parents. Talk to the child. If you are at the scene of an emergency in which the parents are also injured, let the child know that people are caring for their parents, too.

Infants

Birth to One Year

- In your primary assessment, establish your general impression from a distance.
- Ensure an adequate airway. If needed, provide ventilations.
- Protect the head and spine.
- Control your emotions and facial expressions to help reduce the child's fear.
- Provide care to prevent shock. (A small amount of blood loss can cause shock.)

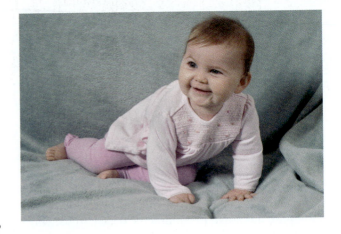

Establishing Responsiveness: The infant should move or cry when gently tapped or shaken. Is he alert, responsive to voice or to pain stimulus, or unresponsive?

Opening the Airway: Use slight head-tilt/chin-lift. (Use the jaw-thrust for possible spine injury.)

Evaluating Breathing: If the infant is responsive but cyanotic and struggling to breathe, or has inadequate breathing, assist ventilations and arrange for immediate transport. If the infant is unresponsive, check for a pulse. If there is no breathing and no pulse, begin CPR.

Rescue Breaths: If the infant has a pulse but is not breathing normally, ventilate once every three to five seconds while watching for chest rise and fall. Ventilate with the mouth-to-barrier technique, using an appropriate pediatric-size barrier, mask or a pediatric bag mask. If there is evidence of airway obstruction, clear the airway.

Clearing the Airway

- Make certain that you have not overextended or underextended the neck. Place a folded towel under the shoulders to keep the head in a neutral position. If this does not open the airway, then:
- For a responsive child, place the infant over the length of your arm face down with the head lower than the trunk. Support the head with your hand placed around the jaw. Support your forearm by placing it on your thigh.
- Deliver five back blows between the shoulder blades with the heel of your free hand.
- Place your free arm on the infant's back and support the back of his head with that hand. Sandwich him between your arms and hands and turn him over. Support your arm on your thigh. Keep the head lower than the trunk and deliver five chest thrusts. If the airway remains obstructed, but the patient is responsive, continue back blows and chest thrusts.
- If the airway remains obstructed and the patient is unresponsive, open the mouth to look for an obstruction.
- Do not attempt blind finger sweeps. You must see the object before you sweep the mouth with your little finger.
- Even if you did not see or dislodge an obstruction, attempt to ventilate. If unable to ventilate, begin chest compressions. After 30 compressions, look for and remove visible obstructions, and attempt to ventilate again. Repeat sequence of compressions and ventilations until the object is removed or EMS arrives.

Continuing Rescue Breathing

- If patient is still not breathing but you gave two successful breaths, begin CPR.

Performing CPR

- If the patient is unresponsive and not breathing normally, assess for a pulse for no more than 10 seconds. If there is no obvious pulse, start compressions. For the infant, the compression site is one finger-width below an imaginary line drawn across the nipples. Compress with the tips of two or three fingers approximately one-third the depth of the chest at a rate of at least 100 per minute. For two rescuers, use overlapping or side-by-side thumbs and compress on the middle third of the sternum just below the nipple line. The remaining fingers encircle the chest and support the back.
- For a single rescuer, deliver two ventilations following each set of 30 compressions. For two rescuers, deliver two breaths every 15 compressions.

Controlling Bleeding

- Use direct pressure as a primary method to control bleeding.
- If bleeding is not controlled, use elevation combined with direct pressure. If bleeding is still not controlled, apply a tourniquet.
- A small amount of blood loss (25 milliliters) is serious. Care for shock.

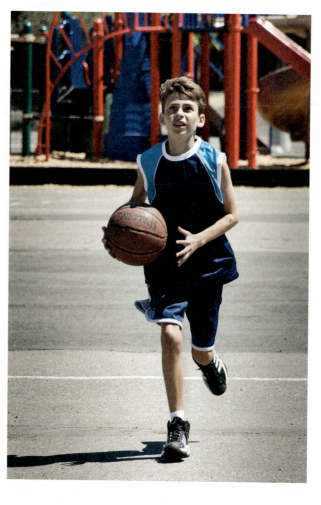

Children

One year to the onset of puberty

- Perform a primary assessment, establish your general impression from a distance.
- Ensure an adequate airway. If needed, provide ventilations as you watch for the chest to rise.
- Protect the head and spine.
- Control your emotions and facial expressions to help reduce the child's fear.
- Evaluate blood loss. Provide care to prevent shock.

Establishing Responsiveness: The child should move or cry when gently tapped or shaken.

Opening the Airway: Use slight head-tilt/chin-lift or jaw-thrust maneuver, as appropriate.

Evaluating Breathing: If the child is responsive but cyanotic or struggling and failing to breathe, assist ventilations and arrange for immediate transport. If the child is in respiratory arrest, open the airway and provide rescue breaths.

Rescue Breaths: If the child has a pulse but is not breathing normally, ventilate once every three to five seconds while watching for chest rise and fall. Ventilate with the mouth-to-mask technique, using an appropriate pediatric-size mask or a pediatric bag mask.

Clearing the Airway

- Make certain that you have the proper head tilt for an unresponsive child. Place a folded towel under shoulders to keep the head in a neutral position. If this does not open the airway, then:
- If the airway remains obstructed and the patient is responsive, perform abdominal thrusts.
- If the airway remains obstructed and the child is unresponsive, begin CPR.
- Do not attempt blind finger sweeps. You must see the object before you sweep the mouth. Use your little finger.
- Even if you did not see or dislodge an obstruction, begin chest compressions. After 30 compressions, look for and remove visible obstructions and attempt to ventilate again. Repeat sequence of compressions and ventilations until the object is removed or EMS arrives.

Performing CPR

- If the patient is unresponsive and not breathing normally, assess for a pulse for no more than 10 seconds.
- Have someone call 911. If you are alone, do CPR for two minutes before calling.
- If there is no obvious pulse, start compressions. For the child, the compression site is on the center of the chest between the nipples. Compress with the heel of one hand approximately one-third the depth of the chest at a rate of at least 100 per minute. Deliver two ventilations every 30 compressions.

Controlling Bleeding

- Use direct pressure as a primary method to control bleeding.
- If bleeding is not controlled, use elevation combined with direct pressure. If bleeding is still not controlled, apply a tourniquet.
- A blood loss of one-half liter (about one pint) is serious. Care for shock.

While assessing and caring for children, you will have to consider and work with the reactions of the parents or primary caregivers. Usually, the responses of a parent or guardian are positive and helpful even while they are concerned. Sometimes parents will react with strong emotional responses that can hinder your care. Both types of reactions are natural.

Ask the anxious caregiver to help you with tasks such as holding and reassuring the child, holding a dressing in place, holding the oxygen mask, or assisting with any other device you need to use in your care of the child. If this does not work to calm the parent, have a friend, neighbor, or other Emergency Medical Responder distract the parent with questions about the child's history or with getting the child's toy, favorite blanket, or clean clothes.

Some children who are seriously ill or injured are recuperating or being cared for at home while attached to medical equipment. These children may be on special monitors, have special tubes in their throats or abdomens, have intravenous lines containing medications, or be in special traction units.

You do not have to learn how to operate all the different types of special equipment, nor are you expected to. The parent will know how to manage the equipment. Your concern will be how to help the child, and the parent can assist you in providing care. Ask the parents what they need you to do and how. Then help the parents do it.

Sometimes this special equipment malfunctions and, again, the parent may be anxious and unsure. Calm the parents, and remind them that they have had training and that you will do what you can to help as they give you instructions. If the parents still hesitate, ask them to contact the child's doctor or the medical supply company that provided the equipment. Most of these companies will have emergency contact numbers and staff on call 24/7 to assist with equipment emergencies.

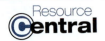

Complete an interactive animation to learn more about special considerations of pediatric patients.

infant ▶ a child between that ages of birth to one year.

toddler ▶ a child between the ages of one and three years old.

school age ▶ a child between the ages of 6 and 12 years of age.

adolescent ▶ a child between the ages of 12 and 18 years old.

IS IT SAFE?

The fontanels of a young infant are soft spots where the bones of the skull have not grown together. These areas are not quite as fragile as some may believe. Although you certainly should not poke and prod or apply firm pressure to these areas, they can be gently palpated without causing harm to the infant.

Age, Size, and Response

You will find that you instinctively treat infants and children differently from adults. You will know that an infant needs to be handled and cared for differently than a toddler, and that a toddler is spoken to and cared for differently than a school-age child or a teenager. Through proper training and experience, you will become familiar with the age ranges, mental and physical development, and varying needs of pediatric patients so you can assess and care for them appropriately.

You have already learned that for the purpose of performing CPR, pediatric patients are classified as infants (up to one year) and as children (one year up to the onset of puberty). After that, CPR is performed on them the same as it is performed on an adult.

When assessing and caring for pediatric patients, keep the following developmental categories in mind (Table 23.1):

- *Infants.* Babies from birth to one year old are considered to be **infants**.
- *Toddlers.* **Toddlers** are from one to three years old.
- *Preschool.* Children ages three to six are called preschool children.
- *School-age.* Usually in elementary school, **school-age** children are 6 to 12 years old.
- *Adolescents.* Usually in middle and high school, **adolescents** are 12 to 18 years old.

Each of the developmental stages requires a slightly different approach to assessment. However, there will be times when you are unable to determine the age of an infant or a child. Some are large or small for their age, and parents may not be there to help you. You will have to estimate age based on the physical size, emotional responses, interaction with you, and language skills.

Special Considerations

You already realize that infants and children are not the same as adults in size, emotional maturity, and responses. You should be aware that there are important anatomical differences as well. Consider the following important differences and comparisons.

Head and Neck

A child's head is proportionately larger and heavier than his body. The body will catch up with the size of the head at about age six. Because of the size and weight of the head, the child can be considered top heavy and is more likely to land head first in a sudden fall or stop.

TABLE 23.1 | Developmental Characteristics of Infants and Children

AGE GROUP	CHARACTERISTICS	ASSESSMENT AND CARE STRATEGIES
Newborns (birth to one month)	Infants do not like to be separated from their parents.	Have the parent hold the infant while you examine him.
Infants (birth to one year)	They have minimal stranger anxiety. They are used to being undressed but like to feel warm, physically and emotionally. The younger infant follows movement with his or her eyes. The older infant is more active, developing a personality. They do not want to be "suffocated" by an oxygen mask.	Be sure to keep the infant warm. Also, warm your hands and stethoscope before touching the infant. It may be best to observe the infant's breathing from a distance, noting the rise and fall of the abdomen for normal breathing and the chest for respiratory distress, the level of activity, and the infant's color. Examine the heart and lungs first and the head last. This is perceived as less threatening and therefore less likely to cause crying. A pediatric nonrebreather mask may be held near the face to provide blow-by oxygen.
Toddlers (one to three years)	Toddlers do not like to be touched or separated from their parents. They may believe that their illness is a punishment for being bad. Unlike infants, they do not like having their clothing removed. They frighten easily, overreact, and have a fear of needles and pain. They may understand more than they communicate. They begin to assert their independence. They do not want to be "suffocated" by an oxygen mask.	Have a parent hold the child while you examine him. Assure the child that he was not bad. Remove an article of clothing, examine the toddler, and then replace the clothing. Examine in a toe-to-head approach to build confidence. (Touching the head first may be frightening.) Explain what you are going to do in terms he can understand. (Taking the blood pressure may be a "squeeze" or a "hug on the arm.") Offer the comfort of a favorite toy. Consider giving him a choice: "Do you want me to look at your belly first or your feet first?" A pediatric nonrebreather mask may be held near the face to provide blow-by oxygen.
Preschool (three to six years)	Preschoolers do not like to be touched or separated from their parents. They are modest and do not like their clothing removed. They may believe that their illness is a punishment for being bad. They have a fear of blood, pain, and permanent injury. They are curious, communicative, and can be cooperative. They do not want to be "suffocated" by an oxygen mask.	Have a parent hold the child while you examine him. Respect the child's modesty. Remove an article of clothing, examine him, and then replace the clothing. Have a calm, confident, reassuring, and respectful manner. Be sure to offer explanations about what you are doing. Allow the child the responsibility of giving the history. Explain as you examine. A pediatric nonrebreather mask may be held near the face to provide blow-by oxygen. Do not lie. Explain that what you do to help may hurt.
School age (6 to 12 years)	This age group cooperates but likes their opinions heard. They fear blood, pain, disfigurement, and permanent injury. They are modest and do not like their bodies exposed.	Allow the child the responsibility of giving the history. Explain as you examine. Present a confident, calm, and respectful manner. Respect the child's modesty. Do not lie. Explain that what you do to help may hurt.
Adolescent (12 to 18 years)	Adolescents want to be treated as adults. They generally feel that they are indestructible but may have fears of permanent injury and disfigurement. They vary in their emotional and physical development and may not be comfortable with their changing bodies.	Although they want to be treated as adults, they may need as much support as children. Present a confident, calm, respectful manner. Be sure to explain what you are doing. Respect their modesty. You may consider assessing them away from their parents. Have the physical exam done by an Emergency Medical Responder of the same sex as the patient if possible. Do not lie. Explain that what you do to help may hurt.

Always handle the head of the newborn with caution because of the fontanels (soft spots). The largest soft spot, the one on top of the head, does not close completely until about 18 months of age. This soft spot is flat when the infant is quiet, and you may see it pulsate with each heartbeat. If the soft spot is sunken, the child may have lost a lot of fluids (dehydration) because illness has caused inadequate fluid intake or diarrhea and vomiting. If the soft spot is bulging, it may indicate that there is increased pressure inside the skull. This can be due to brain swelling from trauma or from an illness such as meningitis. Because the fontanels also can bulge when the infant is agitated and crying, they should be assessed when the infant is quiet.

In any head injury, look for blood and clear fluids leaking from the nose and ears, just as you would in adults.

When infants and small children suffer head injuries and also show signs of shock, suspect and assess for internal injuries as well.

The Airway and Respiratory System

The airway and respiratory systems of the infant and child are not fully developed. The tongue is large relative to the size of the mouth, and the airway is narrower than the adult airway and thus more easily obstructed.

When a child is lying on his back, the shape of the head may cause the airway to flex forward and close. Place a folded towel under the child's shoulders to help keep the head in line with the body and the airway open (Figure 23.2) There are some unique points to remember about children's breathing. Infants are obligate nose breathers. That is, they prefer to breathe through their nose. Make sure the nostrils are clear of secretions so the infant can breathe freely. Remember that the child's windpipe (trachea) is also softer, more flexible, and narrower than an adult's windpipe, and it will obstruct easily. Overextending a child's neck during airway management can cause the trachea to collapse and obstruct the airway.

Chest and Abdomen

Because the diaphragm is the major muscle of breathing, you will see more movement in the abdomen than in the chest. But the chest is more elastic, so when the child's breathing is labored or distressed, chest movement is obvious in the muscles between the ribs and in the muscles above the sternum around the neck and shoulders. The use of the accessory muscles for breathing is important to note and indicates the child is in urgent need of medical care.

The child's less developed and more elastic chest has both disadvantages to and advantages over an adult's chest. In a crushing mechanism of injury, the bones of the child's chest may not break, but they will flex. The disadvantage of this is that the more flexible chest offers less protection to the vital organs underneath (the heart and lungs). In the physical exam, the mechanism of injury is important and will help you determine possibility of internal injury, especially if there is no obvious external injury. Some signs to look

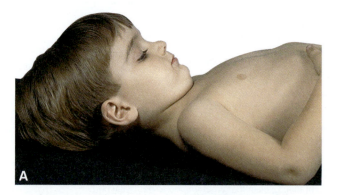
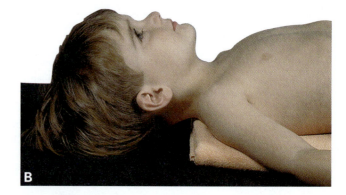

Figure 23.2 • (A) When an infant or young child is supine, the head will tip forward, obstructing the airway. (B) To keep the airway aligned, place a folded towel under the shoulders.

for are loss of symmetry (unequal appearance on both sides of the chest), unequal chest movement with breathing, and bruising over the chest.

Injury to the abdomen can result in tenderness, distention, and rigidity just as it can in adults. The abdominal muscles are not as well developed as they are in the adult and offer less protection. The abdominal organs (especially the liver and spleen) are large for the size of the cavity and are more susceptible to injury. A child who has a blunt abdominal injury can bleed out within minutes. Injury that causes distention or swelling can restrict movement of the diaphragm muscle and make it difficult for the child to breathe.

Pelvis

The child can lose a large amount of blood into the pelvic cavity as a result of trauma to the pelvic girdle. If you suspect hip or pelvis injury, monitor vital signs for shock just as you would in the adult and arrange for transport to a medical facility as soon as possible. Check for bleeding or bloody discharge from the genital area. Do not rock the hips to check for instability.

Extremities

Assess for circulation, sensation, and motor function in the distal extremities. Assess circulation by checking the pulse and capillary refill. Capillary refill is checked by pressing briefly and gently on the hand, foot, forearm, or lower leg. You do not have to press the tiny nail bed. Pressing on the skin will push blood out of the area, cause it to briefly whiten (blanch), and then suddenly refill when pressure is released. Capillary refill time should be less than two seconds.

Injuries that cause soft-tissue swelling or displaced or broken bones can restrict circulation. Always check both pulses and capillary refill in injured extremities. If you should apply a splint or other immobilization device, recheck circulation, sensation, and motor function after the splint is in place.

Children's bones are less developed and more flexible, and will bend and splinter before they break. Provide care for injury sites where there are signs and symptoms of painful, swollen, and/or deformed extremities, especially at any joint.

Children have growth plates at the ends of each long bone. A growth plate is developing tissue and the weakest area of a growing bone. A child who seriously injures a joint is likely to damage the growth plate, which determines the future length and shape of the mature bone. Growth-plate injuries may be the result of falls, competitive sports, recreational activities, and even overuse. Pay special attention to a child who complains of pain or who has swelling or deformity in any joint.

Body Surface Area

Infants and children have a large amount of total surface area (skin) in proportion to total body mass. The large surface can easily lose heat and cause the pediatric patient to become chilled, or hypothermic, even in an environment in which an adult feels comfortable. It is important to keep infants and children covered and warm, especially if there is trauma and blood loss or illness and fluid loss.

Blood Volume

The smaller the patient, the less blood volume the patient has. The newborn may have slightly less than 12 ounces, or about a cup and a half of blood, and cannot afford to lose much. As children grow, their blood volume increases. By age eight, they will have about two liters (roughly one-half gallon) of blood. Moderate blood loss in an adult may not concern you if it is easily controlled, but the same amount of blood loss in an infant or small child can be life threatening.

Vital Signs

Pulse and respiratory rates vary with the size of the child. The smaller the child, the higher the rates are. Table 23.2 lists pulse and respiratory rates for infants and children.

IS IT SAFE?

Never make an assumption that a child is stable or otherwise healthy based on just one set of vital signs. The signs and symptoms of children and infants must be continually assessed for changes. Those changes will reveal important trends in the child's condition.

TABLE 23.2 | Pulse and Respiratory Rates

AGE	AVERAGE PULSE RATE (PER MINUTE)	AVERAGE RESPIRATORY RATE (PER MINUTE)
Newborn (birth to one month)	120–160	30–50
Infant (one month to one year)	80–230	25–30
Toddler (one to three years)	80–130	20–30
Preschool (three to six years)	80–120	20–30
School age (6 to 12 years)	70–110	15–30
Adolescent (12 to 18 years)	60–105	12–20

Blood pressure also varies in children and depends on their sex, age, and height. Boys have slightly higher blood pressure than girls do. Taller children have higher blood pressure than shorter children. The following factors will influence blood pressure readings:

- *Time of day.* Blood pressure fluctuates during waking hours and is lower during sleeping hours.
- *Physical activity.* Blood pressure is higher during and immediately after exercise or activity, such as running, playing ball, or jumping rope, and it is slower during inactive periods, such as reading, coloring, or watching television.
- *Emotional moods or feelings.* Blood pressure fluctuates when the child is afraid, angry, stressed, or happy.
- *Physical condition.* The blood pressure will rise or fall based on the type of illness or an injury.

If you are trained to take blood pressure, use the appropriate size cuff when you take a child's blood pressure. It should cover about one-half of the child's upper arm. Cuffs that are too small or too large may give inaccurate readings. Although there are so many factors that can affect a child's blood pressure, you can still determine an appropriate systolic range by using some simple calculations:

- To determine the upper limit of a child's systolic blood pressure, multiply the child's age in years by 2 and add 90: (age × 2) + 90 = upper limit of systolic blood pressure.
- To determine the lower limit of a child's systolic blood pressure, multiply the child's age in years by 2 and add 70: (age × 2) + 70 = lower limit of systolic blood pressure.

It is not necessary to measure a blood pressure on a child younger than the age of three in the prehospital setting.

Assessment of Infants and Children

Scene Size-up

Size up the scene just as you would a scene involving an adult, but approach slowly so you do not frighten the child. Determine scene safety and the number of patients involved in the emergency. Determine the mechanism of injury or the nature of illness. Prepare for patient care by putting on appropriate personal protective equipment. If you think you may need additional resources, call for them immediately.

Primary Assessment

General Impression

Forming a general impression involves looking at the child and the environment as you approach. Quickly gather critical information that will help you decide whether to hurry or take your time. From a short distance or from across a room, you can see if the child is alert, struggling to breathe, crying, quiet and listless, or unresponsive to your approach. Is the skin pale, bluish, or flushed? How is the child interacting with the environment, with those around him, and to you as you approach? What is the child's body position? From those clues, you can get a general impression of the child's status. In children, the general impression is an important indicator of the severity of illness.

Pediatric Assessment Triangle

A very effective tool used for establishing a general impression of a pediatric patient is known as the **pediatric assessment triangle (PAT)** (Figure 23.3). The PAT assessment tool utilizes three criteria to help make a quick determination as to the seriousness of the child's condition during the general impression. When combined with other signs and symptoms as well as the experience of the Emergency Medical Responder, it can be a very effective for quickly forming an accurate first impression. The three criteria of the PAT are as follows:

- *Appearance.* As you enter the scene and approach the patient, quickly assess the child's appearance. Is he alert and looking around? Is his behavior consistent for his age and the environment? A toddler will likely look frightened and may be crying at the sight of the EMS crew entering his home or the scene. This would be normal behavior for this age child. On the other hand, a child who is motionless and listless might be quite ill and feeling so poorly that he shows no concern for what is going on around him. Characteristics to consider when evaluating appearance of an ill or injured child are muscle tone, interactivity, consolability, gaze, and speech or cry.

OBJECTIVES

3. Explain various techniques that can be employed to maximize successful assessment of the pediatric patient.

4. Explain the components of the pediatric assessment triangle.

pediatric assessment triangle (PAT) ▶ a tool used to perform a general impression of a pediatric patient; the elements of the PAT are appearance, work of breathing, and circulation (perfusion).

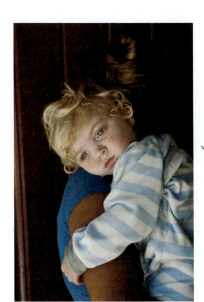
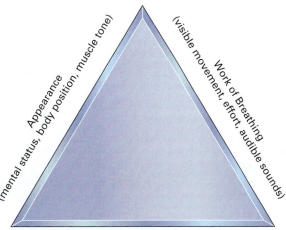
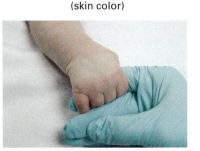
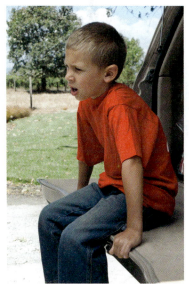

Appearance
(mental status, body position, muscle tone)

Work of Breathing
(visible movement, effort, audible sounds)

Circulation
(skin color)

Figure 23.3 • Pediatric assessment triangle.
(American Academy of Pediatrics)

Pediatric Assessment Triangle

While you may be concerned that you will not remember the components of the PAT, rest assured that this is simply a tool to help you organize your initial impression of the child. The goal of your rapid assessment is to determine if there is an immediate life threat. If there are no life threats, you will want to know if the child is "sick" or "not sick." "Sick" means that he or she has a condition that could quickly worsen. However, "not sick" does not mean he or she does not need EMS and medical evaluation.

work of breathing ▶ the effort that is required for a person to breathe.

retractions ▶ the inward movement of the soft tissues between the ribs when a child breathes in.

- *Work of breathing.* The term **work of breathing** refers to the effort that is required for a person to breathe. Normally, a child displays little to no work when breathing is normal. When a child is hypoxic or in distress, the work of breathing will increase and become more obvious. Typically, this can be seen as you approach the child. You will see obvious movement of the chest and abdomen with each breath, nasal flaring, and possibly retractions.

  Retractions are the inward movement of the soft tissue between the ribs when a child breathes in. They are a sign of significant distress. You also may hear sounds such as stridor or wheezing as the child breathes. These, too, are strong signs of an ill child. Note that you must bare the chest to see retractions.

- *Circulation.* This refers to how well the child is perfusing as evidenced by the presence of pulses and the color of the skin. Notice the general color of the skin. Compare the arms and legs with the trunk of the body. All areas should be an even shade of pink. For dark-skinned patients you will look for pink tissues inside the mouth and at the nail beds. Notice if the skin is mottled or blotchy, pale, or cyanotic (bluish). You also must check capillary refill time at the extremities as well as the trunk of the body. A delayed capillary refill time anywhere on the body is a possible sign of serious illness.

Once you reach the child, you can quickly determine mental status using the AVPU scale. Is the child alert? Is he responsive to your voice or only to a painful stimulus, such as squeezing his shoulder? Or is he unresponsive? Is he oriented to person, place, and time? An infant or a very young child is not able to answer questions about his name, where he is, or what day it is; however, parents or caregivers can explain if the child's actions are as they would normally expect them to be.

Next, quickly assess the child's ABCs. If the child is crying, you may assume that he has an airway and adequate breathing and circulation. For the quiet or unresponsive child, check the airway. Is it open? Check breathing. Is the child breathing normally or with effort? What is the rate? Is chest expansion adequate and equal? Are there noises such as grunting or a high-pitched sound (stridor) associated with the child's respiratory efforts? Is the skin cyanotic, indicating low oxygen levels? Check circulation. Is the pulse strong and regular? Is there any bleeding?

For all children, you will want to find out: Is the skin warm and dry, indicating normal circulation? Or is it cool and clammy, suggesting blood loss and shock? What skin areas are most accessible for you to determine cool and clammy skin? Is capillary refill time less than two seconds? Care for the life-threatening conditions that affect the ABCs first. Remember that the unresponsive child needs immediate care.

When you determine priority of transport, you will recognize the high-priority infant or child patient as one with:

- Displays a poor general impression
- Has an altered mental status
- Has an airway problem
- Exhibits respiratory distress or inadequate breathing
- Has a possibility of developing shock
- Has evidence of bleeding that may soon result in shock

Managing the Airway

The airway is your first concern in the care of any patient. Always ensure that the airway is open and clear and that the patient is breathing adequately or is receiving appropriate ventilations and supplemental oxygen when necessary. Follow local protocols.

Opening the Airway

When a child lies on his back, the tongue may fall to the back of the throat much like in an adult. Remember that with an infant or child the tongue is larger in relation to the body and can more easily obstruct the airway. Also, when lying on his back, the larger head of the infant may cause the head to flex or bend forward and close off the airway. In small children, if you are not careful when opening the airway, you may cause hyperextension or bend the head too far back, which also can close off the airway. You must be sure to align the head and neck or place it in a neutral position so that the airway is open.

As noted previously in this chapter, you can easily position the infant or small child correctly by placing a towel under the shoulders. Check for breathing before repositioning the head. Then, if necessary, perform a slight head-tilt or a jaw-thrust maneuver to assess breathing and provide ventilations.

continued

KEY POINT ▼

An infant's tongue, as well as a hyperflexed or hyperextended head, can easily obstruct the airway.

FIRST ON SCENE

After radioing for an ambulance and notifying dispatch of the description and direction of the suspect vehicle, Bryn quickly flips the car radio to loudspeaker mode. "Attention! This is the police! Is anyone injured?" She speaks clearly into the mic. Her voice bounces off the surrounding buildings and echoes into the distant concrete canyons of the city's west side. People are cautiously standing up all around the intersection, looking around with wide eyes.

There is no indication of other injuries, so Bryn turns her attention to the baby. She gently removes the child from the arms of the sobbing woman and sets the bundle onto the hood of her patrol car. The baby cries weakly as she unwraps the blanket and examines the little pale body. There is a ragged wound to the child's lower abdomen and a small round hole in the lower back. Blood flows steadily from both wounds, and Bryn cradles the baby in one arm as she runs to the trunk of the patrol car to get the Emergency Medical Responder bag.

Clearing and Maintaining the Airway

If air does not enter easily or the chest does not rise when providing rescue breaths, reposition the head and try again. If you still have no success in ventilating the patient, perform 30 compressions. Then check the mouth to see if there is an obstruction. If you see one, sweep the mouth with the little finger of your gloved hand. Do not perform blind finger sweeps.

If there are fluids in the airway, clear them by sweeping the mouth with a gauze pad or by suctioning. Check with your instructor to see if Emergency Medical Responders are allowed to use suctioning equipment in your area. If so, your instructor will provide you with training. You also may be able to use nasopharyngeal and oropharyngeal airways in the infant and child patient. Again, your instructor will let you know and give you appropriate training.

IS IT SAFE?

Do not perform blind finger sweeps when trying to clear an airway obstruction.

Providing Oxygen

In some jurisdictions, and for some EMS agencies, training Emergency Medical Responders in oxygen delivery is optional. If you are allowed to provide oxygen to patients, your instructor will have the appropriate equipment and train you how and when to use it with pediatric patients.

The oxygen requirement for children can be more than that of adults. A low oxygen level (hypoxia) causes serious physical reactions in children. It can affect the heart rate, slowing the pulse and reducing oxygen circulating to tissues. This in turn affects the brain, decreasing oxygen to cells and causing altered mental status and tissue death.

Providing oxygen may be a vital part of the emergency care procedures used in caring for children. However, it may be difficult to deliver in the prehospital setting. Children

Blow-by Technique

When administering oxygen by the blow-by technique, avoid blowing the oxygen directly into the child or infant's face. It can frighten the pediatric patient and in the case of the infant can cause him to hold his breath, which could worsen respiratory status.

may resist having a mask placed over the face, and the flow of oxygen may even cause children to hold their breath. The Emergency Medical Responder can still provide oxygen to children who need it by using a blow-by technique.

To perform the blow-by technique, hold, or have the parent hold, the oxygen tubing or the pediatric nonrebreather mask about two inches from the child's face. The oxygen will enrich the area in front of the face as it blows by and the child inhales (Figure 23.4). Oxygen tubing can be pushed through the bottom of a paper cup and provide oxygen effectively. The advantage to this method is the child will likely be curious about the cup and hold it to his face to examine it or try to drink from it. At the same time the child is receiving oxygen, he also will calm down because he has something of interest to keep his attention. Do not use a Styrofoam cup because it could crumble and particles can blow into the child's face, eyes, and airway.

If the patient is not breathing, provide rescue breaths. For infants, provide rescue breaths at a rate of one breath every three to five seconds using a pediatric-size pocket face mask or a bag-mask device of the correct size. Remember the following steps when ventilating:

- Breathe less forcefully through the pocket face mask. Watch for the chest to rise. Ventilate slowly so as not to cause stomach distention.
- Excessive force is not needed with the bag-mask device. Watch for the chest to rise.
- Use a properly sized face mask to get a good mask-to-face seal.
- Do not use flow-restricted, oxygen-powered ventilation devices (demand valves) on infants and children.
- If ventilations are not successful, perform the procedures for clearing an obstructed airway. Then try to ventilate again.

Secondary Assessment

After completing your primary assessment, focus on getting a history and conducting a physical exam. Those steps may be done at the scene with the responsive patient and

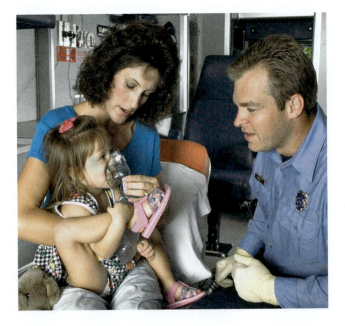

Figure 23.4 • Hold the oxygen mask close to the child's face to provide blow-by oxygen.

while you are waiting for the ambulance to arrive. Normally, infants or very young children will not respond to your questions, but children older than two or three years will be able to answer questions requiring a yes/no answer. They also can tell you or point to where it hurts. Otherwise, parents or other caregivers, such as babysitters or teachers, will have to give you information about the child's history and how he became sick or hurt.

While you are getting a general impression of the child, decide if he is seriously injured or sick. For any child who is, perform a rapid assessment just as you would do for an adult:

- *Patient with significant mechanism of injury (MOI).* Maintain manual in-line stabilization of the head and spine while performing a primary assessment. Inspect and palpate each body area. Get baseline vital signs and, if possible, get a history.
- *Unresponsive patient.* Maintain manual in-line stabilization of the head and spine while performing a primary assessment. Inspect and palpate each body area. Get a history if possible from those at the scene. Get baseline vital signs.

If your general impression leads you to decide that the child is responding or acting normally, then perform a secondary assessment:

- *Trauma patient with no significant MOI.* Determine the chief complaint. Inspect and palpate the area. Get baseline vital signs. Gather a history that focuses on the injury and events that caused the injury.
- *Responsive medical patient.* Determine the chief complaint, or the nature of illness. Gather a history of the events leading up to the illness and the illness itself. Focus your physical exam on the area of complaint, or inspect and palpate the part of the body involved. Get baseline vital signs.

Physical Exam

Now that you have completed a focused assessment, you may have time to perform a more detailed physical exam. This exam is similar to what you do for an adult, except for the frightened or crying infant or young child, it is performed in reverse order (toe to head). This will give the child an opportunity to get used to you and your touch, if he has not done so during the short focused assessment.

In a medical situation, examine the child in more detail from toe to head, while he is in the parent's lap or being held by a trusted caregiver. In a trauma situation with no significant MOI, let the parent or other trusted caregiver help comfort the child while you begin your exam.

Always explain to the child and parent what you are doing, and make sure that both understand. Most young children are used to being dressed and undressed and examined by their doctors and will not be embarrassed. As they get older, children are more modest and have learned that strangers should not touch them. Only remove or rearrange clothing that must be moved for you to determine what is wrong with the child during your exam. Then replace it when you have examined that part of the body.

Trauma patients with a significant MOI or unresponsive medical patients who require a rapid assessment are usually unresponsive or too critically injured or ill to know or care where you start your assessment. Stabilize the head and neck before you reposition the head to assess the ABCs in a trauma case, and then follow the steps described above.

Reassessment

You are never finished with your patient until he has been turned over to an equal or higher level of medical care. This means that when you finish your secondary assessment, you will start again. This is called the reassessment, and it will continue until EMT or ALS personnel arrive. The status of a child can change rapidly and frequently, so reassess mental status, maintain airway, monitor breathing, check pulse, and reevaluate skin color, temperature, and condition. Take and record vital signs every five minutes for unstable patients and every 15 minutes for stable patients. Continue to monitor the effects of interventions, provide appropriate care, and give emotional support.

5. State the most common cause of cardiac arrest in the pediatric patient.

10. Explain the assessment and management of the following emergencies in pediatric patients: (a) upper airway obstruction, (b) lower reactive airway disease, (c) seizures, and (d) shock.

IS IT SAFE?

Emergency Medical Responders should consider all respiratory disorders in children as serious and take action immediately. Respiratory distress and low oxygen levels in children are the primary causes of cardiac arrest not related to trauma.

KEY POINT ▼

Never perform a blind finger sweep on an infant or a child, and never perform abdominal thrusts on an infant.

Managing Specific Medical Emergencies

Many of the specific medical emergencies listed here have been described in detail in other chapters. Much of the care you will provide to infants and children is similar to what you would provide to adults.

Respiratory Emergencies

Emergency Medical Responders do not usually receive the in-depth training for determining different respiratory illnesses and causes of airway and breathing problems in pediatric patients. This section lists some common causes, covers general signs and symptoms, and describes the general management of respiratory emergencies in pediatric patients (Figure 23.5).

Guidelines for the assessment and emergency care of a pediatric patient with any respiratory emergency are summarized in Figure 23.6. It is important to note that *the most common cause of cardiac arrest in infants and children is respiratory arrest*. Identifying and caring for a respiratory problem early can minimize the chances of cardiac arrest.

Airway Obstruction

You may want to review the signs and symptoms and the management of partial and complete airway obstruction for pediatric patients in Chapter 8. Continue to review and practice them during and after your training. This will enable you to act quickly to ensure an open airway and adequate breathing for all patients. Because the steps of relieving an obstructed airway in infants are different than for adults, practice the steps of back blows and chest thrusts frequently so that you can perform them quickly and effectively. Remember that the unresponsive child needs immediate care.

Difficulty Breathing

There are many types of airway and respiratory infections and conditions that cause airway and breathing problems. A simple cold can plug the nose and make breathing difficult, but the nose can be easily cleared by blowing or suctioning. A respiratory infection

Figure 23.5 • Signs of early respiratory distress.

SIGNS OF EARLY RESPIRATORY DISTRESS

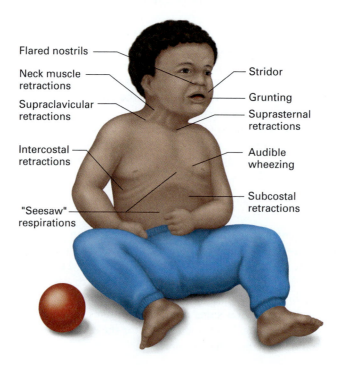

Flared nostrils

Neck muscle retractions

Supraclavicular retractions

Intercostal retractions

"Seesaw" respirations

Stridor

Grunting

Suprasternal retractions

Audible wheezing

Subcostal retractions

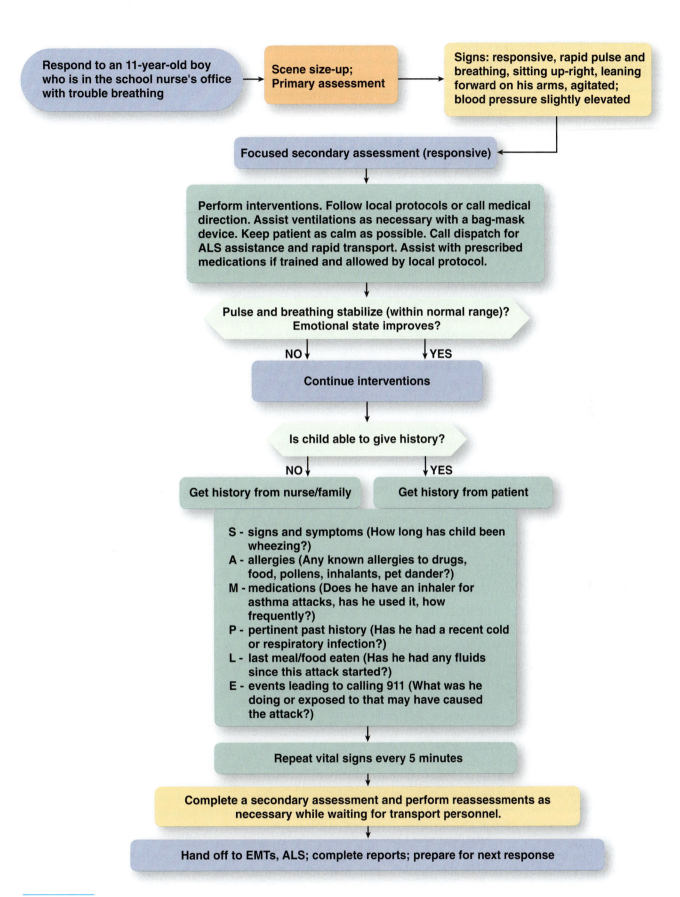

Figure 23.6 • Algorithm for the emergency care of pediatric patients with respiratory emergencies.

OBJECTIVES

5. State the most common cause of cardiac arrest in the pediatric patient.

10. Explain the assessment and management of the following emergencies in pediatric patients: (a) upper airway obstruction, (b) lower reactive airway disease, (c) seizures, and (d) shock.

croup ▶ an acute respiratory condition common in infants and children that is characterized by a barking type of cough or stridor.

epiglottitis ▶ swelling of the epiglottis that may be caused by a bacterial infection; may cause airway obstruction.

IS IT SAFE?

When caring for a patient with suspected croup or epiglottitis, *do not* attempt to examine the mouth by placing a tongue blade or bite stick in the mouth. Doing so could cause rapid swelling of the tissues of the throat and upper airway. This could lead to complete airway obstruction. If you see a child presenting with signs and symptoms of croup or epiglottitis, call for transport immediately and keep the child comfortable and calm.

KEY POINT ▼

Whenever possible, listen for evidence of wheezing. A child with a history of asthma who is in respiratory distress and who is not wheezing is at serious risk of respiratory failure.

---

can cause swelling of the respiratory tract or blocking by mucous secretions, making it difficult to breathe.

Another respiratory problem that occurs in some infants involves periods of time when they will stop breathing and then start up again on their own. This period of interrupted breathing is known as *apnea*. In almost all cases, apnea occurs while sleeping. For this reason, it is called *sleep apnea*. Some cases of sleep apnea are related to airway obstruction, while others are associated with failure in the central nervous system to stimulate respiration during sleep. The relationship between apnea and sudden infant death syndrome (SIDS) is still under study.

Respiratory Infections

Upper respiratory tract infections are very common in infants and children. One such infection is known as **croup**, and any infant or child with noisy respiration and a hoarse cough may have it. Croup is an infection caused by a virus and affects the larynx (voice box), trachea, and bronchi. It usually causes the tissues in the upper airway to become swollen, restricting airflow.

A less common problem that can affect the respiratory status of a pediatric patient is known as **epiglottitis**. It occurs when the epiglottis (the flap that closes over the trachea while swallowing) becomes inflamed. Epiglottitis can have a sudden onset in what seems to be an otherwise healthy child. Suspect this respiratory emergency if the child develops a rapid fever, has cold-like symptoms, has difficulty swallowing, and is drooling. Children with epiglottitis also will sit upright in a *tripod position* (leaning forward with arms braced on the edge of the bed or chair) with the chin thrust out and the mouth wide open. You will notice that they will use the muscles in their upper chest and those around their shoulders and neck to breathe. This effort to breathe is very tiring for the child. The Emergency Medical Responder must act quickly. Although rare, epiglottitis is considered life threatening.

Because it may be difficult to determine what type of respiratory emergency an infant or a child is having, consider any airway problem or breathing difficulty a life-threatening emergency. Call for transport immediately. Provide oxygen as soon as possible using a blow-by technique if you cannot get the child to accept a face mask or a nasal cannula. Do not place anything in the child's mouth (a tongue depressor, for example) in an attempt to examine the airway. Probing the mouth can cause spasms that will further close the airway. Avoid any actions that might agitate or stimulate the child.

Signs and symptoms of respiratory distress include the following:

- Wheezing or a high-pitched harsh noise, or grunting
- Exhaling with abnormal effort
- Breathing that is faster or slower than normal, is inadequate, and requires assisted ventilations and oxygen
- Use of accessory muscles to breathe
- Child holding a tripod position
- Drooling
- Nasal flaring
- Cyanosis (late sign)
- Capillary refill of more than two seconds (late sign)
- Slow heart rate (late sign)
- Altered mental status (late sign)

Asthma is also a respiratory condition common to children. It can become life threatening if left untreated. Most children who have asthma use a medication or inhaler prescribed by their doctors. Parents or caregivers call for assistance for a child with asthma if the signs and symptoms are new and unfamiliar, do not respond to at-home care, or the child is not responding to the usual prescribed treatment. Signs and symptoms of asthma occur when the small airways in the lungs go into spasm and constrict or become too narrow for air to pass through. Something the child eats or breathes or unusual excitement may trigger the attack.

Signs and symptoms of asthma include:

- Shortness of breath
- Wheezing that can be heard with a stethoscope and possibly without
- Obvious respiratory distress with easy inhalation and forced expiration
- Cough
- Faster than normal breathing rate
- Increased heart rate
- Sleepiness or slowed response
- Bluish (cyanotic) tint to the skin, especially around the lips and eyes

Provide emergency care to the pediatric patient who has difficulty breathing and the above signs and symptoms by following these steps:

1. Act calmly and with assurance, which will help calm and reassure the child and the parents or caregiver. For mild distress, the child will be agitated. For severe distress, the child will be exhausted and unable or unwilling to move. Signs of sleepiness and slow response mean low oxygen levels.

2. Place the child in a sitting position. The child will likely have taken a position of comfort that makes it easy for him to breathe, usually a tripod position (leaning forward and bracing himself on his forearms).

3. Administer oxygen. (Follow local protocols.) Ask the child to breathe in normally but to blow out air forcefully, as if blowing out the candles on a birthday cake or blowing up a balloon. Show the child how and breathe with him.

4. If you are allowed to assist in giving medications, help the parents or caregiver administer the child's medication. Check local protocols and always call for medical direction before assisting a patient with medications. (See Appendix 2.)

5. Have the parents or caregiver contact the child's physician.

6. Arrange for transport by ambulance. A severe and ongoing asthma attack that is not relieved by medication and oxygen may be *status asthmaticus*, a very serious and life-threatening condition.

In cases of respiratory distress, provide oxygen by a pediatric-size nonrebreather mask (Figure 23.7) or by using the blow-by technique. For severe distress and respiratory arrest, provide assisted ventilations with a pediatric-size bag mask and supplemental oxygen and call for support (Figure 23.8).

Always allow the child to assume a comfortable position. The alert child will naturally find the position in which it is easiest to breathe. Remember, if you are not trained to use oxygen or do not carry it, call for transport at the first sign of respiratory distress in children.

Seizures

A seizure will cause a sudden change in mental status as well as sensation, behavior, or movement. The more severe forms of seizure cause violent muscle contractions called *convulsions*. Seizures may be the result of high fever, epilepsy, infections, poisoning, low blood sugar (hypoglycemia), or head injury. They also may occur when the brain does not receive enough oxygen because of inadequate blood circulation (shock) or inadequate oxygen in the blood (hypoxia). In some cases, there is no known cause. Many children suffer seizures, but they are rarely life threatening. Seizures caused by fever

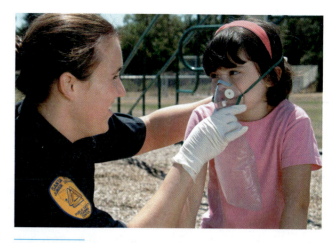

Figure 23.7 • For respiratory distress, provide oxygen with a correctly sized pediatric nonrebreather mask placed on the child, or use the blow-by method.

OBJECTIVE

10. Explain the assessment and management of the following emergencies in pediatric patients: (a) upper airway obstruction, (b) lower reactive airway disease, (c) seizures, and (d) shock.

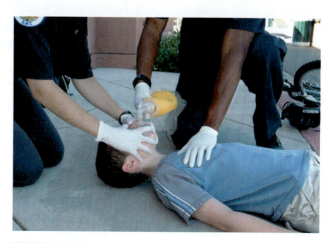

Figure 23.8 • If respirations are inadequate, provide assisted ventilations with the bag-mask device.

(**febrile** seizures) should be taken seriously. If a child is having prolonged or multiple seizures and has an altered mental status, consider it a life-threatening emergency and call for transport immediately.

In many cases, a patient's seizures stop before EMS arrives. After a seizure, it is normal for children to be either lethargic (drowsy) and difficult to arouse or agitated and combative. Look for signs of illness or injury and question the child or family about symptoms. Also get the following information:

- Has the child had prior seizures? How long did they last? What part of the body was affected?
- Has the child had a fever?
- Has the child had an injury or fall in which the head may have been struck?
- Is the child taking any medications, specifically medication for seizures?
- Did the child's skin (nail beds and mucous membranes) change from its normal color to bluish or grayish, indicating low oxygen (hypoxia)?

Any child who has had a seizure must have a medical evaluation. Arrange for transport as soon as possible. In the meantime, provide the following emergency care steps:

1. Maintain an open airway and insert nothing in the mouth.
2. Look for evidence of injury suffered during the seizure.
3. If you do not suspect spine injury, position the child on his side.
4. Be alert for vomiting.
5. Provide oxygen or assisted ventilations with supplemental oxygen, if allowed to do so.
6. Monitor breathing and altered mental status.

Altered Mental Status

Any medical or trauma emergency that affects the brain can cause an altered mental status. Examples include low blood sugar (hypoglycemia), poisoning, infection, head injury, decreased oxygen levels, shock, and seizures. As you assess the child, note the mechanism of injury or nature of illness, which will give clues to causes of the child's mental status. Look for signs of poisoning (ingested, inhaled, or absorbed), and ask family members or teachers if there is a history of diabetes or seizure disorder. Take and monitor vital signs, which can indicate shock as a cause. While observing and examining the child, you may notice signs of sleepiness, confusion, agitation, or listlessness.

As you gather information, perform the following emergency care steps:

OBJECTIVE

10. Explain the assessment and management of the following emergencies in pediatric patients: (a) upper airway obstruction, (b) lower reactive airway disease, (c) seizures, and (d) shock.

1. Maintain an open airway, but protect the spine in cases of trauma. If necessary, ventilate the patient.
2. Provide oxygen as soon as possible by nonrebreather mask, or assist ventilations with a bag-mask device and supplemental oxygen.
3. Place the patient in the recovery position if there is no indication of spine injury. Care for shock.
4. Arrange to transport as soon as possible.

Shock

Common causes of shock in infants and children include losing large amounts of fluid from diarrhea and vomiting, blood loss, and abdominal injuries and other trauma. Shock from fluid loss occurs quickly in infants and is a serious emergency. Call for transport immediately. Although not as common, shock also can be caused by allergic reactions, poisoning, and, rarely, cardiac-related problems.

The child's body can compensate for shock for a long time, but the body's compensating mechanisms can suddenly fail. This failure is called *decompensated shock*. It occurs when the body can no longer function or compensate for low blood volume or lack of perfusion of oxygenated blood to the brain. As a result, the child has an altered mental

KEY POINT ▼

In the adult, shock typically develops more gradually, and the signs tend to be easier to recognize. In the child, you must suspect and anticipate shock and begin caring for it immediately, even before you see definite signs of it.

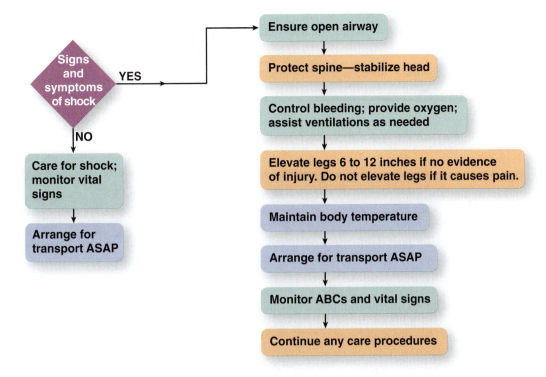

Figure 23.9 • Algorithm for the emergency care of pediatric patients with signs of shock.

status and the blood pressure drops (hypotension). When a child goes into the decompensated shock stage, signs and symptoms of shock can develop rapidly and include:

- Rapid heart and respiratory rate. (Both heart rate and respiratory rate will reflect the course of shock.)
- Weak or absent pulse
- Delayed capillary refill
- Decreased urine output (information from parents), which indicates dehydration
- Altered mental status
- Pale, cool, clammy skin
- Sunken fontanels

Provide the following care in your management of the sick or injured infant or child who has evidence of shock (Figure 23.9):

1. Ensure an open airway, but protect the spine in cases of trauma. Provide ventilations, if necessary.
2. Provide oxygen by nonrebreather mask or assist ventilations by bag-mask device with supplemental oxygen as per local protocols.
3. Control any bleeding and dress wounds.
4. Elevate the legs if there is no trauma or suspected spine injury.
5. Maintain body warmth, but do not overheat.
6. Arrange to transport as soon as possible.
7. While waiting for EMT personnel to arrive or while en route, continue to monitor airway, breathing, and vital signs and continue any care.

Fever

The body's normal response to many childhood diseases and infections is a high temperature or fever. But the rise in body temperature also may be caused by heat exposure, by a noninfectious disease problem, and even by childhood immunization shots. The parents

Fever

Frequently, rescuers are called for "child not breathing" only to be met with a crying child who is reported to have had a seizure and then stopped breathing. This is the most common presentation of a febrile seizure. The child may appear perfectly fine upon your arrival. However, it is vital that the child receives a medical evaluation to exclude any serious cause of the fever.

probably monitored their child's temperature and can report the temperature readings taken before you arrived. Try to find out how high the fever is and how rapidly it rose. Increased temperature is not necessarily what causes a seizure, but a rapid rise in body temperature can cause one.

A fever with a rash, long bouts of diarrhea and vomiting, little intake of fluids, or a fever that rose rapidly with or without seizure are all indications that a potentially serious medical condition may be present. Call for transport as soon as possible.

It is not necessary to try to take a temperature. If the skin feels very warm to touch, report this finding along with skin color and condition. A child with a high fever will likely be flushed (red) and dry. A mild fever may quickly elevate to a high fever and become a life-threatening problem.

If the child is hot to the touch and there is a history of fever reported by the parent or caregiver, take the following steps if your local protocols allow (Figure 23.10):

- Undress the child down to underwear or diaper, but do not allow him to become chilled. Many parents still believe that feverish children must be bundled up so they will not become chilled or so they will sweat out a fever. All this clothing retains the heat of the fever.
- Cover the child with a towel soaked in tepid (not cold) water if the fever is the result of heat exposure. If the child starts to shiver, stop the cooling process and cover with a light blanket.
- Place damp, cool cloths on the child's forehead.
- Call for the transport of any child who has had a seizure. If the child is seizing, monitor airway and breathing.
- *Never* submerge a child in cold water.
- *Never* use rubbing alcohol for cooling. It can be absorbed in toxic amounts through the child's skin.

Be cautious about cooling a fevered child. You can cause hypothermia or reduced body temperature. Wet towels and sheets cool rapidly and become cold, which causes the child to shiver and become chilled.

Hypothermia

Children lose a lot of body heat through their heads. The surface area of the child's head is proportionately larger than the rest of the body. The large head radiates and loses heat when it is uncovered. When the head is exposed, the body will make every effort to keep the brain warm and functioning, so it sends heat from other parts of the body to the head. Because the child cannot conserve heat well, it will not take long to use up any reserves and develop hypothermia. Keep the head covered to prevent heat loss when caring for infants and children in cool environments.

Children's bodies are unable to regulate temperatures as well as adult bodies can, even in normal room temperatures (68°F, or 20°C). Most children do not have much fat stored under their skin and cannot conserve heat. They can become chilled through the environment, injury, or illness, including:

- Exposure to cool weather and water
- Damp or wet clothes, or removal of clothes for medical evaluation

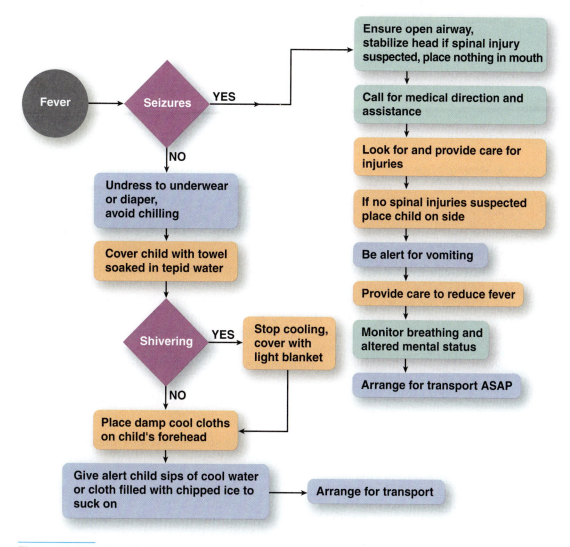

Figure 23.10 • Algorithm for the emergency care of pediatric patients with signs of fever.

- Alcohol or drugs, which dilate peripheral vessels
- Low blood sugar (hypoglycemia)
- Brain disorder or head trauma that affects the temperature regulation mechanism of the body
- Severe infection
- Shock

When you look for a mechanism of injury or try to determine the nature of illness, also think about conditions that can cause overcooling of the child. In a cold environment, warm the child by stripping off any wet clothing and by wrapping him in a blanket. Be sure the head is covered.

Diarrhea and Vomiting

The child can lose large amounts of needed body fluids through vomiting and diarrhea, which are normal reactions to illness (and sometimes to certain ingested poisons). This fluid loss is called *dehydration*. Infants are more susceptible to dehydration than adults are because the infant has such a small circulating blood volume to start with. For example, think about losing one cup of fluid during an illness. This would be insignificant to an adult, whereas the total circulating blood volume in a newborn is only a cup and a half.

Suspect that a child is dehydrated if he has been feverish for some time, if he has been vomiting without taking in any fluids, or if he has had diarrhea for several days. As the child loses fluids through vomiting and diarrhea and cannot replace them, the fluid balance in the body is disturbed. A balance of fluids-in to fluids-out is needed to maintain muscle and organ function. Shock can result when large amounts of fluids are lost, even if the fluid is not blood.

If you suspect a child is dehydrated, do the following:

1. Monitor the airway.
2. Position the child so the airway will not be obstructed if the child vomits. Elevating the legs may help if the patient is showing signs of shock.
3. Monitor respirations and administer blow-by oxygen as per local protocols.
4. Check vital signs. If they indicate shock, arrange to transport immediately.
5. If possible, save some vomit for hospital personnel to examine.

Poisoning

Part of a child's learning experience includes exploring and tasting things. This can sometimes lead to exposure to or ingestion of poisonous substances. Poisons can affect any or all of the body's systems and can rapidly threaten the life of a child. Much of your assessment and care will be the same as for an adult. Know your local protocols for contacting medical direction or a poison control center if there is any indication or suspicion that a child has been exposed to a poison. Be aware that some poisons may be considered hazardous materials, which will require response by specialized personnel trained to handle them.

Drowning

The child who has been submerged in water may still be alive or clinically dead (no breathing and no heartbeat) but not biologically dead (brain cells are still alive). Many patients have been revived after more than 30 minutes of submersion in cold water. Children have been successfully revived more often than adults in these situations. When caring for a possible drowning patient:

1. Make sure the airway is clear and free of fluids.
2. Provide artificial ventilations or CPR as necessary.
3. Protect the spine in cases where the near drowning was the result of a diving or boating incident.
4. Get the patient to a warm and dry environment away from wind to prevent or care for hypothermia. Remove wet clothing.
5. Place the child in the recovery position to prevent aspiration. Administer high-concentration oxygen (as per local protocols).
6. Obtain a baseline set of vital signs.
7. Arrange to transport all drowning patients, even if they have recovered and are breathing on their own. It is possible that they will deteriorate hours after they have recovered.

OBJECTIVES

6. Describe the signs and symptoms of sudden infant death syndrome (SIDS).

7. Explain the appropriate steps for management of a suspected SIDS death.

sudden infant death syndrome (SIDS) ▶ the sudden unexplained death of an apparently healthy baby during sleep.

Sudden Infant Death Syndrome (SIDS)

In the United States, **sudden infant death syndrome (SIDS)** claims thousands of infants each year. It is the sudden unexplained death of an apparently healthy baby during sleep. SIDS is most likely to occur in the first three months of life and may occur up to one year of age. Possible causes and theories are still being investigated. It is known that SIDS is not caused by external methods of suffocation, by vomiting, or by choking.

When Emergency Medical Responders arrive, they may see distraught parents with their infant in respiratory and cardiac arrest during the scene size-up. Because Emergency Medical Responders cannot diagnose SIDS, you must immediately start emergency care as you would for any patient in cardiac arrest. Provide resuscitation and arrange transport to the hospital. Assure the parents that everything is being done for the baby. Normally, Emergency Medical Responders will not begin resuscitation if there is obvious stiffening of the body (rigor mortis) or if blood has pooled (lividity) along whatever side the child was lying on. Check with your instructor to find out what your protocols require for this situation. In either case, be sure to provide emotional support to the parents.

Managing Trauma Emergencies

General Care of the Child Trauma Patient

Because of their size, curiosity, and lack of fear due to their inexperience, infants and children are frequent victims of trauma. It is the number one cause of death in people 1 to 18 years of age—as a result of motor-vehicle crashes, drowning, burns, firearms, falls, blunt and penetrating trauma, abuse, entrapment, crushing, and various other mechanisms of injury (Figure 23.11).

When performing a physical exam on a stable, responsive child, you may reverse your assessment order and do a toe-to-head physical exam. For unresponsive or unstable patients, perform the head-to-toe assessment, focus on the ABCs, and determine priority of transport.

When managing injuries in children, keep in mind that their larger head size and weight will make them more prone to head and neck trauma in motor-vehicle collisions, especially if unrestrained. This is also true of bicycle mishaps if children are not wearing helmets, in mishaps in which they are struck, in swimming and diving mishaps, and in sports mishaps. Expect abdominal and pelvic injuries in vehicle crashes in which the child is restrained, and extremity injuries in falls of three times their height or greater.

General emergency care steps for the infant or child trauma patient include the following (Figure 23.12):

1. Ensure an open airway. Manually stabilize the head and neck. Use a jaw-thrust maneuver to open the airway and protect the spine. Place a folded towel under the shoulders to maintain a neutral position for the airway and alignment of the head.

2. Make sure the airway is clear. Suction, if local protocols allow. If necessary, provide ventilations.

3. Provide oxygen by nonrebreather mask or assist ventilations with a bag-mask device with supplemental oxygen as per local protocols.

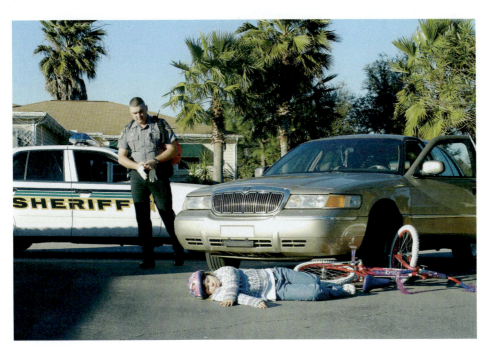

Figure 23.11 • Look for the mechanism of injury.

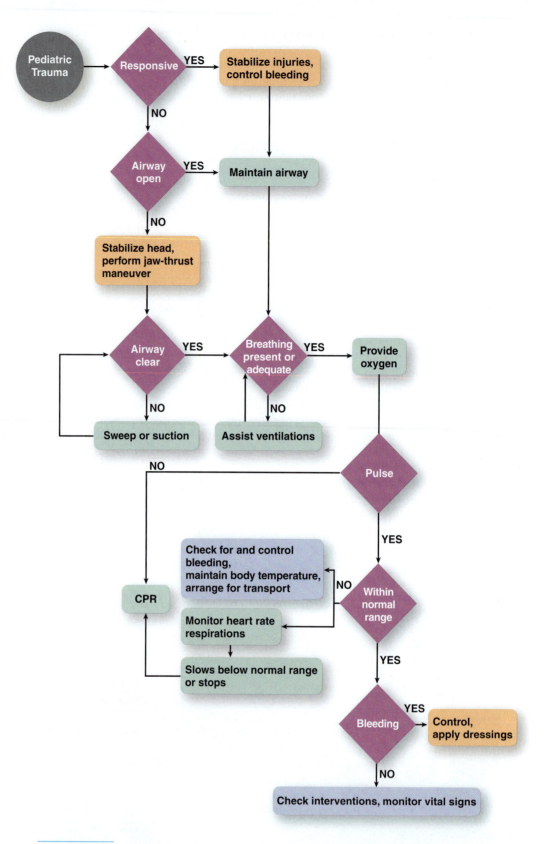

Figure 23.12 • Algorithm for the emergency care of an injured pediatric patient.

4. Control bleeding by applying appropriate dressings.

5. Stabilize suspected fractures.

6. Maintain manual stabilization of the patient's head and neck until the ambulance arrives.

7. Arrange for transport as soon as possible.

8. While waiting for the EMTs to arrive or while en route, perform your detailed and ongoing assessments.

For a summary of the assessment and emergency care of pediatric patients with specific musculoskeletal injuries, see Figure 23.13. For assessment and care of bleeding, shock, and specific soft-tissue injuries, see Figure 23.14.

continued

Burns

Burns in infants and children are assessed somewhat differently than for adults because of the child's proportionally larger surface area and head, and smaller extremities. In the rule of nines, for example, the percentage of body surface area assigned is slightly different: 18% to the head and neck, 18% to the chest and abdomen, 9% to each arm, 18% to the entire back, 23% for each leg, and 1% to the genital area. If you find it is difficult to do the estimations with accuracy while you are trying to quickly care for and stabilize the patient, do not worry about precision. The safest procedure is to estimate quickly and overestimate rather than underestimate the body surface area burned. The younger the child, the more important it is that he is seen in a burn center because of concerns about abuse and long-term morbidity.

Carefully and quickly care for the burned area with dry, sterile, and nonadherent dressings or sheets. Dry dressings will keep air, foreign materials, and dirt off the burn and will help keep the child warm, which will help in preventing shock. Moist dressings may chill the child and could speed the shock response. Follow local protocols for burn management. Arrange to transport the burned child as quickly as possible. Check local protocols for determining the type of cases (degree of severity, respiratory burns) that should be transported to a burn center. Burns are excruciatingly painful, and children are likely to be frantic. Rapid transport is important for obtaining pain relief for the child and care of the burns.

Suspected Abuse and Neglect

The news media have been reporting more stories of child **abuse** and neglect in recent years. These events are not something new. Rather, they have always existed but are now more recognized and reported. Calls involving pediatric patients can be some of the most difficult situations for the Emergency Medical Responder to handle both during and after the call. It is normal to experience strong emotions following a difficult call, but calls involving pediatric patients can be especially difficult emotionally. It is very important to

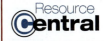

Resource **Central**

Read the fact sheet about child maltreatment to learn more.

OBJECTIVES

8. Describe common signs and symptoms of abuse and neglect.

9. Explain the role of the Emergency Medical Responder in cases of suspected abuse and/or neglect.

abuse ▶ the physical, emotional, or sexual mistreatment of another person.

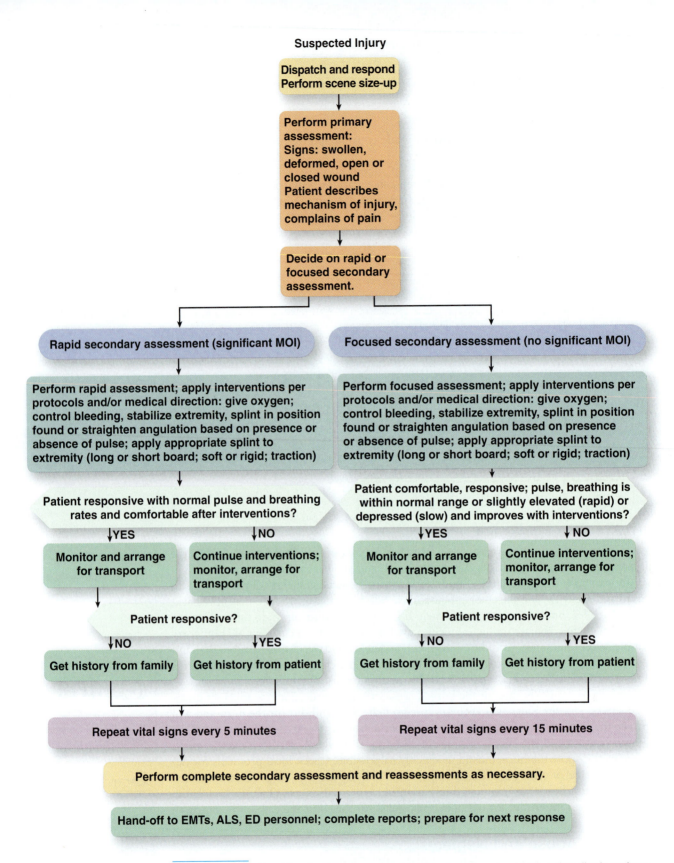

Suspected Injury

Dispatch and respond
Perform scene size-up

Perform primary assessment:
Signs: swollen, deformed, open or closed wound
Patient describes mechanism of injury, complains of pain

Decide on rapid or focused secondary assessment.

Rapid secondary assessment (significant MOI)

Perform rapid assessment; apply interventions per protocols and/or medical direction: give oxygen; control bleeding, stabilize extremity, splint in position found or straighten angulation based on presence or absence of pulse; apply appropriate splint to extremity (long or short board; soft or rigid; traction)

Patient responsive with normal pulse and breathing rates and comfortable after interventions?

↓YES
Monitor and arrange for transport

↓NO
Continue interventions; monitor, arrange for transport

Patient responsive?

↓NO
Get history from family

↓YES
Get history from patient

Repeat vital signs every 5 minutes

Focused secondary assessment (no significant MOI)

Perform focused assessment; apply interventions per protocols and/or medical direction: give oxygen; control bleeding, stabilize extremity, splint in position found or straighten angulation based on presence or absence of pulse; apply appropriate splint to extremity (long or short board; soft or rigid; traction)

Patient comfortable, responsive; pulse, breathing is within normal range or slightly elevated (rapid) or depressed (slow) and improves with interventions?

↓YES
Monitor and arrange for transport

↓NO
Continue interventions; monitor, arrange for transport

Patient responsive?

↓NO
Get history from family

↓YES
Get history from patient

Repeat vital signs every 15 minutes

Perform complete secondary assessment and reassessments as necessary.

Hand-off to EMTs, ALS, ED personnel; complete reports; prepare for next response

Figure 23.13 • Algorithm for the assessment and emergency care of injured pediatric patients with musculoskeletal emergencies.

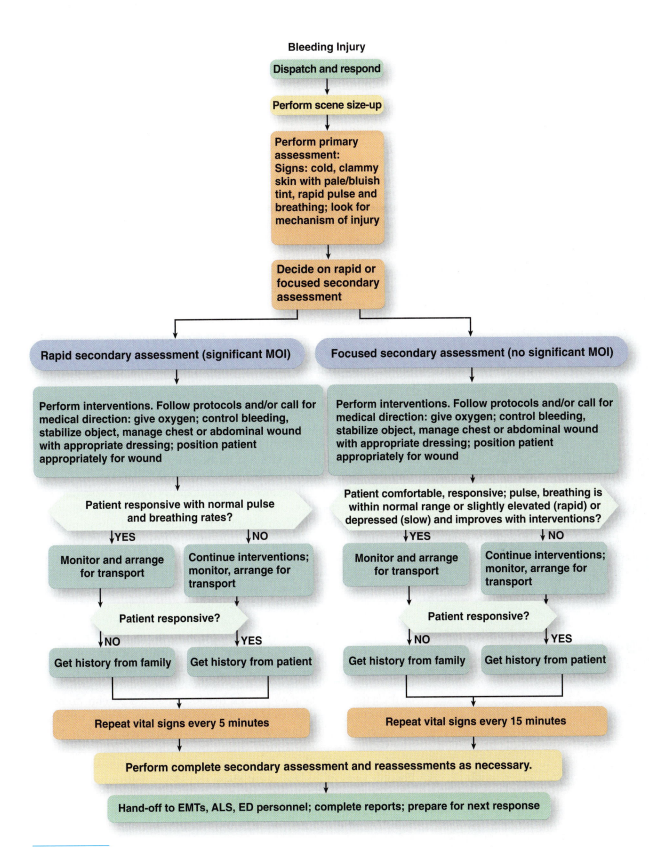

Bleeding Injury

Dispatch and respond

Perform scene size-up

Perform primary assessment:
Signs: cold, clammy skin with pale/bluish tint, rapid pulse and breathing; look for mechanism of injury

Decide on rapid or focused secondary assessment

Rapid secondary assessment (significant MOI)

Perform interventions. Follow protocols and/or call for medical direction: give oxygen; control bleeding, stabilize object, manage chest or abdominal wound with appropriate dressing; position patient appropriately for wound

Patient responsive with normal pulse and breathing rates?

↓YES — Monitor and arrange for transport

↓NO — Continue interventions; monitor, arrange for transport

Patient responsive?

↓NO — Get history from family

↓YES — Get history from patient

Repeat vital signs every 5 minutes

Focused secondary assessment (no significant MOI)

Perform interventions. Follow protocols and/or call for medical direction: give oxygen; control bleeding, stabilize object, manage chest or abdominal wound with appropriate dressing; position patient appropriately for wound

Patient comfortable, responsive; pulse, breathing is within normal range or slightly elevated (rapid) or depressed (slow) and improves with interventions?

↓YES — Monitor and arrange for transport

↓NO — Continue interventions; monitor, arrange for transport

Patient responsive?

↓NO — Get history from family

↓YES — Get history from patient

Repeat vital signs every 15 minutes

Perform complete secondary assessment and reassessments as necessary.

Hand-off to EMTs, ALS, ED personnel; complete reports; prepare for next response

Figure 23.14 • Algorithm for the assessment and emergency care of pediatric patients with bleeding, shock, and soft-tissue injuries.

recognize those feelings and not try to hold them in. It is always a good idea to talk out your feelings with those who can offer support and understanding. If given the opportunity, it is highly recommended that you participate in a formal debriefing for any difficult call. Remember to maintain patient confidentiality. You cannot name the child or family to anyone but medical or juvenile authorities or the police.

You must collect information, perform your assessments, and provide care without making a judgment or expressing your suspicion, distaste, or disbelief. Keep in mind that the abuser also needs help. Remember that your suspicions may be unfounded and that not every injury or sign of possible abuse to a child is the result of actual abuse. It is not your place to accuse the parents or caregiver, because they may not even be the abuser. You will need to check for patterns in responses and reports to confirm your suspicions. Report your concerns and impressions to ambulance personnel, medical direction, social services, the health department, or law enforcement, as required by local protocols. In all 50 states, **mandated reporters** are those designated by law to report cases of suspected abuse or neglect. In most states, EMS personnel are specifically named as mandated reporters. Be aware of your local laws and protocols regarding reporting abuse.

Abuse is the physical or emotional or sexual mistreatment of another person. There are several different forms of child abuse, and they frequently occur in combination (Figure 23.15): psychological abuse, neglect, sexual abuse, and physical abuse.

mandated reporter ▶
individuals designated by law to report cases of suspected abuse or neglect.

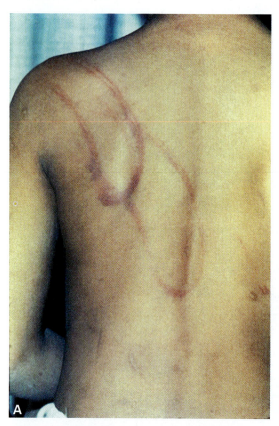

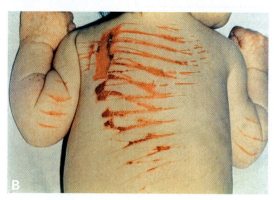

Figure 23.15 • Examples of injuries caused by abuse and neglect. (A) Cord bruise to the back. (B) Cigarette burns to the back.
(© Robert A. Felter, MD)

Psychological Abuse

It may be rare that Emergency Medical Responders are called to care for a patient who has been psychologically abused because there is no physical injury. However, there may be emotional signs and symptoms that may be difficult to assess unless you know the patient.

Psychological abuse includes emotional or verbal abuse that seriously affects the child's positive emotional development, well-being, and self-esteem. Children exposed to psychological abuse may feel rejected, degraded, or terrified. They may be forced into isolation with limited freedom or contact with others. They may be exploited or corrupted and forced to accept the beliefs of another, such as a cult or gang leader. Verbal abuse that affects emotional well-being and self-esteem and causes feelings of rejection or degradation in children includes phrases such as, "You're stupid," "You are no good," "You are not like your sister," "I wish you were never born," or "I hate you." Some parents isolate their children, locking them in closets or not letting them attend school. Cult and gang leaders often exploit the emotions of vulnerable teenagers, making them believe the cult loves them, or the gang gives them power and freedom and their parents do not.

Although psychological abuse can occur alone, victims often suffer other forms of abuse with it, such as sexual and *physical abuse*. The victims of psychological abuse, as well as other forms of abuse, are those with the least power and resources—children and women. Possible signs of psychological abuse include the following:

- Depression
- Withdrawal
- Extreme anxiety
- Low self-esteem
- Feelings of shame and guilt
- Fear
- Lack of normal social skills because of isolation
- Avoidance of eye contact
- Extreme passiveness or compliance
- History or indications of self-harm

- Substance abuse
- Increased tension or anxiety when the abuser is present

Provide care and emotional support by listening to and believing what the child tells you and by expressing your understanding. Let the child know there are people who will help and that you can get help. Arrange to have the child transported to get him away from the abuser, if necessary. Be sure to report your findings to the transport personnel and to social services, the health department, or the police, as required by your protocols.

Neglect

Emergency responses are usually for the obvious traumas that occur in physical and sexual abuse, not for neglect. However, long-term neglect may result in physical deterioration and injury or medical problems. Child **neglect** occurs when parents or caregivers do not provide for any or all of the following basic needs of the child: food and water, appropriate shelter and clothing, medical care, and education.

neglect ▶ failure of parents or caregivers to adequately provide for a person's basic physical, social, emotional, and medical needs.

On arrival, your scene size-up may reveal obvious signs of neglect, such as a child who is dressed inappropriately for the weather; a child who is lean, lethargic, and has signs of dehydration; or an environment with unclean living conditions, particularly where the child sleeps or is confined.

Consider also the circumstances of the family. They may not be able to financially afford to provide for the basic needs of the child or even themselves, and the entire family may need help from social services. Provide appropriate care for the child's illness or injuries and arrange to transport. Follow your protocols for reporting your concerns.

Sexual Abuse

There are many forms of *sexual abuse*, including physical sexual contact or exposure and sexual exploitation by displaying or photographing children for sexual purposes or with sexual intent. Emergency Medical Responders usually receive a call for sexual abuse if the child is injured or showing signs of a sexually related medical condition. A child can be the victim of sexual abuse from a parent or other relative and sometimes from a neighbor, teacher, or other trusted individual.

Do not expect the abuser to admit sexual abuse is the reason for the call. Many excuses and reasons are given for the child who has genital injuries or who has signs and symptoms of sexually transmitted diseases. Continue to act professionally and control your emotions.

When providing care, avoid embarrassing the child or making him feel guilty. Let the child know that you and the people at the hospital will help. Some signs of sexual abuse include:

- Obvious injuries to the genital area, including burns, cuts, bruises, and abrasions
- Rashes or sores around the genitals, discharges (such as seminal fluid), and bleeding from the genital openings or on underclothing
- Information from the child that he was exposed, touched, or assaulted

Be sure to report your suspicions and findings to ambulance personnel or to the appropriate agency, as per local protocols. Use these emergency care steps:

1. Dress wounds and provide other appropriate care for injuries.
2. Save any evidence of sexual abuse, such as soiled or stained clothing. Do not let the child use the bathroom to urinate or defecate. If the child must go to the bathroom, try to collect it in a container for hospital examination. Do not let the child drink any fluids or eat anything. Do not wash the child or let the parent wash the child or change his clothes. (The parent may insist on washing the child and changing his clothing. The child may insist that he must use the bathroom. Be aware that you cannot prevent them from doing so.)
3. Minimize embarrassment by covering the child with a blanket, if necessary.
4. Arrange for transport as soon as possible.
5. Provide emotional support and reassurance. Remember, you are still caring for a child. Try to engage him with toys or age-appropriate conversation or games.

Physical Abuse

Any form of violent, harmful contact with a child or any disfiguring act performed on the child is physical abuse, no matter what the intent of the adult. Some of the indications of physical abuse include the following:

- Outline of marks or bruises that are the size or shape of the object used to strike the child, such as the hand, a belt, strap, rope, or cord
- Areas of swelling, black eyes, loose or missing teeth, split lips
- Lacerations, incisions, abrasions
- Any unexplained bruises, broken bones, or burn marks
- Broken bones, signs of injuries healing incorrectly (misshaped limbs), or a history of numerous broken bones
- Head injuries or indications of closed head injuries that could be the result of violent shaking (bulging fontanels, unresponsiveness), especially in infants and small children
- Bruises—old and new—in various stages of healing
- Abdominal injuries with signs of bruising, distention, rigidity, or tenderness that could be the result of punching or kicking
- Genitalia injuries with lacerations, avulsions, or bleeding
- Bite marks showing the pattern and size of an adult mouth
- Burn marks or patterns caused by cigarettes, hot irons, stove burners; water burns or scalding marks on the legs, such as stocking burns from dipping in hot water, or a hand mark on the buttocks where the child's skin was protected from immersion. The creases at the knees and thighs are also protected when the child flexes his legs while being dipped in hot water.

The child's relationship with the parents or a parent's attitude toward the child or the situation may be a clue to abuse. However, these will not always be reliable indicators of the family relationship. Look for the following:

- Story of how the injury occurred that does not match the injury found
- Child who seems afraid to say how the injury occurred
- Child who is obviously afraid of a parent or other person at the scene
- Child who seems to expect no comfort from the parent
- Child who has no apparent reaction to pain
- Parent who does not want to leave you alone with the child
- Parents who tell conflicting stories or change explanations
- Parent who blames the child for being clumsy or accident prone
- Parent who seems inappropriately concerned or unconcerned
- Parent who is angry and is having trouble controlling it
- One parent who appears depressed or withdrawn while the other parent is expressing anger or giving explanations
- Any signs of alcohol or drug abuse
- Any expression of suicide or seeking mercy for their children
- Parent who is reluctant to give the child's history or to permit transport or who refuses to go to the nearest hospital

You must be the child's advocate and convince the parents that the child needs to be seen by a physician because of "the difficulty of determining the seriousness of injuries in the field." Do not accuse anyone of any wrongdoing.

You may respond to a call for an injured child and have no idea that the injury is related to abuse. You may observe that the child and parents relate well and that there is a strong bond between them. There are still abuse indications that will make you suspicious over time, so be alert for:

- Repeated responses for the same child or children in the same house
- Signs of past injuries during your assessment
- Signs of poorly healing wounds
- Signs of burns that are fresh or in various stages of healing
- Many types of injuries on numerous parts of the body

Obvious abuse situations can trigger strong emotions in you. Most people feel it is their duty to protect young children. Your first reactions to an abuse situation may be anger and disgust. However, you should not display these feelings while caring for the child or dealing with the parents or other caregivers. Providing necessary care for the child's injuries, clearly documenting objective findings, and alerting the proper authorities of your suspicions are appropriate actions.

If you suspect abuse and the parent or caregiver will not allow the child to be transported, call for law enforcement assistance.

Shaken-Baby Syndrome

Another type of abuse is **shaken-baby syndrome**. It is a form of child abuse that occurs when an abuser violently shakes an infant or small child, creating a whiplash-type motion that causes acceleration-deceleration injuries. The intent, usually, is not to harm the baby. Rarely, the syndrome may be caused accidentally by tossing the baby in the air or jogging with the baby in a backpack. It is not a result of gentle bouncing.

Infants and children have large, heavy heads, weak and not fully developed neck muscles, and space between the brain and the skull to allow for growth. The skull is also soft and pliable and not yet strong enough to absorb much force. During violent shaking, the brain will rebound against the inside of the skull and bruise, swell, and bleed, which causes increased pressure. Shaking also can cause injury to the neck and spine and to the eyes, causing loss of vision.

If you are called to the scene of a sick or injured child, ask the parent or caregiver questions to obtain a history. Look for signs and symptoms of illness or injury in your assessment. A shaken baby may have no obvious signs of trauma, such as bruising, bleeding, or swelling. The history and some of the signs and symptoms of shaken-baby syndrome may include the following, which may also be indications of other illnesses:

- Change in behavior
- Irritability
- Lethargy or sleepiness
- Decreased alertness
- Unresponsiveness
- Pale or bluish (cyanotic) skin
- Vomiting
- Convulsions (seizures)
- Not eating normally
- Not breathing

Shaken-baby syndrome is a serious emergency. Call for transport immediately for any child with the above signs and symptoms. While waiting for them to arrive, ensure that the baby has an airway, is breathing, and has a pulse. Perform rescue breathing or CPR as needed and provide oxygen, if you are trained and allowed to do so. If the child is vomiting, protect and clear the airway. Be sure to turn the infant as a unit, keeping the head in line with the body. If the infant is having seizures, protect him from further injury.

Safety Seats

Many safety seats are not installed correctly; and children are often not secured properly by the safety straps and harnesses. Any movement of the seat or the child can throw both forward in a crash. As a result, the child receives internal injuries, which emergency care providers may not be able to initially detect. Usually, the child's body will compensate for these internal injuries and bleeding, which can lull the rescuers into thinking the child is unharmed and stable.

Any vehicle crash should lead you to suspect that the child has been injured, even if you do not see any damage to the safety seat. If the child is still secured to the car seat, leave him there and carefully assess him in place. If there are any issues with the ABCs, then maintain manual stabilization of the child's head, remove from the seat, and provide care as appropriate (Table 23.3).

shaken-baby syndrome ▶ a form of child abuse that occurs when an abuser violently shakes an infant or small child, creating a whiplash-type motion that causes acceleration-deceleration injuries.

TABLE 23.3 | Child Safety Seats

ISSUES	FACTS
Installation and child security	Too many safety seats are not installed correctly, and children often are not secured properly by the safety straps and harnesses.
Restrictions on care	Emergency Medical Responders and other emergency care providers cannot adequately provide airway management care, maintain an open airway, or provide bag-mask resuscitation on a child who is immobilized in a safety seat.
Position of the child	A child's torso in a safety seat is in a flexed position because the seat is designed that way. Spinal immobilization straightens and extends the spine from the cervical spine (the neck) to the sacrum (the part of the spine between the hip bones). Leaving the child in a safety seat continues to stretch the spine in a curved position rather than in a straight, extended position.
Injuries to the child	If an infant or small child of any age is riding in the forward-facing position, the crash forces likely caused the child's body to flex forward extremely (hyperflexion), especially if the seat was installed improperly or the harness securing the child was too loose. This sudden forward flexion causes injury to the cervical spine.
Protection for the child	Children up to age four and up to 40 pounds may be too large for the child safety seat to support the head and protect them properly. If the child's head extends above the top edge of the seat back, the head may hyperextend (be forced extremely backward) in a crash. At the same time, the body is thrust forward. All this sudden and extreme motion stretches the ligaments and muscles of the spinal column, causing severe injuries.
Car seat damage and stability	The safety seat (especially an improperly installed one) involved in a vehicle crash is likely to be damaged, although the damage may not be noticed even on close inspection. A damaged seat will not adequately immobilize and support the child. Furthermore, manufacturers state that child safety seats are not designed to be used as immobilizing devices. Using the safety seat for purposes other than the manufacturer intended places the liability for further patient injury on emergency care providers.
Transport considerations	Safety seats cannot be properly secured in the ambulance. Furthermore, if the ambulance is involved in a collision en route to the hospital, the safety seat cannot endure the forces of another crash. There are enough reports of ambulance crashes while en route to the hospital with patients to cause concern. A second crash may further weaken the effectiveness of the safety seat and leave the child, who is immobilized in it, unprotected. However, many ambulances are now carrying child safety seats in the event they must transport uninjured children to the hospital with their injured parents. The child safety seats are secured in the captain's chair.

There are many types of child safety seats, but each provides the same safety functions if properly used. Emergency Medical Responders should not hesitate to act to immobilize and provide initial airway care for a child, even if they are not familiar with the safety seat they find at a crash site. Use the following guidelines if you must extricate an infant or a child from a safety seat, but do not perform these steps unless you have learned and practiced them under the supervision of your instructor:

- Do a quick visual inspection of the vehicle interior. Did the crash force the safety seat from its position, even slightly? Was the safety seat in the rear or front vehicle seat? Was the safety seat a rear-facing or forward-facing seat? Is there structural damage to the seat?
- Throughout the assessment and immobilization process, be sure that someone maintains manual stabilization of the infant's or the child's head.
- Assess the patient for the ABCs. Assess for injuries.
- If the safety seat has a protection plate over the patient's chest, remove it (cut the straps securing it, if necessary) to assess the chest. (Before performing chest compressions, remove the infant onto an immobilization device.)
- As you assess the patient, check for loose straps, which would have provided little protection. Extricate the child onto an immobilization device, which can then be secured to the ambulance stretcher (Scan 23.2).

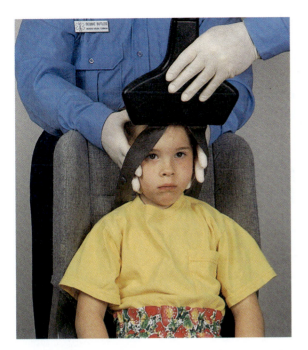

23.2.1 | Rescuer 1 stabilizes car seat in upright position and applies manual head/neck stabilization. Rescuer 2 prepares equipment, then loosens or cuts the seat straps and raises the front guard.

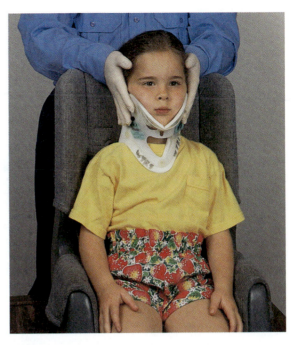

23.2.2 | Cervical collar is applied to patient as Rescuer 1 maintains manual stabilization of the head and neck.

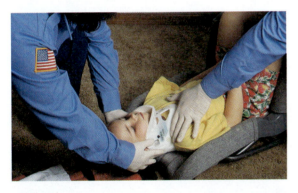

23.2.3 | As Rescuer 1 maintains manual head/neck stabilization, Rescuer 2 places child safety seat on center of backboard and slowly tilts it into supine position. Both rescuers are careful not to let the child slide out of the chair. For the child with a large head, place a towel under area where the shoulders will eventually be placed on the board to prevent head from tilting forward.

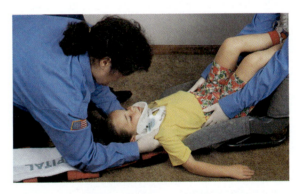

23.2.4 | Rescuer 1 maintains manual head/neck stabilization and calls for a coordinated long axis move onto the backboard.

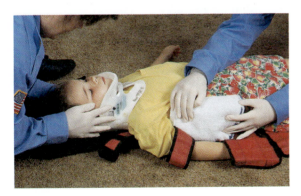

23.2.5 | Rescuer 1 maintains manual head/neck stabilization. Rescuer 2 places rolled towels or blankets on both sides of the patient.

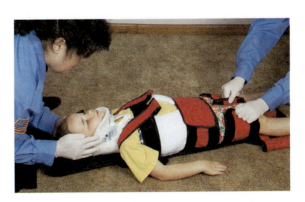

23.2.6 | Rescuer 1 maintains manual head/neck stabilization. Rescuer 2 straps or tapes patient to board at level of upper chest, pelvis, and lower legs. Do not strap across abdomen.

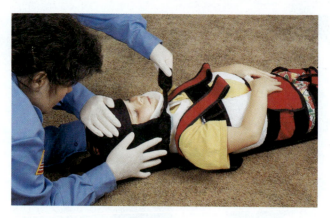

23.2.7 | Rescuer 1 maintains manual head/neck stabilization as Rescuer 2 places rolled towels on both sides of head, then tapes head securely in place across forehead and maxilla (jaw bone) or cervical collar. Do not tape across chin to avoid putting pressure on neck.

WRAP-UP

FIRST ON SCENE

The scene is suddenly awash with flashing emergency lights, and both police officers and firefighters scatter around the intersection checking on people and securing the area. Bryn describes the child's wounds to the medical crew, who quickly give the mother an oxygen mask to hold near the baby's face and usher her to the back of the ambulance.

"It's good that he's crying," the paramedic says to the mother as he helps her into the ambulance. "But we need to get him over to the university right away."

He then turns to Bryn, just before closing the back doors, and says, "You did a great job, officer. Perfect." Bryn nods and waves weakly.

As the ambulance moves quickly across 43rd Street and down Buchanan, Bryn sits down on the bumper of her patrol car. "We caught the shooters, you know," a voice says, startling her. She looks up and sees the shift sergeant standing on the sidewalk, looking at her and the bloody exam gloves she is still wearing.

"How's the little one going to be?" he asks, stepping closer and putting a hand on her shoulder.

"I hope he'll be okay," she answers, standing up. "I mean, I think I did everything I was supposed to."

"You did just fine." He smiles. "Go ahead and head back to the station and relax. We'll all debrief when we're done here."

CHAPTER REVIEW

Summary

- Assessment and emergency care of infants and children is basically the same as for adults. However, you must consider the special characteristics of the pediatric patient's anatomy, physiology, and emotional responses when assessing and caring for them.

- Infants breathe through the nose. If it is obstructed, they may not immediately open their mouths to breathe. Be sure to clear the nostrils of secretions.

- When managing the airway of an infant, make sure the large head is in a neutral position, neither hyperflexed nor hyperextended. Place a folded towel under the infant's or the child's shoulders to maintain the spine and the airway in neutral alignment.

- Care for respiratory distress in infants and children immediately. For respiratory distress, provide oxygen with a pediatric-size nonrebreather mask or by using the blow-by technique. Follow local protocols.

- For severe distress and respiratory arrest, provide assisted ventilations with the appropriate device, such as a pocket face mask or pediatric bag-mask device and supplemental oxygen.

- Children tolerate high fevers better than adults do, but a fever that rises rapidly can cause seizures. Arrange to transport the feverish child as soon as possible. Also arrange to transport the child who is vomiting and has diarrhea.

- Care for shock early. In an infant or child, signs and symptoms of shock mean it has progressed and is in the late stages. If you suspect that shock may result from the mechanism of injury or nature of illness, provide emergency care immediately.

- Because of their size, curiosity, and a lack of fear due to their inexperience, infants and children are frequent victims of trauma. When assessing and providing emergency care, keep in mind that their larger head size and their weight make pediatric patients more prone to head and neck trauma.

- Be calm, professional, and discreet about suspicions of abuse or neglect in the presence of caregivers. Be an advocate for the child, and remember your obligation to report any suspicions to the proper authorities.

Take Action

CHILD ADVOCATE

As much as one would like to think it doesn't happen, more and more stories on the abuse and neglect of innocent children are reported nearly every day. All 50 states have laws and statutes defining those called "mandatory reporters," individuals who are identified by vocation or profession who are legally obligated to report cases of suspected abuse or neglect. While all 50 states do indeed address the subject and define who a mandatory reporter is, each has a slightly different definition. Your job with this activity is to use the Internet to search for the definition and requirements related to mandatory reporters in your state. You can begin your search by going to the U.S. Department of Health and Human Services, Administration for Children and Families, at www.acf.hhs.gov.

First on Scene Run Review

Recall the events of the "First on Scene" scenario in this chapter and answer the following questions, which are related to the call. Rationales are offered in the Answer Key at the back of the book.

1. What information would you want from the dispatcher about the scene?

2. Did Bryn do everything she could for the baby? Describe what she did or did not do.

3. Was it a good idea to have the mother help? Explain your answer.

Quick Quiz

To check your understanding of the chapter, answer the following questions. Then compare your answers to those in the Answer Key at the back of the book.

1. The techniques used for the assessment and care of children are the same as for adults with certain modifications. Those modifications reflect the patient's differences in age and:

   a. physical and intellectual development.
   b. physical development and emotional response.
   c. emotional response and sex of the child.
   d. emotional response and language skills.

2. The most appropriate approach when assessing the pediatric patient is to:
   a. remain at eye level, explain each step of the exam, and be truthful.
   b. remain at eye level, move to a quiet location, and perform the exam.
   c. move to a quiet location, perform the exam, and call parents.
   d. remain at eye level, and perform the exam while telling jokes.

3. When assessing infants younger than one year, you must ensure an adequate airway. You must also:
   a. protect the head, and provide care to prevent shock.
   b. protect the head and spine, and provide care to prevent shock.
   c. protect the head and neck, but do not become too emotional.
   d. protect the head and trunk, but do not become too emotional.

4. If you need to clear the airway of an unresponsive infant, you should:
   a. open the mouth and perform a finger sweep.
   b. provide chest thrusts as quickly as possible.
   c. open the mouth, give two slow breaths, and perform a finger sweep.
   d. open the mouth, look for obstructions, and perform a finger sweep if you see one.

5. If you need to perform CPR on an infant, the proper location for chest compressions is:
   a. two finger widths below the imaginary nipple line.
   b. one finger width below the imaginary nipple line.
   c. three finger widths below the imaginary nipple line.
   d. in the center of the chest between the nipples.

6. You are caring for a responsive child who is cyanotic and struggling to breathe. You should first:
   a. perform a finger sweep.
   b. arrange for immediate transport.
   c. begin rescue breathing.
   d. give two breaths and begin CPR.

7. If parents or guardians are present and their emotional response to the child's injury hinders your ability to properly care for the child, do all of the following EXCEPT:
   a. ignore them.
   b. ask them to assist you with your tasks.
   c. have someone tactfully remove them from the scene.
   d. have a friend, neighbor, or other EMS responder distract them with questions.

8. When examining a child, the strategy that may be perceived by the child as LEAST threatening is to first examine the:
   a. head and neck and then the rest of the body.
   b. head, neck, chest, and then the rest of the body.
   c. heart and lungs, and then the rest of the body.
   d. legs and chest, and then the neck and head.

9. All of the following statements are true for a child from three to six years of age (preschool) EXCEPT that they:
   a. do not like to have their clothing removed.
   b. have a fear of blood, pain, and permanent injury.
   c. believe illness or injury is punishment for being bad.
   d. do not care if they are separated from their parents.

10. All of the following are characteristics of children from 6 to 12 years of age EXCEPT that they:
    a. believe their illness or injury is a punishment for being bad.
    b. are modest and do not like to have their bodies touched.
    c. have a fear of blood, pain, disfigurement, and permanent injury.
    d. are cooperative but like to have their opinions heard.

11. The fontanels on an infant's head do not completely close until about _____ months of age.
    a. 15
    b. 16
    c. 18
    d. 12

12. All of the following are unique to a pediatric patient's breathing EXCEPT:
    a. infants are generally nose breathers.
    b. there is more respiratory movement in the chest than abdomen.
    c. they have a less developed and more elastic chest than adults have.
    d. the trachea is softer, more flexible, and narrower than an adult's.

13. Which one of the following statements about children is NOT true?
    a. They have a larger skin surface area in proportion to total body mass.
    b. They have a constant blood volume regardless of age.
    c. Normal vital signs vary with the size of the child.
    d. Blood pressure will vary depending on age, sex, and height.

14. All of the following are common medical emergencies for the pediatric patient EXCEPT:
    a. respiratory emergencies.
    b. altered mental status.
    c. heart attacks.
    d. seizures.

15. Several different forms of child abuse that usually occur together are sexual, physical, and:
    a. psychological.
    b. neglect.
    c. social.
    d. mental.

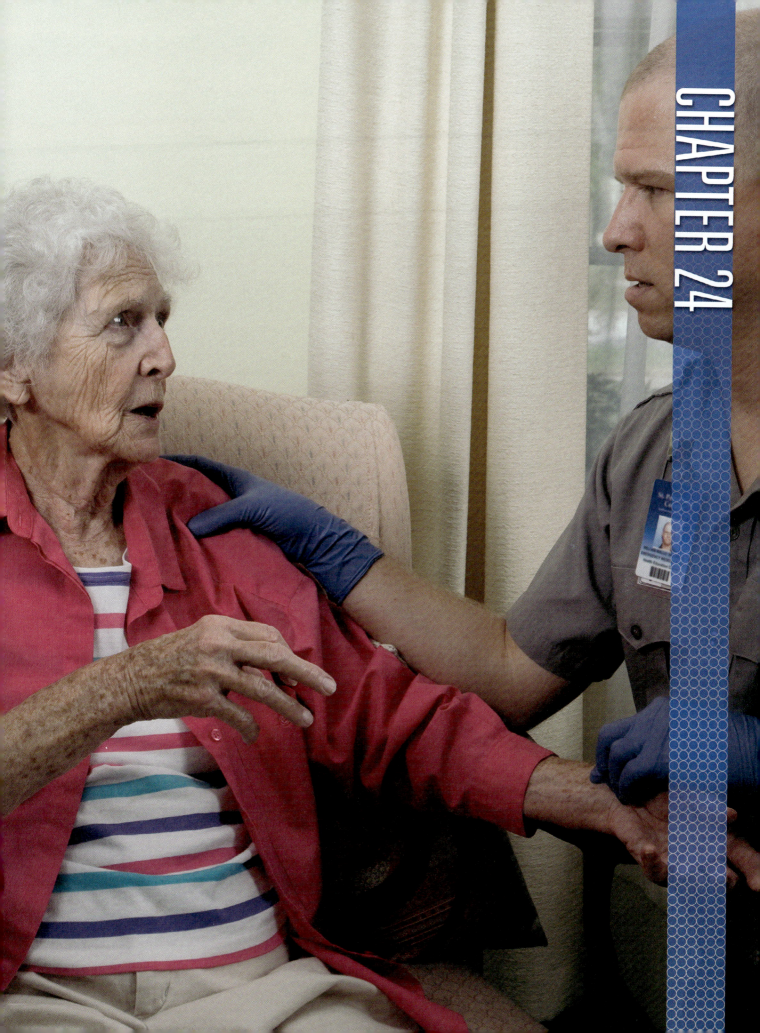

CHAPTER 24

Special Considerations for the Geriatric Patient

EDUCATION STANDARDS • Special Patient Populations—Geriatrics, Patients with Special Challenges

COMPETENCIES • Recognizes and manages life threats based on assessment findings of a patient with a medical emergency while awaiting additional emergency response.

CHAPTER OVERVIEW This chapter introduces the special considerations necessary in assessing and providing care for elderly patients. There are currently more than 35 million elderly people in the United States, and that number is expected to more than double in the next two decades. More and more often, you will find yourself providing care for them. Remember that although people are living healthier lifestyles, age-related changes in anatomy and physiology do make the elderly more susceptible to certain illnesses and injuries.

The term *geriatric* refers to people who are elderly, typically over the age of 65. This chapter uses the terms *geriatric* and *elderly* interchangeably to refer to this growing population.

OBJECTIVES

Upon successful completion of this chapter, the student should be able to:

COGNITIVE

1. Review the major stages of lifespan development of the adult patient. (See Chapter 4.)
2. Define the following terms:
   a. Alzheimer's disease *(p. 554)*
   b. elder abuse *(p. 555)*
   c. elder neglect *(p. 555)*
   d. elderly *(p. 547)*
   e. geriatric *(p. 547)*
   f. self-neglect *(p. 555)*
3. Describe the general characteristics commonly associated with geriatric patients. *(p. 548)*
4. Describe some of the most common age-related physical changes found in geriatric patients. *(p. 550)*
5. Describe the common medical problems of geriatric patients. *(p. 554)*
6. Explain the unique challenges that can arise when assessing and caring for the geriatric patient. *(p. 553)*
7. Describe changes in the approach to care when caring for geriatric patients. *(p. 554)*
8. Describe common signs and symptoms of abuse and neglect. *(p. 555)*
9. Explain the role of the Emergency Medical Responder in cases of suspected abuse and/or neglect. *(p. 555)*

PSYCHOMOTOR

10. Demonstrate the ability to properly assess and care for the geriatric patient.
11. Demonstrate various techniques that can be employed to maximize successful assessment of the geriatric patient.

AFFECTIVE

12. Value the role of the Emergency Medical Responder with respect to patient advocacy.

Security Officer Tom Morales taps the steering wheel of his small car and waits for the light to turn green. He has less than seven minutes to get over to the Meadow Glen Apartments and lock up the pool area or else he is going to be running behind on his nightly route. Just then he hears the roar of a motorcycle engine from somewhere followed by the squeal of tires. He looks around at the other cars waiting on different sides of the intersection. Suddenly his small car shudders and he hears the sound of crushing metal. "What the heck?"

He looks over his right shoulder and sees a large black motorcycle wobble past his passenger window and slide sideways into the middle of the intersection, showering bright sparks into the air. The motorcycle comes to rest on its side with the driver, a small woman, crumpled next to it. Tom grabs his orange Emergency Medical Responder jump bag, hurries into the intersection, and shuts off the still blaring motorcycle.

"Are you okay?" he says to the woman, who has her face buried in the crook of her leather-clad elbow. Her shoulders shake as if she is sobbing, making her black helmet — painted with Egyptian hieroglyphics — tap on the ground. He notices that the woman's left leg is resting at an odd angle on the pavement as he gently touches her shoulder. At his touch, she lifts her face from the sleeve of her leather jacket and turns toward him. She is very old, and she is not crying. She is laughing.

Understanding Geriatric Patients

There is a common misconception that most **elderly** people are usually ill, hard of hearing, and altered in their mental state to the point of not being able to provide reliable information to caregivers. You should understand that this is not true. The vast majority of the elderly lead healthy, active lives and are able to communicate clearly and effectively with those around them (Figure 24.1). Why the misconception, then? Most likely it is because people who are

elderly ▶ a term used to describe a person age 65 or older.

KEY POINT ▼

The term **geriatric** refers to people over the age of 65. The term *elderly* is another word commonly used to describe this population.

geriatric ▶ of or relating to an elderly person.

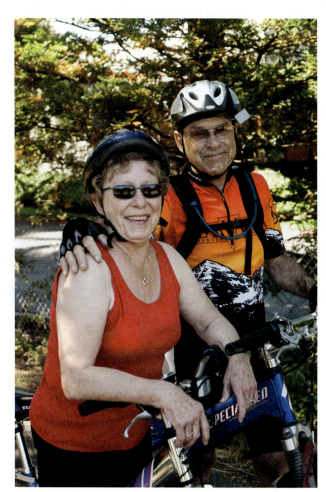

Figure 24.1 • The vast majority of the elderly lead healthy, active lives.

KEY POINT ▼

Appropriate care of elderly patients involves understanding the physical, emotional, and financial difficulties commonly experienced by this growing group.

healthy and active rarely require EMS assistance. So when EMS providers are summoned to help an elderly person, the calls frequently come from extended-care facilities where chronically ill and/or mentally altered geriatric patients are cared for. You should not let frequent calls to these types of facilities distort your view of the geriatric population as a whole.

The majority of elderly patients are as healthy and lucid as you are. However, there are some important differences that you should keep in mind when dealing with elderly patients. Those differences include unique life experiences and the accompanying concerns that come with aging and the reality of their own mortality. The differences also include anatomical and physiological changes.

Characteristics of Geriatric Patients

OBJECTIVE

3. Describe the general characteristics commonly associated with geriatric patients.

Even though geriatric patients, their bodies, and their specific illnesses grow more unique as they age, there are certain generalizations that are fairly consistent across this segment of the population. Being familiar with the following general areas will greatly assist you in understanding your geriatric patients.

Multiple Illnesses

Elderly patients are just as likely to suffer from the same illnesses and disorders as everyone else, but their bodies are less able to defend against them and recover afterward. This results in multiple simultaneous illnesses. Elderly people commonly have multiple medical conditions, illnesses, or diseases at one time. This number tends to increase as the elderly patient ages. Multiple illnesses create a unique challenge for the emergency responder who is assessing the geriatric patient. The patient may be displaying signs and symptoms from a variety of illnesses, with none of them appearing to be anything specific. Do not worry. It will not be your job to diagnose the patient. It usually takes a physician examining the geriatric patient and ordering a battery of lab tests before a diagnosis can be made. Your job is simply to perform a thorough patient assessment and care for the primary complaint as best as you can.

KEY POINT ▼

When taking an elderly patient's medical history, make sure to ask if the patient is taking a prescribed medication as directed. Just because the patient states that he has medications does not mean that he has been taking them as prescribed.

Medications

Directly related to the presence of multiple illnesses, elderly patients take numerous prescription and over-the-counter (OTC) medications each day. Actually, patients age 65 and older take an average of 4.5 medications per day. Incorrect medication usage (sometimes caused by forgetfulness or confusion about instructions) can create numerous problems, from overdosing to underdosing. Overdosing will result in toxic medication levels in the patient's system. Underdosing can cause the patient's illness or disease process to get worse (Figures 24.2 and 24.3).

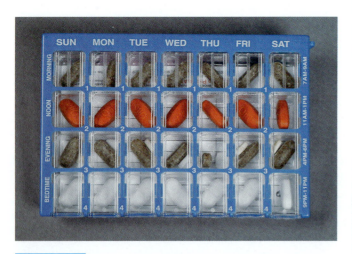

Figure 24.2 • Many elderly people use a pill organizer to help them remember when to take their medications.

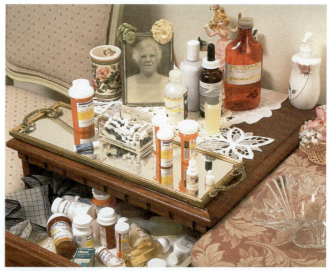

Figure 24.3 • It can be challenging to keep track of multiple medications.

Medications

Most elderly individuals receive some form of ongoing health care for their chronic conditions. This often involves multiple physicians from different specialties who sometimes do not coordinate their care. When this happens, the patient is at risk of suffering complications from the interactions of their medications. Sometimes the drug interactions increase the risk of injuries such as falls. Being aware of these unique challenges prepares you to better understand the patient's signs and symptoms.

Another common cause of medication misuse is due to the cost of prescription medications. Elderly patients on fixed incomes may cut their medications in half or take them only every other day in an attempt to get them to last longer than prescribed.

Mobility

Regular exercise is very important. It can help keep aging patients healthy and mobile. However, it is common for some elderly persons to live increasingly sedentary lifestyles. This can be due to illnesses such as arthritis, medications that cause excessive tiredness, or even the fear of injury as their ability to move about becomes more difficult. Having limited mobility can cause many problems for the elderly person, such as (Figure 24.4):

- Isolation
- Poor nutrition
- Depression
- Difficulty using the bathroom
- Loss of independence
- Higher likelihood for falls or other injuries

Difficulties with Communication

You will find that many geriatric patients have some age-related sensory changes. It is normal for elderly people to experience a lower sensitivity to pain or touch, an altered sense of smell or taste, a certain amount of hearing loss, and impaired vision or blindness. Any of those can affect your ability to assess and communicate with the patient. See Table 24.1 for some ideas about how to effectively communicate with an elderly patient.

Incontinence

Not necessarily caused by aging, several factors predispose elderly persons to the inability to retain urine or feces. Diseases such as diabetes, illnesses that cause diarrhea, and certain medications all can contribute to incontinence. Studies indicate that between 15% and 60% of all elderly people suffer from some form of incontinence. Understand that it is important for you *not* make a big deal out of a geriatric patient's incontinence. The need to help maintain the dignity of any patient is important, but for elderly patients, in particular, respect and dignity are extremely vital.

Confusion or Altered Mental Status

An important thing to remember when you encounter an elderly patient who seems confused or is presenting with an

IS IT SAFE?

You must be especially careful when moving or lifting elderly patients because it is much easier to accidently cause pain or even injure them. Be sure to communicate your intentions thoroughly before lifting or moving them.

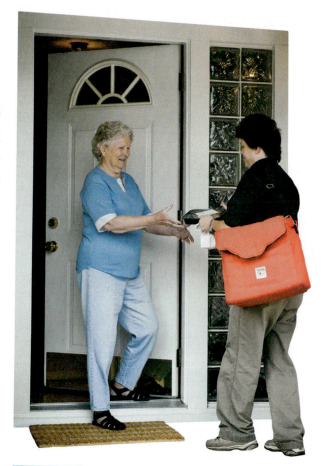

Figure 24.4 • Meals on Wheels helps ensure that elderly people receive nutrition by providing home delivered meals.

TABLE 24.1 | Age-Related Difficulties with Communication

DIFFICULTY	STRATEGY
Poor vision	Position yourself directly in front of the patient so you can be seen.
	Put your hand on the arm of a blind patient so he knows where you are.
	Locate the patient's glasses, if necessary.
Decreased hearing	Speak clearly. Check hearing aids. Write notes.
	Try letting the patient wear a stethoscope and speak into the head like a microphone.
Inability to speak clearly	Ask the patient to put dentures in (or adjust them), if possible.

altered mental status is to try to determine if this is normal behavior for the patient. You want to avoid placing too much importance on a patient's confused state if this is the norm for him.

Age-Related Physical Changes

Although age-related changes can be determined by genetics and begin at the cellular level, they are greatly affected by lifestyle and environment. As anyone can see by looking around in his or her own community, the aging process can differ greatly from person to person. There are, however, some general age-related changes that will be fairly consistent throughout the older population. It is important for Emergency Medical Responders to understand the basics of these changes and how they can impact the assessment and care process (Figure 24.5).

Respiratory System

As early as the age of 30, without regular exercise, the lungs will begin the aging process with decreased ability to ventilate properly. Aging creates many changes in the respiratory system. For example, the mechanism that helps the body detect low levels of oxygen in the blood becomes increasingly less efficient over time. This means that a geriatric patient may become severely hypoxic before the body realizes it and attempts to compensate. Aging also leads to a decrease in the number of cilia in the airway, exposing the elderly person to more respiratory illnesses, such as pneumonia. Other respiratory changes due to aging include:

- Reduced strength and endurance of respiratory muscles
- Decreased chest wall flexibility
- Loss of lung elasticity
- Collapse of smaller airway structures

As with any patient, it is important that you continually assess and maintain the geriatric patient's airway.

Cardiovascular System

Much of what affects the cardiovascular system seems related to lifestyle. Aging, however, does seem to affect it to a certain degree as well. Some of the age-related changes in the cardiovascular system include:

- Enlargement of the left ventricle, which can decrease the amount of blood moved by the heart

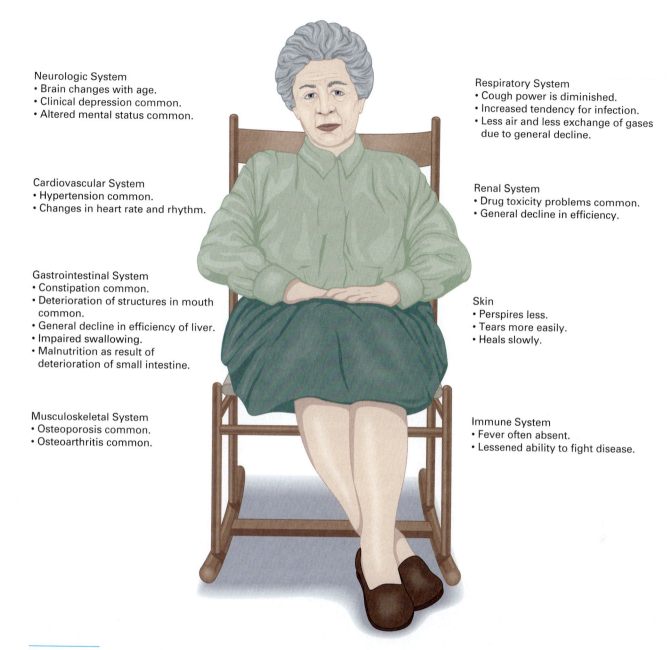

Neurologic System
• Brain changes with age.
• Clinical depression common.
• Altered mental status common.

Cardiovascular System
• Hypertension common.
• Changes in heart rate and rhythm.

Gastrointestinal System
• Constipation common.
• Deterioration of structures in mouth common.
• General decline in efficiency of liver.
• Impaired swallowing.
• Malnutrition as result of deterioration of small intestine.

Musculoskeletal System
• Osteoporosis common.
• Osteoarthritis common.

Respiratory System
• Cough power is diminished.
• Increased tendency for infection.
• Less air and less exchange of gases due to general decline.

Renal System
• Drug toxicity problems common.
• General decline in efficiency.

Skin
• Perspires less.
• Tears more easily.
• Heals slowly.

Immune System
• Fever often absent.
• Lessened ability to fight disease.

Figure 24.5 • Common changes in the body systems of the elderly.

• Stiffening and elongation of the aorta, making it more susceptible to tearing
• Degeneration of the heart's electrical system, causing dysrhythmia
• Loss of elasticity in the blood vessels, which can result in high blood pressure and poor circulation

In addition, medications prescribed to elderly patients for heart conditions can prevent effective compensation for blood loss. Geriatric trauma patients who have lost a good amount of blood should be treated for shock even if their signs and symptoms do not indicate it.

Nervous System

Aging has been shown to affect a person's nervous system in a few key areas. First, the brain loses about 10% of its overall weight between the ages of 20 and 90 years.

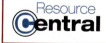

Watch a video to learn more information about geriatric cognition.

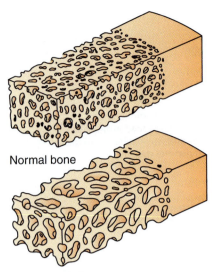

Normal bone

Osteoporotic bone

Figure 24.6 • During the aging process, osteoporosis causes a reduction in the quality of bone, making the skeletal tissue more brittle and less elastic.

Although this does *not* mean that elderly patients are less intelligent than younger ones (no relationship between brain size and intelligence has ever been found), it does mean that there is more room for destructive bleeding inside the skull following a blow to the head. Also, aging causes a substantial decrease in the overall number of nerve fibers and the speed at which the impulses travel across them. Those deteriorations mean that elderly patients may experience some of the following changes over time:

- Decreased reaction times
- Difficulty with recent memory
- Psychomotor slowing

As you examine the geriatric patient, assess for sluggishness, confusion, or any mental status that appears below the level of full coherence. An altered mental status can indicate a wide range of illnesses and injuries, from infection and medication overdose to brain attack (stroke) and head trauma, all of which are very serious conditions. It is important that you summon advanced medical care for any elderly patient who presents with an abnormally altered mental status.

Although it may not be uncommon for an elderly person to seem agitated, confused, or have a decreased level of consciousness, always assume that he or she is normally coherent and mentally sharp until you can determine otherwise by questioning caregivers, spouse, or family members. If you operate on the assumption that a patient is normally altered, you may fail to properly address an underlying medical problem.

Although not directly related to the physical effects of aging on the nervous system, it is worth mentioning here that depression is a common condition found among elderly patients. In fact, suicides, or suicide attempts, are not unusual in the 65 and older segment of the population, especially among males. Be alert for signs of depression, such as poor hygiene, poor eating habits, and disorderly living environments.

Musculoskeletal System

Age-related changes in the musculoskeletal system can lead to changes in posture, range of motion, and balance. Some elderly people can even lose up to three inches of overall height due to deterioration of the discs between the vertebrae and osteoporosis (Figure 24.6). Osteoporosis is the loss of minerals from bones. That loss causes the bones to soften and become weak, making the elderly more susceptible to falls. Once they fall, the injuries can be very severe. Also keep in mind that age-related changes in the spine can result in curvatures, which can affect your ability to manage a patient's airway or effectively immobilize him following an injury.

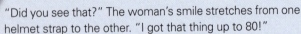

continued

FIRST ON SCENE

"Did you see that?" The woman's smile stretches from one helmet strap to the other. "I got that thing up to 80!"

"Ma'am." Tom places his hands on either side of the black helmet and tries to hold the woman's bobbing head in place. "You may have injured yourself. Please don't move." He can hear sirens growing louder from down Porter Street.

"The leg's a bit sore, but other than that I feel great! I didn't hit anybody, did I?"

"Well, I think you actually hit my car."

Her eyes narrow and she lowers her voice, "Don't you worry. My Richard always kept plenty of insurance on the vehicles."

"Ma'am, right now I'm just worried about you. Please just lie there and hold still. I can hear help coming."

The woman exhales roughly and lets her head rest on Tom's gloved hand. "You know," she touches her left leg with a shaky hand. "This leg is really starting to hurt quite a bit. Can you straighten it out for me?" Tom looks over and sees that the woman's pants are growing dark over the spot where her leg appears to be angulated.

Integumentary System (Skin)

Because of its prominence on the body, age-related changes to the skin are going to be the most obvious to you as an Emergency Medical Responder. As people grow older, their skin loses its elasticity and thickness, causing it to be easily torn or injured. You also may notice dark areas of pigment on the skin, usually called "age spots" or "liver spots." The skin of a geriatric patient may be dry and flaky due to a decrease in the production of oils. The ability to perspire tends to decrease as well, making heat-related emergencies more common and the onset of shock harder to recognize. As skin grows thinner and weaker, cell reproduction slows down, so that not only are skin injuries worse among the elderly, but healing times also can be greatly extended.

Assessment of Geriatric Patients

Your assessment of a geriatric patient will follow the same basic path as any other patient assessment, with a few additional considerations. As always, make sure you begin by taking appropriate BSI precautions.

Scene Size-up

In addition to ensuring that the scene is safe to enter, for geriatric patients you also should survey the environment for evidence of the following:

- Inadequate food, shelter, or hygiene
- Lack of a working heating or cooling system
- Potential fall hazards
- Conditions that suggest abuse or neglect (Figure 24.7)

When you approach the patient, always focus on her instead of caregivers or family members who may be present. This will show the patient you respect her as a person and will give her a sense of control over the situation. If the patient is seated or lying on a bed, position yourself at the patient's level and make eye contact before introducing yourself (Figure 24.8). Another way to show respect to the patient is to use her title and last name, such as "Mrs. Becker." Avoid using generic nicknames such as "dear," "sweetie," or "honey." Also avoid using an elderly person's first name (unless you are asked to use it); doing so could be considered rude or disrespectful. If appropriate, offer to shake the patient's hand during the introduction. This builds rapport while also giving you the ability to check the patient's skin signs and mobility in an unobtrusive way.

Primary Assessment

As with all patients, you will perform a complete primary assessment as the first step in the assessment process. As you approach the patient, make note of his position. Is he sitting up and alert, or is he lying in bed and unresponsive? The patient who is sitting up and aware of his surroundings clearly has a patent airway and is breathing. The patient who presents as unresponsive will require a more aggressive ABC check before you can move on to your secondary assessment.

Confirm that the patient has a clear airway and is breathing with an adequate rate and tidal volume. Confirm that he has an adequate pulse and that there are no immediate threats to life before moving on to your secondary assessment.

OBJECTIVE

6. Explain the unique challenges that can arise when assessing and caring for the geriatric patient.

KEY POINT ▼

Due to an increased risk of tuberculosis in nursing home patients, consider using a HEPA mask as part of your personal protective equipment (PPE).

KEY POINT ▼

Most states have laws that require Emergency Medical Responders to report suspected cases of geriatric abuse and neglect. Make sure that you are familiar with your local requirements.

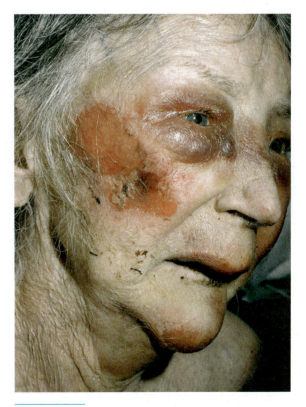

Figure 24.7 • When you encounter evidence of trauma, consider the possibility of abuse until proven otherwise.

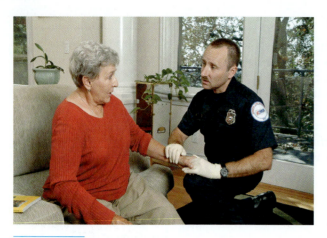

Figure 24.8 • Position yourself at the patient's level, make good eye contact, and speak slowly and clearly.

OBJECTIVE

7. Describe changes in the approach to care when caring for geriatric patients.

KEY POINT ▼

Geriatric patients often do not reveal problems behind the chief complaint because they either fear the loss of independence or they consider the illness "normal" for their age. The best way to determine the patient's chief complaint without getting too much information about unrelated conditions is to ask, "Why did you call today?" or "What is different about how you feel today?"

OBJECTIVE

5. Describe the common medical problems of geriatric patients.

Alzheimer's disease ▶ a progressive, degenerative disease that attacks the brain and results in impaired memory, thinking, and behavior.

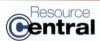

View a video to learn more about Alzheimer's disease.

Obtaining a History

Unlike the majority of younger patients, gathering a medical history on an elderly person may take quite a bit of time. You will find it helpful to first obtain the patient's medications (prescription and over-the-counter) and then ask why each is taken. Also be aware of the patient's surroundings. Are there medical identification tags or stickers? Oxygen supplies? Is there anything else that would indicate a medical condition? If you are unsure about a patient's answers to your questions, try to verify the information he or she gives you with a reliable source such as a caregiver.

The Physical Exam

The following considerations are important when examining a geriatric patient:

- Handle elderly patients gently.
- Histories and exams can easily tire elderly patients.
- Always explain what you are going to do before you do it.
- Anticipate numerous layers of clothing (due to problems with temperature regulation).
- Respect the modesty and privacy of elderly patients.

Remember that some geriatric patients may deny or minimize symptoms during the physical exam. Often this is because they fear being hospitalized and losing their independence, if the extent of their condition is "discovered."

Common Medical Problems of Geriatric Patients

As we age and our bodies become less efficient, illnesses become more common. The average geriatric patient may be taking several different medications to help minimize the effects of those illnesses related to age.

Illnesses

Common illnesses among the elderly include pneumonia, chronic obstructive pulmonary diseases, cancer, heart failure, aneurysm, high blood pressure, brain attack (stroke), dementia, Parkinson's disease, diabetes, bleeding in the stomach, esophagus or intestines, urinary tract infections, and reactions to medications. Due to the thinning of skin, a decreased ability to perspire, and muted physical sensations, heat- and cold-related emergencies are also common among geriatric patients.

Another illness that affects over 5 million elderly in the United States is **Alzheimer's disease**. Alzheimer's is a progressive, degenerative disease that attacks the brain and results in impaired memory, thinking, and behavior. Deaths due to Alzheimer's are on the rise and increased over 46% between the years 2000 and 2006. Alzheimer's can last from 3 to 20 years. As it progresses, the patient is less able to properly care for his or her own needs, often resulting in self-neglect.

Injuries

Trauma caused by falls is the leading cause of injury death among the elderly. The weakening of bones, deterioration of skin integrity, and loss of blood vessel flexibility all combine to make injuries much more severe for geriatric patients. Add to that the medications taken by many elderly persons, including those that can prevent clotting and make controlling bleeding extremely difficult. In those cases, you can have a relatively minor injury for a young patient actually causing serious injury or even death for an elderly one.

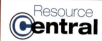
From the Medical Director

Bleeding Control

Many of the medications prescribed include those that can prevent clotting and as a result make controlling bleeding extremely difficult.

As an Emergency Medical Responder, you should be an advocate for injury prevention among the elderly. As you are responding to the homes of geriatric patients, you should always be looking for potential dangers, such as unsecured rugs, loose handrails, unsafely stacked items, and so on, and make a caregiver or family member aware of the safety concerns.

Elder Abuse and Neglect

According to the Center of Excellence on Elder Abuse and Neglect at the University of California at Irvine, elder and dependent adult abuse is the mistreatment or neglect of an elderly person or disabled adult. As mentioned earlier, an elderly person is anyone over the age of 65. A dependent adult is anyone between the ages of 18 and 64 who is physically, developmentally, or emotionally disabled.

Elder neglect is defined as the abandonment or the deprivation of basic needs such as water, food, housing, clothing, or medical care. There is another form of abuse unique to this population called self-neglect. **Self-neglect** is characterized by the inability or unwillingness to provide or care for oneself. Self-neglect can be a deliberate act on the part of the elderly person, who has purposely given up or intentionally stopped caring for themselves. It also can be the result of an inability to properly care for oneself due to illness, dementia, or physical limitations.

Elder abuse comes in many forms as well, including:

- *Physical abuse*, such as hitting, pushing, causing unnecessary pain, intentional misuse of medication, causing injury, and unauthorized restraint
- *Sexual abuse*, such as inappropriate exposure, inappropriate sexual advances, inappropriate sexual contact, sexual exploitation, and rape
- *Emotional or verbal abuse, such as humiliation, threats of harm or abandonment, isolation, non-communication, intimidation*
- *Financial abuse, such as undue influence to change legal documents, misuse of property, and theft or embezzlement*

The signs of abuse and neglect are not always obvious and sometimes difficult to identify. In many cases, the injuries or circumstances can be blamed on the normal characteristics of aging, such as dementia, coexisting illnesses, and more frequent falls.

Some clues that you might discover during your physical exam that may be indications of abuse or neglect include:

- Sores, bruises, or other wounds
- Unkempt appearance
- Poor hygiene
- Malnutrition
- Dehydration

Advocate for the Elderly

As an Emergency Medical Responder you have a duty to serve as an advocate for your patients, especially those patient populations that may not be able to care or advocate for themselves. When caring for the elderly, be especially diligent when obtaining a history and performing your physical exam. Be sure to evaluate for signs and symptoms that may not necessarily pertain to the chief complaint. Common signs of suspected abuse:

- Unrealistic or vague explanations for injuries
- An obvious delay in seeking care

KEY POINT ▼

Remember that a fall often has more than one cause. When assessing an elderly fall patient, be sure to thoroughly investigate the exact cause of any fall and interview anyone who may have witnessed the event.

IS IT SAFE?

An elderly patient who has suffered an injury has a greater likelihood of developing hypothermia, even in an environment that you would consider mild or warm. Carefully monitor body temperature and ensure that the patient is kept warm at all times.

elder neglect ▶ the neglect by caregivers of the needs of an elderly person, usually one who is disabled or frail.

self-neglect ▶ **a condition whereby an individual fails to attend to his or her own basic needs, such as hygiene, appropriate clothing, medical care, and so on.**

elder abuse ▶ the physical, sexual, or emotional abuse of an elderly person, usually one who is disabled or frail.

OBJECTIVES

8. Describe common signs and symptoms of abuse and neglect.

9. Explain the role of the Emergency Medical Responder in cases of suspected abuse and/or neglect.

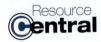
- Unexplained injuries (past or present)
- Poor interaction between patient and caregiver

Much like any suspected case of abuse or neglect, you have an obligation to carefully and thoroughly document your findings objectively and report all cases of suspected abuse or neglect to the proper authorities. All 50 states have specific guidelines for the reporting of elder abuse and neglect, and your instructor can provide you with the details for your state.

WRAP-UP

FIRST ON SCENE

Within minutes, the intersection is bustling with firefighters in turnout pants and dark T-shirts, along with several serious-looking police officers. The ambulance arrives moments later, its siren trailing off to silence about two blocks before it reaches the scene. A bald firefighter with a large mustache takes over holding the patient's head while several others begin gently straightening her body on the pavement. Tom stands and stretches his back before quickly pointing at the patient's leg. "I think it looks broken. Make sure to be careful with it."

"We've got it, thanks," comes the reply from one of the firefighters. By now the patient is no longer smiling, but biting her lower lip and clawing at the pavement each time the group of firefighters straightens body parts.

Once the woman is secured to the board and lifted onto the ambulance gurney, the bald fireman walks over to where Tom stands giving information to a police officer. "You did a real good job by taking care of the C-spine right away." He pats Tom on the shoulder. "A lot of people would've jumped right to dealing with the busted leg."

"Thanks." Tom smiles, feeling his face redden. He wants to say more, but before he can think of anything, the firefighter has already disappeared into the fire truck across the intersection. About 20 minutes later, Tom gets back into his car, intent on finally locking up the pool area at the Meadow Glen Apartments. Only now, as he rests his hand on the jump bag in the passenger seat, he isn't quite so concerned about running behind.

CHAPTER REVIEW

Summary

- The assessment and emergency care of geriatric patients can sometimes be challenging due to normal age-related changes in the human body.

- Many geriatric patients have multiple illnesses, take numerous prescription and over-the-counter medications, have problems with mobility, and may have issues of incontinence.

- The respiratory system can experience a reduction in strength and endurance of the muscles that assist in breathing, a loss of lung elasticity, and collapsing of the smaller airway structures, all of which contribute to respiratory challenges.

- The circulatory system can be affected by a thickening of the walls of the heart, a reduction in the effectiveness of the heart's conduction system, and a loss of elasticity of the blood vessels, which can cause everything from reduced cardiac output and dysrhythmia to aneurysms that can burst.

- Age-related deterioration of the nervous system can cause slowing of psychomotor functioning, decreased reaction times, forgetfulness, and loss of sensation and coordination, which is often the cause of falls among the elderly.

- Osteoporosis and degeneration of the musculoskeletal system can cause bone weakness and general instability, which

can lead to falls and serious injuries. You also will notice degeneration-related curvature of the spine in some elderly patients, which makes immobilization and airway maintenance a challenge.

- Age changes the skin in several important ways. The skin becomes thinner and weaker, more susceptible to tears and injuries, and yet due to sluggish cellular regeneration, it can be very slow to heal.

- When assessing a geriatric patient, remember to look for things in the patient's environment such as unsafe conditions, nonworking heating and cooling systems, and signs that may indicate abuse or neglect.

- Be respectful when physically examining a geriatric patient, ensuring modesty and privacy.

- Elder abuse can come in many forms, including physical, emotional, sexual, and financial.

- As an Emergency Medical Responder you have a legal duty to report suspected cases of abuse and neglect to the appropriate authorities.

Take Action

GETTING TO KNOW YOU

As a young person, it may be impossible to truly understand what it feels like to get old. However, we do believe you can strive to better understand the struggles and frustrations that the elderly face as a result of the aging process. For this activity, identify someone in your life that is above the age of 65 and perhaps close to 80 if possible. Make an appointment to sit down with

the person and discuss, from a medical standpoint, what the aging experience has been like. You should explain this is part of your new training as an Emergency Medical Responder. If possible, ask to be allowed to perform a patient assessment, including a history and vital signs. Your goal is to better understand the feelings, struggles, and frustrations that come with age and care for an elderly person who may become ill or injured.

First on Scene Run Review

Recall the events of the "First on Scene" scenario in this chapter and answer the following questions, which are related to the call. Rationales are offered in the Answer Key at the back of the book.

1. How would Tom make the scene safe?

2. How should Tom assess the person after he was holding the head?

3. What information should Tom give to the firefighters?

Quick Quiz

To check your understanding of the chapter, answer the following questions. Then compare your answers to those in the Answer Key at the back of the book.

1. Geriatric patients often are less able to defend against illness and may take much longer to recover when they do become ill. This often results in:

   a. multiple simultaneous illnesses.
   b. forgetting doctor appointments.
   c. taking the wrong medications.
   d. hearing loss.

2. The average geriatric patient takes _____ medications per day.

a. 2.5
b. 3.0
c. 4.5
d. 10.0

3. Which one of the following can cause a patient's illness or disease process to become worse?

a. Overdosing
b. Underdosing
c. Dementia
d. Incontinence

4. The loss of mobility is a common complaint among the elderly and can lead to other problems, such as:

a. skeletal fractures.
b. hearing loss.
c. depression.
d. nearsightedness.

5. The inability to retain urine or feces is called:

a. dementia.
b. aphasia.
c. priapism.
d. incontinence.

6. When assessing a geriatric patient who has an altered mental status, you must:

a. do your best to keep him awake and alert.
b. determine if his mental state is normal.
c. determine if he has had any recent surgeries.
d. find out from family if he can walk.

7. All of the following are ways the respiratory system is affected by the aging process EXCEPT:

a. increased strength of respiratory muscles.
b. decreased flexibility of the chest.
c. collapse of the smaller airways.
d. loss of elasticity.

8. The aging process can cause a degeneration of the heart's electrical system, which can lead to:

a. hearing loss.
b. vision loss.
c. dysrhythmia.
d. stroke (brain attack).

9. Age-related changes in the musculoskeletal system can lead to changes in posture, range of motion, and:

a. awareness.
b. medication usage.
c. mental status.
d. balance.

10. Most states have laws that require Emergency Medical Responders to report suspected cases of:

a. dementia.
b. abuse and neglect.
c. Alzheimer's disease.
d. overdose.

11. You have been called to the home of an elderly person and discover that she is refusing care. She states that she just wants to be left alone. You observe that the patient lives alone, is wearing only undergarments, and has multiple open sores and bruises over her body. These are most likely the signs of:

a. abuse.
b. neglect.
c. self-neglect.
d. Alzheimer's

12. While caring for an elderly patient, he shares with you that his caregiver frequently leaves him alone in his bedroom for days and refuses to respond to his calls for assistance. This may be a form of what type of abuse?

a. Physical
b. Emotional
c. Financial
d. Sexual

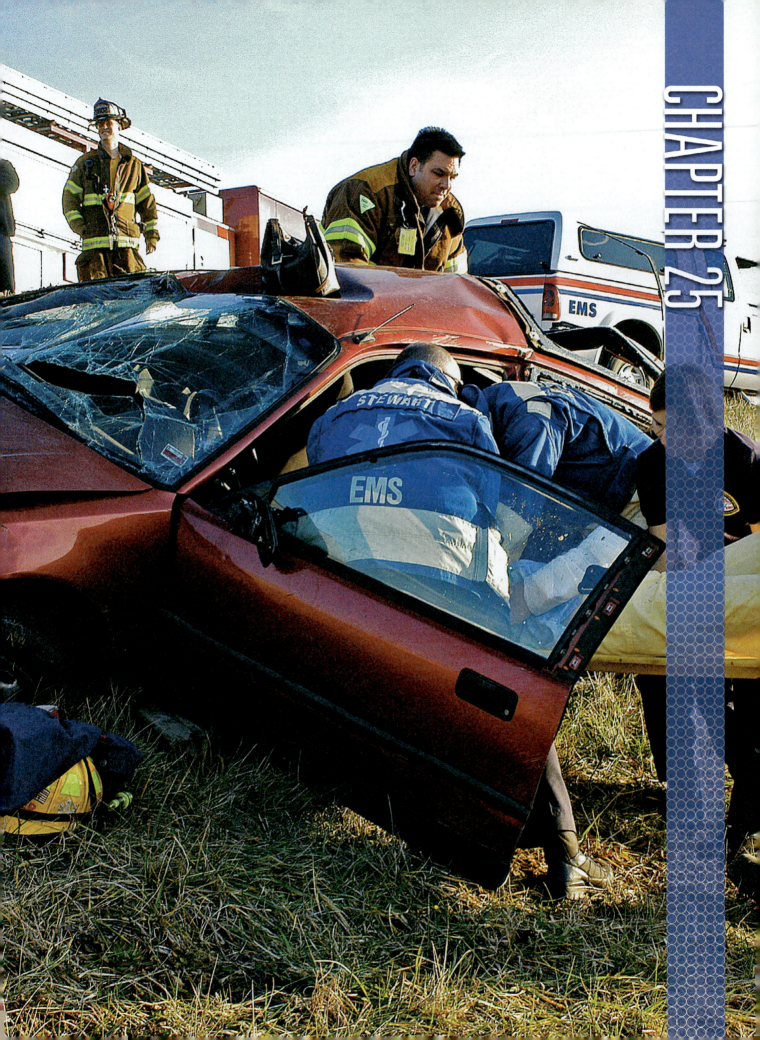

CHAPTER 25

Introduction to EMS Operations and Hazardous Response

EDUCATION STANDARDS
- EMS Operations—Principles of Safely Operating a Ground Ambulance, Hazardous Materials Awareness, Vehicle Extrication

COMPETENCIES
- Knowledge of operational roles and responsibilities to ensure safe patient, public, and personnel safety.

CHAPTER OVERVIEW

Emergency Medical Responders are just one component of an EMS system that functions and responds 24 hours a day, every day of the year. These operations include many services involving a wide range of skills. Emergency Medical Responders provide basic services, such as responding to minor illnesses and injuries. They also are prepared for more serious medical and trauma incidents, such as helping Emergency Medical Technicians (EMT) and Advance Life Support (ALS) personnel, such as Advanced Emergency Medical Technicians (AEMT) and Paramedics, in monitoring and providing care for critically injured patients at vehicle crashes, building fires, and other hazardous scenes and multiple-casualty incidents.

Learning what steps to take, what care to provide, and what assistance to give, and performing these tasks in cooperation with other personnel and services in the system are all part of EMS operations.

OBJECTIVES

Upon successful completion of this chapter, the student should be able to:

COGNITIVE

1. Define the following terms:
   a. cold zone *(p. 576)*
   b. complex access *(p. 566)*
   c. due regard *(p. 564)*
   d. extrication *(p. 567)*
   e. hazardous materials *(p. 575)*
   f. *Hazardous Materials: Emergency Response Guidebook (p. 575)*
   g. HAZWOPER *(p. 575)*
   h. hot zone *(p. 576)*
   i. placard *(p. 576)*
   j. simple access *(p. 566)*
   k. warm zone *(p. 576)*

2. Describe the common equipment necessary to appropriately respond to an emergency. *(p. 563)*

3. Describe common devices used at the scene of an emergency to keep personnel and the scene safe. *(pp. 565)*

4. Explain the importance of keeping all equipment serviceable and ready at all times. *(p. 563)*

5. Describe the phases of an emergency call. *(p. 563)*

6. Explain the appropriate use of lights and sirens when responding to or from an emergency scene. *(p. 564)*

7. Explain the concept of due regard when responding in an emergency vehicle. *(p. 564)*

8. Explain the role of the Emergency Medical Responder during extrication operations. *(p. 565)*

9. Describe common hazards during vehicle extrication operations. *(p. 565)*

10. Differentiate various methods for gaining access to an entrapped patient. *(p. 566)*

11. Differentiate simple vs. complex access as it pertains to patient extrication. *(p. 566)*

12. Explain the role of the Emergency Medical Responder at a hazardous materials incident. *(p. 575)*

13. Describe the common signs of a potential hazardous materials incident. *(p. 575)*

14. Differentiate the purpose of the cold, warm, and hot zones at a hazardous materials incident. *(p. 577)*

PSYCHOMOTOR

15. Demonstrate the ability to identify and manage common hazards at a simulated emergency response.

16. Demonstrate the process for proper cleaning and de-contamination of equipment following a simulated emergency response.

17. Demonstrate how to use the *Emergency Response Guidebook* appropriately to identify a suspected hazardous material.

AFFECTIVE

18. Value the importance of always being ready and prepared for an emergency response by keeping equipment serviceable and ready for a response.

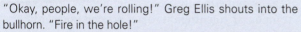

FIRST ON SCENE

"Okay, people, we're rolling!" Greg Ellis shouts into the bullhorn. "Fire in the hole!"

Greg is the safety supervisor for Legend Studios. He watches as the small army of technicians and pyrotechnicians all don safety goggles and squint against the anticipated propane explosion. It is a cool, dark night; and once the flood lights are doused, shrouding the five-story-tall, fabric blue screen in total darkness, the only light still visible on the film set is the bobbing tip of somebody's cigarette.

After a full minute of dark silence, somebody swears loudly and yells for the lights. The generators cough and sputter to life; and, as the floodlights warm, they grow steadily brighter, until the entire set is illuminated in harsh, white light.

"What's the problem, McQueeny?" Greg walks over to the pyrotechnician hovering above the control box.

"I don't know," the man says. "It should have gone." He is interrupted by a deafening rushing sound, like a tornado passing directly overhead, and jets of flame erupt like large, boiling clouds from the pressure valve at the far end of the pipe system.

The explosion immediately superheats the night air and sends the crew scattering in all directions as the monstrous blue screen catches fire. The flames race up the fabric, sending burning bits fluttering down behind them.

"Shut it off!" Greg shouts, as he tries to avoid the flames floating down from the sky like glowing snowflakes. "Everybody run!"

The lead pyrotechnician succeeds in shutting the main propane valve, but it is too late. The blue screen is fully engulfed and raining fire down onto a bank of large propane tanks on a nearby concrete pad. Greg dials 911 on his cell phone as he and the crowd of technicians run east along the main studio access road.

Safety

Your first consideration at any emergency scene is your own safety. To ensure it, you must learn to follow *standard operating procedures (SOPs)*, limit your actions to your training level, and use the proper equipment and the required number of trained persons for any task (Figure 25.1). SOPs are specific and different for every department, service, and jurisdiction. SOPs outline how you will function operationally within your own organization.

There will always be risks associated with emergency responses, but EMS personnel must minimize those risks by learning which ones can be controlled before acting. You must be able to develop a "risk vs. benefit analysis" mentality. Meaning, does the risk related to your actions on the scene have a measurable benefit? There is a fine line between aggressiveness and recklessness. This is the "gray" area of risk management and decision-making that *all* of us in emergency services are responsible for. Always remember: Some risks you can avoid, some risks you can pass off to other agencies, and some risks you have to face.

EMS is a dangerous profession, but one that demands effective management of risk. For example, you have no control over the chance that a drunk driver could crash into you as you provide care at the scene of a traffic collision. But by using proper warning devices (for example, reflective triangles, cones, or flares), positioning response vehicles properly to divert traffic, and by positioning your own vehicle properly, you can minimize your risks of being injured by passing cars (Figure 25.2).

At any emergency scene, the following rules must always be followed:

- Prior to approaching the patient, be certain it is safe to do so. If there is a hazard, make sure you can control it before you approach. If you cannot control a hazard, wait for assistance.

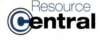

Resource Central

Learn more about roadside vehicle safety and emergency vehicle safety.

KEY POINT ▼

Many types of emergencies require specialized training and equipment to operate safely. If you are not properly trained you must stay clear and call for the appropriate resources.

KEY POINT ▼

You must maintain a healthy respect for risk, and always be evaluating the risk vs. benefit of any hazardous action you undertake.

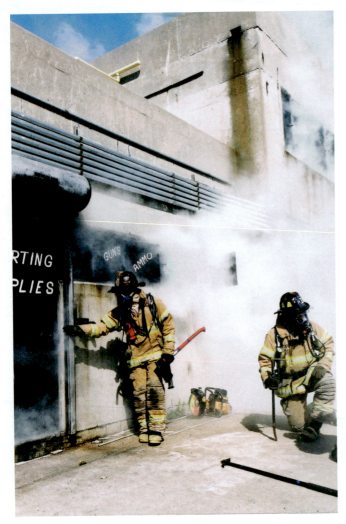

Figure 25.1 • Ensure the safety of you and your crew before entering the scene.
(© Craig Jackson/In the Dark Photography)

- Use the protective gear appropriate for the situation and for which you are certified or qualified to wear. Examples include firefighting turnout gear, hazmat suit, eye protection, and gloves. All emergency responders are now required by law to wear an approved high-visibility safety vest. On November 24, 2008, a new federal regulation (23 CFR 634) went into effect mandating that anyone working in the right-of-way of a federal-aid highway must be wearing high-visibility clothing that meets the requirements of ANSI/ISEA 107, 2004 edition, class 2 or 3. This requirement applies to *all* emergency responders.
- Legally and ethically, you are limited by your level of training. If you attempt to act beyond your level of training, you may risk injury to yourself, cause harm to the patient, or add to the extent of the incident
- When you call dispatch, describe the incident so that the needed personnel and equipment may respond as soon as possible.

The Call

Emergency Medical Responder responsibilities at motor-vehicle collisions will vary, depending on the type of agency, jurisdiction, regulations, and SOPs. You must be prepared to perform your duties on any emergency call (Figure 25.3). You have a legal and ethical responsibility to always be prepared to respond to an emergency. Therefore, one of your first duties at the beginning of every shift is to thoroughly check all equipment and confirm it is in working order.

All EMS responses progress through several phases. These phases may differ slightly, depending on the level of care you provide. For Emergency Medical Responders, the

Figure 25.2 • There are many ways you can make the scene safer once you arrive.

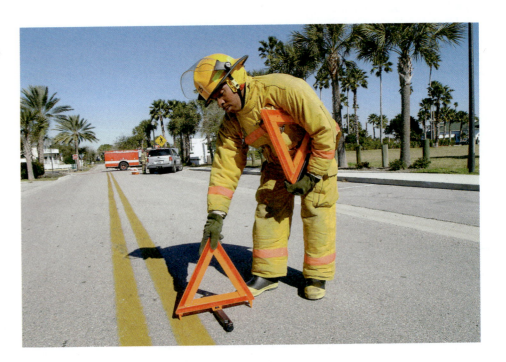

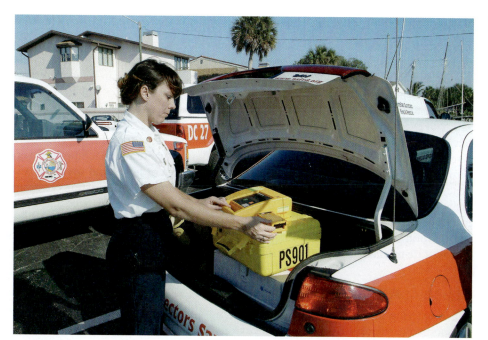

six phases of an emergency call include preparation, dispatch, en route to the scene, arrival at the scene, transferring patients, and after the emergency.

Phase 1: Preparation

Being prepared means having the proper training, tools, equipment, and personnel:

- *Medical supplies.* Make sure your unit is stocked with medical supplies such as personal protective equipment (PPE), airways, suctioning equipment, artificial ventilation devices (pocket face masks, bag masks), and basic wound-care supplies (dressings, bandages).
- *Nonmedical supplies.* Check for other necessary items such as personal safety equipment (helmets), flares, flashlights, fire extinguisher, blanket, simple tools (screwdrivers, hammer, spring-loaded punch), and area maps.
- *Equipment.* Be sure to check that all special equipment is on your unit and operating properly, that any malfunctioning equipment is replaced or repaired, and that all supplies are restocked. Check the engine compartment and fluid levels of your vehicle (fuel, oil, transmission, windshield washer). It is also important to check the emergency equipment, including flashing lights, sirens, and radios, at the beginning of every shift or on a daily basis.
- *Personnel.* Ensure that the appropriate number of personnel are on duty and will be able to respond with you or can be dispatched to assist you, if necessary.

Phase 2: Dispatch

Be familiar with your dispatch or communications system and what procedures you follow when dispatched. Note any information the dispatcher gives you about the call.

Most dispatch systems have a central dispatch or communications center with 24-hour access. Dispatch centers are staffed with personnel specially trained to dispatch the most appropriate units. Many dispatch centers are training their personnel in Emergency Medical Dispatch programs so they may provide pre-arrival instructions to the caller over the telephone while EMS personnel are responding.

All dispatchers are trained to gather as much information from the caller as possible and relay that information to responding units. The nature of the call, the location of the incident or the patient, the number of victims, and the severity of illness or injury, as well as any other special problems that responders might encounter at the scene, are all important pieces of information and must be relayed to responding personnel.

OBJECTIVES

2. Describe the common equipment necessary to appropriately respond to an emergency.

4. Explain the importance of keeping all equipment serviceable and ready at all times.

5. Describe the phases of an emergency call.

KEY POINT ▼

More often than not, the information received from dispatch can be incomplete or incorrect. Always expect the unexpected when responding to what would otherwise appear a routine dispatch.

6. Explain the appropriate use of lights and sirens when responding to or from an emergency scene.

7. Explain the concept of due regard when responding in an emergency vehicle.

due regard ▶ the appropriate care and concern for the safety of others.

Phase 3: En Route to the Scene

Emergency Medical Responder duties continue while en route to an emergency scene and include more than simply finding the location on the map. State vehicle codes give special privileges to operators of emergency vehicles when responding to an emergency. However, these privileges do not relieve the operator from the responsibility of keeping everyone's safety in mind. You must always operate an emergency vehicle with **due regard** for the safety of everyone on the road. Failure to do so is risky and may result in fines and penalties from local law enforcement. Emergency lights must be on for all emergency responses. Sirens should be used when traffic is an issue and when approaching and traveling through intersections. Some jurisdictions require the use of lights and sirens for all emergency responses. Your ability to drive defensively and anticipate the actions of other drivers will help ensure a safe response. You must communicate with dispatch and keep them informed of any delays you may encounter while en route. Be sure you have the essential information on the call, such as location, potential hazards, and number of patients. Do not hesitate to check back with the dispatcher if you need more information.

Phase 4: Arrival at the Scene

When arriving at the scene, be extra alert and approach cautiously. Look for hazards. Position your response unit where you have access to it but where it will not interfere with access to the scene by other responders. A good rule of thumb if you are the first on scene is 50 feet before the scene with emergency lights or flashers activated. Remember to always keep your eye on traffic. Do not become a victim yourself. Whenever possible, always position your vehicle as if there were a hazardous materials spill; that is, upwind and uphill from the crash scene.

Notify the dispatcher of your arrival. Because dispatchers can only communicate what they are given from the reporting party, you may have to provide additional information once you arrive on scene, such as:

- Actual location of the incident if it is different from what was given on dispatch
- Type of incident and the need for additional resources (utility company, air medical helicopter, law enforcement)
- Number of victims

Size up the scene to ensure that it is safe. Do your best to identify any hazards before entering. Put on your PPE, including your approved, federally mandated reflective vests. As you approach, look for the mechanism of injury in trauma scenes or determine if it is a medical emergency.

Always stabilize vehicles before entering them or attempting to extricate any patients. Determine if it is a multiple-casualty incident and, if so, determine the approximate number of patients. Evaluate patients quickly to determine if they are high or low priority. Do you need to move patients immediately? Can it be done safely? Will you need more assistance? Let the dispatcher know what additional resources you are going to need as soon as possible.

Phase 5: Transferring Patients

Emergency Medical Responders help lift, carry, and load patients on appropriate devices and assist in preparing the patient for transport. While doing so, be sure to use appropriate lifting and moving procedures. You also need to provide the transporting personnel

From the Medical Director

Arriving at the Scene
Always consider the possibility of hazardous materials when positioning vehicles. When in doubt, use the Emergency Response Guidebook *to identify potential hazards.*

with an accurate account of the patient's status. If practical, provide them with written documentation of your assessment findings.

Phase 6: After the Emergency

The phases of emergency calls are cyclic. Once a call is finished, prepare for the next call, including cleaning and disinfecting equipment, restocking supplies, and refueling the emergency vehicle. You also should complete paperwork and file reports, participate in debriefing, and, finally, notify the dispatcher that you are back in service.

Motor-Vehicle Collisions

Once you ensure your own safety, your main duty at the scene of an emergency is to provide patient care. At the scene of a motor-vehicle collision, however, you may have other duties to perform before you can reach the patients. Your responsibilities at the scene may include:

- Making the scene safe, ensuring no one else is hurt as they approach
- Requesting additional resources as appropriate
- Gaining access to patients
- Freeing trapped patients
- Evaluating patients and providing emergency care
- Moving patients who are in danger from fire, explosion, and other hazards
- Determining which patients may be moved so that you can reach and provide care for another more critically injured patient

Many Emergency Medical Responders are injured each year as they attempt to help at vehicle collisions. They are struck by another vehicle when they do not take initial steps to make the scene safe. Your first step is to secure an area around the scene so you can work safely. Remember to maintain a risk vs. benefit mentality.

Law enforcement officers and firefighters must follow their department's SOPs on vehicle collisions. However, if you are an Emergency Medical Responder without a special course in collision-scene procedures, use the items listed here as guidelines or follow your local protocols. Because each collision scene is unique, you will need to proceed with caution, carefully observe the scene, and decide what actions to take to control it. Follow these steps:

1. Position your vehicle approximately 50 feet before the scene. Turn on your vehicle's emergency flashers. You may want to use your headlights to light up the scene. If so, be sure to angle your vehicle so that it does not blind oncoming drivers.

2. Make certain that you have parked in a safe location. Look for fuel spills and fire. If you are downhill from the scene, fuel may run in your direction. Check the wind direction. Will the wind carry smoke or fire to where you have parked?

3. If your jurisdiction or agency has SOPs for positioning your unit and using warning lights, follow those guidelines. If you turn off the unit, you cannot leave your warning lights on because the battery will be drained of all power and you will be unable to start your vehicle.

4. Set out emergency warning devices, such as cones, flashing lights, or flares, to warn others. On high-speed roads, place one of those devices at least 250 feet from the scene. On low-speed roads, set one of the devices at least 100 feet from the scene. Add at least 25 feet to those distances if the scene is on a curved road.

5. As you approach, check the scene again for safety. Is there fire, leaking fuel or gases, unstable vehicles, or downed electrical wires? If any of those conditions are present, make certain to request the appropriate resources to mitigate the hazards. If a power line is down, get the nearest pole number so you may request that power be turned off. You may need fire services and a rescue squad at the scene. Some jurisdictions automatically dispatch units for motor-vehicle collisions.

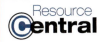

Resource Central

Learn more about ambulance cleaning and disinfection.

OBJECTIVES

8. Explain the role of the Emergency Medical Responder during extrication operations.

9. Describe common hazards during vehicle extrication operations.

KEY POINT ▼

There are thousands of people injured and even killed while attempting to assist at the scene of an vehicle collision. Make certain you ensure your safety before attempting to care for patients.

IS IT SAFE?

For example, as you approach the scene of a vehicle collision, perform a "windshield survey," meaning from the inside of your vehicle get a 360-degree general impression of the scene through all windows. Look carefully for signs of fluid spilling from any of the vehicles. Avoid driving through or parking over the spills or in the path of a fluid as it spreads. Consider all fluids as potentially flammable. Even if you think it might only be radiator coolant, it could still be mixed with fuel and ignite at any time. Be very aware of changing conditions.

OBJECTIVE

3. Describe common devices used at the scene of an emergency to keep personnel and the scene safe.

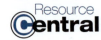
OBJECTIVES

10. Differentiate various methods for gaining access to an entrapped patient.

11. Differentiate simple vs. complex access as it pertains to patient extrication.

simple access ▶ a form of access to entrapped patients that does not require specialized tools or equipment.

complex access ▶ a form of access to patients that requires tools and specialized equipment.

6. As you approach, observe the scene for clues. How many patients can you see? Could someone have been thrown from a vehicle? Could someone have walked away from the scene? Do you see signs indicating that children were in the vehicle (bottles, toys, school books, car seats)? Are there signs that a pedestrian or bike rider was involved? Have someone alert the dispatcher and report the number of possible patients.

7. If the scene is safe, stabilize the vehicle by chocking the wheels, gain access to the patients, perform your assessments, and begin care on those who appear to be most critical.

Remember to evaluate risk vs. benefit. Do not approach or attempt to gain access to victims if the scene is not safe. If you cannot control traffic, if electric lines are down, if there is fire at the scene, or if there are fuel or hazardous material spills, you are in danger. Call the dispatcher for additional resources for any of those conditions. If you are not trained to deal with fires, electricity, or hazardous materials, protect yourself and stay uphill and upwind from any spills. An Emergency Medical Responder's first priority is personal safety. Your primary duty is to provide patient care at a safe scene. Do only what you have been trained to do.

Upright Vehicle

In most traffic collisions, the vehicles involved remain upright and are generally safer to approach than overturned vehicles. Even though the vehicles appear to be stable, with little chance of rolling or sliding away from the at-rest position, it is still necessary to take the safety precaution of stabilizing the vehicle.

Always evaluate vehicle stability when you assess the scene. As you look for traffic hazards, electrical hazards, spilled fuel, and fire, also see if there is any chance that the vehicle may roll away or flip over. Make sure vehicles are in "park" and the ignition is turned off, if you have immediate access. You may find the following situations:

- *Hills or slight inclines.* The vehicle may have come to rest on a surface that slants enough to allow forward or backward roll. To keep the vehicle from rolling, place wheel chocks, spare tires, logs, rocks, or similar objects under one or more wheels.
- *Slippery surfaces.* Ice, snow, or oil can produce a slippery road surface. If available, sprinkle dirt, sand, ashes, or kitty litter, or place newspapers around the wheels and chock the wheels to reduce the chances of slipping.
- *Tilted vehicle.* Even upright vehicles may be tilted to one side by their position or by the terrain. Do not work beneath a tilted vehicle or on the downhill side of one. Chocking the wheels may prevent the vehicle from tilting over, but tying the vehicle in place is safer. If strong rope is available, tie lines to the frame of the car (not the bumper) in front and back or to both sides. Then secure the lines to large trees or poles, guardrails, or heavier stable vehicles while waiting for fire services to arrive.
- *Stacked vehicles.* Part of one vehicle may be resting on top of another vehicle. There are several ways to stabilize them: chock the wheels of both vehicles; insert tires, lumber, blocks, or similar sturdy items between the road surface and the vehicles; or use line or rope to tie and secure both vehicles.

Vehicle Access

Never try to enter or work around a vehicle until you are certain that it is stable. Once you stabilize a vehicle, there are two access methods to use for reaching a patient: **simple access** and **complex access**. Simple access does not require equipment. Complex access requires tools and special equipment, which also calls for additional training. In most cases, you will approach an upright, stable vehicle and reach the patient by simple access. If the doors and windows are closed, there are four ways to gain access to the patients:

- *Open the doors.* Many people drive without locking the doors. However, many new models automatically lock once they reach a speed of 5 mph. Some lock when the driver puts the transmission in "drive." Check all the doors, including side and rear doors on vans and hatchbacks, before trying another entry method. If all doors are locked, one of the occupants may be able to unlock a door. "Try before you pry."

- *Enter through a window.* If doors are locked or jammed, the patient may be able to roll down a window. If not, you will have to break a window. When you begin using tools to access patients, the process becomes more complex. Remember, you must wear the proper PPE for vehicle **extrication** as you will be placing yourself in danger with sharp objects. Helmet, eye protection, gloves, and turnout coat and pants are recommended.

- *Pry open the doors.* This method is very time-consuming and not very practical given the technology available today. Access through windows is usually more practical.

- *Cut through the metal.* The only other access when entry through doors and windows is not possible is cutting through vehicle roofs, trunks, and doors. This entry method takes special tools that Emergency Medical Responders do not usually carry unless they are also members of fire services. If you cannot gain access through a door or window, it may be possible to cut around the lock of a door using a sharp tool (chisel or strong screwdriver) and a hammer.

extrication ▶ the coordinated removal of entrapped patients from vehicles and structures.

Your instructor will teach you how to use these entry methods if they are Emergency Medical Responder skills in your jurisdiction.

Keep in mind that speed is sometimes crucial when you need to reach patients in a vehicle. Precious time is lost if you have to return to your vehicle to retrieve tools. Take all tools with you as you approach a vehicle. Many simple tools will help you gain access to a vehicle, including screwdrivers, chisels, hammers, pliers, wire, washers, and pry bars. Some Emergency Medical Responder tool kits include commercial "Slim Jims" for unlocking doors and spring-loaded center punches for breaking glass. Access with tools and special equipment is considered complex because it takes time, planning, and sometimes special training; and it requires taking additional safety precautions to protect yourself and the patient.

KEY POINT ▼

Don't forget to try the obvious when attempting to access an entrapped patient. Try all doors and windows before deciding to break glass or cut into a vehicle.

Unlocking Vehicle Doors

Special commercial tools for unlocking doors may be part of your Emergency Medical Responder kit. You might be able to unlock doors of older vehicles by slipping a commercial tool known as a "Slim Jim" between the window and the door. You also might be able to pry open the window with a wood wedge or pry bar and slip a wire coat hanger inside the window (Scan 25.1). Opening newer locks using these methods might be impossible, depending on the manufacturer. Some cars have a dead-bolt system that cannot be unlocked with special tools. Those types of locks are designed to unlock on impact and allow rescuers to gain access. If you cannot unlock or open a door, gain access through a window.

Before you attempt to unlock a door, confirm that all doors are indeed locked and windows are up, preventing access any other way. Also be sure occupants on the inside cannot unlock it.

Check the doors for damage. A severely damaged door may not open easily even if you do unlock it. If all doors are damaged, be prepared to break glass and gain access through the window. Look in the windows to see if the car has buttons in the armrest. It will not be easy to unlock doors with this type of locking device. Vehicles with electric locks and windows cannot be unlocked if the battery is disabled.

Gaining Access Through Vehicle Windows

To gain rapid access to patients who are unresponsive or unstable when the doors are locked, use a spring-loaded center punch on the rear or side windows. A heavy hammer may work, but it requires that you aim carefully and strike forcefully (possibly several times), which may shatter and spray glass. Always wear PPE, especially goggles and gloves, when breaking glass.

At the scene of a collision, most people consider breaking the windshield of a vehicle first if they cannot gain access through the doors. However, this is the wrong approach. Windshields are made of laminated safety glass, which has great strength. Even when

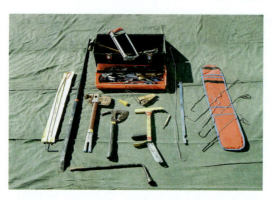

25.1.1 | Various tools can be used to help unlock vehicle doors in older vehicles (check model years):

- Wire hook
- Straight wire
- Slim Jim (or similar device)
- Screwdriver
- Flat pry bar

  An oil dipstick or a keyhole saw may be used to help force up a locking button.

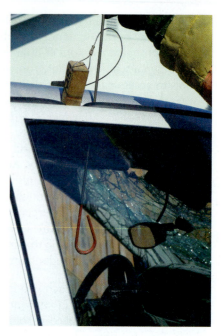

25.1.3 | For flat-top locks, use a hooked wire. Snag the locking button and pull upward.

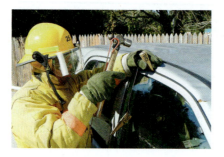

25.1.2 | For framed windows, pry the frame away from the vehicle body with a wood wedge and insert a wire hook.

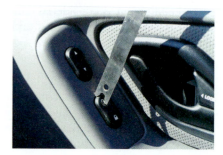

25.1.4 | For rocker or push-button locks on the door panel or on the armrest, use a straight wire and press the lock open.

shattered, the glass will still cling to an inner plastic layer. All cars have laminated safety glass windshields. Many foreign cars have this type of glass in all windows of a vehicle. If it is necessary to remove windshields, Emergency Medical Responders should leave that task to personnel trained in this rescue technique.

Rear and side windows are usually made of tempered glass. When this glass is broken, there is no plastic layer to hold the pieces. Tempered glass will not shatter into sharp pieces or shards. Instead, this glass will shatter into small, rounded pieces and will often drop straight down into the vehicle, if you break it in a corner with a spring-loaded center punch. The small glass pieces can cut, but the cuts are usually minor.

If you must use a hammer, do not bash the center of the glass with it, or you will send pieces throughout the entire passenger compartment.

When gaining access through a vehicle window, you should (Figure 25.4 and Figure 25.5):

1. Make certain the vehicle is stable. If possible, have the driver turn off the ignition.
2. Confirm that all doors and windows are locked and secure.
3. Protect yourself by wearing gloves and eye protection.

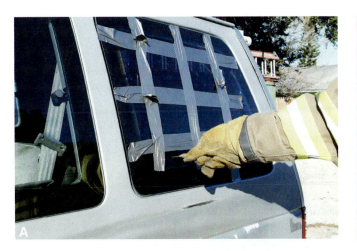
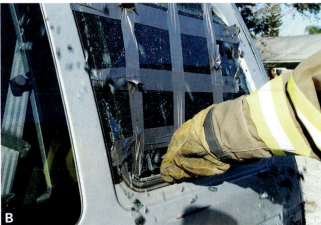
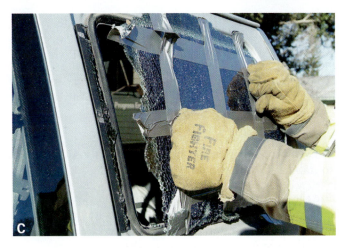

Figure 25.4 • To break a window: (A) Place duct tape across the window to help keep the glass intact after breaking. (B) Use a spring-loaded center punch in one of the corners to break the glass. (C) Once the glass is broken, remove it from the frame.

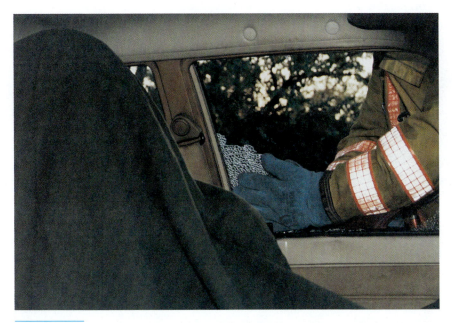

Figure 25.5 • Cover the patient with a blanket prior to breaking any glass. This will prevent the patient from being hit with broken glass.

4. If possible, select a window that is away from the patient. Place one gloved hand flat against the window, resting the heel of your hand on the corner of the door. Place the spring-loaded center punch between two fingers in one of the lower corners of the window, as close to the door as possible. Press the center punch with your other hand. When the window breaks, the hand pressing the center punch will not go through the window.

5. After breaking the window, reach in and try to open the door. You may only have to unlock the door to open it. Often, jammed doors that will not open from the outside will open from the inside.

6. Turn off the vehicle ignition, place the transmission in "park," and set the parking brake.

7. After breaking the glass, the door still may remain jammed. You still must gain access to your patient. Again, you must utilize proper PPE. If not equipped with this equipment, wait for fire or rescue personnel.

Overturned Vehicle

Do not try to right an overturned vehicle. Even if you have enough help to turn the vehicle upright, moving it can cause further injury to the occupants. Stabilize the overturned vehicle while waiting for fire service units and before you try to reach the occupants. Always look for fuel spills, battery acid, and other chemical hazards around an overturned vehicle.

Vehicle on Its Side

If you find a vehicle on its side and have some simple equipment, take the following precautions to stabilize it. You should (Figure 25.6):

1. Stabilize the vehicle with items such as tires, blocks, lumber, wheel chocks, cribbing, rocks, or similar available materials. Place the items between the road surface and the roofline. Also place stabilizing items between the road surface and the lower wheels, if the wheels are not resting on the road surface.

Figure 25.6 • Stabilize the vehicle before attempting to gain access to the patients. This may require specialized training. Do only what you have been trained to do.

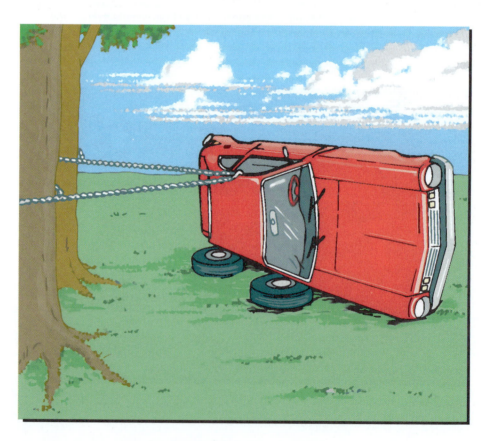

2. If the vehicle is still unstable, use strong rope or line to tie the vehicle to secure objects.

3. Attempt to gain access to occupants of the vehicle. Entry through a door is dangerous because the door may be seven feet or more off the ground and your weight will move the vehicle as you climb on it. It also will be difficult to open the door with the vehicle on its side. Your first and more sensible entry point will be through a window. The rear window is the best approach to take. Never attempt access to a damaged interior through broken glass without adequate protective clothing and equipment.

4. If you open a door, tie it securely open. Do not use a prop. Props can slip or be knocked away, causing the door to slam on you or the occupants.

Patients Pinned Beneath Vehicles

When a patient is pinned beneath a vehicle, call for a rescue squad immediately. Never place yourself in danger by reaching or crawling into the area where the patient is pinned. If it appears that the scene is too dangerous, Emergency Medical Responders can perform certain procedures to move the vehicle and free the patient, but this is often risky. Follow your department's SOPs in these situations.

A jack or pry bar and blocks can be used to raise a vehicle, which will enable rescuers to move the patient from beneath the vehicle. When lifting one side of the vehicle off the patient, be sure you are not causing the other side of the vehicle to press on another part of the patient (for example, his legs). With enough help, you may be able to lift the vehicle off the patient. In any attempt to raise a vehicle off a pinned patient, others must shore up the vehicle as you raise it so that it will not slip or fall back onto the rescuers or the patient. Use blocks, tires, lumber, or similar sturdy items at the scene. Do not attempt to enter the space to remove the victim until the entire vehicle is stable.

Patients Trapped in Wreckage

You may find patients with their arms, legs, or heads protruding through the window. Before trying to free them, you should use blankets to shield any patients who are still in the vehicle, while other rescuers continue to open the vehicle to provide better access and extrication. Use pliers, hammer claws, or a knife to carefully break or fold away glass around the patient's extremity.

When patients are trapped inside crushed vehicles, you must wait for special power tools and skilled rescue personnel. Trained personnel can quickly and easily free or disentangle patients from the wreck.

Emergency Medical Responders working on vehicles with occupants pinned inside often will be able to free some patients by way of the following:

- Remove wreckage from on top of and around the patient.
- Carefully move a seat forward or backward.
- Carefully lift out a back seat.
- Remove a patient's shoe to free a foot, or cut away clothing caught on wreckage.
- Cut seat belts, but be sure to properly support the patient during the cutting and after the tension has been released.
- Follow manufacturer and agency guidelines for working around vehicles with deployed and undeployed airbags. Check the steering wheel beneath the deployed airbag for damage indicating that the patient might have struck it. Airbags may also activate in the front seat passenger area, and some more recent models have side air curtains.

In any attempt to free patients from vehicles, you must consider the immediate need for quick access. If immediate access and patient movement is necessary to save a life, make every attempt to reach the patient. If the patient's life is not at risk but immediate movement will cause further injury, then leave the patient in place until more highly trained personnel respond to the scene.

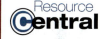

Learn about vehicles with airbags during emergencies.

IS IT SAFE?

Most late-model cars and trucks have airbags in the steering column as well as several other locations within the passenger compartment. It is possible for the airbags to deploy after a collision has occurred. Many EMS and fire personnel have been injured when an airbag deployed while they were attempting to care for a patient. Consider this risk before deciding to enter a vehicle involved in a collision.

During the wait talk to the patient, to offer reassurance and explain why you are taking precautions. While you are talking to the patient, begin your primary assessment and provide oxygen while another Emergency Medical Responder stabilizes the head. If you must move the patient before more advanced care personnel arrive, make every attempt to maintain stabilization of the patient's spine during the move. Once EMTs and other EMS personnel arrive, report your patient assessment findings and provide them with any assistance they need, such as taking vital signs, controlling bleeding, gathering special equipment, or loading and lifting the patient.

Building Access

Gaining access to a patient in a locked building may require special skills and tools outside the range of Emergency Medical Responder duties. There are many types of gates, doors, windows, and locks that restrict access to buildings. In addition to access problems, older buildings may have many hidden and unsuspected dangers. Security devices will present special barriers. Guard dogs will limit or halt your actions until they are contained.

Emergency Medical Responders are not expected to know how to open or destroy locks or have all the tools needed for the variety of windows, doors, and gates found in buildings. Unless you are trained in fire and rescue operations, you are not expected to know how to enter and make your way safely around an empty or abandoned building.

Follow the guidelines below for gaining access to patients inside any type of building (homes, offices, stores, schools). You will be expected to:

- Request additional resources, if necessary.
- Try opening and entering through open doors or windows first.
- Look for a key under mats or in mailboxes.
- Ask bystanders and neighbors if they have a key.
- Break glass to unlock doors or windows.

Follow your SOPs regarding notification of law enforcement prior to and following any forcible entry.

If you know or see that someone inside needs immediate care, do not try to gain access before calling for help. Your efforts to gain entry may fail, and you will need help as soon as possible. Call the dispatcher and request additional resources immediately.

While waiting for help, try different entry points. Try to open a door. If the door is locked, try opening a few low windows on your way to finding a second door. If the second door is locked, break the glass in a window or a door and enter as quickly but as safely as possible. Do not attempt to break through doors or windows made of large sheets of tempered glass. Some newer buildings and homes may have been constructed with Lexan resin (a type of plastic) or a special type of laminated glass that is designed to resist the forces of hurricanes and the debris carried by high winds. Those materials are extremely difficult to break and can bounce a hammer back into your face. Do not try climbing up walls or posts to reach a high window. Do not try to gain access to a window by walking across the roof. Call and wait for special rescue personnel who will have the appropriate equipment.

When attempting to break a window, you should:

1. Make certain that the patient is not lying near the other side of the glass.
2. Use a hammer or similar blunt object to strike the glass near one of its edges (Figure 25.7). A nightstick or an aluminum flashlight will break most window glass. If you do not have tools, use a rock or a similar solid object to strike the glass.

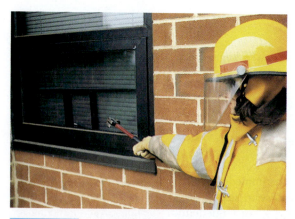

Figure 25.7 • When doors and windows are locked, you may have to break a window to gain access.

3. Carefully clear all glass from the frame and reach in to unlock the door or window.

4. Make certain that you are stepping onto a safe floor. Be sure that you do not have an unusual drop when entering. Take a moment to visually inspect the floor for damage or poke the floor for signs of weakness.

Hazards

Fire

Television and movies have led people to believe that they should enter burning buildings or run up to burning vehicles to save victims. This is a dangerous tactic. Those in the fire service are highly trained at their jobs. They are given special equipment and use special strategies to fight fires, which minimizes the risks to their safety. Firefighting requires special training, protective clothing, the right equipment, and usually more than one firefighter.

If you are a member of the fire service, follow SOPs for rescuing victims from vehicle and structure fires. If you are in law enforcement and have special training in rescuing victims from vehicle and structure fires, do only what you have been trained to do using proper PPE. If you are an Emergency Medical Responder without firefighting training, do not risk your life to approach a fire and provide care.

Motor-vehicle collisions do not usually produce fire, and most emergency calls to buildings do not involve fire. However, those events do occur, and you must be prepared to protect yourself. Your own safety is the first priority. Emergency Medical Responders with no training or little experience at fighting fires must follow the rules listed below to ensure their safety:

- Never approach a vehicle that is in flames. Using blankets, sand, or a fire extinguisher is appropriate if you know how to evaluate the fire and the danger of explosion and if you have protective clothing and know how to attack a fire. If you do not have the proper training to perform those tasks and do not have the necessary protection, stay clear. Make sure that the dispatcher knows there is a fire.
- Never attempt to enter a building that is obviously on fire or has smoke showing. Even a small fire can spread toxic fumes throughout the structure. If you enter, look and smell for signs of fire. Remember that fire could be hidden within the walls, floors, and ceilings.
- Never enter a smoky room or building or go through an area of dense smoke.
- Never attempt to enter a closed building or room giving off grayish-yellow smoke. Opening a door to this building or room will cause a back draft, which is a condition that immediately increases the intensity of the fire and can cause an explosion due to the sudden increase in oxygen supply.
- Do not work by yourself or enter a building unless others know that you are doing so. If you are injured or trapped, you are an unknown victim who may not be found until it is too late.
- Always feel the top of a door before opening it (Figure 25.8). If it is hot, do not open it. (Doorknobs and handles may also be hot.) If the door is cool, open it slowly and cautiously and avoid standing in its path as you open it.
- Never use the elevator if there is a possibility of a fire in a building. The elevator shaft can act as a flue and pull flames, hot toxic gases, and smoke into the shaft. Also, the fire can cause an electrical failure, which could trap you in the elevator.
- If you find yourself in smoke, stay close to the floor and crawl to safety. If possible, cover your mouth and nose with a damp cloth.

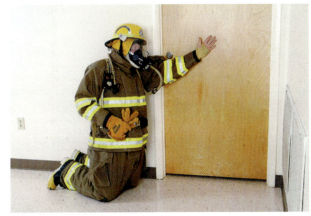

Figure 25.8 • Always check the temperature of the door with the back of your hand before opening. If it is hot, do not enter.

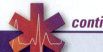

As Greg is waiting for his cell phone call to be routed to the local dispatch center, he grabs two of the fleeing technicians. "I need you guys to go down to the north entrance and make sure nobody gets onto the studio property." The men immediately jog off down the road toward the studio's only other gate.

"City fire dispatch, how can I help?" A man's voice comes onto the line.

"Yes, my name is Greg, and I'm calling from Legend Studios over here on Cornell Boulevard. There's a fire on the exterior west side of our main soundstage building, and there are five or six large propane tanks in the danger zone."

After answering several questions from the dispatcher, Greg hangs up and turns to the lead pyrotechnician, who is staring back at the burning building expectantly. "Hey, McQueeny." Greg takes a notepad and pen from his pocket. "Is there anything at all over in that area other than propane? Any chemicals or other flammable stuff? The fire department will need to know as soon as they get here."

Natural Gas

If you notice the odor of natural gas at any scene, move patients away from the area, keep bystanders away from the scene, alert dispatch so that other services can be activated, and request that gas in the area be shut off or diverted.

The smell of natural gas in a building is a signal for immediate action. Evacuate the building and call dispatch to report the odor of gas. If the gas is coming from a bottled source, do not try to turn off this source unless you have experience with this type of gas system. You can vent the area by opening windows and doors as you leave. Do not enter an area to rescue a patient. You must wear a self-contained breathing apparatus (SCBA) and be trained to handle such emergencies. Remember there is always a danger of fire or explosion from simple acts such as turning on or off a light switch or even from the spark of an appliance turning on. Play it safe and request the help you will need.

Electrical Wires and Aboveground Transformers

If electrical wires are down at a scene and block your pathway to a patient, or if they are lying across a car, do not attempt a rescue. As you approach a scene with downed wires, position your vehicle at least a pole away from the downed wires. If the power is restored, the wires can whip and arc in a circle as wide as their free length, which can be to the next pole (Figure 25.9).

Figure 25.9 • When arriving on scene, position your vehicle at least one utility pole away from the damaged pole.

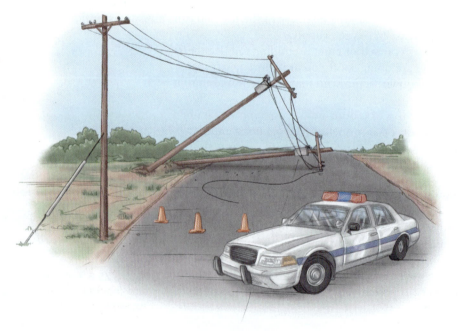

Never assume that power lines are dead or that a dead line will stay dead. Consider all downed lines as live. Do not be fooled by the fact that lights are out in the surrounding area. Even if lights are off all around you, the wire blocking your path may be live or could be re-energized as you pass by. Call or have someone alert dispatch to call the power company and request that the power be turned off. Even if you believe the power has been turned off, it is still best to wait for trained rescue personnel to arrive.

Many newer communities have underground electrical wires with access through an aboveground splice box or transformer. These aboveground transformer boxes are usually green, mounted on concrete pads, and often hidden by shrubbery. It may not be safe to approach a vehicle that has collided with an aboveground transformer box. Alert dispatch immediately and ask for special rescue assistance.

If victims are in a car that is touching a downed wire or is near one or has crashed into an aboveground transformer, tell them to stay in the vehicle and avoid touching any metal parts. If the victims have to leave the vehicle because of fire or other danger, you must tell them to jump clear of the car without touching it and the ground at the same time. If they touch both simultaneously, they will complete a circuit and may be electrocuted.

Hazardous Materials

There may be hazardous chemicals and other materials at the scene of an emergency. If so, do not attempt a rescue or perform patient care. No responders should enter a hazardous materials area unless they are trained to do so.

The possibility of **hazardous materials** incidents exists at every industrial site and every farm, truck, train, ship, barge, and airplane emergency incident. When responding to an emergency at these sites, assume that there are unsafe hazardous materials until their presence can be ruled out. When in doubt, stay clear and keep others clear of a hazardous material spill until trained rescuers arrive. Hazardous material response teams, usually referred to as hazmat teams, consist of personnel with specialized training that goes beyond the scope of this text but may be required by your service or department. This specialized training is regulated by the Occupational Safety and Health Administration (OSHA) Code of Federal Regulations. The regulations on how hazardous materials responders are to be trained and how hazardous materials are to be managed is *OSHA 29 CFR 1910.120* Hazardous Waste Operations and Emergency Response, commonly referred to as **HAZWOPER**. (See Table 25.1.)

Emergency Medical Responder Responsibilities

Your role as an Emergency Medical Responder in a hazardous material situation is to first protect yourself and others around the scene. All emergency response vehicles should carry a current copy of the U.S. DOT's **Hazardous Materials: Emergency Response Guidebook**. At a hazardous material incident, refer to the guidebook for information on the chemical or substance and the perimeter of the safe area.

In general, your responsibilities are: recognition and identification, notification and information sharing, isolation, and protection.

Recognition and Identification
Recognition and identification are the first and most essential safety factors at a hazardous material scene. The following are factors that must be evaluated upon the arrival at these incidents:

- Occupancy/location
- Container shape
- Markings and colors
- Placards and labels
- Shipping papers and Material Safety Data Sheets (MSDS)
- Human senses

Notification and Information Sharing
Contact dispatch immediately with a description of the incident so you can get the appropriate help on the way. Advise the dispatcher of your position and stay on the line until

TABLE 25.1 | OSHA CFR 1910.120		
HAZWOPER REQUIREMENTS		
• Written SOPs and a response plan		
• Use of the Incident Command System		
• Presence of a Safety Officer		
• Use of minimum PPE such as positive-pressure self-contained breathing apparatus (SCBA) and full turnout gear		
• Presence of backup personnel and emergency medical support		
FIVE LEVELS OF HAZMAT TRAINING		
• *First Responder Awareness:* Persons who may witness or discover a chemical release and will notify proper authorities, secure the area and establish command.		
• *First Responder Operational:* Initial responders who are dispatched to releases or potential releases of chemicals and who function in a defensive fashion without attempting to stop the leak or coming into close proximity to the product.		
• *Hazardous Materials Technician:* To respond in a more aggressive fashion, these responders are trained to use chemical protective equipment and are normally members of a hazardous materials team.		
• *Hazardous Materials Specialist:* A responder who has more in-depth knowledge than a technician and serves as a team leader.		
• *Incident Commander:* A responder who will assume command of an incident scene beyond the level of the first responder.		

you are told to disconnect. Ask and wait for information about the danger of the materials and for directions as to what you should do until the hazmat teams arrive. Make certain you give your name and callback number.

If, for some reason, you cannot contact the dispatcher, call one of the following:

CHEM-TEL on its 24-hour toll-free number at 800-255-3924 (for the United States and Canada)

CHEMTREC on its 24-hour toll-free number at 800-262-8200 (for the United States and Canada)

When possible, provide the following information:

- *Nature and location of the problem,* an estimate of when the spill occurred, and if there are other possible hazardous materials near the scene
- *Type of material* (gas, liquid, dry chemical, or a radioactive solid, liquid, or gas) and an estimate of how much material is at the scene
- *Name or identification number of the material.* Look for labels or placards that are visible from your safe point. Use binoculars to help in reading this information.
- *Name of the shipper or manufacturer.* From a safe point or with binoculars, look for names on railroad cars, trucks, or containers. Ask bystanders, drivers, or railroad or factory personnel.
- *Type of container.* Is the material in a rail car or a truck? Is it in open storage, covered storage, or housed storage? Is the container still intact, or is liquid leaking, gas escaping, or a powder spilled? Report if the material is stable or if it is flaming, vaporizing, or blowing into the air.
- *Weather conditions.* Rain and wind are major concerns because they will carry hazardous materials to and contaminate other locations.
- *Estimate of the number of possible victims* both in the hot zone (closest to the spill) and around the hot zone (in circles farther from the spill).
- *Other significant problems at the scene,* such as fire, crowds, and traffic

placard ▶ a sign used to display information pertaining to the contents of transport containers.

hot zone ▶ the area of a hazardous incident that is immediately surrounding the spill or release.

warm zone ▶ a designated area at a hazardous materials incident where decontamination of people and equipment occurs.

cold zone ▶ a designated area associated with a hazardous materials incident that is well beyond the incident and where patients are cared for and placed into ambulances for transport.

You may not be able to obtain and report most of this information, but any information you can provide is important to the responding units.

A major source of information at a hazardous material scene is the standard materials placard required by the U.S. DOT (Figure 25.10). This **placard** is on the vehicle, tank, or railroad car. The numbers, symbols, and colors provide information about the material in the container. Be aware that vehicles transporting hazardous materials insert placards into brackets. They may be made of metal or plastic and are hinged so they can be flipped to indicate a different cargo. During transportation or the incident, the placard may flip and show a different material. If possible, check with the driver, who must have a Material Safety Data Sheet (MSDS) on each hazardous material carried, to determine that the placard is correct.

An MSDS will provide you with the following important information:

- Chemical and common names
- Physical and chemical properties
- Physical hazards
- Health hazards
- Primary routes of exposure
- Exposure limits
- Safe handling procedures
- Emergency and first-aid measures
- Contact person or company

Some hazardous material transporters use placard stickers, which can be peeled off when the load is delivered. The driver applies another sticker for a different load of hazardous materials.

Refer to the U.S. DOT's *Hazardous Materials: Emergency Response Guidebook*. You also may want to become familiar with the National Fire Protection Association's (NFPA's) "Standard 473 Competencies for EMS Personnel Responding to Hazardous Materials Incidents."

Isolation and Protection

For isolation of the incident you may have to assist with the setup of *safety zones*. A **hot zone** (danger), to keep all people out of the contaminated area, a **warm zone** for decontamination procedures, and establishment of a **cold zone** (safe, which should be on the same level as and upwind from the hazardous material incident) that can be used for patient assessment, treatment, and transport.

Be aware that below-grade areas, such as ditches, trenches, and basements, will often have low-oxygen environments. Many gases are heavier than oxygen and will settle in low areas. The safe zone must not be downhill or downwind from the scene or on a high point that may be exposed to vapors if the wind shifts. Avoid low spots, streams, drainage fields, sewers, and sewer openings where spills may flow and fumes may collect.

Remember, the assistance of establishment of both hot and warm zones by an Emergency Medical Responder should be associated with appropriate OSHA-approved training and PPE.

Access to the zones must be controlled with an entrance point that has only one way in, called the "access corridor." The exit point from the hot zone to the warm zone for decontamination is called the "decontamination corridor." This corridor leads to the safe zone or cold zone that the Emergency Medical Responder is allowed to assess, treat, and transport patients. The cold zone is also the area where the command post is located. This is where the Incident Commander coordinates resources to manage the incident. (See Figure 25.11.)

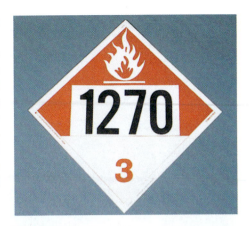

Figure 25.10 • A typical DOT hazardous materials placard.

OBJECTIVE

14. Differentiate the purpose of the cold, warm, and hot zones at a hazardous materials incident.

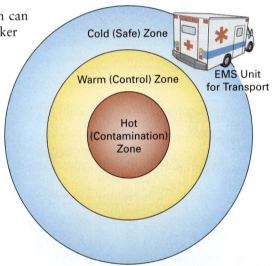

Hot (Contamination) Zone

Contamination is actually present.
Personnel must wear appropriate protective gear.
Number of rescuers limited to those absolutely necessary.
Bystanders never allowed.

Warm (Control) Zone

Area surrounding the contamination zone.
Vital to preventing spread of contamination.
Personnel must wear appropriate protective gear.
Lifesaving emergency care is performed.

Cold (Safe) Zone

Normal triage, stabilization, and treatment performed.
Rescuers must shed contaminated gear before entering the cold zone.

Figure 25.11 • Examples of the safety zones at a hazardous materials incident.

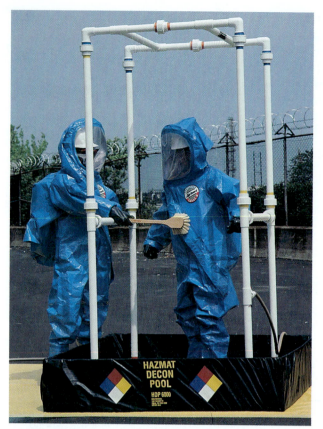

Figure 25.12 • The decontamination of a fellow rescuer.

Decontamination of Hazardous Materials

Decontamination is a chemical or physical process used to remove and prevent the spread of contaminants from an emergency scene to prevent harm to living beings and/or the environment. The best method to accomplish decontamination is to prevent contamination.

Decontamination (decon) is preformed in the warm zone by specially trained personnel. Remember, as an Emergency Medical Responder, you must remain in the cold zone and begin patient treatment and assist with transport there. It is important to note that people, equipment, and the environment are important elements that will need to be decontaminated before you come into contact with them. Keep in mind that there are different types of contaminated people at these scenes. The Emergency Medical Responder must consider all persons in the warm and hot zones contaminated. Both protected responders and victims are to be considered contaminated until proper decon is performed. In the cold zone the Emergency Medical Responder must recognize that victims may be both ambulatory (can walk) and nonambulatory (not able to walk). If there are contaminated victims associated with the hazmat scene, notify receiving health-care facilities of incoming patients and relay that proper decontamination has been conducted at the scene. Inform them of the chemical or substance that the patient was exposed to and of their condition, including vital signs. (See Figure 25.12.)

Managing Patients

Remember, all contaminated victims must remain in the hot zone until the hazmat team decontaminates them and brings them to the warm zone for decon, then to the cold zone for care by EMS personnel. If a victim of a hazardous material incident leaves the hot zone, you must first protect yourself from exposure. Victims may have chemicals on their bodies and clothing that could be harmful to you. *Do not* attempt to care for these patients unless you have the proper protection.

Initial care includes getting the victims into fresh air and flushing with water any contaminated areas, such as the skin, clothing, and eyes for at least 20 minutes, unless the material is dry lime. If dry lime is involved, brush away excess dry lime first, then flush with water. Remove contaminated clothing and jewelry as you flush the patient with water. Once the patient is flushed, use blankets to protect him from the environment and to maintain body temperature.

Victims may be able to wash themselves, or you may wash the victims. Use a small-diameter hose and make sure the victim stands in a large tub, small wading pool, or similar collection container so the contaminated rinse water does not run off into nearby sewers or streams. The hazmat team will manage all of the contaminated water by collecting it for transport and disposal. Perform wash operations uphill and upwind from the site, if possible. Do not place yourself at risk. If it is necessary to provide artificial ventilations, use an appropriate barrier device. Use resuscitation devices with one-way valves so contaminants do not blow back into your mouth or face.

The best thing for you to do at a hazardous material incident is to request the appropriate resources (Figure 25.13) and remain in the cold zone until the patient can be safely treated.

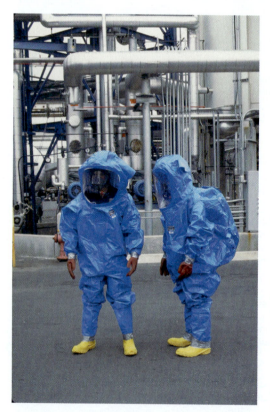

Figure 25.13 • The appropriate response to a hazardous materials incident requires specialized training and equipment.

Radiation Incidents

Stay clear of collisions involving radioactive materials. Your first duty is to protect yourself from exposure. Your next step should be to request the appropriate resources from a safe area away from the scene.

Look for radiation hazard labels (Figure 25.14). Stay upwind from any containers having these labels. Follow the same basic rules as you would when dealing with any hazardous material. The greater the distance you are from the source and the more objects that appropriately shield you from the source (concrete, thick steel, earth banks, heavy vehicles), the safer you will be.

When you are dispatched to hazardous material and radiation incidents, position your vehicle at a safe distance. Do not approach the scene unless you are specially trained to do so and are wearing the appropriate protective equipment (turnout coat, pants, boots, gloves, fire-resistant hood, helmet). Your PPE will provide some protection from most types of radiation, but be aware that it does not protect you enough to work close to a high-level radiation source for any period of time.

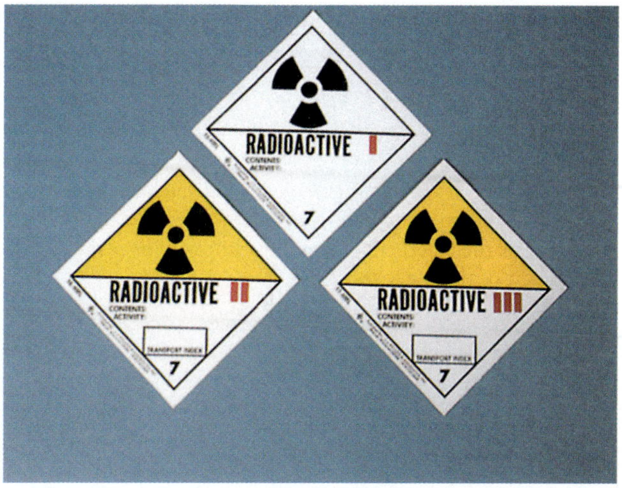

Patients may be exposed to radiation, contaminated by it, or both. A patient who is exposed (not contaminated) was in the presence of radioactive material, but the material did not actually touch his clothing or body. Exposure to radiation may be harmful to the patient, but he is not radioactive and cannot pass on the exposure to you. However, the actual source of the radiation can be harmful to you. If the patient is still in the area of the radiation source, you must wait until the hazmat team brings him to the safe area.

Patients are contaminated when they come in contact with radiation sources, which may be gases, liquids, or particles. The radioactive materials may be on a patient's clothes, skin, or hair and will contaminate you when you touch the patient during assessment or care. The hazmat team will have to decontaminate the patient before you can provide care. Do not attempt to clean or care for radiation patients until they are in a safe area and are decontaminated.

Figure 25.14 • Examples of typical radiation hazard placards.

WRAP-UP

FIRST ON SCENE

Within minutes, the city streets leading to the studio have been closed by law enforcement, and fire services is cooling the propane tank battery with a jet of water from a distant truck. After about 15 minutes, the fabric of the blue screen has burned completely from the large, rectangular frame, and except for drifting gray ash and rapidly dissipating smoke, there is no sign of the once raging fire.

"Well, Greg." The Incident Commander puts his hand on the safety officer's shoulder. "You couldn't have done anything better than you did: evacuating, blocking the two access points, and letting us know exactly what we were up against. You did a real fine job managing a pretty hazardous situation."

"Thank you." Greg smiles briefly. "Next time I'm only going to make one change."

"What's that?" The IC pulls his orange vest off.

"Next time we do a shot like this," Greg says, "I'm going to have you guys already standing by."

CHAPTER REVIEW

Summary

- The phases of a typical emergency call include: preparation, dispatch, en route to the scene, at the scene, transfer of care, and after the emergency. You must know your responsibilities for each of these phases.

- As an Emergency Medical Responder, your first priority is your own safety. Before approaching a patient, make sure the scene is safe. Call for additional resources as soon as possible.

- Do not attempt to provide patient care in or around unstabilized vehicles or try to right overturned vehicles.

- Attempt to reach patients by simple access first, such as doors and windows. Wait for properly trained personnel if complex access is required.

- Remove patients from vehicles only when there is danger or if lifesaving care is required.

- If you smell natural gas, do not approach. Only trained personnel should shut off gas or electricity. If electrical wires are touching a vehicle, have passengers stay in the vehicle and instruct them to avoid touching any metal objects inside the vehicle. If they must get out, warn them to jump clear without touching the vehicle and the ground at the same time.

- There are five levels of hazmat training: awareness, operational, technician, specialist, and commander. In many areas, emergency responders must be trained to the awareness level.

- An important hazmat reference tool that should be carried on all emergency vehicles is called the *Hazardous Materials: Emergency Response Guidebook*. You should become familiar with how to use this valuable resource.

- Hazmat incidents are organized into zones. The hot zone is the area immediately surrounding the incident. The warm zone is a safe distance from the incident and where decontamination operations occur. The cold zone is well beyond the incident and where patients are cared for and placed into ambulances for transport.

Take Action

HAZMAT RIGHT AT HOME

Most people have little understanding of how many hazardous materials surround them each and every day. When things are operating properly, large quantities of hazardous materials are being transported all around them, and they have little awareness until something goes wrong. For this activity, conduct a thorough inventory of your immediate environment right there at home. Take a look in all the usual places, such as under the kitchen sink and in the garage, as well as not-so-obvious places, such as the home office or bathroom. Write down the name of anything that comes in a commercial container, everything from drain cleaner to Wite-Out (correction fluid).

Next, use the power of the Internet to locate a material safety data sheet for each of those products. A simple search such as "MSDS for liquid paper" will quickly bring up a link to the appropriate MSDS. Now review the third section on the MSDS, "Hazard Identification," for the problems this product can cause if the body becomes exposed. Then review the fourth section to learn the appropriate first-aid measures for the specific product.

Having a good understanding of the products right in your own home and what to do should someone ingest or become exposed to them will make you a better prepared Emergency Medical Responder.

First on Scene Run Review

Recall the events of the "First on Scene" scenario in this chapter and answer the following questions, which are related to the call. Rationales are offered in the Answer Key at the back of the book.

1. What precautions could Greg have taken before shouting?

2. What information could Greg give the dispatcher?

3. How might the *Emergency Response Guidebook* have come in handy?

Quick Quiz

To check your understanding of the chapter, answer the following questions. Then compare your answers to those in the Answer Key at the back of the book.

1. The best way to approach a hazardous scene is to:
   a. do only what you feel comfortable doing.
   b. wear protective gear only if needed.
   c. make safety your first consideration before entering.
   d. get as close as possible to assess the scene.

2. The phases of an emergency call in order are:

  a. preparation, dispatch, en route to scene, arrival at scene, transfer of patient, after the emergency.

  b. dispatch, en route to scene, arrival at scene, transfer of patient, after the emergency.

  c. preparation, dispatch, en route to scene, arrival at scene, transfer of patient, en route to hospital.

  d. dispatch, en route to scene, arrival at scene, preparation, transfer of patient, after the emergency.

3. When arriving at a motor-vehicle collision scene, the best place to position your vehicle is:

  a. 50 feet before the scene with lights on.

  b. as close to the scene as possible with lights off.

  c. 500 feet beyond the scene with lights on.

  d. near other responding emergency vehicles.

4. When evaluating the stability of a vehicle before attempting to enter and care for patients, look for common hazards such as slippery surfaces, hills or slight inclines, and _____ vehicles.

  a. sturdy or stacked

  b. tilted or damaged

  c. parked or damaged

  d. tilted or stacked

5. Which one of the following best defines both simple access and complex access?

  a. Neither simple access nor complex access requires specialized tools.

  b. Simple and complex access both require special equipment.

  c. Simple access sometimes requires special equipment; complex access often does.

  d. Simple access does not require equipment, though complex access does.

6. There are four ways to access a patient in a vehicle with closed doors: enter through a window, pry open a door, cut through the metal, and:

  a. call an emergency locksmith.

  b. open the unlocked door.

  c. remove the engine and enter through the dash.

  d. wait until another responder opens a door.

7. The best way for the Emergency Medical Responder to manage a vehicle that is overturned is to:

  a. upright the vehicle, if enough help is available.

  b. upright the vehicle before gaining access to patients.

  c. never upright a vehicle because it can cause further injury to the patients inside.

  d. never upright a vehicle because it can cause further damage to the vehicle.

8. When a patient is pinned beneath a vehicle:

  a. attempt to upright the vehicle yourself.

  b. call for a rescue squad immediately.

  c. stabilize the vehicle and then attempt to upright it.

  d. call for a rescue squad and then attempt to upright it.

9. When you must enter a locked building to gain access to a patient in need of immediate care:

  a. enter the building and then call for help.

  b. enter the building, stabilize the patient, and then call for help.

  c. attempt to enter the building, but if you fail, call for help.

  d. request additional resources, then attempt to access the building.

10. Specialized training is needed to manage fire, as well as:

  a. natural gas.

  b. downed power lines and hazardous materials.

  c. vehicle extrication and rescue.

  d. all of the above.

11. All of the following emergency responders are required to wear a high-visibility vest while working on a highway EXCEPT:

  a. firefighters.

  b. EMS providers.

  c. law enforcement officers.

  d. dispatchers.

12. If you find yourself needing to exit a smoke-filled environment, you should:

  a. stay close to the floor and crawl to safety.

  b. run out of the building.

  c. stop, drop, and roll.

  d. not exit until you find the patient.

13. The patient treatment area and the command post are located in what zone of a hazmat incident?

  a. Hot

  b. Warm

  c. Blue

  d. Cold

14. In radiation incidents, it is okay to follow the same basic rules related to what other hazardous scene?

  a. Natural gas

  b. Downed power lines

  c. Hazardous materials

  d. Vehicle extrication

15. A safety feature of tempered glass is that it will not:

  a. break.

  b. shatter.

  c. crack.

  d. melt.

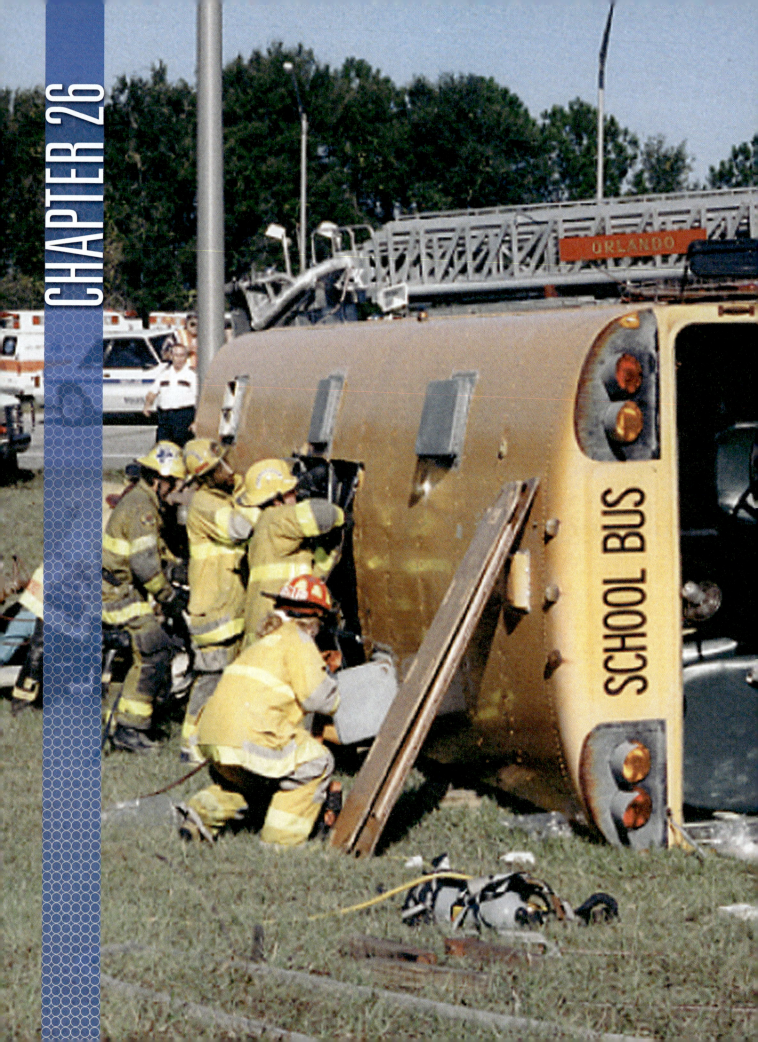

Introduction to Multiple-Casualty Incidents, the Incident Command System, and Triage

EDUCATION STANDARDS • EMS Operations—Incident Management, Multiple Casualty Incidents

COMPETENCIES • Knowledge of operational roles and responsibilities to ensure safe patient, public, and personnel safety.

CHAPTER OVERVIEW This chapter discusses the role of the EMS system and that of the Emergency Medical Responder in emergencies involving multiple victims. Multiple-casualty incidents can be caused by anything, including vehicle collisions, hurricanes, and terrorist events such as those that occurred on September 11, 2001.

OBJECTIVES

Upon successful completion of this chapter, the student should be able to:

COGNITIVE

1. Define the following terms:
   a. incident command system (ICS) *(p. 585)*
   b. incident commander *(p. 585)*
   c. JumpSTART pediatric triage system *(p. 591)*
   d. multiple-casualty incident (MCI) *(p. 584)*
   e. national incident management system (NIMS) *(p. 586)*
   f. START triage system *(p. 588)*
   g. triage *(p. 587)*
2. Explain the criteria that defines a multiple-casualty incident. *(p. 584)*
3. Describe common causes of multiple-casualty incidents. *(p. 584)*
4. Explain the role of the Emergency Medical Responder in the multiple-casualty situation. *(p. 585)*
5. Explain the key principles and structure of an incident command system. *(p. 585)*
6. Explain the key principles of triage at a multiple-casualty incident. *(p. 587)*
7. Differentiate patient priorities related to triage. *(p. 588)*
8. Explain the assessment criteria of the START triage system. *(p. 588)*
9. Differentiate primary and secondary triage. *(pp. 590)*

PSYCHOMOTOR

10. Demonstrate the ability to properly categorize patients of a simulated multiple-casualty situation.

AFFECTIVE

11. Recognize the importance of patient priorities during a multiple-casualty event.

Westside Mall security guard Gus Garban looks at his watch and then leans on the polished wooden banister that borders the mezzanine level of the huge downtown shopping center. He watches as the crowds down on the main level bustles from store to store, swinging noisy plastic shopping bags and chatting on cell phones. It is like every other Saturday afternoon at Westside.

Gus stretches his back and walks toward the escalator that would take him down and out toward the mall's main entrance. If he doesn't wander out and check the marble entryway to the mall every few hours, it gets too crowded with loitering kids and then he'll be dealing with everything from customer complaints to fights. It is definitely better to be proactive.

Just as he steps off of the escalator, it happens. A thunderous explosion from the far end of the mall sends screams and a boiling black cloud of smoke toward him. "Hey, Ted!" Gus yells into his shoulder mic. "We just had an explosion of some kind at the north end of the mall! Call 911 right away!"

"Already on it!" comes the static-filled reply.

Gus tries to see through the wall of rancid smoke, which is rising slowly toward the high ceiling of the shopping center. The mall's automated evacuation message is echoing through the enormous building. He is surprised to see the smoke fade quickly, helped by the large vent fans located on the roof of the mall. As it does, Gus just stands and stares at the scene before him.

Shattered glass, colorful clothing, and people are scattered all over the tile floor at the end of the mall. Those who can move hurry past him to the clean and undamaged part of the mall. The rest, perhaps 15 or 20 people, just lie motionless on the floor, smoking, bleeding, and possibly dead.

Gus's stomach tightens as he realizes that he is to be the first responder on this horrendous scene. He takes a deep breath and moves toward the closest nonmoving person.

Multiple-Casualty Incidents

If taken literally, the definition of a **multiple-casualty incident (MCI)** is any emergency with more than one victim (Figure 26.1). Although MCIs do indeed involve more than one victim, a more realistic definition is any emergency that involves multiple victims and overwhelms the first responding units.

An MCI can be the result of many different types of incidents. Examples of common causes of MCIs are vehicle collisions that involve multiple vehicles, earthquakes, floods, large explosions, and building collapses.

Most fire services, rescue squads, and ambulances are prepared and capable of managing a scene with more than one patient. However, can they manage a scene with three or four? How about five or six? What if the victims are all critical and need immediate transport? It is important for the Emergency Medical Responder to remember that MCI definitions vary from one community to another. In the simplest definition, an MCI may be described as an incident that reduces the effectiveness of the traditional emergency response because of number of patients, special hazards, or difficult rescue (Table 26.1).

In most cases, it is up to the first emergency personnel on the scene to make a judgment call and declare an MCI. If they feel that they can manage the number of patients

Figure 26.1 • Multiple-casualty incidents require the resources of many agencies.

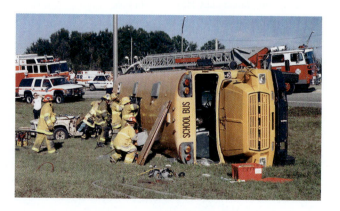

TABLE 26.1 | Multiple-Casualty Incidents

- *Low-Impact Incidents*—manageable by local emergency personnel
- *High-Impact Incidents*—stresses local EMS, fire, and police resources
- *Disaster, Terrorism Incidents*—overwhelms regional emergency response resources

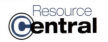

with the resources immediately available, then an MCI may not be declared. If they cannot manage the number of patients, then an MCI is declared and an incident command system (ICS) is put into action.

The role of Emergency Medical Responders at an MCI will vary depending on several factors, such as when they arrive at the scene, the type of agency for whom they are working, and their specific level of training. Emergency Medical Responders who are first on scene may be dedicated to making the scene safe and keeping bystanders from becoming injured. Thus, they may not immediately become involved in patient care. For those who arrive after the scene has been made safe, their role will likely involve the triaging of patients. (Triage is discussed later in this chapter.) Other roles for the Emergency Medical Responder include treatment of patients and assisting with the transport of patients to appropriate receiving facilities. Other duties may include the setting up of landing zones if medical helicopters are used for patient evacuation.

OBJECTIVE

4. Explain the role of the Emergency Medical Responder in the multiple-casualty situation.

Incident Command System

The **incident command system (ICS)** is a model tool for the command, control, and coordination of resources at the scene of a large-scale emergency involving multiple agencies. It consists of procedures for organizing personnel, facilities, equipment, and communications.

The first formal incident command systems were formed as a result of a mandate from Congress to analyze the aftermath of a devastating series of wildfires in Southern California in the early 1970s. Since then, EMS, fire, and police agencies across the United States continue to develop and implement such plans utilizing ICS.

The incident command system is based on well-established management principles of planning, directing, organization, coordination, communication, delegation, and evaluation. ICS is flexible enough to accommodate a single-agency or single-jurisdiction emergency, as well as multiagency or multijurisdictional events. ICS is dynamic in nature and employs a top-down modular structure that can be scaled to any size event. The **incident commander** is the person responsible for all aspects of the emergency response and establishes the structure and requests resources necessary for the event. The incident commander is typically a senior fire department officer.

Some of the modules that might be included in a typical incident command system are: command, operations, planning, logistics, and finance. Under each of the major modules is a complex list of responsibilities related to that functional group. For example, under operations, the Emergency Medical Responder, due to his medical training, may be assigned to the medical branch that is a functional group under this area of responsibility.

It is easy to imagine how chaos can occur when so many different agencies and departments respond to a single large-scale emergency. Designing and implementing an organized approach to such an event will ensure a more positive outcome for both the rescuers and the victims. See Figure 26.2 for an example of the EMS portion of a large incident management system.

incident command system (ICS) ▶ a model tool for the command, control, and coordination of resources at the scene of a large-scale emergency involving multiple agencies. Also known as *incident management system*.

OBJECTIVE

5. Explain the key principles and structure of an incident command system.

incident commander ▶ the person responsible for all aspects of an emergency response.

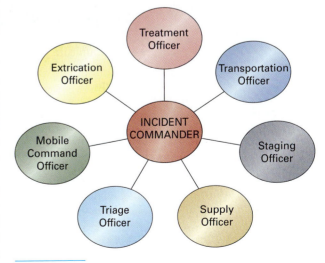

Figure 26.2 • The incident commander delegates duties to the various group officers.

National Incident Management System

national incident management system (NIMS) ► a system that utilizes a unified approach to incident management and standard command and management structures, with an emphasis on preparedness, mutual aid, and resource management.

In response to the increased terrorist threat in the United States, the Federal Emergency Management Agency (FEMA) has developed its own incident management system, which is known as the **national incident management system (NIMS)**. In 2004, the incident command system was included as part of that system to ensure more efficient operations at all emergency responses scenes. NIMS was developed so that federal, state, local, and tribal resources can respond more efficiently to natural disasters and emergencies, including acts of terrorism. NIMS teaches a unified approach to incident management, standard command and management structures, and emphasis on preparedness, mutual aid, resource management, and, most important, common terminology among agencies. Training in NIMS and ICS within emergency response agencies is required to receive federal funds (grants) for equipment, supplies, and personnel.

FEMA offers several free online instructional courses pertaining to both incident command systems and the new NIMS. You can find these courses and many others at the FEMA Web site.

Learn more about NIMS.

The Medical Branch

The branch of the ICS that the Emergency Medical Responder commonly functions in is called the *medical branch*. This branch involves the designation and coordination of elements such as triage, treatment, and transport of patients.

As you arrive on the scene, you will be given a specific assignment based on the needs of the incident. At a large-scale event, the Emergency Medical Responder may be assigned to one of the three functional areas (groups within the medical branch). These areas are triage, treatment, and transport. Emergency Medical Responders will be assigned to those areas and will report to group leaders who report up the chain of command to the medical group supervisor, who reports to the medical branch director. The medical group supervisor will be the group leader's link to the medical branch director for information sharing and resource allocation.

The first responders to arrive at the scene will assume the role of the triage and set up one or multiple triage divisions according to the size of the event.

Triage Group

The triage group usually is composed of the first responders on scene. They perform the following functions:

- Determine the location of triage areas.
- Conduct primary triage and ensure that all patients are assessed and sorted using appropriate START triage protocol. (START is discussed later in this chapter.)
- Communicate resource requirements with the medical group supervisor.
- Communicate with the treatment group leader to allow for movement of patients into the treatment division for prehospital care by the members of the treatment group.

> ### From the Medical Director
>
> #### The Medical Branch
>
> *The Emergency Medical Responder is critical to the effective function of the medical branch because in most cases there are many more Emergency Medical Responders than EMTs and paramedics. Be prepared to perform multiple functions, such as triage and movement of numerous patients, and refrain from spending too much time with any one patient unless instructed to do so by the medical branch manager.*

Treatment Group

Patients are moved from the triage group to the treatment group, where they are cared for by other EMS providers. This group is usually marked with the same color-coded indicators that match the patients' acuity level as indicated with their triage tag. The markers are often marked with flags or tarps using red, yellow, green, or black. The responsibility of the members of the treatment group are as follows:

- Determine the location for treatment group.
- Coordinate with the triage group to move patients from the triage area to treatment areas.
- Maintain communications with the medical group supervisor.
- Reassess patients, conduct secondary triage to match patients with resources.
- Direct movement to the transport division.

Transport Group

The transport group coordinates transportation of victims to appropriate facilities for definitive treatment. Some important functions of this group are to determine the availability of receiving medical facilities. Some of the primary responsibilities of this group are:

- Manage patient movement and accountability from the scene to the receiving hospitals.
- Work with the treatment group to establish adequately sized, easily identifiable patient loading area.
- Designate an ambulance staging division.
- Maintain communication with medical group supervisor.

Medical Staging

The accountability of medical resources and equipment is one of the most challenging aspects of an MCI. With the assistance of individuals assigned to the operations group, the medical branch director can effectively meet the needs of the triage, treatment, and transport groups. The following are considerations related to staging of medical resources and equipment:

- Location designated to collect available resources near incident area
- Whether several staging divisions will be required
- Should be easy for arriving resources to locate
- Whether staging division will need to be relocated as the situation dictates

OBJECTIVE

6. Explain the key principles of triage at a multiple-casualty incident.

triage ▶ a method of sorting patients for care and transport based on the severity of their injuries or illnesses.

Triage

Triage is one of the primary aspects of emergency care at a multiple-casualty incident. When there are many victims at an emergency, it is nearly impossible to provide care to all those who need it when they need it. So a system called **triage** has been developed to help identify those victims who are most in need of immediate care. Triage is a process for sorting injured people into groups based on their need for or likely benefit from immediate medical care. Triage is used in hospital emergency departments, on battlefields, and at emergencies when there are multiple victims and limited medical resources (Figure 26.3).

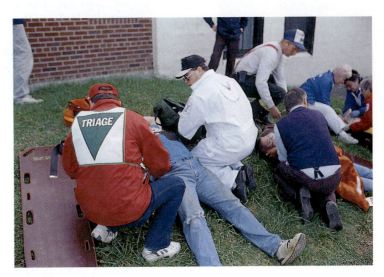

Figure 26.3 • At the scene of a multiple-casualty incident, triage is the system used to identify victims who are most in need of immediate medical care.

Triage

Your natural tendency may be to evaluate each patient as you normally would. However, in a multiple-casualty scenario, your purpose is to rapidly identify all patients who need immediate care. This means that there are some victims you must quickly determine as dead without performing a comprehensive examination. Rest assured that you will save more lives by not missing those who can survive with rapid treatment than you will lose if you spend all your time assuring yourself that a victim is dead.

Because Emergency Medical Responders are first on the scene, they must be able to triage patients and initiate care rapidly. When additional EMS personnel arrive, Emergency Medical Responders pass on information, continue to help complete the triage process, and help provide care to the worst patients first. You cannot begin to provide care to patients randomly. You must begin caring for those patients who have the highest priority based on their condition. You will need to make brief notes on each patient while you are performing triage.

OBJECTIVE

7. Differentiate patient priorities related to triage.

IS IT SAFE?

Triage is not an easy task. In an MCI, you will be expected to triage as many patients as possible without providing the care they need. It is not unusual for experienced providers to triage patients until they come to one that really needs lifesaving care. At that point, they stop triaging and begin caring for the patient as they see fit. This is not always the best thing for all patients. Triaging is about saving as many patients as possible with the available resources.

OBJECTIVE

8. Explain the assessment criteria of the START triage system.

START triage system ▶ a system that uses respirations, perfusion, and mental status assessments to categorize patients into one of four treatment categories; letters stand for Simple Triage and Rapid Treatment.

Triage Priorities

Triage is simply a process of sorting patients into categories and prioritizing their medical care and transport based on the severity of their injuries and medical condition. This process is used commonly at the scene of multiple-casualty incidents. When there are more victims than there are rescuers, the process of triage helps ensure that the most critical but still salvageable patients are cared for first. This practice allows responding personnel to do the most good for the most number of injured patients.

For many MCIs, there may be a delay before additional help is on scene. If the emergency is large enough or in a remote area, an hour or more may pass before there are enough rescuers present to render care for all patients. So triage is also used to determine the order of transport for patients. Patients who appear to have serious medical- or trauma-related problems—such as heart attack, shock, major injuries, and heat stroke—must be transported quickly, while patients with minor injuries or illnesses are transported later.

Some jurisdictions have Emergency Medical Responders use triage tags for patient information (Figure 26.4). Even if you do not carry the tags, you should be familiar with them in case you are called to help when others are using triage tags. Use one triage tag per patient, and leave the tag attached to the patient so that others arriving at the scene can have immediate access to information. Do not delay the triage process by making elaborate notes.

Triage Process

There are several triage systems. Each uses slightly different criteria for classifying patients. Use the specific triage system and classifications that your jurisdiction has adopted.

START Triage System

One variation of a triage system that is common in the fire service and EMS is the **START triage system** developed by the Newport Beach, California, Fire and Marine Department and Hoag Hospital. The letters START stand for Simple Triage and Rapid Treatment. START is based on the rapid assessment of patients using the following three criteria: respirations, perfusion, and mental status (RPM). Patients are classified into one of four categories and are tagged and with the denoted color-coded tag indicator: immediate (red), delayed (yellow), minor (green), and deceased (black) (Figure 26.5).

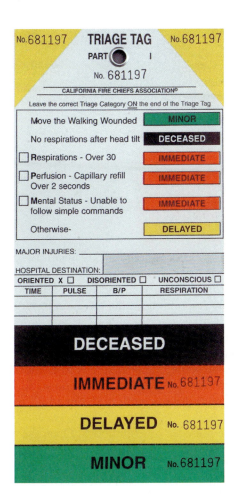

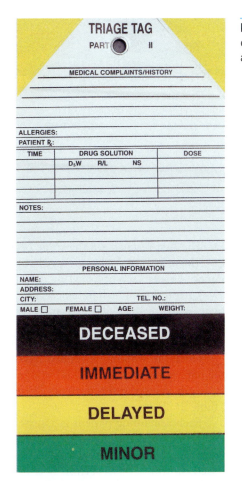

Figure 26.4 • An example of a standard triage tag, front and back.

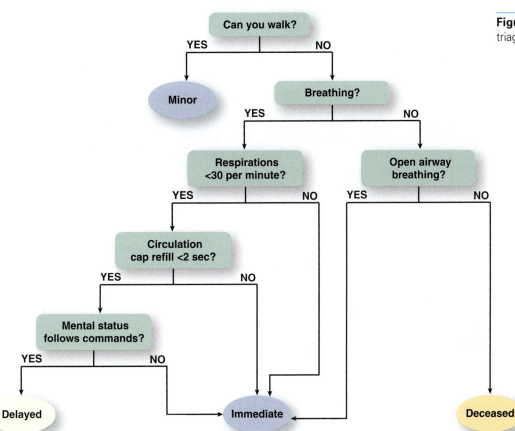

Figure 26.5 • The START triage algorithm.

TABLE 26.2 | START Triage System

	IMMEDIATE	DELAYED	MINOR	DECEASED
Respirations	>30 per minute	<30 per minute	<30 per minute	Absent
Perfusion	Capillary refill >2 seconds or radial pulse absent	Capillary refill <2 seconds or radial pulse present	Capillary refill <2 seconds or radial pulse present	Absent
Mental status	Unable to follow commands	Able to follow commands	Able to follow commands	Absent

Read more about START Triage.

The first rescuers on the scene begin the triage process and quickly identify and separate those patients who are probably the least injured. They are initially classified as minor. This is accomplished by directing all the walking wounded to a specific location away from the immediate emergency scene. By responding to the direction to move, patients who are able will move and therefore self-triage into the minor category, at least initially. It is important not to send these patients too far away because some of them may be able to assist with the care of more injured patients.

Once the walking wounded have exited the scene, the next step is to begin triaging the remaining patients. START triage recommends you to "start where you stand." That is, begin assessing the patients closest to you and work your way out to all patients (Table 26.2).

Each remaining patient is assessed for the presence of respirations. Open the airway and check for breathing. If the patient takes a breath, he is tagged immediate. If he is not breathing, he is not salvageable and is tagged deceased. All respiratory rates are estimates based on quick observation. It is not necessary to take actual rates during the triage process.

Here is a brief overview of how a patient might be tagged based on respiratory status:

- No respirations: dead or non-salvageable (black).
- Respirations above 30 per minute: immediate (red tag). No further assessment needed.
- Respirations below 30 per minute: assess perfusion.

OBJECTIVE

9. Differentiate primary and secondary triage.

Patients who were identified as ambulatory can assist in keeping the airway open for an unresponsive patient. If other patients cannot help, use items on the scene to position the head and maintain the airway. It is important to understand that patients will constantly be reassessed as time and resources permit. When a patient is first identified and triaged, this is referred to as *primary triage*. When a patient is relocated to a treatment area, he or she will immediately be re-triaged by the treatment team. This is referred to as *secondary triage*.

KEY POINT ▼

When working with the START triage process, it is good to know that all unresponsive breathing patients are automatically categorized as immediate.

Responsive patients with respirations less than 30 per minute are assessed for perfusion status. Check the breathing patient's radial pulse. The presence of a radial pulse indicates a systolic blood pressure of at least 80 mmHg. Any patient with a radial pulse is assumed to have adequate perfusion. Therefore, assessment of mental status is the next step before categorizing the patient. Any patient without a radial pulse is assumed to have inadequate perfusion and is tagged immediate.

Some triage systems use capillary refill to assess perfusion. However, it is often unreliable because of many variables, such as age, sex, and environment. If your protocols require that you check capillary refill, the following criteria will guide you: If capillary refill is greater than two seconds or the radial pulse is absent, categorize the patient as immediate and move on to the next patient. If capillary refill is less than two seconds and the patient has a radial pulse, continue to assess mental status.

During the perfusion assessment, if you find major bleeding, do what you can to attempt to control the bleeding. Have the patient or one of the walking wounded hold direct pressure over the wound. Elevate the legs of any patient with no radial pulse and keep him in this position.

The final step in the START triage process requires assessment of the patient's mental status. This is accomplished by determining if the patient can follow simple commands, such as "open and close your eyes" or "squeeze your fingers." If the patient is able to follow simple commands, he is categorized as delayed and you will move on to the next patient. If the patient is unable to follow simple commands, he is categorized as immediate and you will move on to the next patient.

continued

FIRST ON SCENE

The first person that Gus checks on is dead. That is bad, and he has to force himself to continue on. Luckily, the next five are alive. Some are hurt pretty seriously, but they are definitely alive. Of the last 10—those who were obviously closest to the blast—he only finds a pulse in three. He takes the blue permanent marker from his shirt pocket and writes "Red," "Yellow," or "D" on each person's forehead.

He is amazed at how quickly the triage training from his last Emergency Medical Responder class comes back to

him. He is just returning to the first "Red" person to reassess him when a group of police officers moves systematically through the mall doors.

"I didn't have any tags, so I wrote on their foreheads," Gus shouts as the officers stand, unmoving, near the mall entrance. "What are you all waiting for? These people need help!"

"Step away from the area, son," a police officer orders. "Go over by the escalator until we can clear the scene."

JumpSTART Pediatric Triage System

The START triage system works well for rapidly assessing adults, but rescuers need to use different criteria to assess pediatric patients in multiple-casualty incidents. Using the START system, a respiratory rate of less than 30 breaths per minute in adults is a good sign, while a rate faster than 30 breaths per minute indicates a problem. Small children, especially crying infants, will normally have a respiratory rate greater than 30 breaths a minute. A child with a respiratory rate of eight breaths per minute would be categorized delayed using the START system, when actually he is in respiratory failure and should be categorized immediate.

There are similar assessment problems when checking circulation in children. Adults usually have circulatory failure followed by respiratory arrest. Children have respiratory failure followed by circulatory failure, meaning that a nonbreathing child could still have a pulse. But the START system would categorize the child with no respirations as deceased. START also uses capillary refill as an assessment tool, and it can be a useful assessment for children in normal environments. However, the reliability of capillary refill as an assessment tool varies with age, sex, and the environment, and measuring it requires good lighting. The JumpSTART system does not recommend using capillary refill for assessing perfusion.

When checking mental status in children, there is a broad range of responses possible, depending on the child's age. Infants will not be able to obey commands. Small children do not have the developmental ability to respond appropriately to commands. However, rescuers can check for signs of mental status using the AVPU scale (alert, responsive to voice, responsive to pain, or unresponsive).

To meet the needs of children involved in MCIs, Dr. Lou Romig, Medical Director for the South Florida Regional Disaster Medical Assistance Team, developed a special triage system for pediatric patients, the **JumpSTART pediatric triage system** (Figure 26.6). JumpSTART can be used on children from 12 months to eight years of age, although rescuers can use it on older children as well. The age ranges were determined by several criteria. Children from 12 to 18 months are beginning to walk and can be sorted

JumpSTART pediatric MCI triage system ▶ a specialized pediatric triage system designed for patients from one to eight years of age.

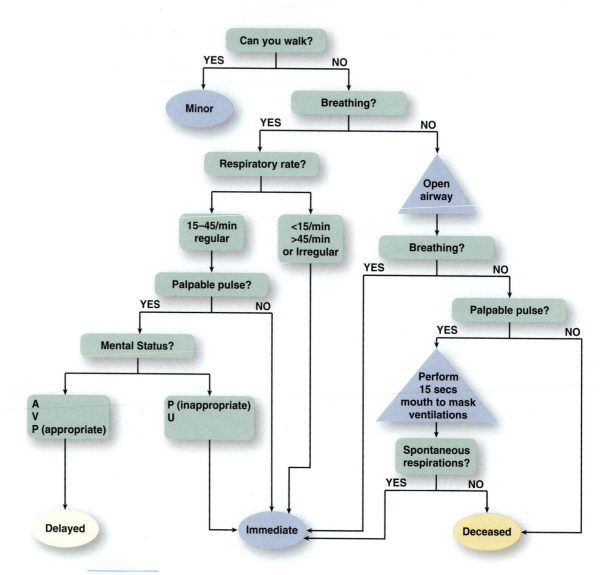

Figure 26.6 • The JumpSTART pediatric triage algorithm.

as "walking wounded," or ambulatory patients. Children older than eight years of age have airway anatomy and physiology similar to that of an adult.

Dr. Romig suggests that if the patient looks like a young adult, use START, and if the patient looks like a child, use JumpSTART.

The assessment categories for the JumpSTART system are the same as for the START system: respirations, perfusion (peripheral pulses), and mental status (AVPU). The steps for JumpSTART are as follows:

1. Move all children who are able to walk to an area set aside for minor injuries. There, rescuers perform a secondary triage, including respirations, pulse, and mental status. Infants who are not yet walking are assessed during initial triage, using the JumpSTART steps, or in the secondary triage area, if someone carries them there. Infants and children who are ambulatory (able to walk), have respirations, perfusion, and appropriate mental status, and have no significant external injury are categorized as minor.

   In an MCI, it is possible to have a child with special health-care needs. He may not be ambulatory and also may have chronic respiratory problems and elevated respiratory rates. Assess the special needs child the same as you would an infant. It may be difficult to assess mental status because of the child's special health-care or developmental status. Look for the child's parent or caregiver to get information if this person is present and uninjured.

2. Assess nonambulatory children for the presence or absence of spontaneous breathing. If there is breathing, assess the respiratory rate. (See step 3.) Open the airway of any child who is not breathing or who is not breathing for more than 10 seconds. Clear a foreign body airway obstruction only if you see it. If the child begins to breathe spontaneously with an open airway, categorize the child as immediate and move on to the next patient.

    If the child does not begin spontaneous breathing when you open the airway, palpate for a peripheral pulse (radial, brachial, or pedal). If there is no peripheral pulse, categorize the patient as deceased, and move on to the next patient.

    If the child does not begin spontaneous breathing when you open the airway, and the child has a pulse, ventilate the patient five times using an appropriate barrier device.

    Giving breaths is considered the "jumpstart" part of the pediatric triage system. Children may stop breathing or have a period of not breathing (apnea) but still maintain a pulse. The START system would categorize the nonbreathing child as deceased, but the JumpSTART system modifies the process to include a pulse check for the nonbreathing child and five ventilations if there is a pulse. The ventilation is meant to jumpstart the child's breathing.

    However, if ventilations do not trigger spontaneous respirations, categorize the child as deceased and move on to the next patient. If the child begins to breathe spontaneously, categorize the child as immediate and move on without providing further ventilations. It is possible that the child may not be breathing when another rescuer arrives to begin secondary triage. This rescuer will determine the appropriate intervention based on the number of patients and the number of rescue personnel.

3. In this step, all patients have spontaneous respirations. If the respiratory rate is 15 to 45 breaths per minute, proceed to step 4 and assess perfusion. If the respiratory rate is slower than 15 (slower than one breath every four seconds) or faster than 45 breaths a minute or very irregular, categorize the child as immediate and move on.

4. In this step, all patients have adequate respirations. Assess perfusion by palpating peripheral pulses on uninjured limbs. Check peripheral pulses rather than capillary refill because of the many variables that affect accuracy. If the child has palpable peripheral pulses, assess mental status (step 5). If there are no peripheral pulses, categorize the patient as immediate and move on.

5. In this step, all patients have adequate ABCs. Check the child's mental status by using a rapid AVPU assessment. Keep in mind that the developmental age of the child will affect results. If the child is alert, responds to your voice, or responds appropriately to pain (localizes the pain, or knows where you are pressing or grasping, and withdraws or pushes you away), categorize the patient as delayed. If the child does not respond to your voice and responds inappropriately to pain (makes a noise, moves sporadically, or does not localize the pain), shows "posturing" (decorticate, with arms curled onto the chest toward the midline of the body; or decerebrate, with arms stiff at the sides and hands flexed away from the body), or is unresponsive, categorize as immediate and move on. You have learned about the significance of the injuries and how to provide care for patients with these signs and symptoms throughout your Emergency Medical Responder course.

When you are faced with multiple casualties at critical incidents, also be aware of your mental and physical stress levels. Critical incident stress debriefing (CISD) sessions or other qualified psychological support should be available after a disaster or unusual emergency to address the needs of rescuers who may have been influenced by the scene and the stress generated in providing emergency care.

Gus sits on the frozen escalator for what seems like an eternity as the mall slowly fills first with police officers and then with people in large, clumsy bomb suits. Finally, the firefighters and EMTs are allowed in to quickly carry out the wounded shoppers. The deceased ones, the ones on which Gus had written "D," are left sprawled on the beige tiles where they fell following the explosion.

Gus rubs his eyes and notices that his white uniform shirt is now covered in bloody smears and dark, pungent ash. He is taking it off when a police officer approaches him. "Let's get you out to the treatment area, son."

"Oh, I'm not hurt." Gus rolls his shirt into a ball and puts it under his arm.

"That's fine," the officer says, jabbing his thumb toward the main mall doors. "Let's just have you looked at, okay?"

Gus can't think of any good reason to stay in the mall or to ever come back for that matter, so he walks to the door and, without looking back, walks out into the late afternoon sun. He is immediately overwhelmed by the number of emergency vehicles and rescuers, hustling around on the marble entryway. He shades his eyes from the sun and sees crowds of people, some with cameras, being held back by police barricades on the far side of the street.

"Are you the one who did the triaging in there?" A gruff voice startles Gus and he spins around.

"Uh, yes, sir," he answers, seeing an older firefighter with a white helmet on.

"You did a real fine job." The man smiles, reaches out, and shakes Gus's hand. "I bet you saved some lives in there."

Summary

- While relatively rare, multiple-casualty incidents (MCIs) can easily overwhelm the first responding units at the scene. It is up to those first units to quickly request additional resources and begin to establish command over the incident.

- An incident command system, or incident management system, is a tool used to manage overall control of large scenes involving many resources and multiple agencies.

- Triage is the sorting of patients based on the severity of their injuries or illnesses. The goal of triage is to save as many patients as possible using the available resources.

- Triage systems vary by jurisdiction, but they generally use a three- or four-category system. Typical categories include:

immediate for the most critical but salvageable patients, *delayed* for those less critical but still in need of care, *minor* for those who are generally ambulatory at the scene, and *deceased* for those who show no signs of life.

- One variation of a triage system is the START system—a Simple Triage and Rapid Treatment program that uses respirations, perfusion, and mental status assessments to categorize patients into one of four treatment categories.

- A variation of the START triage system designed specifically for pediatric patients is called the JumpSTART system, which takes into account the unique needs and presentation of pediatric patients.

Take Action

VOLUNTEERS NEEDED

Multiple-casualty incidents can be some of the most frightening and rewarding events to ever be a part of. While they are rare, if you are involved in EMS long enough, you are certain to have your chance to respond to one. One of the best ways to begin to get a glimpse at how these events unfold is to volunteer for a local MCI drill in your area. Fire departments, hospitals, and

EMS agencies frequently conduct MCI drills as a way to prepare for the real event. There is a huge need for volunteers to play victims at those events. Contact your instructor or local EMS agency to offer your services at the next MCI drill. You will probably discover that there are several of the drills conducted each year in your area or region.

First on Scene Run Review

Recall the events of the "First on Scene" scenario in this chapter and answer the following questions, which are related to the call. Rationales are offered in the Answer Key at the back of the book.

1. In an explosion, what is your first priority?

2. In triaging, how do you prioritize the patients?

3. What information do you want to give the arriving firefighters?

Quick Quiz

To check your understanding of the chapter, answer the following questions. Then compare your answers to those in the Answer Key at the back of the book.

1. A multiple-casualty incident (MCI) involves _____ victims.
   a. more than one
   b. more than two
   c. fewer than 10
   d. fewer than 100

2. An incident management system is a tool for the command, control, and _____ of resources at the scene of a large-scale emergency involving multiple agencies.
   a. constant monitoring
   b. care of victims
   c. coordination
   d. concerns of safety

3. The triage system was developed to assist in determining those victims needing:
   a. standard care.
   b. immediate transport.
   c. immediate care.
   d. long-term care.

4. Triage is a process of sorting patients into categories and prioritizing their medical care and transport based on:
   a. number of injuries and medical conditions.
   b. age, weight, and height of the patient.
   c. proximity to the mechanism of injury.
   d. severity of injuries and medical conditions.

5. During the triage process, patients will be placed into one of four categories—immediate, delayed:

   a. minor, or non-injury.
   b. minor, or deceased.
   c. non-injury, or deceased.
   d. minor, or walking wounded.

6. In the START triage system, patients are categorized based on an assessment of respirations and:

   a. perfusion and mental status.
   b. blood pressure and mental status.
   c. perfusion and signs of shock.
   d. signs of shock and mental status.

7. Patients may be classified as "walking wounded" if they are able to assist:

   a. in the triage of other patients.
   b. with hazard control.
   c. with the simple care of patients.
   d. in the extrication of victims.

8. The JumpSTART triage system was developed for:

   a. children age 12 months to the teenage years.
   b. children age 12 months to eight years of age.
   c. adult patients younger than 50 years of age.
   d. adult patients older than 50 years of age.

9. The JumpSTART triage assessment categories are:

   a. the same as for the START triage system.
   b. dependent on the age of the pediatric patient.
   c. very different from the START triage system.
   d. dependent on the injuries of the pediatric patient.

10. When determining the order of care for victims of multiple-casualty incidents, it is critical to consider the mechanism of injury and the findings from the:

    a. assessment of mental status.
    b. primary assessment only.
    c. primary and secondary assessments.
    d. secondary assessment only.

APPENDIX 1

Patient Monitoring Devices

EDUCATION STANDARDS • Assessment—Monitoring Devices

COMPETENCIES • Use scene information and simple patient assessment findings to identify and manage immediate life threats and injuries within the scope of practice of the Emergency Medical Responder.

OVERVIEW Assisting advanced-level providers such as the EMTs and Paramedics is an important role of the Emergency Medical Responder. Often the advanced provider is busy with many things at once and the support from an Emergency Medical Responder can greatly enhance the efficiency and quality of patient care. This appendix introduces you to the most commonly used monitoring devices in the prehospital environment. We will also describes the general features of each device and explain how the Emergency Medical Responder can best assist.

OBJECTIVES

Upon successful completion of this appendix, the student should be able to:

COGNITIVE

1. Define the following terms:
   a. blood glucose *(p. 600)*
   b. cardiac monitor *(p. 598)*
   c. end-tidal CO_2 detector *(p. 601)*
   d. glucometer *(p. 600)*
   e. pulse oximeter *(p. 599)*

2. Explain the purpose of a cardiac monitor. *(p. 598)*

3. Describe the procedure for appropriately attaching cardiac electrode pads to a patient. *(p. 599)*

4. Explain the purpose of a pulse oximeter. *(p. 599)*

5. Explain the two values that a pulse oximeter monitors. *(p. 599)*

6. Differentiate normal and abnormal values displayed by the pulse oximeter. *(p. 599)*

7. Explain the factors that might cause a pulse oximeter to provide inaccurate readings. *(p. 599)*

8. Explain the purpose of a blood glucometer. *(p. 600)*

9. Differentiate normal and abnormal blood glucose values. *(p. 600)*

10. Explain the purpose of an end-tidal CO_2 detector. *(p. 601)*

11. Describe the procedure for using an end-tidal CO_2 detector while ventilating a patient. *(p. 601)*

12. Differentiate and discuss normal and abnormal values displayed by an end-tidal CO_2 detector. *(p. 601)*

PSYCHOMOTOR

13. Demonstrate the proper method for attaching a three- and four-lead monitor to a simulated patient.

14. Demonstrate the proper method for attaching a pulse oximeter to a simulated patient.

15. Demonstrate the proper method for using an end-tidal CO_2 detector when ventilating a simulated patient.

AFFECTIVE

16. Recognize the limitations of monitoring devices.

17. Value the importance of caring for the patient based on all signs and symptoms and not just those being displayed by the monitoring device.

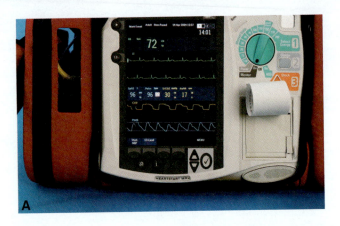

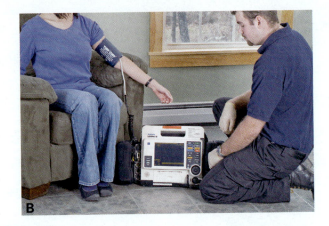

Figure A1.1 • Cardiac monitors. (A) Some heart monitors simply provide an electrical tracing of the heart. (B) More sophisticated monitors can measure blood pressure as well as other things.

Patient Monitoring Devices

Cardiac Monitor

Cardiac monitors come in a variety of shapes and sizes depending on the manufacturer and purpose of the device. Some **cardiac monitors** simply provide an image of the patient's electrocardiogram (ECG) on a screen, while others are far more complex and allow for the monitoring of several signs (Figure A1.1). These monitors are distinguished from automated external defibrillators (AEDs) in that a trained provider is required to interpret and act on the ECG rhythm provided by the monitor. When using an AED, the provider does not need to have any knowledge of cardiology or ECG interpretation: The machine takes care of that part and instructs the provider to either shock or continue CPR.

The typical cardiac monitor used on advanced life support (ALS) ambulances is a multipurpose model that can obtain both 3-lead and 12-lead ECGs, provide varying levels of shocks, and serve as a pacemaker for the patient's heart. Increasing numbers of EMS systems are beginning to use models that can monitor the patient's exhaled carbon dioxide levels, oxygen saturation levels, and automatically take blood pressures.

The main purpose of an ECG monitor is to allow the EMS provider to easily monitor the heart rate and, more importantly, the rhythm. Electrodes placed on the skin pick up the electrical conductions within the heart that occur with every beat. The ECG monitor can reassure the EMS provider that the patient's heart rate is normal or alert him to an acute condition that could require further evaluation and treatment.

Initially, the three-lead monitor is used on the patient, although this requires the placement of four electrodes. The fourth electrode is the ground that allows the electrical circuit to close. The electrical rhythm of the heart portrayed on the ECG screen does not represent the physical motion of blood in and out of the heart, only the electrical conduction. Therefore, pulse and blood pressure must always be checked in conjunction with use of the ECG monitor.

If the patient is having chest pain or other cardiac signs and symptoms, the paramedic may decide to perform a 12-lead ECG. This involves using six extra cables that are placed on the chest wall to provide multiple images of the heart from various angles (Figure A1.2). The main purpose of this is to identify if a heart attack is occurring, and where within the heart it is located.

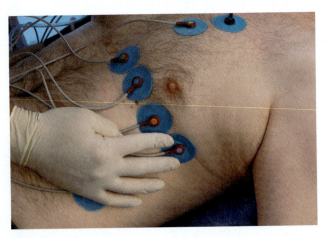

Figure A1.2 • Several electrode pads are placed on the chest to allow the monitor to obtain a 12-lead view of the heart.

The Emergency Medical Responder can assist by connecting the cables to the ECG monitor, snapping electrodes to the ends of each cable, and placing the electrodes on the patient. Most monitors have labels on the end of each cable indicating where on the body they should be placed, such as "LL" for left leg and "RA" for right arm. Some monitors may not have this but instead use a color system. In those cases, the black lead is for the upper left extremity or chest, the red lead is for the lower left extremity or chest, and the white lead is for the right upper extremity or chest.

As a general rule, electrodes should always be placed over muscle or fat tissue, not the more bony areas.

If the patient has excess body hair, this can interfere with electrode placement. Most monitor packs will have a disposable shaving razor to use for clearing the areas where electrodes will be applied.

Another problem occasionally encountered is an extremely diaphoretic patient. The excess sweat can allow the electrodes to slide off of the skin, leading to a poor connection. Be sure to dry the skin thoroughly before attempting to apply the electrodes.

Once the electrodes are placed on the patient and the monitor cables are plugged into the monitor, turn on the monitor and advise the paramedic that the monitor is ready. Occasionally there may be artifact, which is a result of patient or vehicle movement and appears as erratic movement in the ECG baseline rhythm. If the paramedic deems the rhythm acceptable, print a six-second-long strip from the monitor to capture the rhythm.

Follow these steps when applying a cardiac monitor to the patient:

1. Explain to the patient what you are doing and why.
2. Take out ECG cables and electrodes.
3. Attach the three-lead cable to the monitor.
4. Place an electrode in the end of each cable.
5. Expose the patient's extremities or chest as appropriate. Shave excess hair as necessary.
6. Apply the appropriate electrode to each limb, ensuring that all electrodes are firmly adhered to the skin.
7. Turn on the ECG monitor.
8. Observe for artifact, and ensure that the patient is not moving.
9. Print a six-second ECG strip.

Pulse Oximeter

A **pulse oximeter**, or pulse ox for short, is a device that uses infrared technology to determine the percent of a patient's hemoglobin that is saturated with oxygen (Figure A1.3). It does this by determining how much of the infrared and red lights that are shot through a thin area of skin are absorbed by the hemoglobin. Most commonly the finger tip, ear lobe, and toe are used for measurement. The pulse oximeter can be a standalone device, but increasingly it is being incorporated into ECG monitors. The pulse oximeter displays two values: the percentage of oxygen saturation and the heart rate (Figure A1.4). The percentage of peripheral oxygen saturation, often abbreviated as SpO_2, is a valuable clinical tool for monitoring patients with respiratory complaints. A normal saturation is above 97%, although values as low as 90% could be normal for a patient with chronic lung disease such as COPD. Saturations below 90% are never normal and should be corrected quickly with supplemental oxygen.

To obtain accurate baseline saturations, the pulse oximeter should first be applied when the patient is on "room air," meaning not on any supplemental oxygen. Whenever saturation is measured for a patient that is on oxygen, it is important to record what type of oxygen-delivery device was being used and what the flow rate was.

The pulse oximeter device can give false readings in certain circumstances, and the Emergency Medical Responder should be aware of this. The most common reason is nail polish, which will prevent the pulse oximeter probe from shooting the light through the tissue. Any patient with nail polish on should have the polish removed on the finger to be used for monitoring. Most pulse oximeter kits contain nail polish remover for this purpose.

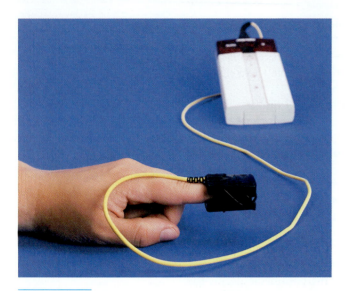

Figure A1.3 • A typical pulse oximeter applied to a patient's finger.

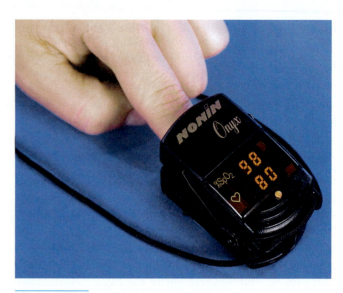

Figure A1.4 • A pulse oximeter will measure and display both oxygen saturation and pulse rate.

Hypothermia is a condition that will give falsely low pulse oximeter readings due to the constriction of blood vessels in the fingers or toes.

Falsely high readings occur in patients exposed to carbon monoxide poisoning, because the carbon monoxide binds to the hemoglobin instead of oxygen. To the monitor, the hemoglobin appears saturated and will display a falsely high reading. However, the reality is that the hemoglobin is saturated with carbon dioxide and the patient will become hypoxic. For use in children, a special probe is used to accommodate for the smaller size.

Follow these steps when applying a pulse oximeter to a patient:

1. Remove the probe from the kit and connect the cable to the device, if applicable.
2. Identify a finger to use for probing and remove nail polish if necessary. Then place the probe on the finger.
3. Turn the device on.
4. Record the percent saturation and heart rate. Confirm the heart rate on the device by taking a radial pulse.

Glucometer

OBJECTIVE

8. Explain the purpose of a blood glucometer.

glucometer ▶ a device used to measure and display the amount of glucose in a given sample of blood.

The **glucometer** is a device that measures a patient's glucose (sugar) level in the blood. It is a portable device that allows rapid testing in the field by the EMS provider or patient (Figure A1.5). Diabetic patients are routinely prescribed glucometers and trained to check and monitor their own blood sugar level at home.

To use the device, a small drop of blood must be obtained for testing. Typically, the patient's fingertip is cleaned and stuck with a small disposable needle called a lancet. A drop of blood is then placed on a chemical test strip, which is inserted into the device either before or after the addition of blood, depending on the model (Figure A1.6). Once the sample is collected, most glucometers will produce the result within 30 seconds. The result is given in milligrams per deciliter (mg/dL), and this is how it is traditionally reported. After use, the chemical strip and lancet are disposable, and the lancet should be placed in a sharps container.

OBJECTIVE

9. Differentiate normal and abnormal blood glucose values.

blood glucose ▶ the level of glucose in the bloodstream and any given time.

Normal **blood glucose** levels range from 80 to 120 mg/dL. Some diabetic patients may run slightly higher or lower, and they will typically inform the EMS provider of this. Hypoglycemia occurs in patients with low blood glucose levels, and can cause altered mental status, lethargy, and eventually unconsciousness and seizures. High blood-glucose levels, or hyperglycemia, also can cause confusion but generally to a lesser extent than hypoglycemia.

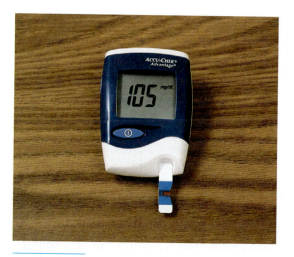

Figure A1.5 • A typical blood glucometer.

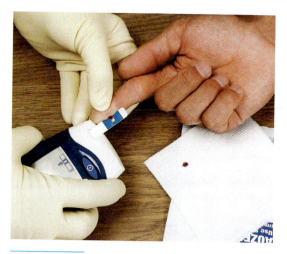

Figure A1.6 • A drop of blood is placed on the test strip and is immediately analyzed by the device.

In many EMS systems, Emergency Medical Responders are not allowed to use a glucometer. This must only be used by EMS providers who are trained and authorized to do so. Always follow local protocol.

End-Tidal Carbon Dioxide Detector

The **end-tidal carbon dioxide (CO_2)** detector measures the amount of carbon dioxide that the patient exhales with each breath (Figure A1.7). The reason it is called the end-tidal CO_2, or $ETCO_2$, is because the number it provides reflects only the amount of CO_2 at the very end of exhalation. More advanced monitors have waveform capnography, which allows the measurement of CO_2 levels throughout the entire ventilatory cycle.

$ETCO_2$ detectors come in a variety of forms, but in EMS they are used primarily to verify proper placement of an endotracheal tube following intubation. Increasingly the detectors are being used on conscious and breathing patients to evaluate for the presence of certain respiratory diseases such as asthma, hyperventilation, and congestive heart failure.

When used in intubation, there are two types of $ETCO_2$ detectors: disposable colormetric devices and digital sensors. The disposable colormetric devices use litmus paper and will change color in the presence of CO_2. The device is small and plastic, and has a port on either side. One side attaches to the endotracheal tube and the other to the

end-tidal CO_2 detector ▶ a device used to detect the presence of CO_2 in the exhaled breath of a patient.

OBJECTIVES

10. Explain the purpose of an end-tidal CO_2 detector.

11. Describe the procedure for using an end-tidal CO_2 detector while ventilating a patient.

12. Differentiate and discuss normal and abnormal values displayed by an end-tidal CO_2 detector.

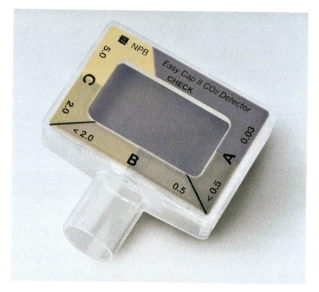

Figure A1.7 • A color-changing (colormetric) end-tidal CO_2 detector.

bag-mask device. Therefore, the detector lies directly in the path of air flow. The paper is purple initially, and will change to gold when it comes in contact with CO_2, indicating the tube placement is correct. The reason is that if the tube is in the trachea, and the lungs are being ventilated, then the gas exchange will cause CO_2 to be exhaled. If the tube is misplaced, such as in the stomach, then no CO_2 will be returned and the color on the detector will not change.

Digital and waveform sensors attach similarly to the endotracheal tube and plug into the $ETCO_2$ monitor or ECG machine, depending on the model. The devices allow continuous monitoring that can be used to evaluate the efficiency of ventilation. A normal $ETCO_2$ level is 35 to 45 mmHg, and when ventilating a patient the provider should aim to keep the level at the low end of this range. If ventilations are being given too rapidly, then the $ETCO_2$ level will drop. If ventilations are too slow, the opposite will occur and CO_2 levels will rise because the patient is not exhaling enough.

In conscious patients, the $ETCO_2$ can be monitored by a cannula-type device. The devices can measure the exhaled CO_2 from the nostril. The waveform can then be interpreted to assist in diagnosing the patient's condition, such as differentiating between an asthma attack and hyperventilation.

Limitations of Monitoring Devices

The increased use of technology in medicine has greatly enhanced diagnostic and treatment abilities, but devices are no replacement for a proper and detailed physical examination. The tools are best used as supplements to traditional examination skills, and can be used to support assessment findings. All of the devices can be fooled by various conditions: carbon monoxide poisoning for the pulse oximeter, poor calibration for the glucometer, and so on. The EMS provider must always take this into account when treating the patient. Any finding on the devices should always be compared to the actual vital signs, patient complaints, and patient appearance. Remember: treat the patient, not the monitor.

APPENDIX 2

Principles of Pharmacology

EDUCATION STANDARDS
- Pharmacology—Principles of Pharmacology, Medication Administration, Emergency Medications

COMPETENCIES
- Uses simple knowledge of the medications that the Emergency Medical Responder may self-administer or administer to a peer in an emergency.

OVERVIEW

NOTE: This appendix is designed to aid Emergency Medical Responders who are being trained to assist patients in taking specific prescribed medications. This training is meant to be a part of a formal training program that is under the guidance and supervision of a Medical Director. All EMS providers who administer or assist patients in administering their own prescribed medications must follow local protocols. Emergency Medical Responders must not attempt to give any medication without specific medical direction.

Pharmacology is the study of drugs, their origins, nature, chemistry, effects, and use. Emergency Medical Responders will assess and care for many patients whose medical history includes the medications they take, and whose problems may be caused by the effects of taking or not taking medications properly. This appendix lists and describes the few medications that Emergency Medical Responders may be carrying and the few prescribed medications you may assist a patient in administering. It also discusses how to give or assist the patient in administering the medications and the effects of the medications on the patients.

Remember that you may only give or assist in giving certain medications under the supervision of medical direction.

OBJECTIVES

Upon successful completion of this appendix, the student should be able to:

COGNITIVE

1. Define the following terms:
   a. actions *(p. 604)*
   b. autoinjector *(p. 610)*
   c. contraindication *(p. 604)*
   d. indication *(p. 604)*
   e. medication *(p. 604)*
   f. side effect *(p. 604)*

2. Describe the indications, contraindications, actions, and side effects of the following medications commonly encountered in the field environment:
   a. activated charcoal *(p. 604)*
   b. epinephrine autoinjector *(p. 611)*
   c. metered-dose inhalers *(p. 608)*
   d. nitroglycerin *(p. 609)*
   e. oral glucose *(p. 606)*

3. List the five "rights" of medication administration. *(p. 612)*

4. Explain the role of the Emergency Medical Responder when assisting a patient with administration of medication. *(p. 612)*

PSYCHOMOTOR

5. Demonstrate the ability to properly assist a patient with the administration of prescribed medication.

6. Demonstrate the ability to properly assist a patient with the administration of an autoinjector.

AFFECTIVE

7. Value the importance of medications being administered as prescribed.

Medications

Emergency Medical Responders may be trained to assist with or administer in the field *oxygen, activated charcoal,* and *oral glucose*. Many Emergency Medical Responders are allowed by their Medical Director to administer those medications under specific conditions and circumstances. Activated charcoal and oral glucose are sold over the counter in most pharmacies and are found in many households.

The other medications described in this appendix must be prescribed by a physician and are usually carried by the patient. They are prescribed *metered-dose inhalers, nitroglycerin,* and *epinephrine autoinjectors*. Depending on the specific EMS system, Emergency Medical Responders may be able to assist a patient in taking any one of these medications with the approval of medical direction and under specific conditions and circumstances.

Indications, Contraindications, Actions, and Side Effects

For each medication, the Emergency Medical Responder must know and understand the specific indications, contraindications, and actions, as well as any expected side effects the medication may have on the patient. After a medication has been administered, it will be important to monitor the patient to see how the drug is affecting him. If taken properly, **medication** will usually ease the ill effects of the medical condition. But if the medication is expired, or the patient's condition is beyond the help of the drug, the medication may be ineffective.

For each drug, there are *indications* for its use. **Indications** are specific signs or symptoms for which it is appropriate to use the drug. For example, nitroglycerin is indicated for patients experiencing cardiac chest pain, and an inhaler is indicated for someone having an asthma attack.

Also, there are contraindications for each drug's use. **Contraindications** are specific signs, symptoms, or conditions for which it is not appropriate to use the drug. For example, nitroglycerin is contraindicated in patients experiencing cardiac chest pain and who have a systolic blood pressure below 100. Since nitroglycerin reduces blood pressure, it is possible to cause the blood pressure to drop too low if it is not above 100 systolic before taking the dose. Administering oral glucose to an unresponsive patient may be contraindicated, since it may cause an airway obstruction.

A medication's **action** is the specific effect it is designed to have on the patient. The action of nitroglycerin is to dilate the vessels. The action of activated charcoal is to bind with the poison, and the action of glucose is to raise the level of sugar in the blood.

Medications sometimes have side effects. A **side effect** is any unwanted action or reaction caused by the drug other than the desired effect. Some side effects are expected and predictable. Nitroglycerin will dilate vessels, not just in the heart but also throughout the body. This may cause a large enough drop in blood pressure to make the patient dizzy or lightheaded. Another common side effect of nitroglycerin is a headache. You must anticipate side effects and document them when they occur, especially before administering a second dose. It is good practice to advise or remind the patient about the possible side effects before administering any medication. This could minimize the chances of any surprises that could further add to the patient's anxiety. If the patient has taken any of these medications before, he probably will know what side effects to expect.

medication ▶ something that treats, prevents, or minimizes the symptoms of disease.

indication ▶ the reason a medication should be administered.

contraindication ▶ a reason that a medication should not be administered to a patient because of the potential for harmful effect.

actions ▶ the intended effect of a drug on the body.

side effect ▶ an action of a medication that is not desired.

Medications Carried on the Emergency Medical Responder Unit

Activated Charcoal

Activated charcoal (Scan A2.1) is not the kind of charcoal you find in the barbecue grill. It is most often found in a slurry form, which is a powder premixed with water for use in the prehospital emergency situation. (Some brands require you to add the

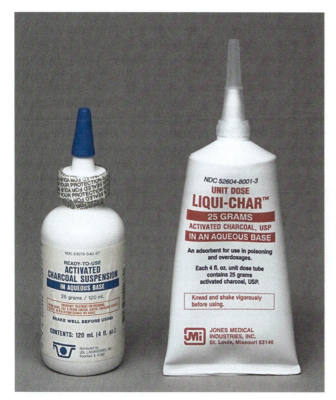

MEDICATION FORM

- | Premixed in water, frequently available in plastic bottle containing 12.5 grams of activated charcoal
- | Powder, which should be avoided in field

DOSAGE

- | Adults and children: 1 gram activated charcoal/kg of body weight
- | Usual adult dose: 25–50 grams
- | Usual pediatric dose: 12.5–25 grams

STEPS FOR ADMINISTRATION

1 | Consult medical direction.
2 | Shake container vigorously.
3 | Since medication looks like mud, patient may need to be persuaded to drink it. Providing a covered container and a straw will prevent the patient from seeing the medication and so may improve patient compliance.
4 | If patient does not drink the medication right away, the charcoal will settle. Shake or stir it again before administering.
5 | Record the name, dose, route, and time of administration of the medication.

ACTIONS

- | Activated charcoal binds to certain poisons and prevents them from being absorbed into the body.

SIDE EFFECTS

- | Causes black stools.
- | Some patients, particularly those who have ingested poisons that cause nausea, may vomit. If patient vomits, repeat the dose once.

REASSESSMENT STRATEGIES

Be prepared for the patient to vomit or further deteriorate. If the patient worsens, provide oxygen as you have been trained to do.

MEDICATION NAME

- | Generic: activated charcoal
- | Trade: SuperChar, Insta-Char, Actidose, Liqui-Char, and others

INDICATIONS

Poisoning by mouth (ingestion)

CONTRAINDICATIONS

- | Altered mental status
- | Ingestion of acids or alkalis
- | Unable to swallow

water.) Activated charcoal is administered to patients who have ingested a poison or who took an overdose of oral drugs or medications. When the patient drinks the activated charcoal slurry, it binds with the poisonous substance and also helps prevent the poison or drug from being absorbed by the body. Follow local protocols for administration.

Oral Glucose

Glucose is a simple sugar found in many common foods such as fruit, bread, and vegetables and is the body's main source of energy. The brain in particular is very sensitive to abnormal levels of glucose and functions poorly without it. A patient with abnormal glucose levels will commonly have an altered mental status.

Glucose levels can be raised by giving oral glucose (Scan A2.2), a form of glucose that comes in a gel or chewable tablet. It is indicated for patients with an altered mental status and a history of diabetes. It is taken orally.

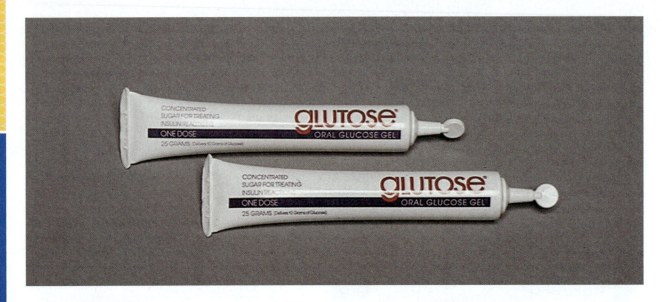

MEDICATION NAME

- | Generic: glucose, oral
- | Trade: Glutose, Insta-glucose, BD Glucose Tablets

INDICATIONS

- | Patient has altered mental status with a known history of diabetes.
- | Patient has taken insulin but no food recently and may have been very physically active.

CONTRAINDICATIONS

- | Unresponsiveness or unable to swallow or otherwise manage own airway
- | Known diabetic who has not taken insulin for days

MEDICATION FORM

Gel, in toothpaste-type tubes; chewable tablets

DOSAGE

One tube; three 5 gram chewable tablets. This dose can be used for both adults and children. Tubes can come in 15, 30, and 45 mg dosages.

STEPS FOR ADMINISTRATION

1 | Ensure signs and symptoms of altered mental status with a known history of diabetes.
2 | Ensure patient is alert enough to swallow.
3 | Administer glucose.
   a. Self-administered into mouth and swallowed.
   b. Place on tongue depressor between cheek and gum.
   OR
   c. Have patient chew one to three tablets.
4 | Perform ongoing assessment.

ACTIONS

Increases blood sugar levels

SIDE EFFECTS

None when given properly

REASSESSMENT STRATEGIES

Continue to monitor the patient's mental status and signs and symptoms. If patient becomes less responsive, discontinue administration. Continue to provide oxygen as you have been trained to do.

To assist in the administration of oral glucose, have the patient hold the tube and instruct him to squeeze small amounts into his mouth and swallow. You want him to ingest the entire tube as quickly as possible but without choking. An alternative method for administration is to apply some of the gel to a tongue depressor and spread it between the patient's cheek and gum. Continue to apply small doses until the tube is empty. The mucous membrane inside the mouth is rich in blood vessels, which quickly absorb the glucose and carry it through the bloodstream. Once the level of glucose is elevated, the patient's condition usually begins to improve.

For tablets, the typical strength is 5 grams of D-glucose (dextrose). This form of glucose passes through the mucosa (lining) of the mouth, esophagus, and stomach so that no special digestion is needed. It does not have to enter the small intestine to be absorbed. The manufacturer's recommended dosage is three tablets, or 15 grams, of D-glucose. *Do not* try to administer glucose tablets to anyone who is unresponsive and unable to manage his own airway.

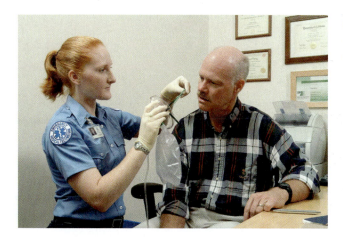

Figure A2.1 • Oxygen is a useful medication for many patients.

The patient should respond quickly to the tablets. Fatigue may remain for various periods of time depending on the patient and how rapidly the blood glucose level fell during the hypoglycemic (low blood sugar) episode. Some patients have feelings of uneasiness that remain for up to one-half hour. Most are able to eat additional foods that help with their symptoms. However, do not allow someone to ingest foods if he has been given glucose and reports nausea. The nausea should subside shortly and, if the patient requests food and remains alert, most protocols for hypoglycemic events allow it.

Oxygen

A drug, 100% oxygen (Figure A2.1) is used to treat patients who have low oxygen levels in their blood because of medical or traumatic conditions. Oxygen and oxygen therapy are described in detail in Chapter 9. If your Emergency Medical Responder unit carries oxygen and oxygen-delivery devices, you must participate in a training program to learn how and when to use them properly. Be sure to follow your jurisdiction's guidelines, protocols, and medical direction.

Prescription Medications

Metered-Dose Inhalers

Many patients have chronic respiratory diseases—such as asthma, emphysema, or bronchitis—that cause the airway passages in the lungs to narrow, or become constricted. Such patients usually carry a device called a *metered-dose inhaler* (Scan A2.3). It typically contains medication called a *bronchodilator.* This medication enlarges, or dilates the airway passages so the patient can breathe easier. The inhaler device holds the medication in an aerosol form, which can be sprayed into the mouth and inhaled.

You must have medical direction to help a patient self-administer this medication. You must also make sure that this medication belongs to the patient and was not lent to him by a well-meaning family member or friend with a similar problem. Also, checking for an expiration date is important since expired medication is less effective.

Nitroglycerin

Nitroglycerin is a chemical that is well known as an explosive, but it also has medical uses. It decreases the workload of the heart while dilating blood vessels. It is effective in relieving certain types of pain, particularly the type caused by a heart condition called *angina pectoris.* Patients who have heart conditions that cause recurring chest pain or who have a history of heart attack may have a prescription for nitroglycerin

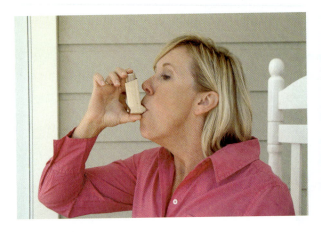

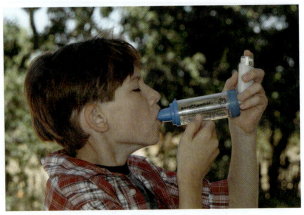

MEDICATION NAME

- | Generic: albuterol, ipratropium, metaproterenol
- | Trade: Proventil, Ventolin, Atrovent, Alupent, Metaprel

INDICATIONS

Meets all of the following criteria:
- | Patient exhibits signs and symptoms of respiratory difficulty.
- | Patient has physician-prescribed inhaler.
- | Medical direction gives Emergency Medical Responder specific authorization to use.

CONTRAINDICATIONS

- | Altered mental status (such that the patient is unable to use the device properly)
- | No permission has been given by medical direction
- | Patient has already taken maximum prescribed dose prior to rescuer's arrival

MEDICATION FORM

Handheld metered-dose inhaler

DOSAGE

Number of inhalations is based on medical direction's order or physician's order.

STEPS FOR ADMINISTRATION

1 | Obtain order from medical direction.
2 | Confirm patient is alert enough to use inhaler.
3 | Ensure it is the patient's own prescription.
4 | Check expiration date of inhaler.
5 | Check if patient has already taken any doses.
6 | Shake inhaler vigorously several times.
7 | Have patient exhale deeply.
8 | Have patient put lips around the opening of the inhaler.
9 | Have patient depress the handheld inhaler when beginning to inhale deeply.
10 | Instruct patient to hold breath for as long as is comfortable so that medication can be absorbed.
11 | Allow patient to breathe a few times and repeat second dose if so ordered by medical direction.
12 | If patient has a spacer device for use with the inhaler (device for attachment between inhaler and patient to allow for more effective use of medication), it should be used.
13 | Provide oxygen as appropriate.

ACTIONS

Dilates bronchioles, reducing airway resistance

SIDE EFFECTS

- | Increased pulse rate
- | Anxiety
- | Nervousness

REASSESSMENT STRATEGIES

- | Monitor vital signs.
- | Adjust oxygen as appropriate.
- | Reassess level of respiratory distress.
- | Observe for deterioration of patient. If breathing becomes inadequate, provide artificial ventilations.

(Scan A2.4). Nitroglycerin is available in several forms, including pill, spray, and paste.

Patients are typically instructed by their physician to take up to three tablets—one every 5 minutes—over a 15-minute period.

You will need to consult medical direction to help administer nitroglycerin or to get permission to give more after the patient has taken three doses. As with the inhaler, be sure to check that the nitroglycerin is actually the patient's medication and that it has not reached the expiration date.

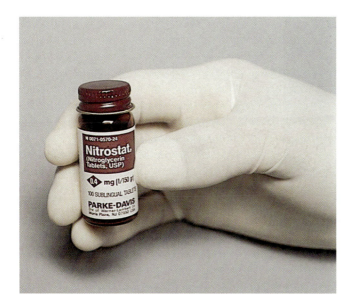

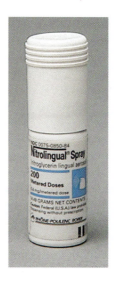

MEDICATION NAME

- | Generic: nitroglycerin
- | Trade: Nitrostat, NitroTab, Nitrolingual

INDICATIONS

All of the following conditions must be met:

- | Patient complains of chest pain.
- | Patient has a history of cardiac problems.
- | Patient's physician has prescribed nitroglycerin.
- | Systolic blood pressure is greater than 100 systolic. (Local protocols may vary.)
- | Medical direction authorizes administration of the medication.

CONTRAINDICATIONS

- | Patient has a systolic blood pressure below 100 mm Hg. (Local protocols may vary.)
- | Patient has a head injury.
- | Patient has already taken the maximum prescribed dose.

MEDICATION FORM

Tablet or sublingual spray

DOSAGE

One dose is equal to 0.4 mg, repeat in three to five minutes. If no relief, systolic blood pressure remains above 100 (local protocols may vary), and if authorized by medical direction, up to a maximum of three doses. Spray is typically prescribed for one metered spray followed by a second in 15 minutes.

STEPS FOR ASSISTING PATIENT

1 | Perform focused assessment for cardiac patient.
2 | Take blood pressure. (Systolic pressure must be above 100; local protocols may vary.)

3 | Contact medical direction if no standing orders.
4 | Ensure right medication, right patient, right dose, right route. Check expiration date.
5 | Ensure patient is alert.
6 | Question patient on last dose taken and effects. Ensure understanding of route of administration.
7 | Ask patient to lift tongue and place tablet or spray dose on or under tongue (while you are wearing gloves), or have patient place tablet or spray under tongue.
8 | Have patient keep mouth closed with tablet under tongue (without swallowing) until dissolved and absorbed.
9 | Recheck blood pressure within two minutes.
10 | Record administration, route, and time.
11 | Perform reassessment.

ACTIONS

- | Dilates blood vessels
- | Decreases workload of heart

SIDE EFFECTS

- | Hypotension (lowers blood pressure)
- | Headache
- | Changes pulse rate
- | Dizziness, lightheadedness

REASSESSMENT STRATEGIES

- | Monitor blood pressure.
- | Ask patient about affect on pain relief.
- | Seek medical direction before re-administering.
- | Record assessments.
- | Provide oxygen as appropriate.

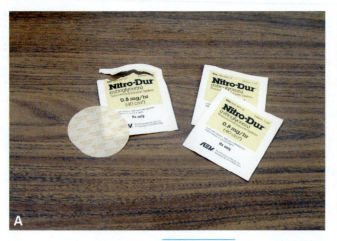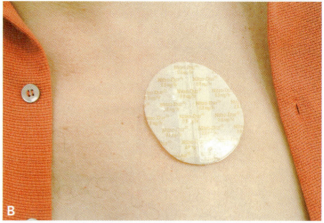

Figure A2.2 • Transdermal nitroglycerin patches may be found applied to the patient's chest, upper arm, or upper back.

The patient may have a bottle of nitroglycerin sublingual spray (such as Nitrolingual Pumpspray). Depending on local protocol, up to three metered sprays may be administered under the tongue within 15 minutes for cases of suspected cardiac chest pain.

The patient may have nitroglycerin transdermal patches (transdermal infusion system). These are for daily application and help prevent angina attacks, but they are not meant to relieve and correct an acute event (Figure A2.2).

Anytime a patient complains of chest pain—whether it persists or not, whether the patient has a history of chest pain or not—arrange for immediate transport to a medical facility.

In recent years, the use of aspirin for the treatment of suspected heart attack has become commonplace in most hospitals and EMS systems. In fact, several pharmaceutical companies have created television and radio commercials encouraging the use of aspirin for this purpose. As an Emergency Medical Responder, you may encounter patients who have recently taken aspirin or who may want to take some while in your care. You must follow your local protocols when assisting any patient with the administration of aspirin.

Epinephrine Autoinjectors

Many people have allergies and will react severely to certain foods, medicines, or the poisons of insect stings or snakebites. Those reactions may be life threatening when they cause the airway to become swollen and blood vessels to dilate. Epinephrine (Scan A2.5) is a medication that can reverse those reactions. It dilates the air passages so breathing becomes easier, and it constricts the blood vessels.

Reactions to allergens can have a very sudden onset, and any reaction that causes breathing and circulation problems must be recognized and treated quickly. The patient must take his prescribed epinephrine immediately.

autoinjector ▶ a type of device used to self-administer some medications by way of needle injection.

Those patients who are aware of their allergies and expect severe reactions generally carry a prescription with them in a device called an **autoinjector**. This is a syringe with a spring-loaded needle that will release and inject epinephrine into a muscle when the patient presses it against his skin (usually in the thigh). If you need to assist the patient in taking epinephrine, first check to see if the injector is prescribed for that patient and get permission from medical direction. Remember to always check the expiration date.

Many diabetic patients now use a pen-type device to inject themselves with insulin. Be sure to check the device carefully before helping with administration.

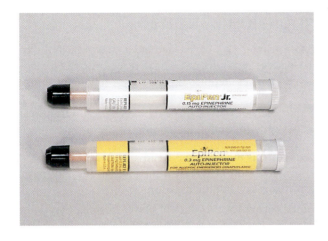

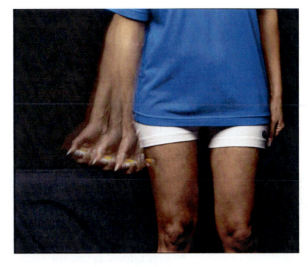

MEDICATION NAME

- | Generic: epinephrine
- | Trade: Adrenalin, Epi-Pen

INDICATIONS

Must meet the following three criteria:
- | Patient exhibits signs of a severe allergic reaction, including either respiratory distress or shock.
- | Medication is prescribed for this patient by a physician.
- | Medical direction authorizes use for this patient.

CONTRAINDICATIONS

No contraindications when used in a life-threatening situation.

MEDICATION FORM

Liquid administered by an autoinjector, which is an automatically injectable needle-and-syringe system.

DOSAGE

Adults: one adult autoinjector (0.3 mg)
Infant and child: one infant/child autoinjector (0.15 mg)

STEPS FOR ASSISTING PATIENT

1 | Obtain patient's prescribed autoinjector. Ensure:
   a. Prescription is written for the patient who is experiencing the severe allergic reaction.
   b. Medication is not expired or discolored (if visible).
2 | Obtain order from medical direction.
3 | Remove cap from autoinjector.
4 | Place tip of autoinjector against patient's lateral thigh, midway between hip and knee.
5 | Push the injector firmly against the thigh until the injector activates.

6 | Hold the injector in place until the medication is injected (at least 10 seconds).
7 | Record activity and time.
8 | Dispose of injector in biohazard container.

ACTIONS

- | Dilates the bronchioles
- | Constricts blood vessels

SIDE EFFECTS

- | Increased heart rate
- | Dizziness
- | Chest pain
- | Headache
- | Nausea
- | Vomiting
- | Excitability, anxiety
- | Pale skin

REASSESSMENT STRATEGIES

1 | Arrange for transport.
2 | Continue focused assessment of airway, breathing, and circulatory status. If patient's condition continues to worsen (decreasing mental status, increasing breathing difficulty, decreasing blood pressure):
   a. Obtain medical direction for an additional dose of epinephrine.
   b. Provide care for shock, including administration of oxygen per local protocols.
   c. Prepare to initiate basic life support (CPR, AED).
3 | If patient's condition improves, provide supportive care:
   a. Continue oxygen.
   b. Provide care for shock.

Rules for Administering Medications

Before you give any of the three medications you may carry (activated charcoal, oral glucose, or oxygen), or before you assist a patient in taking any of the three prescribed medications (metered-dose inhaler, nitroglycerin, or epinephrine), there are a few more things you need to know.

OBJECTIVES

3. List the five "rights" of medication administration.

4. Explain the role of the Emergency Medical Responder when assisting a patient with administration of medication.

You must check the five "rights" that are rules for giving any medication. Often you will have to rely on the patient's word. Ask the following questions:

- *Right patient?* Is this the right patient for this medication? Read aloud the name written on the medication bottle: "Is your name Bob Becker?" If the patient does not have a labeled box or bottle, simply ask if this is his own medication.
- *Right medication?* Is this the right medication for this patient? For example, the patient is having chest pain but hands you a bottle of penicillin, or the patient has strep throat but hands you a bottle of nitroglycerin.
- *Right dose?* Is this the right dose for this patient? The dosage is usually written on the label, but the patient does not always carry the original box or bottle the medication came in.
- *Right route?* Is this the right route for taking the medication? Different types of medications, such as tablets, powders, sprays, gels, slurries, and pastes, are given by different routes—swallowed by mouth, inhaled by mouth, dissolved under the tongue, injected into or absorbed through the skin.
- *Right time?* Is this the right time to be giving the medication? In the case of nitroglycerin, has enough time elapsed since the last dose was given?

Routes for Administering Medications

The way a patient takes a medication has an effect on how quickly the medication enters the bloodstream and begins to relieve the medical condition. Medications are administered by the following routes:

- *Oral or swallowed,* usually in some solid form (a tablet or pill), or in some liquid form (powder dissolved in or mixed with a liquid, such as the activated charcoal slurry)
- *Intramuscular,* or injected into a muscle, like the epinephrine autoinjector
- *Sublingual,* or dissolved under the tongue, like the nitroglycerin tablets
- *Inhaled,* or breathed into the lungs, from an inhaler or oxygen-delivery device such as the medication given for chronic respiratory problems or the oxygen gas given for respiratory distress and for most medical and trauma patients
- *Endotracheal,* or sprayed into a tube inserted into the trachea (windpipe), so it can more directly reach the lungs and be absorbed quickly. (Emergency Medical Responders will not administer medication in this form.)
- *Transdermal patches or transdermal infusion systems,* affixed to the skin by an adhesive backing on one side of the patch. Another chemical is mixed in with the medication, usually a form of alcohol that will carry the medication or drug through the patient's skin into the bloodstream. These patches are slow to react and are not meant for acute attacks such as the onset of chest pain.
- *Intranasal,* or sprayed directly into the nasal cavity through the nostril. Studies have shown that certain medications can be rapidly and effectively absorbed through the nasal mucous membranes and into the bloodstream.

You can see there is a lot to know and understand about medications. Once you do, you will become more confident in giving the ones that you carry and the prescribed ones you can assist patients in taking. Remember, you may only administer or assist with specific medications and then only with medical direction.

Nerve Agent Autoinjectors

The threat of terrorism is an unfortunate reality of the times we live in. EMS systems across the country must anticipate this threat and do what they can to prepare. One of the most likely threats involves the dispersal of a deadly chemical known as a nerve agent. Nerve agents affect the nervous system and cause uncontrolled muscle activity and death.

Because of the strong likelihood that nerve agents may be used by terrorists, many EMS systems have assembled large supplies of an antidote. These antidotes most commonly come as an autoinjector and are designed for self-administration (Figure A2.3). As a member of the EMS team in your region or state, you will likely receive training on the indications and use of the antidote.

The autoinjectors contain two drugs, atropine and pralidoxime (Protopam), and are meant to be utilized by EMS personnel in the event of a terrorist attack involving nerve agents. They are meant for self-administration and for administration to other EMS personnel.

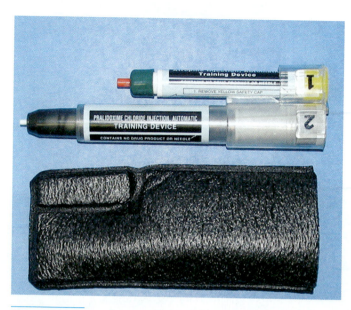

Figure A2.3 • The Mark I autoinjector is used to deliver the antidote for nerve agent exposure.

The administration of the antidote is like any autoinjector and should be injected into the lateral thigh muscle.

APPENDIX 3

Air Medical Transport Operations

EDUCATION STANDARDS

- EMS Operations—Air Medical Transport

COMPETENCIES

- Knowledge of operational roles and responsibilities to ensure safe patient, public, and personnel safety.

OVERVIEW

Many EMS systems across the United States use air medical resources such as helicopters (rotor wing) and airplanes (fixed wing) to transport critically ill and injured patients (Figure A3.1). It is estimated that there are approximately 500,000 patients transported by helicopter and another 150,000 transported by airplane in the United States each year.

Although it is uncommon for an Emergency Medical Responder to be hired to work on an EMS aircraft, your current training can be the first step in becoming qualified to eventually gain employment with an air medical organization. However, as an Emergency Medical Responder, you may be in a position to request a helicopter or at the very least assist in the landing of a helicopter at the scene of an emergency.

OBJECTIVES

Upon successful completion of this appendix, the student should be able to:

COGNITIVE

1. Define the following terms:
   a. fixed wing *(p. 616)*
   b. helipad *(p. 616)*
   c. instrument flight rules (IFR) *(p. 617)*
   d. landing zone (LZ) *(p. 618)*
   e. rotor wing *(p. 615)*
   f. visual flight rules (VFR) *(p. 617)*

2. Describe the common crew configurations within air medical transport. *(p. 615)*

3. Differentiate and discuss the benefits of both fixed-wing and rotor-wing air medical transport. *(p. 615)*

4. Describe the two types of rotor-wing air medical transport missions. *(p. 615)*

5. Explain the common criteria for choosing air medical transport over ground transport. *(p. 617)*

6. Differentiate between visual and instrument flight rules. *(p. 617)*

7. Describe the characteristics of an appropriate helicopter landing zone. *(p. 618)*

8. Explain the safe principles of working around aircraft at the scene of an emergency. *(p. 619)*

PSYCHOMOTOR

9. Demonstrate and discuss the ability to establish an appropriate helicopter landing zone.

AFFECTIVE

10. Recognize the value of air medical transport when utilized properly.

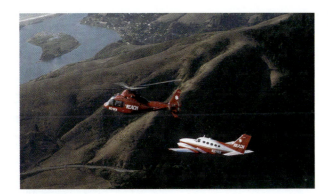

Figure A3.1 • Both helicopters and airplanes are used in EMS today.
(© Reach, Inc./Tony Irvin)

Crew Configurations

The majority of EMS aircraft being flown in the United States are staffed with a nurse and a paramedic. The following is a list of other common medical crew configurations:

- Nurse and nurse
- Doctor and nurse
- Nurse and respiratory therapist
- Paramedic and paramedic

The specific crew configuration is often determined by local regulations or the type of patient being cared for. These configurations are common for both helicopters and planes.

Air Medical Resources

Rotor-Wing Resources

The term **rotor wing** refers to the helicopter. Most EMS helicopters fly two types of missions: the *scene call* and the *interfacility transport (IFT)*. The scene call is made when a helicopter is requested to respond to the scene of an emergency, such as a vehicle collision or a near-drowning incident at a lake or the beach. In those cases, the helicopter is requested to respond to the scene just as a ground ambulance might. If all goes well, the helicopter will land near the patient, allowing the medical crew to exit the aircraft, begin caring for the patient, and prepare him for transport (Figure A3.2).

The interfacility transport (IFT) occurs when a patient is already at a hospital but needs to be transported to another hospital. In most cases, the patient is in need of a higher level of care than the sending hospital is capable of providing. For example, a patient with significant trauma transported by ground ambulance to a hospital five minutes away may need to be transported to the regional trauma center 60 miles away. An interfacility transport by aircraft would be required.

There are many different types of EMS helicopters in use today. They differ in many ways, including size, shape, number of engines, and how high or fast they can fly (Figure A3.3). Regardless of size or performance capabilities, EMS helicopters all share one very important characteristic—they are designed to carry critically ill or injured patients. The vast majority of helicopters are configured to carry just one patient lying on a stretcher. Although some can carry two patients, the ability to provide care while in flight is greatly minimized due to the limited space. Because a helicopter can fly from hospital pad to hospital pad, it is ideal for short transports (under 200 miles).

OBJECTIVE

2. Describe the common crew configurations within air medical transport.

IS IT SAFE?

Helicopter-scene call operations are very risky. It is important to use an experienced person to help choose an appropriate landing zone and assist with landing the helicopter.

rotor wing ▶ helicopter.

OBJECTIVES

3. Differentiate and discuss the benefits of both fixed-wing and rotor-wing air medical transport.
4. Describe the two types of rotor-wing air medical transport missions.

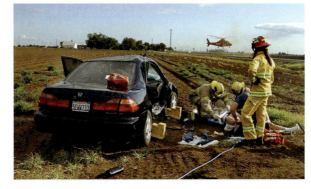

Figure A3.2 • In many cases, a helicopter can land right at the emergency scene.
(© Reach, Inc./Rick Roach)

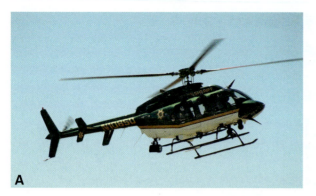

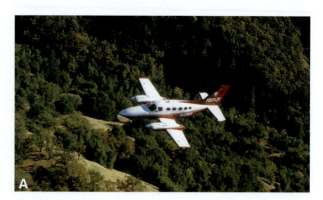

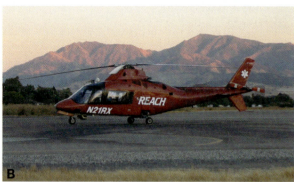

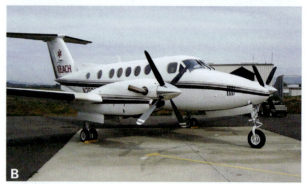

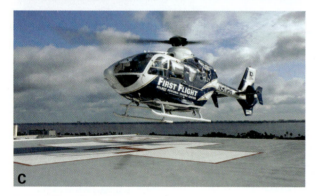

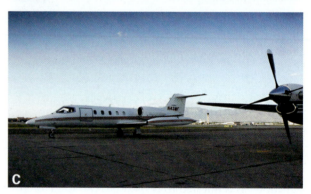

Figure A3.3 • EMS helicopters come in many shapes and sizes: A. Bell 407, B. Agusta 109, and C. Eurocopter EC 135.
(© Reach, Inc.)

Figure A3.4 • Fixed-wing aircraft (airplanes) are used for longer transports: A. Cessna 421 (© Reach, Inc./Tony Irvin); B. KingAir B2000 (© Reach, Inc.); and C. Lear Jet. (© Med Flight Air Ambulance)

Fixed-Wing Resources

fixed wing ▶ an airplane.

helipad ▶ a designated location for the landing of a helicopter, typically at a hospital or airport.

Like helicopters, **fixed-wing** resources (airplanes) vary in size and performance capabilities as well and include jets, turboprops, and piston-driven aircraft (Figure A3.4). The reason to choose an airplane over a helicopter is most often distance. Airplanes can fly much faster and farther than the typical helicopter, due largely to their ability to carry much more fuel. The airplane is ideal when there is no **helipad** at either the sending or receiving hospital and the two hospitals are more than 200 miles apart. Unlike the helicopter, the airplane is only capable of performing interfacility transports. This is because it is not feasible for an airplane to land at the scene of an emergency. It can, however, land at an airport and meet a waiting ambulance.

Note that all fixed-wing transports require a ground ambulance at each end of the transport. One ambulance will be necessary to bring the patient from the sending hospital to the airport and another to take the patient from the receiving airport to the receiving hospital.

Requesting Air Medical Resources

In most cases, it is the first responding units that determine the need for a helicopter response. This is why it is important for you as an Emergency Medical Responder to become familiar with the air medical resources in your region and understand their capabilities and limitations.

In most cases, a helicopter is appropriate whenever expedient transport is necessary or advanced providers are required. Most helicopter medical personnel receive specialized training over and above their counterparts on an ambulance or in a hospital. This training gives them an advanced scope of practice and allows them to deliver medications and perform procedures beyond those of the typical nurse or paramedic.

Most EMS systems that have air medical resources will have specific protocols and/or guidelines for deciding when it is appropriate to activate an air resource. The protocols often define specific patient types such as severe trauma and critical medical, or they may also define areas of the region that are remote and thus may take hours for a typical ground ambulance transport. It is important that you familiarize yourself with your local protocols for the use of air medical resources.

Just because you request a helicopter does not mean that one will respond. EMS helicopters are a limited resource, and many things can prevent them from responding to your request. They could be committed to another emergency and therefore may be unable to respond to your request, or there could be weather in the area of the scene or at the receiving hospital that would prevent the pilot from completing the transport safely and legally.

Air medical transport may not be the most appropriate mode of transport for a victim of a hazardous materials incident. Despite proper decontamination, the risk of exposure for the medical crew and pilot is too great in the confined space of the aircraft.

Visual Flight Rules

All pilots must operate aircraft based on specific and clearly defined rules established by the Federal Aviation Administration (FAA). The ability to fly any particular mission will depend on at least two factors: the training and capabilities of the pilot, and the design and configuration of the aircraft. It is safe to say that most EMS aircraft operate under what are known as **visual flight rules (VFR)**. This means that conditions along the intended route must be clear and free of weather such as fog or clouds. A VFR mission can be flown day or night so long as there is no significant weather anywhere along the intended route of flight.

Instrument Flight Rules

Many EMS air medical programs have specially trained pilots and specially configured aircraft so they can accept a request for transport even when the weather is bad. The rules that must be followed are called **instrument flight rules (IFR)**. Being IFR capable allows the pilot to fly into and through known weather along the route of flight. There are limitations as to the type and extent of weather an IFR pilot can fly in. For instance, there must be at least some visibility on the ground for the pilot to take off and land safely. In conditions where the fog is so thick that the pilot cannot see more than a few hundred yards, he or she may decline the request due to extreme weather conditions.

Note that there are many more requirements that must be met for a team to safely complete a patient transport under IFR rules. The planning and preparation for an IFR flight may include extra weather checks and additional fuel, which can add to the time it takes to launch and get to the scene or hospital.

What Happens After a Request Is Made?

EMS flight programs use specially trained dispatchers called Flight Communication Specialists. It is the Communication Specialist who receives the request for transport, provides an ETA (estimated time of arrival) to the caller, and relays the request to the flight crew in the form of a dispatch. Once the flight crew receives a dispatch, several events

OBJECTIVE

5. Explain the common criteria for choosing air medical transport over ground transport.

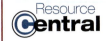

Learn more about air medical services.

OBJECTIVE

6. Differentiate between visual and instrument flight rules.

visual flight rules (VFR) ▶ rules defined by the Federal Aviation Administration regarding the operation of aircraft when weather is not a factor.

instrument flight rules (IFR) ▶ rules defined by the Federal Aviation Administration regarding the operation of aircraft in inclement weather.

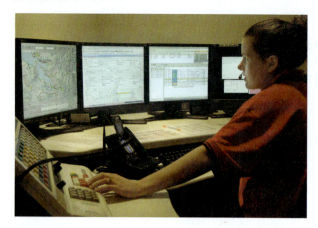

Figure A3.5 • Flight Communication Specialists are responsible for dispatching and tracking EMS aircraft on each mission.

must take place prior to the launch of the aircraft. The pilot will perform a weather check and confirm that weather conditions along the intended route of flight are within acceptable minimums. The medical crew will gather any needed equipment and head to the aircraft. In many programs, a specific risk assessment is performed prior to each flight to ensure the highest level of safety (Figure A3.5).

If the weather is acceptable and the medical crew has everything they need, all crew members approach the aircraft and perform a series of specific preflight safety checks prior to engine start and launch. If all goes well, they will be in the air and headed to their destination within minutes.

Occasionally, there will be factors that require the team to decline a request. Some of the most common reasons a crew might decline a request are poor weather conditions, mechanical failure, or patient size and weight.

The Landing Zone

Selecting an Appropriate Landing Zone

OBJECTIVE

7. Describe the characteristics of an appropriate helicopter landing zone.

landing zone ▶ a temporary location for the landing of a helicopter, typically at the scene of an emergency.

One of the characteristics that make helicopters so versatile is their ability to land nearly anywhere. The term *nearly* is used here because helicopters do need a clear, flat space to set down. An appropriate space for a helicopter to land has several important characteristics and is referred to as a **landing zone (LZ)**. The following characteristics are simply general guidelines and may differ slightly from program to program. It is best to learn the specific requirements of the programs operating in your area (Figure A3.6). Characteristics of a good landing zone include:

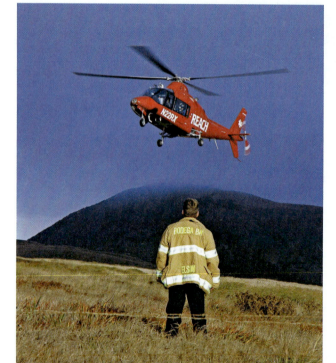

Figure A3.6 • To ensure a safe landing, an Emergency Medical Responder should assist in the landing process. (© Reach, Inc.)

- As close to the incident as possible
- 100 feet × 100 feet for daytime use, or 125 feet × 125 feet for nighttime use
- Little or no slope
- Free of dry sand or dirt and loose debris
- Free of utility wires near or around the site
- Free of tall trees or poles around the site
- Free of roaming animals

One of the most important things you can do as an Emergency Medical Responder at the scene where a helicopter has been requested is to provide the dispatch center with accurate GPS coordinates (latitude and longitude). If the flight crew can simply find the scene from the air based on your coordinates, they may be able to see other areas near the scene that could serve as ideal landing zones.

Once an LZ has been selected, it is important to perform a quick checklist and report the findings to the flight crew. The acronym HOTSAW is a common tool used to remember this LZ checklist:

H — *Hazards.* Be sure the area is free of obvious hazards such as loose debris and traffic.

O — *Obstacles.* Confirm that there are no obstacles such as tall trees, poles, or wires.

T — *Terrain.* Ensure that the area selected is firm and even.

S — *Slope*. Ensure that the area is as flat as possible.

A — *Animals*. Check to see that there are no roaming animals in the area.

W — *Wind*. Estimate wind speed and direction and relay that information to the flight crew.

If the area chosen for the LZ is a dirt surface, try to wet the area down prior to landing. This will avoid a dust storm caused by the downwash from the rotor blades. An excessive amount of dirt or snow can cause the pilot to lose site of the ground, which can be very dangerous.

In most instances, a single person will be designated as the landing officer for the aircraft. This person should maintain radio contact with the flight crew during the entire landing phase whenever possible. He should stand at one side of the LZ and wave his arms to signal to the flight crew that he is the landing officer. It is important for the landing officer and others to wear proper eye and ear protection whenever working around a helicopter. Remove any hats or other loose clothing that could be blown off during the landing or departure.

If the helicopter is to land at night, *never* shine any kind of light, such as a flashlight, at the aircraft. This could temporarily blind the pilot, which could have catastrophic consequences. In most cases, the lights of your emergency vehicle will be all the pilot needs to locate the scene.

Once the aircraft is safely on the ground, maintain direct eye contact with the pilot or other flight crew members. Do not approach the aircraft until someone from the flight crew has specifically directed you to do so.

Safety Around the Aircraft

Depending on several factors, the pilot may decide to shut down at the scene or remain "hot" with the rotors spinning. Regardless of the circumstances, follow these important guidelines when working around an aircraft at an LZ:

- Never approach an aircraft unless specifically directed to do so by the flight crew.
- Never shine any light at the aircraft.
- Never walk behind an aircraft, regardless of whether or not it is shut down.
- If on a slight slope, never approach the aircraft from the uphill side.
- Always remove your hat before approaching the aircraft.

OBJECTIVE

8. Explain the safe principles of working around aircraft at the scene of an emergency.

Introduction to Terrorism Response and Weapons of Mass Destruction

EDUCATION STANDARDS

• EMS Operations—Mass-Casualty Incidents Due to Terrorism and Disaster

COMPETENCIES

• Knowledge of operational roles and responsibilities to ensure safe patient, public, and personnel safety.

OVERVIEW

The U.S. government defines **terrorism** as "the use of force or violence against persons or property to intimidate or coerce a government, the civilian population, or any segment thereof to further political or social objectives." For years the people of the United States remained somewhat insulated from the effects of terrorists and terrorism, since they only viewed such events on the news. Terrorism is no longer something that only happens in distant countries.

In recent years, the use of weapons of mass destruction and the effects of terrorism have hit home with incidents such as the bombing of the Federal Building in Oklahoma City, the spread of anthrax through the U.S. Postal Service, and the events of September 11, 2001, in New York (Figure A4.1), Washington DC, and Pennsylvania.

OBJECTIVES

Upon successful completion of this appendix, the student should be able to:

COGNITIVE

1. Define the following terms:
   a. biological agent *(p. 622)*
   b. chemical agent *(p. 622)*
   c. chemical antidote autoinjector *(p. 622)*
   d. nerve agent *(p. 622)*
   e. nuclear/radiological agent *(p. 621)*
   f. terrorism *(p. 621)*
   g. weapons of mass destruction *(p. 621)*
2. Describe the signs and symptoms of a nuclear/radiological exposure. *(p. 621)*
3. Describe the signs and symptoms of a biological agent exposure. *(p. 622)*
4. Describe the signs and symptoms for the following types of chemical agent exposures: nerve agent, vesicant agent, cyanogens agent, pulmonary agent, riot control agent. *(p. 622)*
5. Describe the role of the Emergency Medical Responder at a weapons of mass destruction incident. *(p. 624)*

PSYCHOMOTOR

6. Demonstrate the procedure for administering a chemical antidote autoinjector to yourself and a fellow EMS provider.

AFFECTIVE

7. Recognize the importance of personal safety when working at the scene of a suspected terrorist incident.

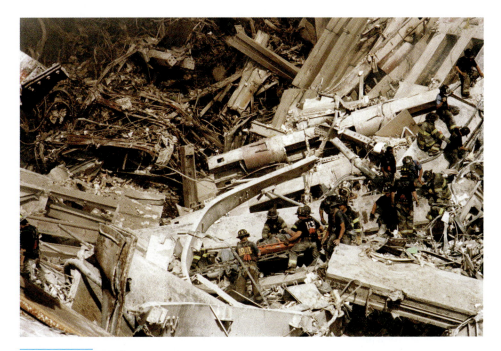

Figure A4.1 • World Trade Center, September 2001.
(© David Turnley/Corbis)

Incidents Involving Nuclear/ Radiological Agents

Until recently, the potential for a terrorist organization to obtain or develop **weapons of mass destruction** such as nuclear devices was thought to be minimal. With the growing supply of nuclear waste on a worldwide scale and the developing technology of third-world countries, the likelihood of a nuclear threat by a terrorist organization is ever increasing.

There are two types of potential nuclear incidents. One is the possible detonation of a nuclear device, and the other is the detonation of a conventional explosive incorporating nuclear material. A plausible scenario involves the second example above. It involves the detonation of a *radiological dispersal device (RDD)*, which would spread radioactive material throughout a wide area surrounding the blast site. Another example involves the detonation of a large *explosive device* (such as a truck bomb) near a nuclear power plant or radiological cargo transport.

Nuclear incidents emit three main types of radioactive particles/rays: alpha, beta, and gamma.

- *Alpha particles* are the heaviest and most highly charged of the nuclear particles. They are easily stopped by human skin but can become a serious hazard to reproductive organs if ingested or inhaled.

- *Beta particles* are smaller and travel much faster and farther than alpha particles. Beta particles can penetrate through the skin but rarely reach the vital organs. While they can cause burns to the skin if exposure lasts long enough, the biggest threat occurs when they are ingested or inhaled into the body. Beta particles also can enter the body through unprotected open wounds.

- *Gamma rays* are a type of radiation that travels through the air in the form of waves. The rays can travel great distances and penetrate most materials, including the human body. Acute radiation sickness occurs when someone is exposed to large doses of gamma radiation over a short period of time and can cause symptoms such as skin irritation, burns, nausea, vomiting, high fever, and hair loss.

terrorism ▶ the use of force or violence against persons or property to intimidate or coerce a government, the civilian population, or any segment thereof to further political or social objectives.

nuclear/radiological agent ▶ a substance containing radioactive material in quantities large enough to threaten human life.

weapon of mass destruction ▶ a weapon that can bring significant harm and kill large numbers of humans and cause great damage to manmade structures, natural structures, or the environment.

OBJECTIVE

2. Describe the signs and symptoms of a nuclear/radiological exposure.

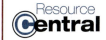

Learn about the role of the Department Homeland Security. Also find out more about blast injuries.

Incidents Involving Biological Agents

Biological agents pose one of the most serious threats due to their accessibility and ability to spread rapidly. The potential is also very high for widespread casualties. Biological agents are most dangerous when either inhaled (spread through the air) or ingested (through contaminated food or water supplies).

Signs and symptoms of biological agent exposure will vary by the specific agent involved, but some of the more common include:

- Fever
- Headache
- Breathing difficulty
- Nausea
- Vomiting
- Diarrhea

There are four common types of biological agents: bacteria, rickettsia, viruses, and toxins:

- *Bacteria* are single-celled organisms that can quickly cause disease in humans. Some of the more common bacteria used for terrorist activities are anthrax, cholera, the plague, and tularemia.
- *Rickettsia* are smaller than bacteria cells and live inside individual host cells. An example of rickettsia is *Coxiella burnetii*, which is the organism that causes Q fever.
- *Viruses* are infectious agents that require a living host to survive. The most common viruses that have served as biological agents include smallpox, Venezuelan equine encephalitis, and Ebola.
- *Toxins* are substances that occur naturally in the environment and can be produced by an animal, plant, or microbe. They differ from biological agents in that they are not manufactured. The four common toxins with a history of use as terrorist weapons are botulism, staphylococcal enterotoxin (SEB), ricin, and mycotoxins. Ricin has been used in several well-publicized incidents in the United States and Japan. It is a toxin made from the castor bean plant, which is grown all over the world.

Incidents Involving Chemical Agents

The primary routes of exposure for **chemical agents** are inhalation, ingestion, and absorption or contact with the skin, with inhalation being the most common. The classifications of chemical agents include nerve agents, vesicant (blister) agents, cyanogens agents, pulmonary agents, and riot-control agents.

Nerve Agents

Nerve agents disrupt the nerve impulse transmissions throughout the body and are extremely toxic in very small quantities. In some cases, a single small drop can be fatal to an average human being. Nerve agents include sarin (GB), which has been used against Japanese and Iraqi civilians; soman (GD); tabun (GA); and V agent (VX). These are liquid agents that are typically spread in the form of an aerosol spray.

In the case of GA, GB, and GD, the first letter *G* stands for the country (Germany) that developed the agent. The second letter indicates the order in which the agent was developed. In the case of VX, the *V* stands for venom and the *X* represents one of the chemicals that make up the compound. These agents resemble water or clear oil in their purest form and possess no odor. Sometimes small explosives are used to spread them, which can cause widespread death. Many dead animals at the scene of an incident may be an outward warning sign or detection clue.

biological agent ▶ any bacterium, virus, or toxin that could be used in biological warfare to cause death.

OBJECTIVE

3. Describe the signs and symptoms of a biological agent exposure.

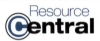

Learn more about anthrax and smallpox.

chemical agent ▶ any noxious substance used in chemical warfare to cause widespread death.

nerve agent ▶ a toxic substance that is inhaled or absorbed through the skin and has harmful effects on the nervous and respiratory system.

OBJECTIVE

4. Describe the signs and symptoms for the following types of chemical agent exposures: nerve agent, vesicant agent, cyanogens agent, pulmonary agent, riot control agent.

Early signs of nerve agent exposure are:

- Uncontrolled salivation
- Pupil constriction (miosis)
- Urination
- Defecation
- Tearing

Other later signs and symptoms include:

- Blurred vision
- Excessive sweating
- Muscle tremors
- Difficulty breathing
- Nausea, vomiting
- Abdominal pain

Many EMS systems have large supplies of antidote for nerve agent exposure. They are often self-administered by way of a **chemical antidote autoinjector**. See Appendix 2 for more information on the antidote for nerve agents.

chemical antidote autoinjector ▶ a method for the self-administration of a chemical antidote, primarily nerve agents.

Vesicant Agents

Vesicant agents are more commonly referred to as blister or mustard agents due to their unique smell. They can easily penetrate several layers of clothing and are quickly absorbed into the skin. Mustard (H, HD, HN) and Lewisite (L, HL) are common vesicants. Although less toxic than nerve agents, it takes only a few drops on the skin to cause severe injury.

The signs and symptoms of vesicant exposure include:

- Reddening, swelling, and tearing of the eyes
- Tenderness and burning of the skin followed by the development of fluid-filled blisters
- Nausea, vomiting
- Severe abdominal pain
- After about two hours, victims will experience runny nose, burning in the throat, and shortness of breath

Cyanogens

Cyanogens are agents that interfere with the ability of the blood to carry oxygen and can cause asphyxiation in victims of exposure. Common cyanogens are hydrogen cyanide (AC) and cyanogens chloride (CK). All cyanogens are very toxic in high concentrations and can lead to rapid death. Under pressure, these agents are in liquid form. In their pure form, they are a gas. Cyanogens are common industrial chemicals used in a variety of processes, and all have an aroma similar to bitter almonds or peach blossoms. Signs and symptoms of cyanogens exposure include:

- Severe respiratory distress
- Vomiting
- Diarrhea
- Dizziness, headache
- Seizures, coma

It is essential that victims of exposure be quickly moved to fresh air and treated for respiratory distress.

Pulmonary Agents

Pulmonary agents are sometimes called *choking agents*. They directly affect the respiratory system, causing fluid buildup (edema) in the lungs, which in turn causes asphyxiation similar to that seen in drowning victims. Chlorine and phosgene are two of the most common of these agents and are commonly found in industrial settings. Chlorine is a familiar smell to most people. Phosgene has an aroma of freshly cut hay. Both of these chemicals are in a gaseous state in their pure form and are stored in bottles or cylinders. Signs and symptoms include:

- Severe eye irritation
- Coughing
- Choking
- Severe respiratory distress

Riot-Control Agents

Riot-control agents include both irritating and psychedelic agents, both of which are designed to incapacitate the victim. For the most part, they are not lethal. However, under certain circumstances irritating agents have been known to cause asphyxiation. In some individuals, psychedelic agents have been known to cause behavior that can lead to death.

Common irritating agents include mace, tear gas, and pepper spray. These agents will typically cause severe pain when they come in contact with the skin, especially moist areas such as the nose, mouth, and eyes.

Signs and symptoms of exposure to irritating agents include:

- Burning and irritation in the eyes and throat
- Coughing, choking
- Respiratory distress
- Nausea
- Vomiting

Psychedelic agents include lysergic acid diethylamide (LSD), 3-quinuclidinyl benzilate (BZ), and benactyzine. These agents alter the nervous system, causing visual and aural hallucinations and severe changes in thought processes and behavior. The effects can be unpredictable, ranging from overwhelming fear to extreme belligerence.

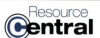

Read more information about terrorism.

Role of the Emergency Medical Responder

Terrorist attacks are meant to cause fear, and they are likely to occur when they are least expected. Having a high index of suspicion and recognizing the outward warning signs of a possible terrorist attack is of utmost importance for the first units on scene. Donning the appropriate personal protective equipment (PPE) early will minimize the chances of all emergency responders becoming victims themselves.

Firefighters are probably the best prepared of all Emergency Medical Responders because of the wide range of duties they are trained and expected to perform. Ambulance personnel are probably the least equipped to respond to a terrorist attack because their personal protective equipment is primarily designed to minimize exposure to body fluids and aerosolized droplets from coughing patients.

Without the proper training and equipment, Emergency Medical Responders are likely to become victims if they enter the scene too quickly. In most cases the best action will be to recognize the danger as soon as possible and retreat to a safe distance from the scene.

Note that many terrorists will set a secondary device that is meant to incapacitate or kill responders. The devices may be set to go off minutes to hours after the first one. By doing this, terrorists will be sure that the device will go off while rescuers are caring for patients who were injured by the first one. Make sure that the scene is truly safe before entering.

Decontamination

Decontamination is the process by which chemical, biological, and/or radiological agents are removed from exposed victims, equipment, and the environment (Figure A4.2). Regardless if the incident is a hazardous-materials release or an intentional terrorist act, prompt decontamination can be the single most important aspect of the operation to minimize exposure and limit casualties.

Depending on the size and scope of the incident, Emergency Medical Responders may be asked to assist with the decontamination process. If not a part of the decontamination process, they will certainly play an important role in the emergency care given to patients after coming out of decontamination. It will be important for Emergency Medical Responders assisting at such an event to continue to wear the appropriate PPE even after a victim has been decontaminated. This will minimize any contamination from residual agents remaining on the victim or equipment.

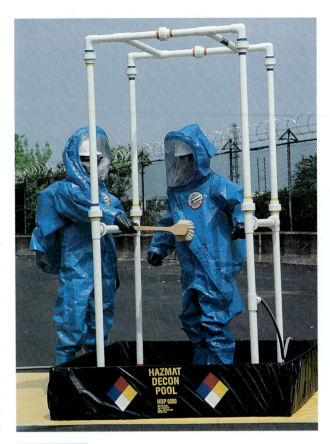

Figure A4.2 • Decontamination must occur before any patients can be properly cared for.

Chapter 1

Quick Quiz

1. c
2. a
3. b
4. d
5. d
6. b
7. c
8. a
9. a
10. b

Rationale for First on Scene Run Review

1. The dispatcher is in need of pertinent information to relay to the emergency responders, who must be prepared and able to treat the patient accordingly. Examples would include but are not limited to what the problem is, the patient's age, signs and symptoms, location of the patient, if any first aid is being rendered, and if the caller needs any guidance to help the patient until the Emergency Medical Responders arrive.

2. They should have personal protective equipment to protect themselves against any body fluids. They also should have basic equipment to help the patient, including but not limited to oxygen, airway adjuncts, a bag-mask device, an AED, and bleeding-control materials.

3. It is important to do a scene size-up along with determining the patient's chief complaint so you are able to treat the patient appropriately. This way you can be the patient's advocate and do what is best for him. For example, you can transfer information to the EMT, Paramedic, or hospital staff. Also, consideration should be given with respect to the patient's privacy.

4. It is important to know and follow local protocols and standing orders that are set forth by your jurisdiction's Medical Director. This will ensure proper care for the patient.

Chapter 2

Quick Quiz

1. b
2. c
3. d
4. b
5. d
6. d
7. b
8. c
9. a
10. b

Rationale for First on Scene Run Review

1. Possible reasons that Anthony wanted to leave the scene may include a fear of being sued, or perhaps a fear that he did not have the skills necessary to treat the individual.

2. The first priority would be the unresponsive male in the middle of the road because he has been ejected from a vehicle and likely suffered the most significant mechanism of injury. The second patient in the car must be extricated before being treated.

3. You should never leave the scene after treatment is started because this could be considered abandonment. The only time you can leave the scene is when you realize that no one else is around to call for help. In this instance, Anthony could have gone for help if no one else was there.

4. The information you need to give the ambulance crew is the position that the unresponsive person was found in and what you have done for him so far. You should also give the crew the information on the girl in the car, what you saw, and what her condition is.

Chapter 3

Quick Quiz

1. b
2. a
3. c
4. d
5. c
6. a
7. a
8. d
9. c
10. c
11. b
12. a
13. b
14. d

Rationale for First on Scene Run Review

1. You should always ask permission when you go to provide care for an individual because if he or she does not want your help, this would be called battery.

2. He did the right thing by not controlling the bleeding because he did not have proper BSI. You must always consider your personal safety first. The patient had hepatitis, which would be contagious if he had any open wounds or sores on his hands.

3. Jake could have given the patient dressings to apply direct pressure herself. He also could have had someone get the first-aid kit while someone else called 911.

Chapter 4

Quick Quiz

1. c
2. b
3. a
4. d
5. a
6. c
7. b
8. c
9. a
10. d
11. c
12. a
13. d
14. b
15. c
16. d
17. b
18. b
19. c
20. a

Rationale for First on Scene Run Review

1. The five elements of a scene size-up are safety, BSI, MOI/NOI, number of patients, and do I need more help.

2. She stopped the air from entering into the chest, which is a life-threatening condition that takes priority over finishing an assessment.

3. When an individual gets shot in the chest, there are several organs that can be injured. They are the lungs, heart, and the great vessels. This is why while doing your patient assessment, you need to palpate and listen for breath sounds in the chest. With this injury, he sustained a sucking chest wound.

Chapter 5

Quick Quiz

1. a
2. c
3. c
4. b
5. a
6. b
7. d
8. a
9. a
10. d

Rationale for First on Scene Run Review

1. Jesse could make the scene safe by having the first passerby pull off to the side of the road to speak to him and not stay in the middle. Also, he could have pulled his car halfway off the road and onto the shoulder with his hazards on after the accident happened to alert on coming traffic.

2. Jesse could have pulled his car halfway off the road and onto the shoulder with his hazards on to alert oncoming traffic. Also he should have asked the passerby to pull off to the side of the road.

3. Jesse should only remove him if there is a life-threatening condition, such as the patient is not breathing, or imminent danger such as a gas leak, or the vehicle is on fire.

Chapter 6

Quick Quiz

1. c
2. a
3. c
4. d
5. a
6. c
7. d
8. a
9. b
10. a

Rationale for First on Scene Run Review

1. Kaitlyn and Nick did not check for scene safety. The proper way to check would have been to determine if the man answering the door had any weapons or harmful intentions.

2. You must show respect for all cultures and beliefs. You would need to explain to patients your thoughts and how their actions could affect the outcome.

3. Someone from a different culture does not always understand your intentions. You would need to be patient and communicate clearly with him so as to earn his trust.

Chapter 7

Quick Quiz

1. b
2. c
3. d
4. a
5. b

Rationale for First on Scene Run Review

1. Yes. It is possible to add additional information to a report, but you must follow proper protocol for your agency. You must ensure that your documentation gets added to all copies of the PCR.

2. If you still have access to the report you can cross out any errors with a single line and then initial the change. You may add information on additional paper and add it to the report.

Chapter 8

Quick Quiz

1. b
2. a
3. a
4. d
5. c
6. d
7. b
8. c
9. a
10. b
11. c
12. d
13. a
14. d
15. a
16. c
17. d
18. a

Rationale for First on Scene Run Review

1. Yes, Kayla knew that Camille did not have an open and clear airway and needed to be rolled onto her back. You must move someone if there are problems with the ABCs that cannot be addressed in the position in which the person is found.

2. The likely cause of Camille's airway obstruction is her tongue. You must roll her onto her back and perform a jaw-thrust, which will lift the tongue and open the airway.

3. A suspected neck injury should never take priority over an obstructed airway. You can however manage the airway while being mindful of a possible neck injury.

Chapter 9

Quick Quiz

1. b
2. d
3. b
4. d
5. d
6. b
7. d
8. d
9. d
10. c
11. a
12. c
13. c
14. b
15. c

Rationale for First on Scene Run Review

1. Questions you would likely want to ask are: When did the breathing difficulty start? Do you have a history of breathing problems? Can you estimate when you may have run out of oxygen? Did you do anything prior to our arrival?

2. It is very common for patients with COPD to be on low-flow oxygen by nasal cannula full time.

3. The medic needs to know what treatment has been given to the patient thus far, as well as the results of the treatment. Additionally, the medic should be given the patient's history and vitals.

Chapter 10

Quick Quiz

1. c
2. b
3. b
4. a
5. a
6. d
7. a
8. a
9. c
10. b
11. d
12. a
13. a
14. d
15. c

Rationale for First on Scene Run Review

1. Yes, Kim did indeed respond appropriately to Chris's situation. She confirmed that he was unresponsive and immediately called for an ambulance and the AED. She could tell Chris was not breathing because there was no chest rise and fall.

2. Yes, it was the right decision to place the AED immediately. Any patient who is unresponsive, not breathing normally, and who has no pulse should get an AED.

3. The information you should relay is that you were talking to the patient when he collapsed and stopped breathing. You called for help and initiated CPR. You then placed the AED on the patient and shocked him one time. With that, the patient started to respond.

Chapter 11

Quick Quiz

1. a
2. c
3. c
4. b
5. c
6. b
7. c
8. d
9. b
10. c
11. b
12. b
13. c
14. d
15. b
16. c
17. d
18. c
19. c
20. a

Rationale for First on Scene Run Review

1. The signs and symptoms were as follows: He was having a hard time breathing, and he was talking in one-word sentences. His respiratory rate would indicate that he could not catch his breath. He also had some swelling to his ankles, which would indicate that he possibly has congestive heart failure (CHF).

2. First, place him in a position of comfort. Next, place him on a nonrebreather mask for his breathing difficulties and provide reassurance to calm him down and make him feel more at ease. During this time, also obtain his vital signs.

3. When a patient who is short of breath sits up, it takes the pressure off the diaphragm and helps him breathe easier.

Chapter 12

Quick Quiz

1. b
2. d
3. c
4. a
5. c
6. c
7. c
8. b
9. Step 1—c, Step 2—u, Step 3—f, Step 4—p, Step 5—k, Step 6—g, Step 7—r, Step 8—t, Step 9—a, Step 10—v, Step 11—i, Step 12—m, Step 13—n, Step 14—q, Step 15—j, Step 16—b, Step 17—h, Step 18—s, Step 19—o, Step 20—i, Step 21—d, Step 22—e

Rationale for First on Scene Run Review

1. It is always important to ask permission to help an individual, especially if he did not call for help. Unwanted help can be considered battery.

2. You are at a facility where there could be a lot of onlookers, and you would not want the patient to get upset and aggravate his condition.

3. The signs and symptoms this individual was exhibiting are indicative of someone having a heart attack. One of the first things you can do is to make the patient calm and reassure him. Next, place him on oxygen and get any other past medical history that might help you in your treatment.

4. Some possible reasons could be that the patient may be embarrassed to have additional attention drawn his way. Or, he may be scared or in denial that something could be wrong with him.

Chapter 13

Quick Quiz

1. b
2. c
3. b
4. a
5. c
6. d
7. a
8. a
9. b
10. c

Rationale for First on Scene Run Review

1. No matter where you are, you should always check to make sure the scene is safe; you do not want to put yourself in danger. If you are injured, you will be unable to help the person in need.

2. Seeing the chest cavity rise and fall ensures that air is getting to the lungs and there is no blockage. If you do not see chest rise, you should reposition the head and try again.

3. You should inform the paramedics of the following:
   — The fact that this was an unwitnessed cardiac arrest
   — The time CPR was initiated
   — The number of times the AED shocked the patient
   — Whether you got a pulse back at any time

Chapter 14

Quick Quiz

1. b
2. a
3. c
4. a
5. b
6. d
7. b

8. c

9. a

10. c

Rationale for First on Scene Run Review

1. The OPQRST assessment tool should have been used to determine when it started, what provoked it, if there is any severity, and how long has it lasted. Because Scott did ask all of these questions, the answer would be yes.

2. The treatment for this condition would be to have her relax and coach her on slowing her breathing. If that does not work, the appropriate course of action is to place a nonrebreather mask, set at 3 to 4 liters.

3. An ambulance should always be called, because you don't know if you will be able to have this patient control her own breathing.

Chapter 15

Quick Quiz

1. d

2. b

3. a

4. d

5. c

6. b

7. c

8. a

9. d

10. d

11. c

12. c

13. b

14. c

15. a

16. c

17. d

Rationale for First on Scene Run Review

1. The information you would want to obtain would be: When did the seizure start? How long did the seizure last? Does she have a history of seizures, and is she on any medication? If the patient is unresponsive, you should look for medical identification jewelry that could indicate any prior medical history.

2. The treatment would be: Make sure the person has a patent airway and is breathing adequately. Place her in the recovery position in case she vomits.

3. If she takes her insulin and does not eat, this would cause a drop in blood sugar (hypoglycemia), which then could possibly cause a seizure.

Chapter 16

Quick Quiz

1. a

2. c

3. b

4. c

5. a

6. c

7. a

8. a

9. d

10. a

Rationale for First on Scene Run Review

1. Signs and symptoms of heat stroke would be altered level of consciousness and hot, warm, and possibly dry skin. Sometimes the skin can be a little moist. The victim will experience weakness, nausea, vomiting, and sometimes seizures.

2. AJ did not need to ask permission because Melody was unresponsive. AJ is allowed to provide care based on implied consent.

3. AJ would need to tell responders that Melody has an altered level of consciousness, possibly had a seizure, and that they were cooling her off because she had signs of heat stroke.

Chapter 17

Quick Quiz

1. b

2. c

3. a

4. d

5. d

6. a

7. a

8. d

9. b

10. a

11. c

12. d
13. a
14. a
15. b
16. c
17. d
18. b
19. c
20. a

Rationale for First on Scene Run Review

1. The information you would like to receive would be the location of the incident, what happened, if any first aid is being administered, and if someone will be meeting the responder at the call.

2. The individual was conscious and alert. If she did not ask permission, this would be considered battery.

3. It is possible that the skin can be reattached. It would depend on how the first responder handles it in transporting it to the hospital. In transport, you should make sure it is placed in gauze in a Ziploc-type bag on top of ice to keep it cool.

4. You would apply direct pressure and elevation. If the gauze gets saturated, put more on and never remove it. You would then transport to the nearest trauma center.

Chapter 18

Quick Quiz

1. c
2. c
3. a
4. d
5. b
6. c
7. a
8. d
9. b
10. c

Rationale for First on Scene Run Review

1. The information that you will need from dispatch is the location of the call, what happened, if there is any first aid being administered, and if someone will be meeting you at the call.

2. For a patient who is feeling weak or lightheaded, have him lie supine on the ground to avoid passing out.

Also, when a person is in shock, he feels nauseated and cold, so you should cover him to keep him warm.

3. The best way to control bleeding is to apply direct pressure, using a clean dressing, and elevate. If the dressing becomes saturated, apply additional dressings and continue with direct pressure and elevation. Use a tourniquet as a last resort.

Chapter 19

Quick Quiz

1. a
2. a
3. b
4. d
5. b
6. a
7. d
8. c
9. d
10. a
11. d
12. c
13. b
14. c
15. c
16. b
17. d

Rationale for First on Scene Run Review

1. The only reason you would straighten out the leg would be to regain a distal pulse. If you start moving it and the patient is in too much pain, you should stop.

2. Yes. By splinting the leg, you immobilize the bone ends so there will be no further damage. Also, splinting helps to relieve the pain.

3. Ron will want to tell the ambulance crew how the injury occurred, if the patient has lost consciousness, that the leg needed to be straightened to get a distal pulse, and that he applied the splint to help keep it from moving and to make the patient comfortable.

Chapter 20

Quick Quiz

1. d
2. c

3. b

4. b

5. d

6. c

7. c

8. b

9. d

10. b

Rationale for First on Scene Run Review

1. Shelby will want to find out if anyone saw what happened, if the patient lost consciousness, any past medical history, and why an individual was holding the patient's head.

2. The person in need was conscious and alert. Failure to ask can be considered battery.

3. With this type of injury, the patient had the possibility of a spinal-cord injury. You always want to hold the head in-line with the body as to not create further injury. With Shelby's assessment, it became apparent that there was a possibility of a spine injury.

Chapter 21

Quick Quiz

1. a

2. b

3. c

4. b

5. c

6. b

7. a

8. d

9. a

10. b

Rationale for First on Scene Run Review

1. You should obtain OPQRST information from Nico. Ask: When did this pain start? Does anything make it worse? Does the pain radiate anywhere? Rate the pain on a scale of 1 to 10, with 10 being the worst. How long have you had this pain?

2. Place the patient in a position of comfort. Talk to the patient and obtain any past medical history. If you have oxygen, administer it and do a secondary assessment. Be prepared in the event the patient vomits.

3. From the patient's mother you would like to know if Nico had experienced this stomach pain before. If so, what did the doctors state was the cause? You would give the mother information about her son's condition that will calm her down and reassure her that everything is being done properly.

Chapter 22

Quick Quiz

1. a

2. c

3. b

4. c

5. c

6. a

7. d

8. c

9. a

10. b

11. b

12. a

13. b

14. d

15. c

16. c

17. b

18. c

Rationale for First on Scene Run Review

1. You always need to ask permission, even if the husband wants you to help, because the patient may not want you to touch her. If you do touch her without permission, it would be considered battery.

2. When a woman is delivering a baby, there are three stages of labor she goes through: The first stage is dilation of the cervix. The second stage is delivery of the baby. The third stage is delivery of the placenta.

3. You would want to know if this is her first pregnancy. If not, how many times has she been pregnant before? How many children does she have? Has she been receiving prenatal care? Are there any history issues/complications in this or her past pregnancies?

4. The information you would need to record would be the time of birth and the baby's name, if the parents have selected one.

Chapter 23

Quick Quiz

1. b
2. a
3. b
4. d
5. b
6. c
7. a
8. d
9. d
10. a
11. c
12. b
13. b
14. c
15. a

Rationale for First on Scene Run Review

1. The information you would want to obtain from the dispatcher would be: Is the scene safe? What is happening at the scene? Is more backup being sent? Is anyone injured?

2. Bryn did everything she could for the baby by covering the wounds in an effort to control the bleeding before the ambulance arrived. Had this not been done, the baby may not have survived.

3. It is always a good idea to have the parents help if they are able to. The mother holding the baby close to her and talking to her helps to calm the baby.

Chapter 24

Quick Quiz

1. a
2. c
3. b
4. c
5. d
6. b
7. a
8. c
9. d
10. b
11. c
12. b

Rationale for First on Scene Run Review

1. To make the scene safe, Tom would have to stop traffic in all directions at the intersection. To do this, he could have other bystanders help.

2. The only way Tom would be able to assess the patient after he was holding the head is by doing a quick visual scan to see if he could see any life-threatening problems. His first concern is stabilizing the head in case the senior citizen has a spine injury.

3. He should tell the firefighters that she was riding her motorcycle and lost control and went sliding down the road. The patient never lost consciousness, remembers everything that happened, and complained of leg pain after reality set in.

Chapter 25

Quick Quiz

1. c
2. a
3. a
4. d
5. d
6. b
7. c
8. b
9. d
10. d
11. d
12. a
13. d
14. c
15. b

Rationale for First on Scene Run Review

1. In addition to all of the correct steps that Greg took, he could have made sure that the pyrotechnicians had all of the proper safety equipment along with fire extinguishers and that someone was at the shut-off valve to shut off the propane in case anything happened.

2. He should state that someone will meet the fire vehicles at the access points and that there are no known injuries. As of now this is strictly a fire scene call.

3. The *Emergency Response Guidebook* would have come in handy because it would give the individuals at the scene a start on how to evaluate and handle emergencies dealing with propane. It would describe the criteria for evacuation from the site and from the surrounding areas. The guidebook also explains how to handle first-aid emergencies.

Chapter 26

Quick Quiz

1. a
2. c
3. c
4. d
5. b
6. a
7. c
8. b
9. a
10. d

Rationale for First on Scene Run Review

1. Your first priority is scene safety. You would then begin evacuating the mall. Next you would evaluate the scene to determine if you need more help and, if possible, obtain a rough estimate on the number of patients who need help. You would then call 911 and give them all the information so they can dispatch the proper help.

2. The priority of triage is red for immediate, yellow for delayed, green for walking wounded, and black for deceased. The way you determine the priorities is to use the START triage system. You determine respiratory rate, profusion, and mental status.

3. The information you want to give the arriving firefighters is how many patients you have, who has been triaged, and if more help is needed.

GLOSSARY

A

abandonment to leave a sick or injured patient before equal or more highly trained personnel can assume responsibility for care.

ABCs the patient's airway, breathing, and circulation as they relate to the primary assessment.

abdominal cavity the anterior body cavity that extends from the diaphragm to the pelvic cavity.

abdominal quadrants four divisions of the abdomen used to pinpoint the location of pain or injury: right upper quadrant (RUQ), left upper quadrant (LUQ), right lower quadrant (RLQ), and left lower quadrant (LLQ).

abdominal thrusts manual thrusts delivered to create pressure that can help expel an airway obstruction in an adult or child. Also known as *Heimlich maneuver*.

abuse the physical, emotional, or sexual mistreatment of another person.

accessory muscle use the use of the muscles of the neck, chest, and abdomen that can assist with breathing effort.

actions the intended effect of a drug on the body.

adolescent a child between the ages of 12 and 18 years old.

advance directive a document that allows a patient to define in advance what his wishes are should he become incapacitated due to a medical illness or severe injury.

advanced life support (ALS) prehospital emergency care that involves the use of intravenous fluids, drug infusions, cardiac monitoring, defibrillation, intubation, and other advanced procedures.

agonal respirations an abnormal breathing pattern characterized by slow, shallow breaths that typically occur following cardiac arrest.

allergy shock See *anaphylactic shock*.

altered mental status a state characterized by a decrease in the patient's alertness and responsiveness to his surroundings.

Alzheimer's disease a progressive, degenerative disease that attacks the brain and results in impaired memory, thinking, and behavior.

amniotic fluid the fluid surrounding the baby contained within the amniotic sac.

amniotic sac the fluid-filled sac that surrounds the developing fetus.

amputation the cutting or tearing off of a body part.

anaphylactic shock a severe allergic reaction in which a person goes into shock. Also called *anaphylaxis* or *allergy shock*

anatomical position the standard reference position for the body in the study of anatomy; the body is standing erect, facing the observer with arms down at the sides, palms forward.

anatomy the study of body structure.

angina pain in the chest caused by a lack of sufficient blood and oxygen to the heart muscle.

angulated refers to an injured limb that is deformed and out of normal alignment.

anterior the front of the body or body part.

apnea the absence of breaths.

artery a vessel that carries blood away from the heart, typically carrying oxygenated blood.

asthma a condition affecting the lungs, characterized by narrowing of the air passages and wheezing.

asystole no electrical activity in the heart; cardiac arrest. Also called *flatline*.

auscultation the act of listening to internal sounds of the body, typically with a stethoscope.

autoinjector a type of device used to self-administer some medications by way of needle injection.

automated external defibrillator (AED) an electrical device that can detect certain abnormal heart rhythms and deliver a shock through the patient's chest. This shock may allow the heart to resume a normal pattern of beating.

AVPU scale a memory aid for the classifications of mental status, or levels of responsiveness; the letters stand for *alert, verbal, painful,* and *unresponsive*.

avulsion the tearing loose of skin or other soft tissues.

B

bag-mask device an aid for pulmonary resuscitation; made up of a face mask, self-refilling bag, and valves that control the one-way flow of air. Also referred to as a *bag-valve mask (BVM)*.

bag-valve mask (BVM) See *bag-mask device*.

bandage a device used to secure a dressing in place on the body, typically made of cloth or similar material.

base station radio a high-powered two-way radio located at a dispatch center or hospital.

baseline health status a pre-employment medical examination to determine overall health status prior to beginning a job.

baseline vital signs the first determination of vital signs; used to compare with all further readings of vital signs to identify trends.

basic life support (BLS) externally supporting the circulation and respiration of a patient in respiratory or cardiac arrest through CPR.

battery unlawful physical contact.

behavioral emergency a situation in which an individual exhibits abnormal behavior that is unacceptable or intolerable to the patient, family, or community.

biological agent any bacterium, virus, or toxin that could be used in biological warfare to cause death.

biological death occurs approximately four to six minutes after onset of clinical death and results when there is an excessive amount of brain cell death.

birth canal the interior aspect of the vagina.

blanket drag a method used to move a patient by placing him on a blanket or sheet and pulling it across the floor or ground.

blood glucose the level of glucose in the bloodstream at any given time.

blood pressure the measurement of the pressure inside the arteries, both during contractions of the heart and between contractions.

bloody show the normal discharge of blood prior to delivery.

blunt trauma an injury that is caused by the impact with a blunt surface such as the ground or a large object. Also called *nonpenetrating trauma*.

body language communication using the movements and attitudes of the body.

body mechanics the proper use of the body to facilitate lifting and moving to minimize injury.

body substance isolation (BSI) precautions practice of using specific barriers to minimize contact with a patient's blood and body fluids.

BP-DOC a memory aid used to recall what to look for in a physical exam; the letters stand for *bleeding, pain, deformities, open wounds,* and *crepitus*.

brachial pulse the pulse that can be felt in the medial side of the upper arm between the elbow and shoulder.

breach of duty a violation of the basic duty to act; failure to provide care to an acceptable standard.

breech birth a birth in which the buttocks or feet deliver first.

bronchitis a condition of the lungs characterized by inflammation of the bronchial airways and mucus formation; a form of chronic obstructive pulmonary disease (COPD).

burnout an extreme emotional state characterized by emotional exhaustion, a diminished sense of personal accomplishment, and cynicism.

C

capillary refill the return (refill) of blood into the capillaries after it has been forced out by fingertip pressure; normal refill time is two seconds or less.

capillary the smallest of the body's blood vessels.

cardiac arrest the absence of a heartbeat. Also, the ineffective circulation caused by erratic muscle activity in the lower chambers of the heart (ventricular fibrillation).

cardiac compromise a general term used to describe specific signs and symptoms that indicate some type of emergency relating to the heart.

cardiac monitor a device used to display the electrical activity of the heart.

cardiogenic shock a form of shock caused when the heart is unable to pump blood efficiently.

cardiopulmonary resuscitation (CPR) combined compression and breathing techniques that maintain circulation and breathing.

carotid pulse the pulse that can be felt on either side of the neck.

CDC Centers for Disease Control and Prevention.

central nervous system a bodily system that is responsible for many of the body's involuntary functions such as heartbeat, respirations, and temperature regulation; composed of the brain and the spinal cord.

cervix the opening of the uterus.

chain of survival the idea that the survival of the patient in cardiac arrest depends on the linkage of early access, early CPR, early defibrillation, and early advanced life support.

chemical agent any noxious substance used in chemical warfare to cause widespread death.

chemical antidote autoinjector a method for the self-administration of a chemical antidote, primarily nerve agents.

chest compressions putting pressure on the chest to artificially circulate blood to the brain, lungs, and the rest of the patient's body.

chest thrusts manual thrusts delivered to create pressure that can help expel an airway obstruction in an infant or in pregnant or obese patients.

chief complaint the reason EMS was called, in the patient's own words.

chronic obstructive pulmonary disease (COPD) a general term used to describe a group of lung diseases that commonly cause respiratory distress and shortness of breath.

civil law (tort) a body of law that addresses and provides remedies for civil wrongs not arising out of contractual obligations.

clinical death the moment when breathing and heart actions stop.

closed chest injury an injury to the chest that is not associated with an open wound.

closed fracture a broken bone that does not have an associated break in the outer layers of the skin.

clothing drag an emergency move in which a rescuer grabs the patient's clothing near the shoulders and pulls him to safety.

cold zone a designated area associated with a hazardous materials incident that is well beyond the incident and where patients are cared for and placed into ambulances for transport.

communication the activity of conveying information.

compensated shock the condition in which the body is using specific mechanisms, such as increased pulse rate and increased breathing rate, to compensate for a lack of adequate perfusion.

competent properly or sufficiently qualified or capable of making appropriate decisions about one's own health or condition.

complex access a form of access to patients that requires tools and specialized equipment.

conduction pathway the electrical pathway within the heart.

conduction the loss of body heat through direct contact with another object or the ground.

confidentiality refers to the treatment of information that an individual has disclosed in a relationship of trust and with the expectation that it will not be divulged to others.

congestive heart failure See *heart failure.*

consent the legal term that means to give formal permission for something to happen.

continuity of care refers to how each new provider, who is assuming care for a patient, is properly informed of the patient's progression, so he can watch for trends and continue effective treatments.

continuous quality improvement (CQI) a continuous improvement in the quality of the product or service being delivered.

contraindication a reason that a medication should not be administered to a patient because of the potential for harmful effect.

convection the loss of body heat when air that is close to the skin moves away, taking body heat with it.

convulsions uncontrolled muscular contractions.

core temperature the temperature in the core of the body. Typically 98.6° Fahrenheit or 37° Celsius.

cranium the skull.

cravat a triangular bandage that is folded to a width of three to four inches; used to tie dressings and splints in place.

crepitus a grating noise or the sensation felt when broken bone ends rub together.

criminal law the body of law dealing with crimes and punishment.

critical incident stress debriefing (CISD) a process in which teams of professional and peer counselors provide emotional and psychological support to EMS personnel who are or have been involved in a critical (highly stressful) incident.

critical incident stress management (CISM) an in-depth, broad plan designed to help rescue personnel cope with the stress resulting from a highly stressful incident.

critical incident any situation that causes a rescuer to experience unusually strong emotions that interfere with the ability to function either during the incident or after; a highly stressful incident.

croup an acute respiratory condition common in infants and children that is characterized by a barking type of cough or stridor.

crowning the bulging out of the vagina caused by the baby's head during delivery.

cyanosis the bluish discoloration of the tissues caused by a lack of sufficient oxygen in the blood; typically seen at the mucous membranes and nail beds.

D

DCAP-BTLS a memory aid used to recall what to look for in a physical exam; the letters stand for *deformities, contusions, abrasions, punctures and penetrations, burns, tenderness, lacerations,* and *swelling.*

decompensated shock the condition in which the body is no longer able to compensate for a lack of adequate perfusion.

defibrillation the application of an electric shock to a patient's heart in an attempt to convert a lethal rhythm into a normal one.

diabetes usually refers to diabetes mellitus, a disease that prevents individuals from producing enough insulin or from using insulin appropriately.

diaphoresis excessive sweating; commonly caused by exertion or some medical problem, such as heart attack and shock.

diaphoretic See *diaphoresis.*

diaphragm the primary muscle of respiration; divides the chest cavity from the abdominal cavity.

diastolic the pressure that remains in the arteries when the heart is at rest; the resting phase of the heart.

direct carry a carry performed to move a patient with no suspected spine injury from a bed or from a bed-level position to a stretcher.

direct ground lift a standard lift in which three rescuers move a patient from the ground to a bed or stretcher.

direct medical control See *on-line medical direction.*

disaster medical assistance team (DMAT) specialized teams designed to provide medical care following a disaster.

dislocation the pulling or pushing of a bone end partially or completely free of a joint.

distal farther away from the torso.

distention swelling of the abdomen.

dorsalis pedis pulse the pulse located lateral to the large tendon of the big toe.

draw sheet move a method for moving a patient from a bed to a stretcher.

dressing a device used to cover an open wound, typically made of absorbent gauze that may be sterile or nonsterile.

drowning a process resulting in respiratory impairment from submersion in water or other type of liquid.

due regard the appropriate care and concern for the safety of others.

duty to act a requirement that Emergency Medical Responders in the police and fire service, at least while on duty, must provide care according to their department's standard operating procedures.

duty the legal obligation to provide care.

dyspnea difficult or labored breathing; shortness of breath.

E

eclampsia a life-threatening condition characterized by seizures, coma, and eventually death of both the mother and baby.

ectopic pregnancy a condition that occurs when the fertilized egg implants somewhere other than the uterus.

elder abuse the physical, sexual, or emotional abuse of an elderly person, usually one who is disabled or frail.

elder neglect the neglect by caregivers of the needs of an elderly person, usually one who is disabled or frail.

elderly a term used to describe a person age 65 or older.

electronic documentation refers to technology such as computers, PDAs, and cellular phones and their use to document patient condition and care.

emancipated minor a minor whose parents have entirely surrendered the right to the care, custody, and earnings and no longer are under any duty to support the minor.

emergency care the prehospital assessment and basic care for the sick or injured patient; during care the physical and emotional needs of the patient are considered and attended to.

Emergency Medical Dispatcher (EMD) a member of the EMS system who provides pre-arrival instructions to callers, thereby helping to initiate lifesaving care before EMS personnel arrive.

Emergency Medical Responder (EMR) a member of the EMS system who has been trained to render first aid care for a patient and to help EMTs at the emergency scene.

emergency medical services (EMS) system the chain of human resources and services linked together to provide continuous emergency care from the onset of care at the prehospital scene, during transport, and on arrival at the medical facility. In some localities, multiple EMS agencies work together as an EMS network.

Emergency Medical Technician (EMT) a member of the EMS system whose training emphasizes assessment, care, and transportation of the ill or injured patient. Depending on the level of training, emergency care may include starting IV (intravenous) lines, inserting advanced airways, and administering some medications.

emergency move a patient move that is carried out quickly when the scene is hazardous, care of the patient requires immediate repositioning, or you must reach another patient who needs lifesaving care.

emphysema a progressive condition of the lungs characterized by destruction of the alveoli; a form of chronic obstructive pulmonary disease (COPD).

end-tidal CO_2 detector a device used to detect the presence of carbon dioxide in the exhaled breath of a patient.

epiglottis a flap of cartilage and other tissues located above the larynx that help close off the airway when a person swallows.

epiglottitis swelling of the epiglottis that may be caused by a bacterial infection; may cause airway obstruction.

epilepsy a disorder of the brain that causes seizures.

ethics the study of the principles that define behavior as right, good, and proper.

evaporation the loss of body heat through the vaporization of moisture in the form of sweat on the skin.

evisceration an open wound of the abdomen characterized by protrusion of the intestines through the abdominal wall.

exhalation the process of breathing out.

exposure a condition of being subjected to a fluid or substance capable of transmitting an infectious agent.

expressed consent a competent adult's informed decision to accept emergency care provided by an Emergency Medical Responder. Also referred to as *informed consent*.

extremity lift a move performed by two rescuers, one lifting the patient's arms and one lifting the patient's legs.

extrication the coordinated removal of entrapped patients from vehicles and structures.

F

fallopian tube the tube-like structure that connects the ovary to the uterus.

febrile refers to a fever.

fibrillation a disorganized electrical activity within the heart that renders the heart incapable of pumping blood.

firefighter's carry a method used to walk to safety with a patient securely placed over one shoulder.

firefighter's drag a move in which the rescuer straddles the supine patient, secures the patient's hands behind the rescuer's neck, and then crawls to safety while dragging the patient underneath him.

fixed wing an airplane.

flail chest a chest injury characterized by two or more ribs that are broken in two or more places.

focused secondary assessment an examination conducted on stable patients, focusing on a specific injury or medical complaint.

fontanel an area on the infant's skull where the bones have not yet fused together, leaving a soft spot.

Fowler's position a position in which a patient is placed fully upright in a seated position, creating a 90-degree angle.

frostbite localized cold injury in which the skin is frozen.

full term a pregnancy that has achieved a complete gestation of between 38 and 40 weeks.

G

gag reflex a retching action, hacking, or vomiting that is induced when something touches a certain level of the patient's throat.

gastric distention inflation of the stomach.

generalized cold emergency See *hypothermia*.

generalized seizure a type of seizure characterized by a loss of consciousness and full-body muscle contractions.

geriatric of or relating to an elderly person.

glucometer a device used to measure and display the amount of glucose in a given sample of blood.

Good Samaritan laws a series of state laws designed to protect certain care providers if they deliver the standard of care in good faith, to the level of their training, and to the best of their abilities.

guarding the protection of an area of injury or pain by the patient; the spasms of muscles to minimize movement that might cause pain.

H

hazardous materials incident the release of a harmful substance into the environment. Also called a *hazmat incident*.

Hazardous Materials Emergency Response Guidebook: an official printed government resource for the identification of hazardous materials.

hazardous materials materials that are harmful to humans when exposed.

HAZWOPER an abbreviation for hazardous waste operations and emergency response.

head-tilt/chin-lift maneuver technique used to open the airway of a patient with no suspected neck or spine injury.

Health Insurance Portability Accountability Act (HIPAA) a law that dictates the extent to which protected health information can be shared.

heart attack See *myocardial infarction.*

heart failure a condition that develops when the heart is unable to pump blood efficiently, causing a backup of blood and other fluids within the circulatory system. Also may be referred to as *congestive heart failure.*

heat cramps common term for muscle cramps in the lower limbs and abdomen associated with the loss of fluids and salts while active in a hot environment.

heat exhaustion prolonged exposure to heat, which creates moist, pale skin that may feel normal or cool to the touch.

heat stroke prolonged exposure to heat, which creates dry or moist skin that may feel warm or hot to the touch.

Heimlich maneuver See *abdominal thrusts.*

helipad a designated location for the landing of a helicopter, typically at a hospital or airport.

hemodialysis the process of mechanically filtering the blood to remove wastes and excess fluid.

hemorrhagic shock a form of hypovolemic shock that occurs when the body loses a significant amount of blood.

hemostatic dressing a dressing that has been treated with a specialized chemical that when placed onto a wound promotes clotting.

hemothorax blood in the chest cavity.

hot zone the area of a hazardous incident that is immediately surrounding the spill or release.

humidifier a device used to increase the moisture content of supplemental oxygen.

hydrostatic test the process of testing high-pressure cylinders.

hypercarbia an abnormally high level of carbon dioxide in the blood.

hyperglycemia an abnormally high blood-sugar level.

hyperthermia an increase in body core temperature above its normal temperature.

hyperventilation a temporary condition characterized by uncontrolled, rapid, deep breathing that is usually self-correcting; often caused by anxiety but may have more serious causes as well.

hypoglycemia an abnormally low blood-sugar level.

hypoperfusion a condition in which the organs and cells are not receiving an adequate supply of well-oxygenated blood and nutrients. Also known as *shock.*

hypotension abnormally low blood pressure.

hypothermia a general cooling of the body. Also called *generalized cold emergency.*

hypovolemic shock a category of shock caused by an abnormally low fluid volume (blood or plasma) in the body.

hypoxia a condition in which there is an insufficient level of oxygen in the blood and tissues.

I

immediate life threats any condition that may pose an immediate threat to the patient's life, such as problems with the airway, breathing, circulation, or safety.

imminent delivery a delivery that is likely to occur within the next few minutes.

implied consent a legal position that assumes an unresponsive or incompetent adult patient would consent to receiving emergency care if he could. This form of consent may apply to other types of patients (e.g., the mentally ill).

incident command system (ICS) a model tool for the command, control, and coordination of resources at the scene of a large-scale emergency involving multiple agencies. Also known as *incident management system.*

incident commander the person responsible for all aspects of an emergency response.

incident management system See *incident command system.*

indication the reason a medication should be administered.

indirect medical control See *off-line medical direction.*

infant a child between that ages of birth to one year.

infection the condition in which the body is invaded by a disease-causing agent.

inferior toward the feet (e.g., the lips are inferior to the nose).

informed consent See *expressed consent.*

inhalation the process of breathing in. See *inspiration.*

inspiration refers to the process of breathing in, or inhaling. Opposite: *expiration.*

instrument flight rules (IFR) rules defined by the Federal Aviation Administration regarding the operation of aircraft in inclement weather.

interpersonal communication a form of communication where the participants are dependent on one another and have a shared history.

interventions actions taken to correct or stabilize a patient's illness or injury.

J

jaw-thrust maneuver technique used to open the airway of a trauma patient with possible neck or spine injury.

jugular vein distention (JVD) an abnormal bulging of the veins of the neck indicating possible injury to the chest or heart.

JumpSTART pediatric MCI triage system a specialized pediatric triage system designed for patients from one to eight years of age.

L

labor the process the body goes through to deliver a baby.

landing zone a temporary location for the landing of a helicopter, typically at the scene of an emergency.

laryngectomy the total or partial removal of the larynx.

larynx the section of the airway between the throat and the trachea that contains the vocal cords.

lateral recumbent position the patient is lying on his side.

lateral to the side, away from the midline of the body.

liter flow the measure of the flow of oxygen being delivered through a mask or cannula.

log roll a method used to move a patient with a suspected spine injury from the prone position to the supine position.

M

mandated reporter professionals who, in the ordinary course of their work, are required to report (or cause a report to be made) whenever financial, physical, sexual, or other types of abuse or neglect have been observed or are suspected.

manual stabilization using your hands to physically hold the body part and keep it from moving.

mass-casualty incident See *multiple-casualty incident.*

mechanism of injury (MOI) the force or forces that may have caused injury.

meconium the product of the baby's first bowel movement.

medial toward the midline of the body.

mediastinum the structure that divides the two halves of the chest cavity.

medical direction the medical oversight provided for an EMS system or one of its components by a licensed physician.

Medical Director a physician who assumes the ultimate responsibility for medical oversight of the patient care aspects of the EMS system.

medical history previous medical conditions and events for a patient.

medical patient one who has or describes symptoms of an illness; a patient with no injuries.

medication something that treats, prevents, or minimizes the symptoms of disease.

mental status the general condition of a patient's level of consciousness and awareness.

message the thought, concept, or idea that is being transmitted.

midline an imaginary vertical line used to divide the body into right and left halves.

minimum data set the essential information that must be gathered and documented on every patient care report.

miscarriage the spontaneous natural loss of the embryo or fetus before the 26th week of pregnancy.

multiple-casualty incident (MCI) any incident that results in enough patients to overwhelm immediately available resources. Also known as a *mass-casualty incident.*

multisystem trauma trauma to the body that affects multiple organ systems.

myocardial infarction (MI) a condition that results when the blood supply to a portion of the heart is interrupted. Also known as a *heart attack.*

N

nasal airway See *nasopharyngeal airway.*

nasal cannula a device used to deliver low concentrations of supplemental oxygen to a breathing patient.

nasopharyngeal airway (NPA) a flexible tube that is lubricated and then inserted into a patient's nose to the level of the nasopharynx (back of the throat) to provide an open airway. Also called *nasal airway.*

National EMS Education Standards the education and training standards developed by the National Highway Traffic Safety Administration (NHTSA) for all levels of EMS training.

national incident management system (NIMS) a system that utilizes a unified approach to incident management and standard command and management structures, with an emphasis on preparedness, mutual aid, and resource management.

nature of illness (NOI) what is medically wrong with the patient; a complaint not related to an injury.

neglect failure of parents or caregivers to adequately provide for a person's basic physical, social, emotional, and medical needs.

negligence a failure to provide the expected standard of care.

neonate See *newborn.*

nerve agent a toxic liquid that is inhaled or absorbed through the skin and has harmful effects on the nervous and respiratory system.

neurogenic shock a form of distributive shock, resulting from spinal-cord injury.

newborn a baby that is less than 28 days old. Also called *neonate.*

NFPA National Fire Protection Association.

nonrebreather mask a device use to deliver high concentrations of supplemental oxygen.

nuchal cord a condition where the umbilical cord is around the baby's neck during delivery.

nuclear/radiological agent a substance containing radioactive material in quantities large enough to threaten human life.

O

O ring the gasket used to seal a regulator to the oxygen cylinder.

occlusive dressing a dressing that is nonpermeable and will not allow air to pass through.

off-line medical direction an EMS system's standing orders and protocols, which authorize personnel to perform particular skills in certain situations without actually speaking to the Medical Director. Also called *indirect medical control.*

on-line medical direction orders to perform a skill or administer care from the on-duty physician, given to the rescuer in person by radio or by phone. Also called *direct medical control.*

open chest injury an injury to the chest that is associated with an open wound.

open fracture a broken bone with an associated break in the outer layers of the skin.

OPQRST a memory device used for assessing the responsive medical patient; the letters stand for *onset, provocation, quality, region/radiate, severity,* and *time;* usually used during the secondary assessment.

oral airway See *oropharyngeal airway.*

oropharyngeal airway (OPA) a curved breathing tube inserted into the patient's mouth to hold the base of the tongue forward. Also called *oral airway.*

OSHA U.S. Occupational Safety and Health Administration.

ovary the structure that produces the ovum.

overdose an incident that occurs when a person takes in more of a medication or substance than is normal.

ovum the unfertilized egg produced by the mother.

oxygen concentration the amount of oxygen being delivered to a patient.

oxygen supply tubing the tubing used to connect a delivery device to an oxygen source.

P

palpation the act of using one's hands to touch or feel the body.

paradoxical movement movement of an area of the chest wall in opposition to the rest of the chest during respiration; commonly associated with a flail chest.

paralysis the loss of mobility and feeling.

Paramedic a member of the EMS system whose training includes advanced life support care, such as inserting endotracheal tubes and starting IV lines. Paramedics also administer medications, interpret electrocardiograms, monitor cardiac rhythms, and perform cardiac defibrillation.

partial seizure a seizure characterized by a temporary loss of awareness with no dramatic body movements.

patent airway an airway that is open and clear.

pathogen an organism such as a virus or bacterium that causes infection and disease.

patient assessment the gathering of information to determine a possible illness or injury; includes interviews and physical examinations.

patient care report (PCR) a document that provides details about a patient's condition, history, and care as well as information about the event that caused the illness or injury.

pediatric assessment triangle (PAT) a tool used to perform a general impression of a pediatric patient; the elements of the PAT are appearance, work of breathing, and circulation (perfusion).

pediatric patient refers to infants and children. For the purposes of CPR, patients from birth to one year of age are considered infants. Patients from one year old to the onset of puberty are considered children.

pelvic cavity the anterior body cavity surrounded by the bones of the pelvis.

penetrating trauma injury to the body caused by any object that punctures the skin.

perfusion the adequate supply of well-oxygenated blood and nutrients to all vital organs.

peripheral nervous system a bodily system that connects the to central nervous system to the limbs and organs by way of nerves; composed of all the nerves and nerve endings that extend from the spinal cord throughout the body.

personal protective equipment (PPE) equipment such as gloves, mask, eyewear, gown, turnout gear, and helmet that protects rescuers from infection and/or from exposure to hazardous materials and the dangers of rescue operations.

pharynx the throat.

pin index system the safety system used to ensure that the proper regulator is used for a specific gas, such as oxygen.

placard a sign used to display information pertaining to the contents of transport containers.

placenta previa a condition that results when the placenta grows and develops over the cervix.

placenta the organ of pregnancy that serves as the filter between the mother and developing fetus.

pleura the thin, saclike structure that surrounds each lung.

pleural space the potential space that exists between the visceral and parietal pleura in the chest.

pneumothorax air in the chest cavity.

pocket face mask a device used to help provide ventilations. It has a chimney with a one-way valve and HEPA filter. Some have an inlet for supplemental oxygen.

portable radio a handheld device used to transmit and receive verbal communications.

position of function refers to a hand or foot; the natural position of the body at rest.

positional asphyxia refers to death resulting from the securing of a person in the prone position, limiting his ability to breathe adequately. Also called *restraint asphyxia*.

positive pressure ventilation the process of using external pressure to force air into a patient's lungs, such as with mouth-to-mask or bag-mask ventilations.

posterior tibial pulse the pulse felt behind the medial ankle.

posterior the back of the body or body part.

postictal the phase of a seizure following convulsions.

power lift a technique used to lift a patient who is on a stretcher or cot.

preeclampsia a potentially life-threatening condition that affects the mother during the third trimester and is characterized by high blood pressure and fluid retention.

prenatal care the routine medical care provided to a mother during her pregnancy.

pressure gauge the device on a regulator that displays the pressure inside a cylinder.

pressure regulator the device used to lower the delivery pressure of oxygen from a cylinder.

primary assessment a quick assessment of the patient's airway, breathing, circulation, and bleeding to detect and correct any immediate life-threatening problems.

prolapsed cord a condition resulting in the delivery of the umbilical cord prior to the delivery of the baby.

prone the patient is lying face down.

protocols written guidelines that direct the care EMS personnel provide for patients.

proximal closer to the torso.

psychogenic shock a form of distributive shock that results in a sudden, temporary dilation of blood vessels.

public health system local resources dedicated to promoting optimal health and quality of life for the people and communities they serve.

public safety answering point (PSAP) a designated 911 emergency dispatch center.

pulmonary resuscitation a technique by which breaths are provided to a patient in an attempt to artificially maintain normal lung function. Also called *rescue breathing* or *artificial ventilation*.

pulse oximeter a device used to measure and display the percentage of hemoglobin in blood that is saturated with oxygen.

pulse the pulsation of the arteries that is felt with each heart beat.

Q

quadrant an area of the abdomen; used to identify the location of pain during palpation.

R

radial pulse the pulse felt on the thumb side of the wrist.

radiation loss of body heat to the atmosphere or nearby objects without physical contact.

rapid secondary assessment a quick head-to-toe assessment of the most critical patients.

reassessment the last step in patient assessment, used to detect changes in a patient's condition; includes repeating initial assessment, reassessing and recording vital signs, and checking interventions.

receiver the person for whom the message is intended.

recovery position the position in which a patient with no suspected spine injuries may be placed, usually on the left side. Also called the *lateral recumbent position*.

repeater a fixed antenna that is used to boost a radio signal.

rescue breathing the act of providing positive pressure ventilations for a patient who has inadequate respirations.

research the systematic investigation to establish facts.

reservoir bag a device attached to an oxygen-delivery device that temporarily stores oxygen.

respiration the act of breathing; the exchange of oxygen and carbon dioxide that takes place in the lungs.

respiratory arrest the absence of breathing.

respiratory compromise a general term referring to the inability of a person to breath adequately.

respiratory distress refers to breathing that becomes difficult or labored; the body's normal response to not getting an adequate supply of oxygen. Also called *dyspnea*.

respiratory failure a respiratory condition characterized by altered mental status, slow respiratory rate, and shallow tidal volume; occurs when the body's normal ability to compensate for inadequate oxygen fails.

respiratory/metabolic shock a form of shock caused by the disruption of the transfer of oxygen into the cells or the ability of the cells to utilize oxygen.

restraint the process of securing a combative patient's body and extremities to prevent injury to himself or others.

restraint asphyxia See *positional asphyxia*.

retractions the inward movement of the soft tissues between the ribs when a child breathes in.

retroperitoneal cavity the area behind the abdominal cavity that contains the kidneys and ureters.

rotor wing helicopter.

S

SAMPLE history a system of information gathering that allows the rescuer to ask questions about past or present medical or injury problems; the letters stand for *signs/symptoms, allergies, medications, pertinent past medical history, last oral intake,* and *events leading to the illness or injury.*

scene size-up an overview of the scene to identify any obvious or potential hazards; consists of taking BSI precautions, determining the safety of the scene, identifying the mechanism of injury or nature of illness, determining the number of patients, and identifying additional resources.

school age a child between the ages of 6 and 12 years of age.

scope of care See *scope of practice*.

scope of practice the care that an Emergency Medical Responder, an Emergency Medical Technician, or Paramedic is allowed and supposed to provide according to local, state, or regional regulations or statutes. Also called *scope of care*.

Scope of Practice Model a national model that defines the scope of care for all levels of EMS training.

secondary assessment a complete head-to-toe physical exam, including medical history.

self-neglect a condition whereby an individual fails to attend to his or her own basic needs, such as hygiene, appropriate clothing, medical care, and so on.

semi-Fowler's position semi-seated position in which the patient reclines at a 45-degree angle.

sender the person introducing a new thought or concept or initiating the communication process.

sepsis a widespread infection of the body.

septic shock a form of distributive shock caused by a widespread infection of the blood.

shaken-baby syndrome a form of child abuse that occurs when an abuser violently shakes an infant or small child, creating a whiplash-type motion that causes acceleration-deceleration injuries.

shock the failure of the body's circulatory system to provide an adequate supply of well-oxygenated blood and nutrients to all vital organs. Also known as *hypoperfusion*.

side effect an action of a medication that is not desired.

sign something that can be observed or measured when assessing a patient; objective indications of illness or injury that can be seen, heard, felt, and smelled by another person.

simple access a form of access to entrapped patients that does not require specialized tools or equipment.

sling a large triangular bandage or other cloth device that is used to immobilize an elbow and support the forearm.

specialty hospital a hospital with special designation that is capable of providing specialized services such as trauma care, pediatric care, or burn care.

splint any device that is used to immobilize an injured extremity.

spontaneous pneumothorax a sudden collapse of one or more lobes of a lung; not typically associated with trauma.

spotting the discharge of blood during pregnancy.

sprain a partial or complete tearing of the ligaments and tendons that support a joint.

standard move the preferred choice when the situation is not urgent, the patient is stable, and you have adequate time and personnel for a move.

standard of care the care that should be provided for any level of training based on local laws, administrative orders, and guidelines and protocols established by the local EMS system.

standard precautions steps to take to protect against exposure to body fluids.

standing orders the Medical Director's specific instructions for the Emergency Medical Responder, Emergency Medical Technician, or Paramedic to provide care for specific medical conditions or injuries.

START triage system a system that uses respiration, perfusion, and mental status assessments to categorize patients into one of four treatment categories; letters stand for *simple triage and rapid treatment*.

stethoscope a device used to auscultate sounds within the body; commonly used to obtain blood pressure.

stoma any permanent opening that has been surgically made; the opening in the neck of a neck breather.

strain the overstretching or tearing of a muscle.

stress an emotionally disruptive or upsetting condition that occurs in response to adverse external influences; can increase heart rate, raise blood pressure, and cause muscular tension, irritability, and depression.

stressor any emotional or physical demand that causes stress.

stroke a condition that occurs when an area of the brain does not receive an adequate supply of blood. Also referred to as *brain attack*.

sucking chest wound an open chest wound that is characterized by a sucking sound each time the patient inhales.

sudden infant death syndrome (SIDS) the sudden, unexplained death of an apparently healthy baby during sleep.

superior toward the head (e.g., the chest is superior to the abdomen).

supine hypotensive syndrome an abnormally low blood pressure that results when the mother is supine and the fetus puts pressure on the vena cava.

supine the patient is lying face up.

supplemental oxygen a supply of 100% oxygen for use with ill or injured patients.

swathe a large cravat used to secure a sling or splint to the body.

symptoms subjective indications of illness or injury that cannot be observed by another person but are felt and reported by the patient.

systolic the pressure within the arteries when the heart beats; the contraction phase of the heart.

T

tension pneumothorax an abnormal buildup of pressure in the chest cavity.

terrorism the use of force or violence against persons or property to intimidate or coerce a government, the civilian population, or any segment thereof to further political or social objectives.

therapeutic communication the face-to-face communication process that focuses on advancing the physical and emotional well-being of a patient.

thoracic cavity the anterior body cavity that is above (superior to) the diaphragm. Also called *chest cavity*.

tidal volume the amount of air being moved in and out of the lungs with each breath.

toddler a child between the ages of one and three years old.

tourniquet a device use to cut off all blood supply past the point of application.

trachea the windpipe.

tracheal deviation a shifting of the trachea to either side of the midline of the neck caused by the buildup of pressure inside the chest.

track marks small dots of infection that form a track along a vein; may be an indication of IV drug abuse.

transfer of care the physical and verbal handing off of care from one health-care provider to another.

trauma patient one who has a physical injury caused by an external force.

Trendelenburg position a position in which the patient is placed flat on his back with his legs and feet raised.

trending the act of comparing multiple sets of signs and symptoms over time to determine patient condition.

triage a method of sorting patients for care and transport based on the severity of their injuries or illnesses.

trimester three months of pregnancy.

tripod position a body position characterized by the person sitting forward with hands on knees.

U

umbilical cord the structure that connects the baby to the placenta.

unconscious See *unresponsive*.

universal precautions a component of standard precautions that involves the philosophy that all patients are considered infectious until proven otherwise.

unresponsive having no reaction to verbal or painful stimuli. Also referred to as *unconscious*.

uterus the muscular structure that holds the baby during pregnancy.

V

vagina the birth canal.

values the personal beliefs that determine how a person actually behaves.

vein a vessel that returns blood to the heart, typically carrying deoxygenated blood.

ventilation the supplying of air to the lungs. See *pulmonary resuscitation*.

ventricular fibrillation (VF) disorganized electrical activity, causing ineffective contractions of the lower heart chambers (ventricles).

ventricular tachycardia the abnormally rapid contraction of the heart's lower chambers, resulting in very poor circulation. Also called *V-tach*.

visual flight rules (VFR) rules defined by the Federal Aviation Administration regarding the operation of aircraft when weather is not a factor.

vital signs the five most common signs used to evaluate a patient's condition (respirations, pulse, blood pressure, skin, and pupils).

W

warm zone a designated area at a hazardous materials incident where decontamination of people and equipment occurs.

weapon of mass destruction a weapon that can bring significant harm and kill large numbers of humans and cause great damage to manmade structures, natural structures, or the environment.

wheezing a course whistling sound often heard in the lungs when a patient with respiratory compromise exhales. May also be heard on inspiration.

work of breathing the effort that a patient must exert to breathe.

INDEX